Basic Electrocardiology

Peter W. Macfarlane · Adriaan van Oosterom · Michiel Janse · Paul Kligfield ·
John Camm · Olle Pahlm (Eds.)

Basic Electrocardiology

Cardiac Electrophysiology, ECG Systems and Mathematical Modeling

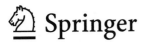 Springer

Editors
Peter W. Macfarlane
University of Glasgow
Glasgow
UK

Adriaan van Oosterom
Radboud University Nijmegen
Nijmegen
The Netherlands

Olle Pahlm
Lund University
Lund
Sweden

Paul Kligfield
Weill Cornell Medical College
New York, NY
USA

Michiel Janse
University of Amsterdam
Amsterdam
The Netherlands

John Camm
St. George's, University of London
London
UK

ISBN 978-0-85729-870-6
DOI 10.1007/978-0-85729-871-3

Library of Congress Control Number: 2011943328

First published in 2010 as part of Comprehensive Electrocardiology, 2nd Edition (ISBN 978-1-84882-045-6)

© Springer-Verlag London Limited 2012

Printed on acid-free paper

Springer is part of Springer Science+Business Media (www.springer.com)

Editors-in-Chief

Peter W. Macfarlane
University of Glasgow
Glasgow
UK

Adriaan van Oosterom
Radboud University Nijmegen
Nijmegen
The Netherlands

Olle Pahlm
Lund University
Lund
Sweden

Paul Kligfield
Weill Cornell Medical College
New York, NY
USA

Michiel Janse
University of Amsterdam
Amsterdam
The Netherlands

John Camm
St. George's, University of London
London
UK

Preface

The first edition of *Comprehensive Electrocardiology* was published in 1989, when e-mail was still in its infancy (!!), and it was never envisaged at that time that a new edition would be prepared. It is probably fair to say that the majority of physicians would have regarded electrocardiography in particular as having reached its maximum usefulness with little additional information to be obtained therefrom. The intervening 20 years have shown how untrue this was.

An update to the book is long overdue. Sadly, some of our former contributors have died since the first edition was published and it is with regret that I note the passing of Philippe Coumel, Rudolph van Dam, Karel den Dulk, Ramesh Gulrajani, Kenici Harumi, John Milliken, Jos Willems and Christoph Zywietz. Where relevant, their contributions continue to be acknowledged but in some cases, chapters have been completely rewritten by new contributors. On the other hand, eight completely new chapters have been added and the appendices restructured.

The publisher felt it would be opportune to produce separate paperback versions of each of the four volumes of the second edition of *Comprehensive Electrocardiology* – hence this book entitled *Cardiac Electrophysiology, ECG Modeling and Lead Systems*.

In some ways, it is inconceivable what has taken place in the field of electrocardiology since the first edition. New ECG patterns have been recognised and linked with sudden death, new prognostic indices have been developed and evaluated, the ECG has assumed a pivotal role in the treatment of an acute coronary syndrome and among many other things, automated ECG interpretation is now commonplace. Significant advances have been made in the field of mathematical modeling and a solution to the inverse problem is now applied in routine clinical use. Electrophysiological studies have taken giant steps over the past 20 years and biventricular pacing is a relatively recent innovation. Electrocardiology has certainly not stood still in the last 20 years. Of course there have been parallel advances in imaging techniques but the ECG still retains a unique position in the armamentarium of the physician, let alone the cardiologist.

For this edition, my previous co editor, Professor T.D. Veitch Lawrie, decided to step aside and I wish to congratulate him on reaching his 91st birthday in September 2011. However, I am pleased that other very eminent individuals agreed to assist with the editing of the book, namely Adriaan van Oosterom, Olle Pahlm, Paul Kligfield, Michiel Janse and John Camm. In the nature of things, some of these co editors undertook much more work than others. For this book, I particularly have to acknowledge the support of Adriaan van Oosterom, who authored four chapters and edited four others. Without his support, this revised version of the material in the first edition would not have been possible. Michiel Janse reviewed the cellular electrophysiology chapters for which I am very grateful.

Locally, I am very much indebted to my secretary Pamela Armstrong for a huge contribution in checking and subediting every chapter which went out from my office to the publisher. This was a Herculean task carried out with great aplomb. I would also like to thank Ms. Julie Kennedy for her contribution to a variety of tasks associated with preparing selected chapters, including enhancements to the English presentation on occasions.

I also wish to thank the publishers Springer for their considerable support throughout. Grant Weston initially commissioned the book and I am grateful to him for his confidence in supporting the preparation of a new edition. Jennifer Carlson and her team in New York also assisted significantly. I am also indebted to Mr. R. Samuel Devanand and his team at SPi Global, in India, for production of the paperback edition.

I again must thank my long suffering wife Irene who has had to fight to gain access to our home PC every night over these past few years!

Comprehensive Electrocardiology aims to bring together truly comprehensive information about the field and *Basic Electrocardiology* provides a strong theoretical foundation to the principles of electrocardiography. A book can never be completely up to date given the speed of publication of research findings over the internet these days but hopefully this publication will continue to be of significant use to readers for many years to come. *Basic Electrocardiology*, together with the other three paperback versions of the other volumes of *Comprehensive Electrocardiology*, contains much information that should be of use both to the practising clinician and the experienced researcher.

Now that this huge effort has been completed and the book is available electronically, it should be much easier to produce the next edition…!!

Peter Macfarlane
Glasgow
Autumn

Table of Contents

List of Contributors

R.C. Barr
Duke University
Durham, NC
USA

Dana H. Brooks
Northeastern University
Boston, MA
USA

Martin Buist
National University of Singapore
Singapore
Singapore

Leo K. Cheng
The University of Auckland
Auckland
New Zealand

Alireza Ghodrati
Draeger Medical
Andover, MA
USA

B. Milan Horáček
Dalhousie University
Halifax, NS
Canada

Michiel J. Janse
University of Amsterdam
Amsterdam
The Netherlands

S.M. Lobodzinski
California State University
Long Beach, CA
USA

Peter W. Macfarlane
University of Glasgow
Glasgow
UK

Rob MacLeod
University of Utah
Salt Lake City, UT
USA

Martyn P. Nash
The University of Auckland
Auckland
New Zealand

A. van Oosterom
Radboud University Nijmegen
Nijmegen
The Netherlands

Tobias Opthof
University Medical Centre Utrecht
Utrecht
The Netherlands

R. Plonsey
Duke University
Durham, NC
USA

Andrew J. Pullan
The University of Auckland
Auckland
New Zealand

Ronald Wilders
University of Amsterdam
Amsterdam
The Netherlands

Antonio Zaza
Universita di Milano-Bicocca
Milano
Italy

Part I

Introduction

1   The Coming of Age of Electrocardiology

Peter W. Macfarlane

P. W. Macfarlane et al. (eds.), *Basic Electrocardiology*, DOI 10.1007/978-0-85729-871-3_1,
© Springer-Verlag London Limited 2012

1.1   Introduction

The history of electrocardiography and vectorcardiography is relatively well established [1, 2]. Indeed, it is now well over one hundred years since the electrocardiogram was first recorded in a human and the 100th anniversary of this event resulted in a number of reviews dealing with the early days of electrocardiography [3–7].

While, in the relatively early days of a new century, it would seem appropriate to look back over developments in the last century, others recently have recently reviewed the present status of the ECG [8] and this author has referred to a renaissance in electrocardiography [9] since the first edition of this book. Electrocardiography has come under increasing pressure in recent years with the advent of new techniques such as echocardiography, which undoubtedly provide information that complements the electrocardiogram. On the other hand, Wellens [10] regretted the fact that younger physicians are increasingly unable to interpret electrocardiograms correctly. He referred to the views of Fisch [11] who had emphasized the fact that the ECG is a noninvasive technique that is inexpensive, simple and reproducible. He might have added that the ECG can be rapidly recorded with extremely portable equipment (the most recent having integral computer facilities as well as wireless or telephone transmission capabilities) and is always able to be derived unlike the echocardiogram, which in some situations cannot be satisfactorily obtained. Of course, the ECG provides unique information that cannot be obtained by any other technique; it is only necessary to think of secondary ST-T changes due to left ventricular hypertrophy and their prognostic importance for proof of this. Furthermore, as Fisch indicated [11], "He who maintains that new knowledge of electrocardiography is no longer possible or contributive, ignores history." This new edition of Comprehensive Electrocardiology proves how prophetic these words were.

Much of the early work in electrocardiography was carried out in Europe, where today there is still considerable development effort being expended, particularly in the field of computer-based electrocardiography (see ❷ Chap. 5 of *Specialized Aspects of ECG*). There is much work elsewhere mainly based around mathematical modeling. A European physician and physiologist, the late Professor Pierre Rijlant wrote an article in 1980 entitled "The Coming of Age of Electrophysiology and Electrocardiography" [12]. It is from this article that the title for the present chapter is drawn, in memory of the contribution of Rijlant, President of the 1958 World Congress of Cardiology, to the field of electrocardiology.

It is questionable where the term "electrocardiology" arose. In 1959, the first of a series of colloquia on vectorcardiography was organized by Kowarzyk and held in Wroclaw in Poland. For many years thereafter, an International Colloquium Vectorcardiographicum was organized, and Rijlant was the driving force and Honorary President of the Organizing Committee. In 1973, the author attended a meeting of the Organizing Committee in Yerevan, Armenia, USSR, at which it was agreed that, from 1974 onwards, the name of the meeting should be changed to the International Congress on Electrocardiology. The first such meeting was organized in Wiesbaden in 1974 and was attended by many prominent researchers including the late Ernst Simonson, well known for his work on the normal electrocardiogram (see ❷ Chap. 1 of *Electrocardiology: Comprehensive Clinical ECG*).

Earlier, in 1968, Zao and Lepeschkin founded the *Journal of Electrocardiology*, which grew in strength under the editorship of Startt/Selvester, who has contributed to ❷ Chap. 4 of *Electrocardiology: Comprehensive Clinical ECG*, and is now being significantly restructured by Wagner, who has also contributed to the same chapter. Lempert [13] in 1976 also commented on the transition from the term "electrocardiography" to "electrocardiology" and pointed out he had used the term "electrocardiology" in his 1961 textbook, written in Latvian, and the 1963 edition written in Russian. (Professor Ruttkay-Nedecky from Bratislava has recently pointed out that J. Martinek used the term "electrocardiology" in 1959 in the title of his paper referring to "electrocardiology in the USA" at a meeting in Wroclaw, Poland, which became the forerunner of the Colloquium Vectorcardiographicum). "Electrocardiography" conjures up a view of 12 leads, perhaps recorded singly on an electrocardiograph. The explosion of technology in recent years and the variety of investigative techniques now available for studying the cardiac electrical activity demands that the relatively newer term of "electrocardiology" be used to encompass the various subject areas associated with the electric and magnetic fields generated by the individual cells of the heart. It is hoped that it will be evident from the contents of this book that the term "electrocardiography" would be inappropriate.

1.2   The Groundwork for Electrocardiography

By the mid-nineteenth century, it was generally agreed that nerves, muscles and so on could be stimulated by artificial electrical generators [11]. The first galvanometer had beeninvented by that time and physiologists were engaged in

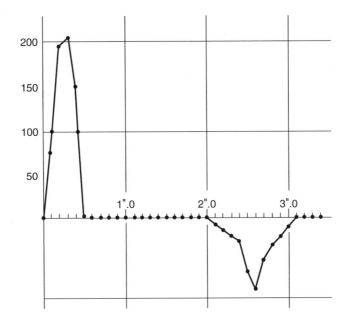

exploring the discharge from electric eels, the flow of current through frogs and the effects of injury. Such work was probably initiated by Galvani [14]. He was criticized by Volta who argued that electrical current was generated only by different metals making contact-the basic work that ultimately led to the development of batteries. It was du Bois-Reymond who continued much of this work as highlighted by Rijlant [12]; in particular he found that action current in muscle was opposite to the direction of a continuous current, which his pupil Hermann showed later was present only following an injury to the muscle [14]. In 1856, Kölliker and Muller [15] demonstrated bioelectric potentials in the frog's heart. As far as is known, this was the first recording of cardiac electrical activity. These authors described a negative deflection that could be measured by a galvanometer prior to each contraction. This confirmed earlier work of du Bois-Reymond in muscle from a guinea pig and a frog. In 1876, Marey used the capillary electrometer invented by Lippmann and photographically recorded the electrical activity of the frog's heart [16]. Engelmann [17] as well as Burdon Sanderson and Page [18] were also among the earliest to plot the potential variation of electrical activity of the heart (❷ Fig. 1.1). It is fascinating to read that in 1879, Burdon Sanderson and Page stated [19]: "We owe most to the labors of Engelmann whose researches on the propagation of the wave of contraction in the ventricles, on the electromotive properties of the resting heart, and on the electrical charges which immediately follow excitation, leave little more to be done."

It is evident that, as is usually the case, a whole series of developments finally led to a "first" – in this case, the first known recording of the human electrocardiogram (❷ Fig. 1.2) by Waller in 1887 [20]. Waller published further observations in 1889 [21] on his dog Jimmie, which is almost as well known as its owner (❷ Fig. 1.3)! The dog was in fact used in many of Waller's studies involving the capillary electrometer (❷ Fig. 1.4).

Besterman and Creese [22] lamented the fact that the contribution of Waller to the development of electrocardiography is often ignored. At the time of his publication of the human electrocardiogram, Waller was lecturer in physiology at St. Mary's Hospital, Paddington, London. The electrical activity of the exposed heart was already known as discussed above, but Waller decided to investigate the possibility of recording potentials from the limbs of animals and from man. Note, however, that the ECG of ❷ Fig. 1.2 was obtained from electrodes on the front and back of the chest. According to Besterman and Creese, the following is attributed to Waller at an informal talk in London in 1915 [22].

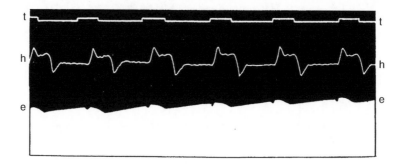

⬛ Fig. 1.2

The first published human electrocardiogram recorded by Waller in 1887. The ECG is represented by the lowest black/white interface (e), which represents the movements of mercury in the Lippmann Electrometer. The tracing denoted (h) records chest-wall movement and essentially is a form of apex cardiogram. The top calibration pulses represent the time (t) in 1s intervals between the onset of each pulse. This ECG was recorded with one electrode, which was strapped to the front of the chest, connected to the mercury column in the electrometer, while the other electrode, on the back of the patient's chest was connected to the sulfuric acid which formed the interface at the top of the mercury column in the electrometer. Note that this ECG did not exhibit atrial activity (After Waller [20]. © Physiological Society, London. Reproduced with permission)

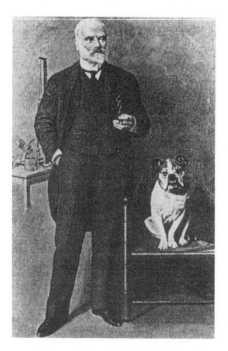

⬛ Fig. 1.3

A photograph of Waller with his dog Jimmie (After Besterman and Creese [22]. © British Medical Association, London. Reproduced with permission)

▶ "I studied the hearts of all sorts of animals and one fine day after leading off from the exposed heart of a decapitated cat to study the cardiogram by aid of a Lippmann electrometer, it occurred to me that it ought to be possible to use the limbs as electrodes and thus lead off from the heart to the electrometer without exposing the heart, i.e., from the intact and normal organ. Obviously man was the most convenient animal to use so I dipped my right hand and left foot into a couple of basins of salt solution, which were connected with the two poles of the electrometer and at once had the pleasure of seeing the

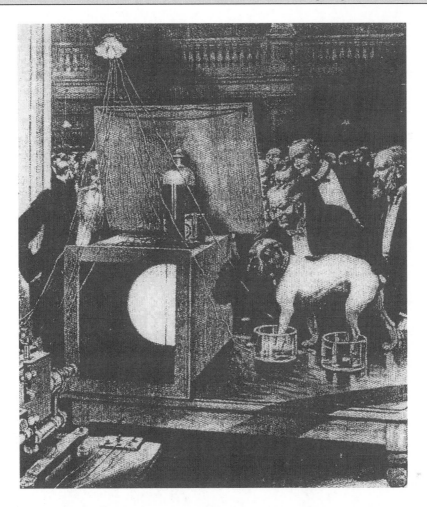

◘ Fig. 1.4
Waller's dog, Jimmie, being used to demonstrate the recording of an electrocardiogram to the Royal Society (Reproduced from Levick JR, An Introduction to Cardiovascular Physiology, 3rd Edition, London, Arnold, 2000)

mercury column pulsate with the pulsation of the heart. This first demonstration was made in St. Mary's Laboratory in 1887 and demonstrated there to many physiologists and among others, to my friend Professor Einthoven of Leiden…During the summer of that year, I made a complete summary of all sorts of leads from the hand and feet and mouth (❯ Fig. 1.5)."

There is an anecdotal story that a question was also asked in the House of Commons concerning the use of Jimmie in experiments where the dog's limbs were immersed in the saline solutions (❯ Fig. 1.4). The questioner asked whether such a procedure should not be prohibited under the Cruelty to Animals Act of 1876. The answer given, reputed to be by the Secretary of State at the time, Mr. Gladstone, suggested that if the Honorable Member who had posed the question had ever paddled in the sea, he would have appreciated fully the sensation obtained from this simple pleasurable experience! [22].

Physiological measurement technicians, or cardiac physiologists as they are now known in the UK, would be interested to know that Waller's early electrocardiograms were recorded photographically on a plate which was mounted on a toy railway wagon running on rails (❯ Fig. 1.6) in order to move the plate across a light beam which cast a shadow on the moving mercury meniscus of the electrometer [4]. Indeed, what would now be called the frequency response of the electrometer was so poor that the recorded deflections did not give an accurate recording of the cardiogram, but mathematical techniques were later used to correct this shortcoming [23].

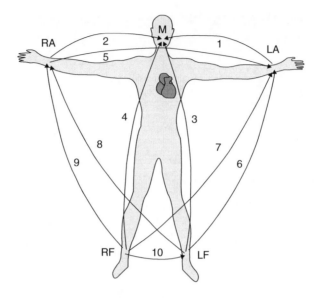

⬛ Fig. 1.5

A schematic representation of the various electrode combinations used by Waller in his early investigations. Note that, in addition to the four limb electrodes, the mouth was used as a fifth electrode. This allowed the derivation of 10 bipolar leads (Adapted from Bioelectromagnetism – Principles and Applications of Bioelectric and Biomagnetic Fields, Oxford University Press, New York, 1995 by J. Malmivuo and R. Plonsey. Reproduced with permission from http://www.bem.fi/book/index.htm)

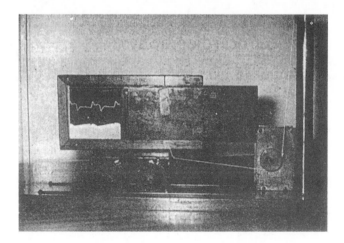

⬛ Fig. 1.6

The train wagon which was used to transport the photographic plate on which Waller recorded electrocardiograms (After Besterman and Creese [22]. © British Medical Association, London. Reproduced with permission)

It is of parochial interest that Waller qualified in medicine at Aberdeen, Scotland in 1878 [4], but he was not Scottish! It is also of historical interest to note that in 1889 in Berlin, he demonstrated the recording of an electrocardiogram on a dog, on a horse linked to equipment inside a building by lengthy recording leads and also on du Bois-Reymond [4].

There would appear to be some controversy as to who was the first to introduce the term "electrocardiogram." Burch and de Pasquale ([1], p. 29) state that it was Einthoven who introduced the term. Snellen ([24], p. l0) states that "the term electrocardiogram was coined by Einthoven."

However, Burchell [6] wrote that in 1912 Einthoven said [25]: "It gives me a special pleasure to bring to remembrance here, that the human EKG was first recorded by a London physiologist, Augustus D. Waller, who also introduced the term 'electrocardiogram' into science." There would therefore seem to be no doubt that Waller first used the term "electrocardiogram."

1.3   The Beginnings of Modern Electrocardiography

It is likely that most cardiologists, if asked about the origins of the electrocardiogram, would state that the Dutch physician Willem Einthoven developed a string galvanometer and thereafter applied it extensively to record the electrical activity of the heart. However, as alluded to in ❷ Sect. 1.2, most advances take place by refinement of earlier work, and it is therefore not surprising to find some controversy over the question of who in fact invented the string galvanometer. According to Cooper [3], the French electrical engineer Ader [26] invented a number of items including amplifier systems. He also developed "a highly sensitive, rapidly moving galvanometer that used a small wire instead of a coil to register electricity" [3]. The device was used to study underwater cables that were being laid at that time for transoceanic telegraphy [1].

Cooper [3] and Burch and de Pasquale [1] indicate that Einthoven, having been dissatisfied with the performance of the Lippmann electrometer, used a different instrument called the Deprez-d'Arsonval galvanometer. This galvanometer utilized a light coil of wire suspended between the poles of a permanent magnet, but Einthoven found that an improved sensitivity could be obtained by replacing the coil by a single fiber (a string). Einthoven then described his new galvanometer, and in that publication [27], acknowledged the Ader galvanometer, which also used a fine wire stretched between poles of a magnet. Cooper [3] suggests that Einthoven's wire was 0.002 mm in diameter, approximately one tenth as thick as that used by Ader. Cooper [3] also points out that one of Einthoven's teachers, Bosscha, had 30 years earlier in his own thesis suggested that a "single needle hanging from a silk thread" would form an appropriate moving part of a galvanometer [28].

Burchell [29] reviewed the controversy. His view was basically that the use of the word "invent" in respect of Einthoven's instrument was justified in the sense that Einthoven's device was an instrument specifically designed for recording the cardiac electrical activity. As such, it would have been feasible to patent it because it allowed recordings to be obtained that were not previously possible. He agreed that it was not "a discovery," and as has been suggested in this chapter, there can be very few situations in the history of scientific development where a new instrument is truly unique.

Notwithstanding the above, it is evident that Einthoven did not invent a galvanometer de novo. His major achievement was to design a device that was sensitive enough to record electrical potentials from the surface of the body. He developed a method of moving a photographic plate falling under gravity at a constant rate, and by directing a beam of light on the galvanometric string, its movements were recorded on the falling plate [1]. Einthoven's first electrocardiograph was extremely heavy, weighing around 600 lb, and required five operators. His first results appeared in 1903 [30].

Einthoven's laboratory was approximately one mile from the local hospital and so he had to develop a method for transmitting the ECG over telephone lines. The methods used and the results obtained are described in a classic paper published in 1906 [31]. At that time, leads I, II and III had been introduced and a variety of different electrocardiographic abnormalities demonstrated. This paper was followed by another classic in 1908 [32]. Burch and de Pasquale [1] state that "Einthoven's paper of 1908 may well be the most important single publication dealing with the subject of electrocardiography for it demonstrated to the medical profession that the electrocardiograph was of practical, as well as theoretic importance."

One of the last papers published by Einthoven and colleagues [33] included the now classic Einthoven triangle, whereby the body was represented in electrical terms by an equilateral triangle. From this, the mean QRS axis could be calculated. In addition, the well-known Einthoven's law was put forward around that time and is mentioned in the paper. In this book, the lead systems of electrocardiography are discussed in ❷ Chaps. 10 and ❷ 11. Axis calculations are highlighted in ❷ Chap. 1 of *Electrocardiology: Comprehensive Clinical ECG*.

In his early papers, Einthoven used the terminology of PQRST to describe the deflection of the electrocardiogram (❷ Fig. 1.7). It was suggested that the letters were selected to leave room for further discoveries such as the U wave, which Einthoven later detected using his string galvanometer. However, Cooper's view [3] was that the letters were chosen to conform with the terminology of mathematicians of the day, and Burchell [29] also supported this notion quoting

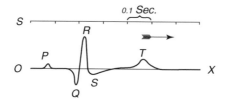

The early notation for the electrocardiogram as proposed by Einthoven. The largest deflection, positive or negative, was termed the R wave (After Einthoven [30]. © Springer, New York. Reproduced with permission)

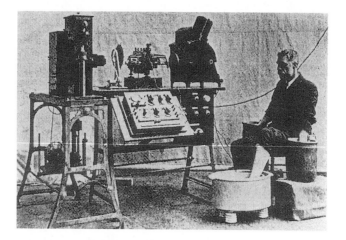

An early commercial version of the electrocardiograph manufactured by Cambridge Scientific Instrument Company of London in 1911. On the left is the camera incorporating the plate falling under gravity, the galvanometer is in the center and on the right is the light source required for the recording (After Br. Med. J. 1950;1: 720. © British Medical Association, London. Reproduced with permission)

Henson [34] who traced the use of PQRST for mathematical reasons back to Descartes. More recently, Hurst has reviewed the naming of all the components of the ECG including the delta and epsilon waves [35]. Gussak et al. [36] also reviewed the J (Osborn) wave.

It is worth noting that Einthoven's galvanometer was developed commercially by the Cambridge Instrument Company (❯ Fig. 1.8) in the UK. Early models found their way into the laboratory of other distinguished electrocardiographers such as Lewis and Wilson. In 1924, 2 years after Waller's death, Einthoven was awarded the Nobel Prize in Medicine for his contribution to electrocardiography.

1.4   Analysis of Cardiac Rhythm

It is relevant to diverge briefly in order to consider parallel work on the study of the rhythm of the heart, because much of the early work in electrocardiography was concerned with this topic. Of course, the study of the rhythm of the heart goes back centuries before the development of electrocardiography, since the rhythmic pulsation of arteries provided an external means of assessing the rhythm of the heart – once it was understood that such pulsation was indeed caused by the beating of the heart. In a historical review of the study of arrhythmias, Scherf and Schott [37] stated that approximately 3,500 years ago there was thought to be a connection between the pulse and the heart. These authors also quoted Read [38] who confidently indicated that a more scientific understanding of the pulse seemed to date in ancient China from about 500 BC. In the same historical review, Hubotter [39] was referenced as indicating that the occurrence of dropped pulse beats was related to prognosis. The more frequent the dropped beat, the higher the number of organs considered to be diseased and therefore the shorter the expected life span.

Not surprisingly, the ancient Greeks and Romans have also been credited with the study of cardiac rhythm. The Greek word *dikrotos* meaning double beating was apparently used by Herophilus (born 300 BC) to describe a dicrotic pulse [40]. Later, in the second century AD, Claudius Galen, a famous medical scholar of that time, introduced the term *eurhythmus* to describe a normal pulse. His original Latin text also used the term *arhythmus* to describe an abnormal pulse, which was further subdivided into three different types. His work remained prominent for over fifteen centuries. A few of his original Latin writings can be found in the review of Scherf and Schott [37].

In order to leap forward in time, it is convenient to link "arrhythmias" with one of the early texts on cardiac rhythm, namely, that by Wenckebach [41] entitled "Arhythmia of the Heart" (❯ Fig. 1.9). The English translation of this Dutch physician's treatise was published in 1904. In his book, Wenckebach acknowledged the contributions of a Scottish physician, Mackenzie, who in 1902 had published his own work on the study of the pulse [42]. At that time he was a general practitioner in the north of England and had spent many years accumulating data on patients with heart disease. What readers may find difficult to imagine is that all of Mackenzie's recordings were made with a polygraph, an instrument which allowed two channels of pressure tracings to be recorded. Mackenzie recorded the arterial and jugular pulsations simultaneously with his homemade instrument. His work at the time was largely ignored, but in 1908 he published a classic paper entitled "Diseases of the Heart" [43] and this brought him much worldwide acclaim.

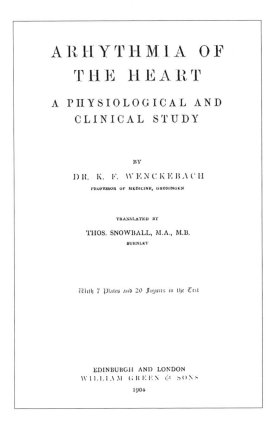

❒ Fig. 1.9

The frontispiece of the English edition of Wenckebach's text on the "Arhythmia of the Heart" published in 1904

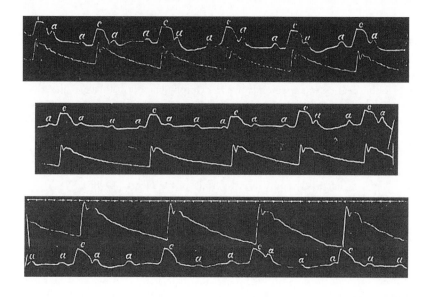

■ Fig. 1.10

Three illustrations of complete heart block recorded from a 66-year-old man: a, atrial contraction; c, carotid pulse. The second trace represents the radial pulse (After MacKenzie [42]. © Pentland, Edinburgh. Reproduced with permission)

An illustration of Mackenzie's tracings is provided in ❷ Fig. 1.10. These were first published in Mackenzie's 1902 book [42] and were reproduced by Wenckebach [41]. The recordings are from a 66-year-old man in "fair health" who was capable of considerable exertion. There was marked variation in heart rate from 23 per min to 42 per min. In the illustration, the small "a" waves represent atrial contraction, while the c waves are indicative of the carotid pulse. The larger waves on the second tracing denote the radial pulse. These recordings illustrate heart block. Wenckebach acknowledged Mackenzie's genius as follows.

▶ "So Mackenzie succeeded in recording the action of all the four chambers in man for the first time, and in establishing beyond doubt the complete heart block, the continued action of the two auricles, and the simultaneous cessation of both ventricles. We are under great obligations to this keen and clever observer for showing how this can be accomplished. A clearer proof for the recurrence of heart-block in persons who were certainly not in the throes of death (Hering) cannot be desired."

Wenckebach also discussed the "conductivity or power of conduction" which he denoted A. Changes in the rapidity of conduction were studied by examining the interval between auricular and ventricular contraction denoted $A_s - V_s$. In reporting another irregularity of conduction, Wenckebach stated the following.

▶ "A great diminution of the conduction power and its consequences can be best demonstrated on a dying frog's heart at the interval $A_s - V_s$.
   As the conduction gradually grows worse and worse, this interval gets always longer; the conduction may become so bad that the ventricle does not begin to contract until just before the next auricular systole. Anyone that had not followed the way in which this phenomenon slowly developed would think that the auricular systole followed the ventricular; in other words, that there was a reversal of the usual order of contraction. But if A continues to grow worse, there finally comes a time when the stimulus is no longer conducted (or not with sufficient strength?), $A_s - V_s = \infty$; in other words, the ventricle does not contract. During the pause that arises through the missing of this systole, however, A will have plenty of time to recover again so far that the next stimulus is again conducted to the ventricle, and it contracts; but after a few systoles have occurred, A is again so much reduced that another beat is missed. In this way a ventricular contraction may continue to be dropped after the same number of systoles for a considerable time, thus producing a regular intermission of the ventricle. A very beautiful example of this missed ventricular systole is given in ❷ Fig. 1.11; the tracing was obtained from a frog's heart and was taken from Engelmann's paper on Conduction of Stimuli [44].

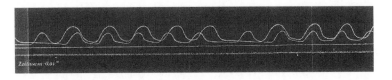

■ Fig. 1.11
The lower amplitude waveform represents atrial contraction, and the larger waveform ventricular contraction, in a frog's heart. Note that the ventricular contraction is missed after the sixth beat. The tracing was first recorded by Engelmann [44] (After Wenckebach [41]. © Green, Edinburgh. Reproduced with permission)

At a later stage of asphyxia, auricular contractions soon drop out in consequence of the defective conduction from the sinus to the auricle. The contractions of the heart are thereby made to appear in groups which may assume a very complicated form from further interference with the conduction power and the other functions. In these cases, we speak of the "periodic" action of the heart and the groups are called after their discoverer "Luciani's periods".'"

There is a great temptation to follow the extract with an exclamation, because what nowadays is referred to as the "Wenckebach" phenomenon was acknowledged by Wenckebach to have been described by others, Again, therefore, there is evidence of the interlinking of the work of many in the advancement and understanding of a field of knowledge.

A complete review of the early work on arrhythmias is beyond the scope of this chapter. It is of interest, however, to mention that a Scot called McWilliam first used the term atrial flutter and in 1887 proposed the concept of ventricular fibrillation [45], a topic that was to interest him, particularly its relationship to sudden death, for 40 years. In 1893, His described the AV bundle [46], a finding which he himself said 40 years later [47] was largely ignored at the time. When electrocardiography became possible, there was of course great interest in the study of cardiac rhythm. Einthoven produced records of ventricular extrasystoles, ventricular bigeminy and atrial fibrillation [31] although it was left to others, notably Hering [48] and Lewis [49] to examine the latter in more detail. Today, our understanding of arrhythmic mechanisms has grown immeasurably through the medium of EPS (electrophysiology study) testing via multiple catheters and perhaps basket electrodes inserted into the heart. The techniques are discussed fully in ❷ Chaps. 2 and ❷ 3 of *Cardiac Arrhythmias and Mapping Techniques* while a variety of arrhythmias is presented in ❷ Chaps. 4–8 of *Cardiac Arrhythmias and Mapping Techniques*.

1.5 Clinical Development of Electrocardiography

By the middle of the first decade of the twentieth century, the Einthoven galvanometer had been developed, the electrocardiogram was beginning to be investigated more extensively and much work on the irregularity of the heart beat had been undertaken using polygraphic methods, which probably arose from the early work of the French physiologist Marey. The first commercial version of the Einthoven electrocardiograph was produced in 1908 by the Cambridge Instrument Company, and other models soon came into use throughout Europe. Interestingly, the first electrocardiograph to be shipped to the United States was developed by Edelmann, who had originally manufactured Einthoven's machine, but because of disagreements over royalty payments, the two had parted company. The Edelmann machine was taken to the USA by Cohn in 1909 after he had spent some time in London working with Mackenzie and one of his junior staff, Thomas Lewis [1]. In the same year, a Russian physiologist Samojloff wrote a short text in German entitled "Elektrokardiogramme" [50]. He had visited Einthoven in Leiden in 1904 and later bought the sixth electrocardiograph to be manufactured by the Cambridge Scientific Instrument Company [51]. Samojloff was a good friend of a Professor Lepeschkin, whose son Eugene remembered spending summer holidays in close proximity to the Samojloff family, as they each had a summer home near Kazan in Russia. Lepeschkin [52] himself later did much fundamental work on electrocardiography and, indeed, married the daughter of Frank Wilson whose unipolar leads have briefly been referenced already [7] and which will be discussed in more detail later. It is fascinating to tie together the various friendships established in the field of electrocardiography, almost as if there had been one large family tree of fellow electrocardiographers! In turn, this leads to some further detail of the extremely distinguished physician later to become Sir Thomas Lewis, whose first work on the mechanism of the heart beat [53] was dedicated to James Mackenzie and Willem Einthoven – a family tree indeed!

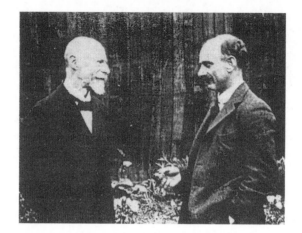

◼ Fig. 1.12

Photograph of Einthoven (left) and Lewis probably taken in 1921 during Lewis' last visit to Leiden (© Museum Boerhaave, Leiden. Reproduced with permission)

Lewis was born in Wales in 1881, and 100 years later a series of editorials was published in the *British Heart Journal* to commemorate his birth [54–57]. Lewis' career was not entirely devoted to electrocardiography, but a large portion of his working life from around 1905 to 1925, when he published the third edition of his now famous textbook, retitled "The Mechanism and Graphic Registration of the Heart Beat" [58], was taken up with the subject. Interestingly, in this edition the former dedication to Mackenzie and Einthoven was removed. In the interim, however, Lewis had formed a strong friendship with Einthoven (❷ Fig. 1.12) and they exchanged much correspondence in the intervening years, as was diligently uncovered by Snellen [24]. Lewis' book of 1925 represented a major advance for electrocardiography. It summarized much of the earlier work on cardiac arrhythmias, but this time ECGs were published in support of the various theories of circus movement, and so on. Electrocardiograms representing hypertrophy with preponderance of one or other ventricle were presented but unfortunately, the now well-publicized ECGs from right and left bundle branch block were wrongly described, that is, what Lewis described as a defect of "the right division of the AV bundle" (❷ Fig. 1.13) was in fact a left bundle branch block. Because the recordings were thought to represent activation principally of the left ventricle, they were called the human "levocardiogram." Conversely, as shown in ❷ Fig. 1.14, the human dextrocardiogram was thought to represent a defect of the left division of the AV bundle. It should be remembered, however, that at that time Lewis was working only with the three limb leads of Einthoven, and even now it would be difficult, given only the three leads of ❷ Fig. 1.14, to say whether the curve truly represented a right bundle branch block or one obtained from a more complex congenital cardiac lesion. Lewis had undertaken much experimental work on dogs in order to prove his conclusions, but it was not until 1929–1931 that the error was corrected by Frank Wilson and colleagues in the USA [59]. In fact, the conclusion that, in left bundle branch block, the principal deflection of the QRS complex would be positive, that is, upwards in lead I, had already been predicted in 1920 by Fahr [60], who had earlier worked with Einthoven.

In the series of editorials [54–57] mentioned above, repeated reference was made to Lewis' book as a classic. That so much of clinical value could have been derived from the available apparatus speaks volumes for the ability and tenacity of those early workers. It is interesting to read the section of Lewis' book [58] on electrodes that were advocated for connecting the patient as shown in ❷ Figs. 1.15 and ❷ 1.16. "A porous inner vessel is filled with warm water, salt and well-washed cotton wool, to give a mixture of porridge-like consistence." In fact, the porous pot was "surrounded by an outer vessel containing saturated zinc sulphate in which was immersed a sheet of zinc to which the leading off wire was soldered." This technique was still in use in the late 1940s. Modern electrode technology is discussed in ❷ Chap. 12.

Lewis was a prolific writer, producing twelve books and over two hundred scientific papers. He was invited by Mackenzie to found the journal *Heart,* which first appeared on 1st July 1909. It is not therefore surprising to find that he had strong views on various matters, and Burchell [54] pointed out Lewis' long campaign "to establish clinical science as a discipline, separate and definable, from both physiology and medical practice." Lewis held the view that

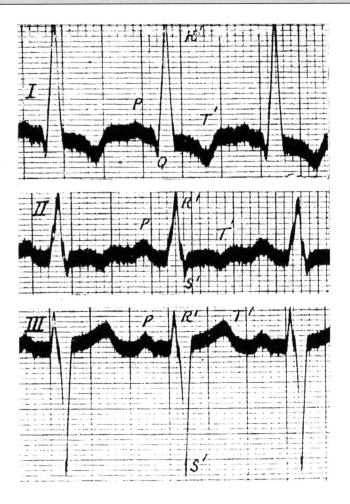

◧ Fig. 1.13

Leads I, II and III (not recorded simultaneously) recorded from a patient who was described by Lewis as having a defect "of the right division of the AV bundle" (After Lewis [58]. © Shaw, London. Reproduced with permission)

"efficient medical practitioners are not scientists" [61]. He discontinued his research into electrocardiography around 1925, perhaps feeling there was not much more of interest, even though the area of myocardial infarction had not been studied.

1.6 The American Connection

As mentioned in ❷ Sect. 1.5, one of the early Edelmann galvanometers found its way to the USA in 1909. Five years later, Frank Wilson, working at the University of Michigan, obtained a string galvanometer manufactured by the Cambridge Instrument Company and became deeply involved with electrocardiography, a research field that was to occupy him for the rest of his academic career. By now the reader should no longer be surprised to learn of one further link in the family tree of electrocardiographers. According to Burch and de Pasquale [1], Wilson was stationed in England during World War I in a rehabilitation hospital under the command of none other than Sir Thomas Lewis! Indeed, his first paper appeared in *Heart,* which was edited by Lewis in 1915 [62].

A glance at the contents list of Lewis' book [58] reveals that only one chapter deals with the morphology of the QRS complex in relation to hypertrophy, aberrant contractions and displaced heart. This represents a small proportion in a book of 38 chapters. The significance of the contribution of Wilson can then be seen in the fact that he concentrated his

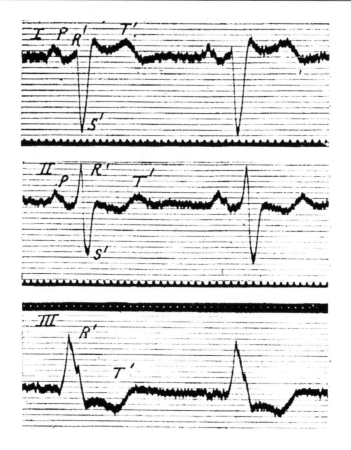

⬛ **Fig. 1.14**

Leads I, II and III recorded from a patient who according to Lewis had a defect in the "left division of the bundle." The time marks each represent 1/30 s (After Lewis [58]. © Shaw, London. Reproduced with permission)

work on the QRS and T morphologies whereas Lewis, often using bipolar chest leads, concentrated heavily on the study of cardiac rhythm.

Although Wilson's initial work appears to have been undertaken in England, Kossmann, in his review of unipolar electrocardiography [7], indicated that Wilson's research in the University of Michigan was based on "a two-string-in-tandem electrocardiograph built by Willem Einthoven and his son." Recordings were at half of normal sensitivity (1 mV = 0.5 cm) in order that two simultaneous recordings could be accommodated on narrow recording film (10 cm wide).

During the 1920s, Wilson and his team undertook a great many studies on correlating the ECG (essentially limb leads I, II and III) with abnormalities such as ventricular hypertrophy and bundle branch block. Some of their work is discussed elsewhere in the book. In particular, the concept of ventricular gradient (❷ Chaps. 5 and ❷ 5 of *Electrocardiology: Comprehensive Clinical ECG*) is still used by many authors today to explain certain phenomena. For example, Abildskov suggests that inequality in the ventricular gradient in different areas of the myocardium may be responsible for ventricular arrhythmias [63]. Nevertheless, it is likely that the major contribution of Wilson will be acknowledged as his "central terminal" with which unipolar chest leads could be recorded. The matter is dealt with fully in ❷ Chaps. 10 and ❷ 11 and will not be reiterated in detail here. In summary, however, the technique allows the potential variation at a single point on the chest to be recorded with respect to a relatively constant reference potential obtained by averaging the potentials of the right and left arms and the left leg.

At this point, it is necessary to consider the confusion that existed around 1930 in terms of the polarity of ECG waveforms. Waller had used a bipolar chest lead in his initial ECG recording of 1887 [20]. However, more extensive

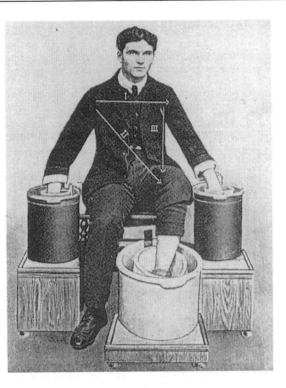

◘ Fig. 1.15
An illustration of an early method of recording the Einthoven limb leads. Further details are in the text (After Lewis [58]. © Shaw, London. Reproduced with permission)

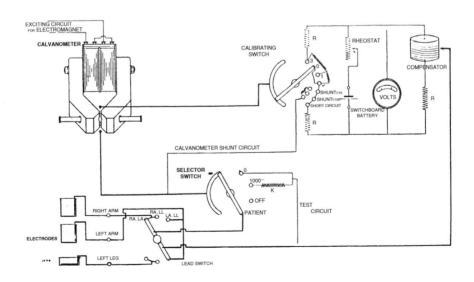

◘ Fig. 1.16
A diagram showing the connections from the electrodes of ❷ Fig. 1.15 to the galvanometer, as in the Cambridge Electrocardiograph

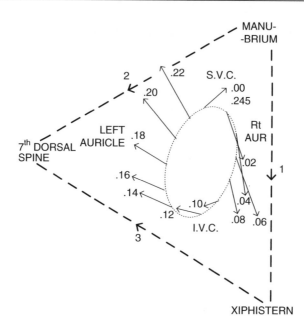

A chest electrode system used by Lewis in his studies of atrial flutter. The connection points for the Einthoven electrodes are shown on the diagram (see text for further explanation). Note also that Lewis used these three leads to calculate the axis of the flutter waves shown in ❷ Fig. 1.18. The direction of the axis is shown at 20 ms intervals. Lewis indicated that "the flutter in this patient depended upon a circulating wave." He regarded this as strong, if not conclusive, evidence "that circus movement is the basis of clinical auricular flutter" (After Lewis [58]. © Shaw, London. Reproduced with permission)

use of chest leads was certainly made by Lewis, and ❷ Fig. 1.17 shows a lead system which he described for recording three bipolar leads from the chest. The notation 1–3 refers to the bipolar leads of Einthoven, but in this case, the left arm lead is connected to an electrode on the xiphisternum, the right arm lead is connected to the manubrium and the left leg is connected to the seventh dorsal spine. Recordings obtained from these leads in a patient with "clinical flutter" are shown in ❷ Fig. 1.18. Einthoven had arranged his galvanometer so that when the left arm connection was relatively positive compared to the right arm connection, an upward deflection was produced by the instrument. In Lewis' system, therefore, the potentials obtained with the connections for lead II and lead III indicate that for the most part the electrode on the spine is relatively positive compared to those on the front of the chest. In fact, in very general terms, the appearances in leads 2 and 3 of ❷ Fig. 1.18 would approximately resemble an inverted V2 used nowadays.

In 1931, Wood and colleagues in Pennsylvania recorded a bipolar chest lead on a patient who had a spontaneous attack of chest pain. The bipolar lead was recorded using the Einthoven lead I connections but the left arm electrode was placed on the back and the right arm electrode was on the precordium "at the cardiac level, just to the left of the midline." This lead configuration was described as lead IV since it was an addition to the three leads of Einthoven. During the attack of pain, lead IV showed marked ST depression in a lead that had essentially a dominant R wave. (It should be noted that Einthoven had always called the most prominent deflection, be it positive or negative, the R wave.) This work was subsequently described by Woolferth and Wood in 1932 [64].

In view of the foregoing comments on polarity, what was recorded at that time as ST depression would nowadays be manifested as significant ST elevation in a lead such as V2.

The use of bipolar chest leads proliferated and various combinations were introduced, e.g., the bipolar chest lead CR had the indifferent electrode on the right arm and the exploring electrode on the chest. Such bipolar chest leads are discussed further in ❷ Chap. 11. In 1960, in a letter to Burch [1], Wood commented that he still used the CR leads although the hospital ECG department had changed to unipolar precordial leads.

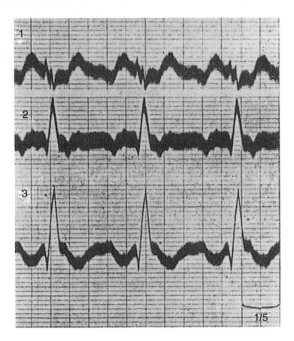

Fig. 1.18

The ECGs recorded with the lead system of ◉ Fig. 1.17 in a patient with "clinical flutter." Note how appearances in leads denoted 2 and 3, which very approximately resemble V_2 and V_3 used nowadays, have the opposite polarity (After Lewis [58]. © Shaw, London. Reproduced with permission)

What was a unipolar precordial lead? As Kossmann has pointed out [7], during all the experimenting with chest leads, a paper of Wilson and colleagues in 1932 [65] largely went unnoticed. By linking the left arm, right arm and left leg through equal resistors to a central terminal, a relatively stable reference potential was obtained with respect to which the potential at an exploring electrode could be measured. The circuit (◉ Fig. 1.19) was also described by Wilson and colleagues in another classic paper in 1934 [66]. Because the potential of the central terminal was essentially constant, the potential difference recorded by the galvanometer reflected the variation at a single point – hence the term "unipolar" lead. Ultimately, these leads became known as "V leads" so that when the exploring electrode was placed on the left arm, the lead was called "VL" (◉ Fig. 1.19). More recently, there has been some discussion [67] on the fact that every ECG lead is bipolar in the sense that the "galvanometer" always measures a potential difference but this author feels that where the potential at one terminal of the galvanometer is essentially constant, the signal generated reflects the potential variation at the other terminal – hence "unipolar" is still an adjective with some meaning even though some would say it was incorrect!

The next stage in the evolution of the unipolar lead was for Wilson's team to specify six precordial positions for the exploring electrode [68]. However, the leads designated V_1 to V_5 covered an area from approximately the fifth rib at the right sternal border to the sixth rib in the left anterior axillary line. The sixth precordial lead was designated VE, where the exploring electrode was placed at the tip of the ensiform process.

In order to try to restore some order from the chaos, a joint group of cardiologists representing the Cardiac Society of Great Britain and Ireland on the one hand and the American Heart Association on the other issued a paper recommending standardization of only one chest electrode position [69]. This paper is very often quoted in error as the definitive recommendation for placement of precordial electrodes. However, it was a second paper, which was published unilaterally later in the same year by the American Heart Association, that did in fact define what are now accepted as the six precordial leads [70]. A further supplementary report was issued by the same committee in 1943 [71].

The story of the American contribution to the development of lead systems (at least for conventional electrocardiography) is completed with the introduction, in 1942, by Goldberger of what became known as the augmented unipolar

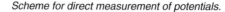

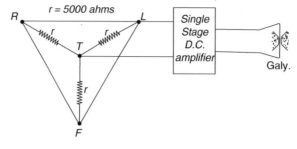

Scheme for direct measurement of potentials.

◻ Fig. 1.19
A diagram of the Wilson central terminal, denoted T. The limb leads are connected through equal resistors to the central point T. In this case, the circuitry for VL is shown (After Wilson et al. [66]. © Mosby, St Louis, Missouri. Reproduced with permission)

limb leads [72]. The modification introduced by Goldberger for recording unipolar limb leads was to remove the Wilson central terminal connection from the limb on which the exploring electrode was placed. In other words, if the exploring electrode were placed on the right arm, the Goldberger terminal, that is, the modified Wilson terminal, would consist only of connections from the left arm and left leg to a central point. It can be shown that the net effect is to augment the potential recorded by VR by 50% exactly (❷ Chap. 11). Thus the term "augmented unipolar limb lead" was introduced. Clearly, there were only three such leads, namely, aVR, aVL and aVF, which could be recorded with this technique.

The development of what is now known as the conventional 12-lead ECG was therefore complete. There were three limb leads I, II and III from Einthoven; three augmented unipolar limb leads aVR, aVL, and aVF from Goldberger's modification of Wilson's central terminal; and six precordial leads V_1–V_6 arising out of the Wilson terminal. The 12-lead ECG is today used everywhere that electrocardiography is practised. Appearances in disease are discussed extensively in ❷ Chaps. 2–10 of *Electrocardiology: Comprehensive Clinical ECG*. Cardiac arrhythmias are discussed separately in ❷ Chaps. 1–8 of *Cardiac Arrhythmias and Mapping Techniques*.

As mentioned above, Einthoven had described the maximum deflection of the ventricular complex as the R wave irrespective of whether it was positive or negative [33]. Lewis, on the other hand, had used Q and S for "downward" deflections even when there was a dominant S wave such as in lead I in right axis deviation [58]. This approach prevailed. The standardization of the precordial leads has also helped to ensure that negative deflections in chest leads resulted in downward displacement, and so on. Pardee [73] suggested that if two upward deflections were present, the first should be designated Ra and the second Rb, but although the concept of both upward deflections being called R waves was accepted, it was subsequently the case that the first R wave was called R and the second R′.

1.7   Vectorcardiography

The concept of a vector is introduced in ❷ Chap. 2, but for the less mathematically inclined it can be summarized as a device for representing an entity such as a force with which would be associated a magnitude and a direction. Almost from the beginnings of electrocardiography, the concept of a vector force was invoked initially by Waller [21] who had produced an isopotential map (see ❷ Sect. 1.10) which suggested that the electromotive force of the heart could be represented by a single dipole, a physical entity which is discussed in ❷ Chap. 2. Later, Einthoven and colleagues in their classic paper of 1913 [33] introduced the concept of measuring the mean electrical axis of the heart, which was represented by a vector (❷ Fig. 1.20). There are a number of ways of calculating such a mean axis (see ❷ Chap. 1 of *Electrocardiology: Comprehensive Clinical ECG*) but, in addition, it should be realized that the concept as illustrated in ❷ Fig. 1.20 allows what might be called an instantaneous axis to be calculated given a knowledge of the potentials in leads I, II and III at the same instant in time. Lewis was also one of the earliest to exploit this idea and, having recorded leads I, II and III singly from a dog whose right bundle had been cut, he plotted the deflections shown in ❷ Fig. 1.21. Thereafter, given the concept of the Einthoven triangle it was feasible to plot a vector for

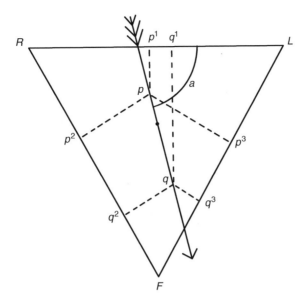

⬛ **Fig. 1.20**
An illustration of the resultant cardiac electromotive force represented by a vector *pq* which makes an angle a with the lead I axis. The projection of the vector on the different leads is denoted p^1q^1, p^2q^2 and p^3q^3 (After Einthoven et al. [33]. © Springer, New York. Reproduced with permission)

successive instants in the cardiac cycle, and these are also shown in ❷ Fig. 1.21. However, although the directions are shown, the magnitude of each vector is apparently constant. Nevertheless, the concept of a vectorcardiogram began to evolve. This work was published by Lewis in his monograph [58] but it had previously appeared in 1916 [74]. It is of interest to note the length of papers published at that time, with this one in particular occupying almost 90 pages.

Burch has reviewed the history of vectorcardiography [2] and he has pointed out that the first publication describing a method for manually deriving "a vectorcardiogram" from standard limb leads was written by Williams and published in 1914 [75]. The methodology is shown in ❷ Fig. 1.22. In this case, however, an amplitude is associated with each vector direction, and if the tips of the vectors had been joined in the correct sequence, an approximate figure-of-eight configuration would have been seen. In fact, this was done shortly afterwards by Mann [76], and the loop thus obtained was called a monocardiogram (❷ Fig. 1.23). It should be emphasized that, at that time, all leads were still being recorded singly and therefore, Lewis, Williams and Mann had to align the three complexes as best as possible. Although Mann subsequently invented a monocardiograph, which according to Burch was developed in 1925 though not described until 1938 [77], the advent of the cathode ray oscilloscope radically changed the approach to displaying loops.

The advantage of the oscilloscope was that two separate leads could be applied to opposite pairs of plates in order to deflect the electron beam in proportion to the strength of the signal on each axis (❷ Fig. 1.24). It should be realized that any two different ECG leads applied to an oscilloscope will produce a loop independent of any vector theory. However, in keeping with the concept of a frontal plane loop, ❷ Fig. 1.24 shows how lead I could be used to produce a lateral component and VF a vertical component that might give an approximate indication of frontal plane vector forces.

Apparently, Schellong in Germany [78], Wilson's team in the USA [79] and Hollmann and Holmann in Germany [80], independently of each other, developed systems for displaying loops. Of these three groups, Schellong was the first to publish loops recorded with the cathode ray oscilloscope. According to Burch [2], Rijlant also used the cathode ray oscilloscope in 1936 but for the display of the scalar electrocardiogram [81]. It can be imagined how the advent of a new tool was eagerly adopted by many laboratories worldwide with the resultant relatively simultaneous publication of results.

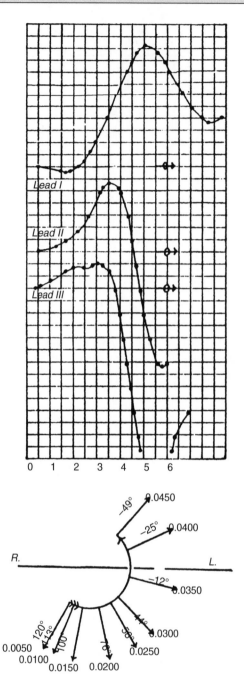

⬛ Fig. 1.21

Leads I, II and III recorded from a dog in which the right division of the bundle had been destroyed. Lewis, who had recorded the leads singly, aligned them as best as possible in order to calculate the frontal plane QRS axis at 5 ms intervals. It can be seen that the vector moves in a counterclockwise direction during the QRS complex (After Lewis [58]. © Shaw, London)

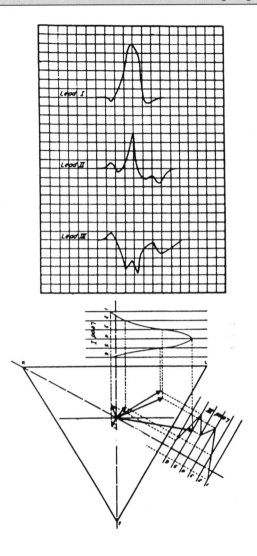

◘ Fig. 1.22
Calculation of the resultant cardiac vector in the frontal plane using leads I and III (After Williams [75]. © American Physiological Society, Bethesda, Maryland. Reproduced with permission)

Although early efforts at constructing loops were in the frontal plane, the use of the oscilloscope allowed other planes to be viewed with relative ease. The concept of a three-dimensional loop in space gradually grew, and a number of lead systems were introduced to derive the components of the resultant cardiac vector, as discussed in ❷ Chap. 2.

1.8   Lead Theory

It would be appropriate at this point to diverge briefly in order to review the development of lead theory and its influence on vectorcardiographic lead systems before concluding this section of the history. The theoretical aspects are considered in detail in ❷ Chap. 10, but it is of relevance at this point to underline the fact that although electrodes may be placed such that a line joining them is along one of the natural axes of the body, it is not necessarily the case that the potential difference measured by them is a true reflection of the component of the cardiac electromotive forces in that particular direction. The whole concept of vectorcardiography was based on deriving a resultant vector given a knowledge of the component

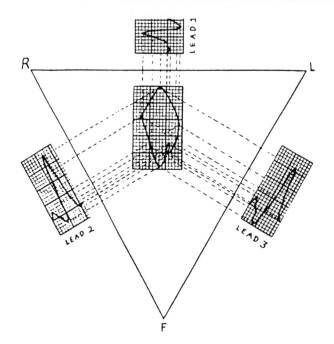

Using a procedure similar to that of ❷ Fig. 1.22, Mann produced the loop which he called a "monocardiogram" (After Mann [76]. © American Medical Association, Chicago, Illinois. Reproduced with permission)

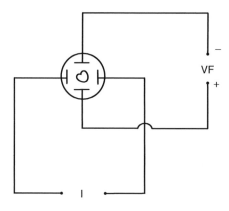

■ Fig. 1.24
A schematic representation showing how two ECG leads applied to opposite pairs of plates of an oscilloscope would deflect the electron beam to produce a loop. The electron beam is deflected in a horizontal direction by an amount in proportion to the amplitude of lead I and is similarly deflected in a vertical direction by VF

forces in three mutually perpendicular directions as shown in ❷ Fig. 1.25. The aim of lead design was therefore to develop electrode configurations that would faithfully measure components in the desired direction.

If a vector alters its magnitude and direction over a period of time, it is feasible to imagine that its tip traces out a path in three dimensional space, as shown in ❷ Fig. 1.26. This illustration also indicates how the loop can be "projected" onto three mutually perpendicular planes to produce 3 two-dimensional loops. In fact, each of these three loops was originally

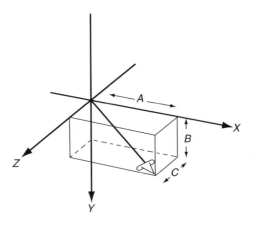

◼ Fig. 1.25

The concept of a resultant vector being derived given a knowledge of its components A, B and C in three mutually perpendicular directions X, Y and Z, respectively. A corrected orthogonal-lead system attempts to derive the components A, B and C

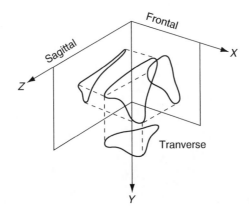

◼ Fig. 1.26

The projection of a spatial loop onto three mutually perpendicular planes. The three planar loops are known collectively as the vectorcardiogram

derived by the methods shown in ❷ Fig. 1.24 and detailed in ❷ Chap. 11; nowadays, computer-assisted methods are used. Wilson and Johnston [82] introduced the term "vectorcardiogram" to describe the three loops of ❷ Fig. 1.26.

A classic series of papers by Burger and van Milaan dealing with lead theory appeared from 1946 to 1948 [83]. These authors showed that in electrical terms, the Einthoven triangle was decidedly not of an equilateral nature (see ❷ Fig. 10.3). Other attempts to study lead characteristics were made using two-dimensional media such that current flow and electrical field could be assessed [84, 85]. For example, ❷ Fig. 1.27 shows flow lines for lead I obtained from a model where the body was represented by a homogenous conducting medium. The same figure also shows the field map of a normal human subject. Note that the current flow is essentially perpendicular to the lead field. McFee and Johnston, in a classic series of three papers [86], elegantly reviewed the theory of electrocardiographic leads.

Separately, at approximately the same time, Frank made use of a tank model of a human torso in which an artificial generator was situated in order to study the effects of different leads. An important outcome was the creation of an image surface [87], which effectively delineated an imaginary torso where lines joining two points bore a true theoretical relationship to the direction of current flow between the two corresponding points on the actual torso. In other

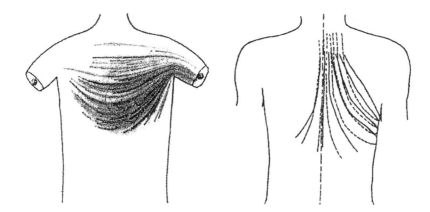

Two-dimensional model studies showing on the left, current flow lines from a lead I configuration and on the right, the corresponding electrical field (After McFee et al. [84]. © American Heart Association, Dallas, Texas. Reproduced with permission)

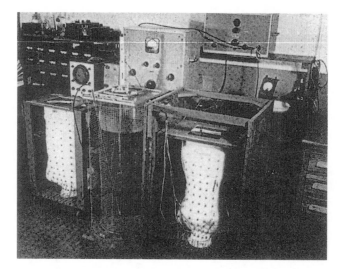

A photograph of Frank's laboratory showing a male and female torso model with electrodes attached. The models are mounted upside down to facilitate accurate positioning of the artificial generator (After Frank E. *Circulation* 1954;9: 723. © American Heart Association, Dallas, Texas. Reproduced with permission)

words, if a bipolar lead were formed by two electrodes, the line joining the two points in image space corresponding to their positions would indicate the direction associated with that lead, that is, the direction in which the component of the resultant cardiac e.m.f. would be measured. Frank's original model with electrodes attached is shown in ❯ Fig. 1.28.

The net result of Frank's studies was the development of a "corrected orthogonal-lead system" which purported to measure the true components of the resultant cardiac vector in three mutually perpendicular directions [88]. This system is probably the most popular lead system for vectorcardiography wherever the technique is still practised. However, it is of interest to note that Burch [2] is somewhat critical of the prominence of the Frank system on account of its susceptibility to repeat variation and the difficulty of applying electrodes properly in all patients, particularly obese women and neonates; he felt that the Equilateral Tetrahedron introduced by Wilson and colleagues [89] was the preferred system.

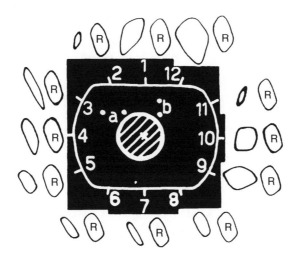

◻ Fig. 1.29

A tank model with an elliptical horizontal cross section in which an artificial electrical generator is positioned at a and b. A nonconducting volume is enclosed within the hatched circle. Different electrode positions are denoted 1 to 12. "Vectorgrams" recorded with the network (see text) are denoted R and essentially have the same configuration whichever group of electrodes is used to record the loop. On the other hand, the corresponding vectorgrams derived without being input via the network show marked variation (After Rijlant [90]. © Academie Royal de Medécine de Belgique, Brussels. Reproduced with permission)

It would seem that if vectorcardiographic systems do continue in existence, it will not be with this system, for which little data is available.

There have been many other systems of vectorcardiography introduced (see ❷ Chap. 11). Rijlant in 1956 proposed the use of a complex electrode array on the body surface consisting of 72 uniformly distributed electrodes. The aim was to link the electrodes together in such a way that they effectively measured potential at an infinite distance from the source assumed to be in a homogenous conducting medium. Such a network minimizes the local or proximity effects. ❷ Figure 1.29 shows how "vectorgrams" derived from the network using different combinations maintain an almost uniform shape, while corresponding loops derived simply from the electrode potentials, not fed via the network, show a variety of configurations depending on the combination of electrodes chosen [90]. Schmitt also made many contributions to theoretical and practical studies in electrocardiography; not least, together with Simonson, he introduced the SVEC III (stereo vector electrocardiography) system [91]. In the author's laboratory, despite extensive experience of 3-lead electrocardiography, it was apparent in the mid-1970s that clinicians were reluctant to move from the 12-lead electrocardiogram. For this reason, a hybrid lead system was introduced [92] to combine the 3 and 12-lead ECGs (see ❷ Chap. 11). This system is no longer used routinely.

Does vectorcardiography have a future? When the hybrid lead system was first described in 1977 at a private meeting, Rautaharju, author of ❷ Chap. 8 of *Specialized Aspects of ECG* of this book, said that it would be the last orthogonal-lead system to be introduced! He was subsequently proved wrong [93, 94], but the substance of his comment is clear. On the other hand, as discussed in ❷ Chap. 11, there are other methods for deriving the orthogonal-lead (or X, Y, Z lead) ECG and hence the vectorcardiogram from the conventional 12-lead ECG. Dower, for example, has long been a proponent of polarcardiography (see ❷ Chap. 13 of *Specialized Aspects of ECG*), which is an alternative form of displaying the orthogonal leads. However, in order to minimize the need for recording both XYZ and 12-lead ECGs, he introduced a method of deriving the 12-lead ECG from the XYZ leads [95]. Essentially, by making use of Frank's image surface, a set of transfer coefficients was derived which allows each of the 12 leads to be expressed as a linear combination of the XYZ leads. Subsequently, there have been several attempts (discussed in ❷ Chap. 11) to adopt the inverse procedure, where the XYZ leads are derived from a linear combination of the conventional 12 leads to give the so-called derived XYZ leads [96–98]. The vectorcardiographic loops derived do not compare exactly with the originals but the discrepancies may prove to be of small consequence. The major advantage of the derived XYZ lead system is that vectorcardiographic loops

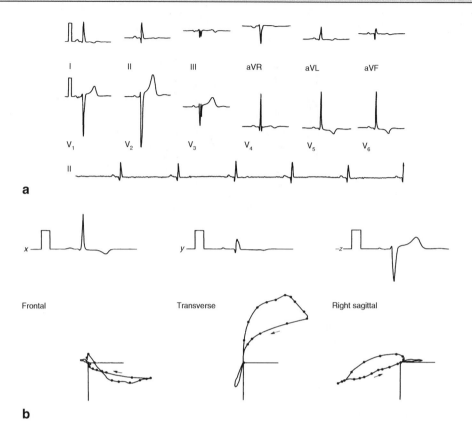

■ Fig. 1.30

12-lead ECG and vectorcardiographic loop derived from the 12-lead ECG (using equations in [96]) in a patient with a history of myocardial infarction. Note that the 12-lead ECG does not show definite evidence of infarction according to classical criteria although RV$_3$ < RV$_2$, yet the clockwise inscription of the loop in the transverse plane is quite abnormal, being consistent with anteroseptal infarction. The low R waves in V$_3$ might be considered as caused by LVH. The patient was a 48-year-old male with severe disease of the right coronary artery and the left anterior descending coronary artery. The cardiothoracic ratio was 0.5

can be obtained without any additional electrodes compared to the 12-lead ECG requirements, and from these loops, information relating to the phase relationships between the leads can be derived. An example is shown in ❷ Fig. 1.30 where the 12-lead ECG does not show clear evidence of myocardial infarction, but where the vectorcardiographic loops with clockwise inscription in the transverse plane are quite abnormal, being consistent with the history of such a clinical abnormality. Dower also developed his EASI lead system [94], so called because of his choice of electrode positions taken from Frank's nomenclature for his own lead system [88]. The EASI lead system is presented in ❷ Chap. 11. With only four electrodes plus a neutral electrode, the 12 lead ECG can be derived.

The development of lead systems certainly does not end at this point and the more recent concept of limited lead systems [e.g., 99, 100]. In this approach, a subset of the chest leads, such as V2 and V5 only, is recorded and the other four chest leads are calculated therefrom. This can be done in different ways and the matter is discussed in ❷ Chap. 11. The opposite of reduced lead systems is body surface mapping but before looking at this technique, it would be appropriate to consider parallel developments in mathematical modeling of the electrical activity of the heart.

It could be said that the first attempt at modeling the electrical activity of the heart was represented by Waller's illustration of the electrical activity on the surface of the body as being of dipolar configuration [101] – see ❷ Fig. 1.31. Einthoven's concept of the mean axis continued the same idea [33] and much work has been done over the intervening years to prove whether or not the single-dipole hypothesis was an adequate representation of what became

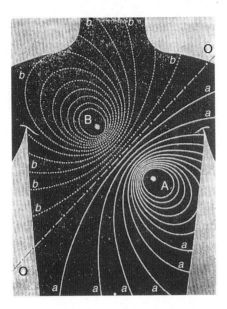

◘ Fig. 1.31
The dipolar distribution of the electrical activity of the heart as described by Waller in 1888. The solid isopotential lines indicate positive potentials and the dashed lines indicate negative potentials (After Waller [101]. © British Medical Association, London. Reproduced with permission)

known as the "equivalent cardiac generator." For example, Geselowitz [102] was one of the earliest to discuss the concept of higher-order components such as the quadrupole. Others including Selvester et al. [103] used a multiple-dipole model of the heart to calculate the appearances of vectorcardiographic loops (❷ Fig. 1.32). Although some of this work was first described in the early 1960s, patient research in the interim has resulted in new concepts for the diagnosis of myocardial infarction, as explained fully by Selvester in ❷ Chap. 4 of *Electrocardiology: Comprehensive Clinical ECG*. The original analogue model of Selvester and colleagues was shortly thereafter transformed into a digital computer model in which simulated myocardial infarction could be studied on the vectorcardiogram [104].

On the other hand, by recording body-surface potentials and using an inverse solution, it is also possible to derive the activities of multiple dipoles as was done for different groups of subjects by Holt and colleagues [105] following on mathematical work undertaken by Lynn and Barnard et al. [106]. Similar work was undertaken in the author's laboratory [107] and ❷ Fig. 1.33 shows a ten-dipole model from which the average dipole strengths during ventricular depolarization for a group of 35 normal adult males have been computed. Using the model, the author's group suggested in 1974 that right ventricular infarction could be detected from reduced dipole activity in the right ventricular dipole areas [108]. This paper was greeted with some scepticism when first presented to the British Cardiac Society.

The topic of the forward and inverse problems of electrocardiography is discussed extensively in ❷ Chaps. 8 and ❷ 9, while other aspects of modeling cardiac cells are discussed in ❷ Chap. 6. This area is still one of considerable activity at the present time and particular emphasis is being put on solutions for calculating the epicardial potential distribution from the body-surface potentials, as discussed in ❷ Chap. 9. Rudy and his team now based in St. Louis, have demonstrated a very high degree of correlation between calculated and measured isopotential maps using sophisticated modeling techniques allied to a detailed knowledge of anatomy determined from magnetic resonance imaging or computed tomography [109]. The technique which they call ECG imaging, or ECGI, is now being applied to localize the site of cardiac arrhythmias [110]. Boyett and colleagues are also developing a complex model of cardiac activation [111] as part of their goal of producing a "virtual heart" with accurate anatomy and electrophysiology.

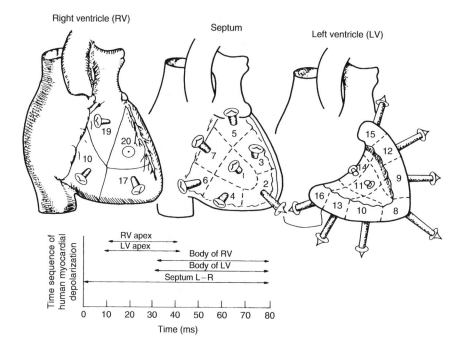

◘ Fig. 1.32

A multiple-dipole model of the heart described by Selvester and colleagues in 1965. The dipoles were activated according to the time sequence shown in the lower part of the diagram and the resultant electrical activity was calculated. From this, vectorcardiographic loops were derived (After Selvester el al. [103]. © American Heart Association, Dallas, Texas. Reproduced with permission)

1.9   Electrocardiographic Mapping

Although Waller [101] had sketched isopotential maps, it was not really until the 1960s that interest grew in mapping the thorax. Prior to that there had been isolated reports on mapping; and perhaps the first body-surface map (❷ Fig. 1.34) was obtained by Nahum et al. in 1951 [112]. However, there is no doubt that Taccardi has been the pioneer in this field and many references to his work can be found in the appropriate ❷ Chap. 10 of *Cardiac Arrhythmias and Mapping Techniques*. He is still active and recently published data on the three dimensional sequence of repolarisation and associated potential fields in the ventricles [113].

There are two facets of body-surface mapping. On the one hand, the technique can be regarded as purely empirical in that the spread of excitation can be studied and correlated with other clinical findings in order to derive diagnostic criteria and to obtain a better understanding of the spread of excitation within the heart. On the other hand, recording of potentials, for example, from over 100 points on the thorax allows a mathematical estimation of the total information content on the body surface and from this can be derived subsets of electrodes which can be used to obtain all information of clinical value while retaining the capability of producing the body surface map for visual display. A few brief historical comments are offered on each of these aspects.

In 1971, Barr, who has co-authored ❷ Chap. 5 of this book, suggested together with colleagues that 24 electrodes was an adequate number for recovering the total information on the thorax [114]. Later, Korneich [115] suggested that nine leads were required to obtain the clinically important information some of which was missing when only the *XYZ* leads were recorded ([105], see ❷ Chap. 11). This result had been obtained after mapping the thorax with a 126-electrode system. A few years later, after extensive mapping of subjects using 192 electrodes, Lux, who has written ❷ Chap. 9 of *Cardiac Arrhythmias and Mapping Techniques* of this book, and his colleagues suggested that the order of 30 electrodes was adequate for deriving the total surface information [116]. This allowed the group to design "a limited-lead" system

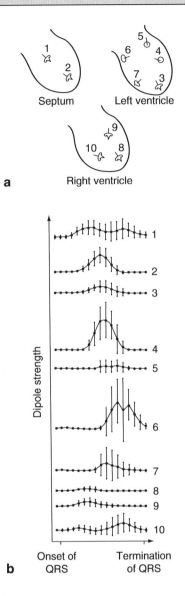

◻ **Fig. 1.33**
In (a), a ten-dipole model of the electrical activity of the heart is shown; (b) shows the average dipole strengths during ventricular depolarization recorded from a group of 35 normal adult males. The standard deviation about the mean values is also shown

of 32 electrodes which they now use routinely. It is thus evident that body-surface mapping techniques have led to the development of newer lead systems.

In addition, however, mapping has contributed other findings. In 1965, Taccardi and Marchetti [117] published a hand-drawn isopotential map that showed clearly the nondipolarity of the surface potential distribution at a selected instant during the QRS complex (❷ Fig. 1.35). They indicated that this multipolar situation lasted for 3–10 ms. These findings had been presented at a meeting on the electrophysiology of the heart, which had been chaired by Rijlant in Milan in October 1963. Finally, in connection with mapping, it would be topical to point out that isopotential mapping is claimed to be superior to the 12 lead ECG in the diagnosis of acute myocardial infarction [118].

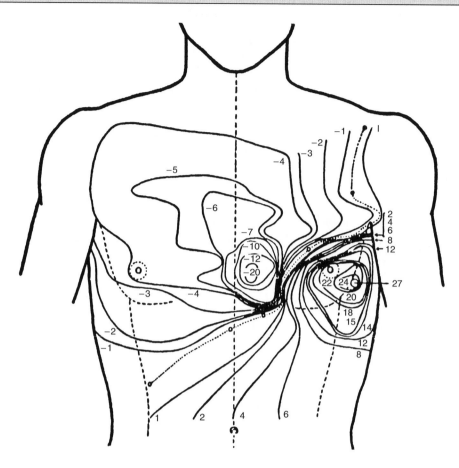

Fig. 1.34

An isopotential map at the instant of time defined by the peak of the R wave in lead I in an 18-year-old male patient. The map was plotted by recording a unipolar lead at various points on the precordium simultaneously with lead I which was used as a time reference. This map was published in 1951 (After Nahum et al. [112]. © American Physiological Society, Bethesda, Maryland. Reproduced with permission)

Various applications of surface mapping are discussed elsewhere in this book. The contribution of body-surface mapping to the field of electrocardiology is ongoing but despite the commercial availability of mapping systems producing attractively colored isopotential maps, it is still true to say, over 20 years after this chapter was first written, that the claimed advantages of mapping per se, as distinct from inverse modeling, have not been readily accepted by the cardiological community at large.

1.10 Activation of the Heart

Studies on the activation of the heart at microscopic and macroscopic level have been in progress from before the start of the twentieth century. The effects of injury had been known at the time of du Bois-Reymond and an article from Burdon Sanderson [119] published in 1900, but possibly displaying data obtained in 1880 according to Burch [1], showed a monophasic action potential recorded from an area of injured myocardium (❷ Fig. 1.36). The first monophasic action potential to be recorded from within a myocardial cell of an intact mammalian heart was reported in 1950 by Woodbury and colleagues [120]. Since then, there has been a dramatic growth in knowledge of the generation of the action potential of individual cells, and in ❷ Chap. 3, the current understanding is explained. Of interest in recent times has been the discovery of M cells by Antzelevitch and co-workers [121] in an isolated dog heart preparation. These cells have a longer

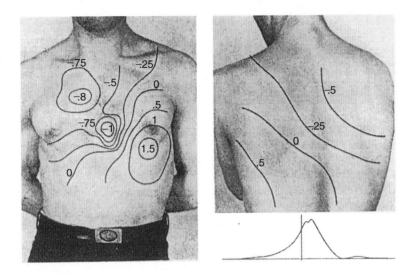

◻ Fig. 1.35
A body-surface map drawn at the instant indicated by the vertical line during ventricular activation. Note the multiple minima in the upper right side of the chest indicating a nondipolar potential distribution (After Taccardi and Marchetti [117]. © Pergamon, Oxford. Reproduced with permission)

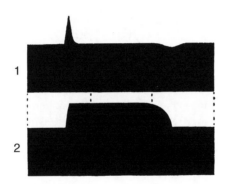

◻ Fig. 1.36
Tracing 1 shows a biphasic action potential recorded from an intact heart, while tracing 2 shows a monophasic action potential recorded from an electrode placed on an area of injured myocardium at the apex of the heart (After Burdon Sanderson [119]. © Pentland, Edinburgh. Reproduced with permission)

action potential than endocardial or epicardial cells (❷ Fig. 1.37). An excellent review of the M cell can be found elsewhere [122]. There is currently some controversy as to the role of M cells, which were at one point said to be responsible for the U wave, a theory which is now discounted. The M cell characteristics are well documented in isolated cells but their characteristics may differ in the intact heart. Rudy has pointed out that there is a difference of 90 ms between the action potential durations of simulated M cells and epicardial cells in isolation but that the difference reduces to 18 ms when the cells are well coupled [123].

In ❷ Chap. 1 of *Cardiac Arrhythmias and Mapping Techniques*, the cellular basis of cardiac arrhythmias is discussed. With the rapid increase of therapeutic preparations for the control of cardiac arrhythmias, there has also been a widespread investigation into the effects of such antiarrhythmic drugs on the action potentials of myocardial cells. An early review of the understanding of action potentials, as well as the role of sodium and calcium ions in the genesis of action potentials, can be found in a symposium on the electrophysiology of the heart [124]. Many well-known European authors contributed to this original work including Grundfest, Girardier, Trautwein, Hecht, Hutter, Corabouf and Wiedmann. This field has also seen an explosion in knowledge in recent years and particularly in the understanding of different

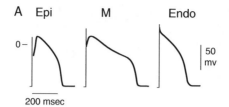

☐ Fig. 1.37

An illustration of the different action potential durations of myocytes isolated from the epicardial (Epi), endocardial (Endo) and M regions of the canine left ventricle (Adapted with permission from Antzelevitch C, Zigmunt AC, Dumaine R. Electrophysiology and Pharmacology of Ventricular Repolarization. In Gussak I, Antzelevitch C (eds). Cardiac Repolarization. Humana Press. 2003)

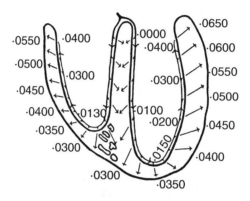

☐ Fig. 1.38

Lewis' conception of the spread of excitation in the human heart derived from a study of the human electrocardiogram as well as a knowledge of canine excitation and its relationship to the canine ECG (After Lewis [58]. © Shaw, London. Reproduced with permission)

ion channels and their role in the generation of cardiac action potentials (see for example [125]). Full details can be found in ❯ Chap. 3.

At the macroscopic level, data on the spread of excitation has continued to accumulate through the years. Lewis in his monograph included a number of illustrations of the spread of excitation in the human and dog hearts, the latter in various experimental situations. ❯ Fig. 1.38 shows Lewis' attempt to describe the spread of excitation in the human heart "with some pretence to accuracy." In fact, Lewis had carefully studied excitation in the dog heart, and by comparing human ECGs with those of the dog, which in turn were correlated with canine activation, he derived the data of ❯ Fig. 1.38. Other notable early contributors to the study of myocardial excitation were Scher and Young [126, 127] as well as the group of Durrer [128] in Amsterdam. The latter group was able to study myocardial activation in the human heart using needle electrodes, and their 1970 paper is an all time classic. One of the authors of that work, namely Janse, has written ❯ Chap. 4 outlining current understanding on the activation of the heart. Important early work in this area was also contributed by Boineau [129] and the group of Spach [130].

Although myocardial activation has been well documented, myocardial recovery is still an area requiring further study, although Abildskov and Burgess have spent much time researching this field [131], particularly in the dog heart. Work still continues in the Salt Lake City lab and Taccardi et al. recently published newer data on repolarization in the dog ventricles [113]. Interesting data on recovery in the human heart was reported by Cowan [132] who studied nineteen patients, fourteen of whom with upright T waves were undergoing coronary artery bypass grafting while the remaining five were having surgery for aortic valve replacement, including four with T-wave inversion. He found that in patients with upright T waves there was an inverse relation between the time of activation and the duration of the monophasic action potential, which he also recorded. As a result, activation and repolarization proceeded in opposite directions. The mean sequence of activation was from the septum to the free wall and from the apex to base, whereas during repolarization the sequence was from base to apex and from the free wall towards the septum. However, in the patients with T-wave inversion, the repolarization sequence resembled that of activation. Thus, it can be seen that there is still much to be explored in the field of cardiac electrophysiology, both at the microscopic and macroscopic levels.

1.11   Arrhythmias, Conduction Defects and Sudden Death

The history of the early work in arrhythmias has been described in ❷ Sect. 1.4, when it was made clear that much information on the pulse obtained from the polygraph was used to infer the nature of the "arrhythmia." How different matters are today, when an average of four intracardiac catheters with multiple electrodes or even basket catheters may be used to determine the precise nature of an arrhythmia, as described in ❷ Chaps. 2 and ❷ 3 of *Cardiac Arrhythmias and Mapping Techniques*. Although Krikler [133] suggested that the first clinical intracardiac recording of the electrical activity of the bundle of His was made in Dundee [134], he also acknowledged earlier intracardiac recordings made in France by Lenegre and Maurice [135] during World War II. However, other earlier recordings of the His-bundle activity had also been made in the dog by Alanis et al. [136] and by Giraud et al. [137] in man. ❷ Figure 1.39 shows one of the earliest (1958)

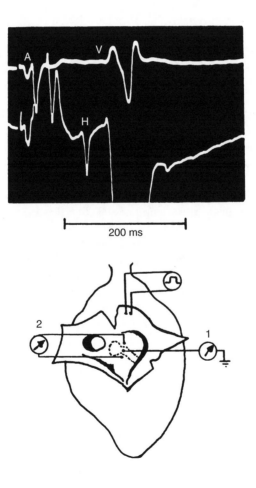

■ Fig. 1.39
A recording made in 1958 of His-bundle activity (H) in a dog. The lower diagram shows the position of the stimulating and recording electrodes. The lower ECG tracing shows the recording from the exploring electrode 1 while the upper tracing shows the bipolar lead 2, when the electrodes were placed 1.5 mm above and below the exploring electrode (After Alanis et al. [136]. © Physiological Society, London. Reproduced with permission)

recordings from the dog. However, it was the work of Scherlag and colleagues [138] that established a standard technique for recording His-bundle activity using an endocardial catheter. About the same time, however, other groups, notably that of Durrer [139] in Amsterdam, had used intracardiac leads for initiating and terminating supraventricular tachycardia and a whole new branch of electrocardiology was opened. The precise mechanisms for arrhythmias could be determined in individual patients and appropriate therapies selected for treatment. ❷ Chaps. 3–8 of *Cardiac Arrhythmias and Mapping Techniques* discuss standard surface electrocardiography for the diagnosis of arrhythmias, and wherever necessary, intracardiac electrocardiography for a more detailed analysis of specific arrhythmias. Additional historical details can be found in ❷ Chap. 2 of *Cardiac Arrhythmias and Mapping Techniques*.

There has been an explosion in clinical electrophysiology in recent years with many cardiologists specialising in this area. With major advances in the use of ablation for treatment of arrhythmias and for disabling accessory pathways, ❷ Chap. 3 of *Cardiac Arrhythmias and Mapping Techniques* is devoted to techniques for intracardiac mapping.

At about the same time as a standard technique for His-bundle recording was introduced, Rosenbaum and colleagues in Argentina introduced their concept of a conduction defect in either of the two main fascicles of the left bundle branch-namely, the anterior and posterior fascicles [140]. The concept of divisional block was not totally new [141], but Rosenbaum et al., on the basis of experimental and clinical data, established the various electrocardiographic patterns for what they called left anterior hemiblock and left posterior hemiblock. In view of the trifascicular nature of the left-sided conducting system (see ❷ Chap. 4), some authors have preferred to use the term "fascicular block" rather than "hemiblock." In 1981, when writing on the occasion of the 100th anniversary of the birth of Lewis [57], Rosenbaum explained that he used Lewis' illustration of the conduction system of a walrus heart (❷ Fig. 1.40) because it clearly demonstrated what Rosenbaum called the "bifascicular character" of the left bundle branch. This is somewhat contradictory to what was stated immediately above in this section and to what is apparent in ❷ Chap. 4. Nevertheless, the point of interest was the reference back to what Rosenbaum called "the gospel." He also went on to recount presenting his ideas in the presence of the late Louis N. Katz who said: "What you have just presented is beautiful; the only problem is that it is not true." Two years later when they met again in San Francisco, Katz told Rosenbaum: "You were right; I was persuaded by having a look at Fig. 1.4 in the Lewis book"! The legend to Fig. 1.4 of Lewis' book, reproduced as the legend to Fig. 1.40, mentions that the further arborization of the two main branches consists of "free strands which cross the cavity." Is this an early demonstration of false tendons that have been suggested as the cause of the wide variation in frontal-plane QRS axis in healthy individuals [142]. Conduction defects are discussed in ❷ Chap. 2 of *Electrocardiology: Comprehensive Clinical ECG*.

If a good example is required of the earlier reference to the comment of Fisch [10] scorning comments to the effect that further developments in electrocardiography are no longer possible, then the recent "discovery" of the Brugada syndrome [143] linking a right bundle branch block type ECG with sudden death is a perfect case in point (❷ Fig. 1.41). This finding has unleashed a major effort to establish genetic links with the ECG appearances and has already been the topic of two consensus reports [144, 145]. By the same token, the long QT syndrome for many years associated with sudden death (and deafness in some cases) has been the subject of much investigation in relation to various genetic abnormalities in certain chromosomes, while over 10 types of long QT have now been described. Much further detail can be found in ❷ Chap. 7 of *Electrocardiology: Comprehensive Clinical ECG*. Conversely, the short QT syndrome, first described in 2000 by Gussak et al. [146] is similarly leading to much research in the way of genotyping. Ott and Marcus recently reviewed the various ECG markers linked with sudden death [147].

1.12   Technical Advances

It must be self-evident that the technical advances throughout the twentieth century almost defy description. With them has come a whole host of new investigative techniques of diagnostic and therapeutic value, only a few of which have been discussed here. No history of electrocardiology would be complete without a brief comment on these newer techniques. Because they are relatively recent in inception, the relevant historical details can generally be found in the various chapters in this book that describe their evolution.

Perhaps one of the most widely appreciated developments of the century has been the microelectronic revolution leading to miniaturized computers with a high processing capacity. Electrocardiography has been one field that has not been left behind by such developments. In the late 1950s, the use of computers for ECG interpretation was first evaluated by Pipberger and colleagues [148] using the orthogonal-lead ECG and by Caceres [149] and his team using the 12 lead

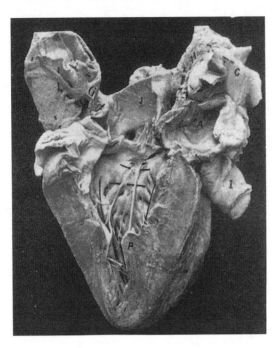

⬛ Fig. 1.40
A specimen in the Royal College of Surgeons Museum, photographed with the kind permission of Professor Keith. The heart of a walrus dissected from the left side. The greater portions of wall of the left ventricle and left auricle (A) have been removed and the aorta has been divided vertically at its base (J) and the left half taken away. The interventricular septum and the cusps of the aortic valve are exposed. The right anterior cusp of the valve is fully exposed and the mouth of the right coronary artery is seen. Directly beneath the posterior end of this cusp (to the right in the figure), the left division of the auriculoventricular bundle enters the ventricle and immediately splits into two chief branches; these branches lie upon two horizontal bristles, over which there has been a very small amount of dissection. The further course of these branches is perfectly clear, the arborization consisting of free strands which cross the cavity; several large branches enter the papillary muscles, the bases of which are seen (P). Two long bristles are placed behind finer branches of the course network. I lies on the inferior cava; G on the pulmonary artery. Note the large collections of nerve tissue at the base of the heart; bristles are placed behind the thick strands at G, H and C (After Lewis [58]. © Shaw, London. Reproduced with permission)

ECG. At that time, large central computers were used for the analysis and at most, leads were recorded in groups of three simultaneously in analog form. In 1964, the author was introduced to electrocardiography by Professor T.D. Veitch Lawrie who, with great foresight, anticipated the role of the computer in this field. By the early 1970s, certainly in the Glasgow Royal Infirmary laboratory, the technique had advanced to the stage whereby a small recording unit could be taken to the bedside to make an analog ECG recording which could subsequently be replayed to a laboratory PDP8 minicomputer for interpretation ([150], ❯ Fig. 1.42). Nowadays, all 12 leads can be recorded effectively simultaneously in digital form using a microprocessor-based electrocardiograph that can produce an interpretation within seconds of the recording being completed (❯ Fig. 1.43). Full details of computer analysis of ECGs can be found in ❯ Chap. 5 of *Specialized Aspects of ECG*.

Computer techniques have also helped to enhance exercise testing as discussed in ❯ Chap. 8 of *Cardiac Arrhythmias and Mapping Techniques*. In particular, the ability of the microprocessor to undertake averaging of the QRST complex in real time represents a significant step forward in improving the quality of data presentation. A word of caution has to be added. Because an average beat represents a collection of beats recorded over a period of time, the trade-off in improved quality possibly has to be set against a small hysteresis in the average beat responding to change in ST-T configuration in particular. Nevertheless, it is now commonplace to use exercise ECG criteria that involve measurement of the ST-T segment 60–80 ms after the end of QRS and this has been greatly facilitated by computer measurement techniques.

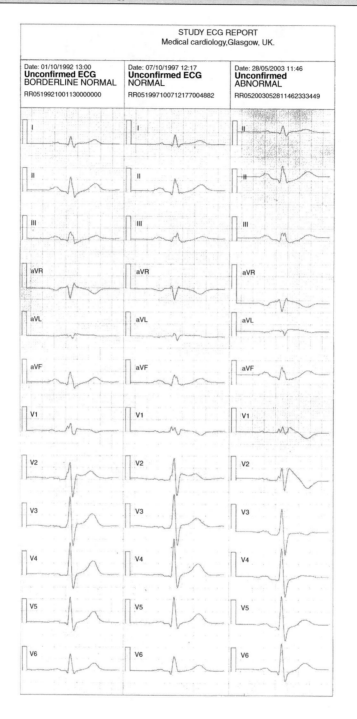

STUDY ECG REPORT
Medical cardiology, Glasgow, UK.

| Date: 01/10/1992 13:00 **Unconfirmed ECG** BORDERLINE NORMAL RR0519921001130000000 | Date: 07/10/1997 12:17 **Unconfirmed ECG** NORMAL RR051997100712177004882 | Date: 28/05/2003 11:46 **Unconfirmed** ABNORMAL RR052003052811462333449 |

⬛ Fig. 1.41

An example of the Brugada pattern with the "shark's fin" appearances seen clearly in V_1 and V_2 in the recording made in 2003 in a 71 year old male. It is important to note that earlier recordings as far back as 1992 do not show such obvious changes

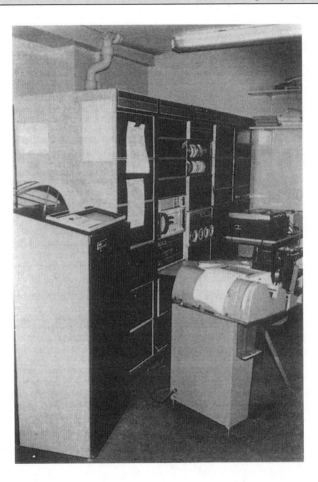

⬤ Fig. 1.42
A PDP8E minicomputer connected to an analog tape recorder (right-hand side) for analysis of three orthogonal-lead ECGs. This 1971 illustration, taken in Glasgow Royal Infirmary, shows probably the first hospital departmental minicomputer system for routine ECG analysis

Advanced signal processing techniques have also led to a greater interest in the concept of microvolt T wave alternans where small beat to beat variations in T wave amplitude can be measured. David Rosenbaum et al. [150] first used cardiac pacing to increase heart rate and induce microvolt T wave alternans, which they demonstrated to be linked to life threatening ventricular arrhythmias. They paced the heart at around 100 beats per minute prior to making recordings but nowadays, patients may be exercised on a bicycle to achieve a similar heart rate at which point the ECG can be analysed for the presence of T wave alternans. However, Klingenheben recently concluded that the predictive efficacy of the test was highly dependent on the population studied [151].

One of the most significant developments in terms of noninvasive electrocardiographic techniques in the second half of the twentieth century has been the rapid advance of Holter electrocardiography. The technique was named after its inventor, Norman J. Holter, who died in 1983. A brief biographical note was published by Roberts and Silver that year [152]. Holter was a scientist with degrees in physics and chemistry. His early interests were related to radiotelemetry used to stimulate the brain of a rat, essentially by remote control, into which a small radio receiver had been implanted. After World War II, Holter established his own research foundation for "trying to broadcast by radio the more obvious electrophysiological phenomena occurring in humans so that they could be free to do something besides lie quietly on a couch." After working with electroencephalograms (EEGs), his team turned their attention to the ECG. According to Roberts and Silver [153], "the first broadcast of an ECG required 85 1b of equipment, which Holter wore on his back and

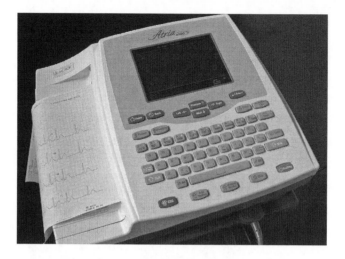

◘ Fig. 1.43

A microprocessor-based portable electrocardiograph (Burdick Atria 6100) with integral interpretative facilities

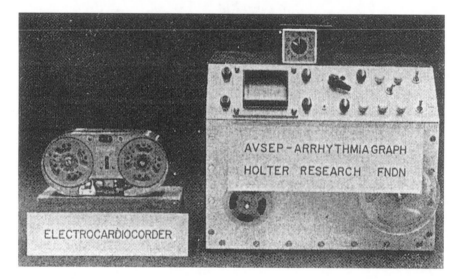

◘ Fig. 1.44

The original electrocardiocorder developed by Holter together with the AVSEP analysis unit (see text for further discussion) (After Holter [155]. © American Association for the Advancement of Science. Washington, DC. Reproduced with permission)

an accurate electrocardiogram during exercise was recorded." MacInnis [154] visited Holter in his laboratory in Helena in Montana and was the first to report on the use of the radiotelemetry technique for monitoring the cardiac patient. The receiving equipment was situated in Holter's office and the patient was free to walk about in the street outside the building.

The miniaturization of equipment continued and the radio receiver became small enough to place in a briefcase into which a tape-recording device was also incorporated. However, this was still somewhat inconvenient and further development resulted in what Holter termed [155] the electrocardiocorder (❷ Fig. 1.44). This was the forerunner of what is nowadays generally called a Holter recorder. The reel-to-reel tape recorder was small enough to be carried in a man's coat pocket or, as suggested by Holter, in a woman's "strap-type handbag." The first recorder was able to operate for 10 h.

Not only did Holter produce the recorder, he developed an analyzer where initially all beats were superimposed on a cathode ray screen in what was called the AVSEP (audio visual superimposed electrocardiogram presentation) technique.

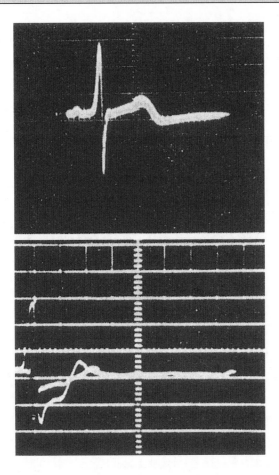

◘ Fig. 1.45
The top waveform shows the superimposition of PQRST cycles in sinus rhythm using the AVSEP technique. The lower tracing shows the same approach in a patient with ventricular bigeminy where two different waveforms can be seen (After Holter [155]. © American Association for the Advancement of Science, Washington, DC. Reproduced with permission)

❯ Figure 1.45 shows the original presentation of Holter. His early paper also introduced the arrhythmiagram, which was essentially a presentation of R-R intervals as shown in ❯ Fig. 1.46. It is also of great interest to note that in his 1961 paper, Holter also presented examples of marked ST depression which he said was evidence of "an attack of angina pectoris in an individual doing forbidden heavy work" (❯ Fig. 1.47). Even allowing for possible shortcomings in the frequency response of the recording system, the ST-T abnormalities do look extremely convincing. Thus from the outset, Holter conceived of his equipment as being of use both for arrhythmia analysis and for the detection of ischemic ST-T changes. This must surely be the first documented Holter ECG evidence of ischemic change.

In their biographical note, Roberts and Silver laid stress on Holter's own belief in serendipity as well as non-goal directed research, that is, the two together could be summarized as discovery by chance. That would seem to be a far cry from today's grant-oriented research teams striving for survival!

The technique of Holter monitoring has opened up a new diagnostic field, while it can also be used to assess the effect of drugs in suppressing arrhythmias. In addition, with modern technology, which mostly involves direct digital recording, accurate ST segment analysis has become possible and this is now of increasing importance in the detection of so-called silent myocardial ischemia and in the evaluation of antianginal drug therapy. Newer concepts such as heart rate turbulence have also evolved from long term ECG recording [156]. Current techniques are discussed in detail in ❯ Chap. 1 of *Specialized Aspects of ECG*.

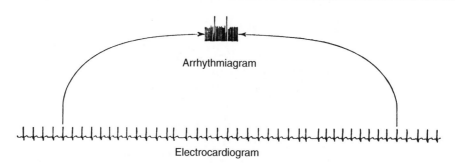

◻ Fig. 1.46

Holter's arrhythmiagram, which is essentially a presentation of R-R intervals. When supraventricular extrasystoles are present, as in this case, the long compensatory pause stands out as the tall spike in the arrhythmiagram (After Holter [155]. © American Association for the Advancement of Science, Washington, DC. Reproduced with permission)

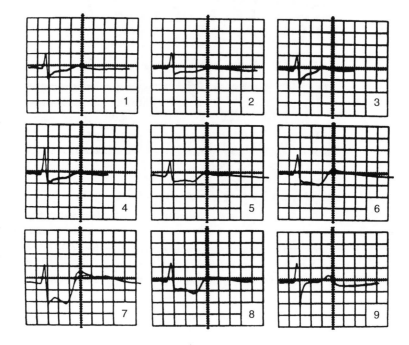

◻ Fig. 1.47

A series of AVSEP patterns showing marked ST-T abnormalities. These were recorded with Holter's electrocardiocorder in 1961 (After Holter [155]. © American Association for the Advancement of Science, Washington DC. Reproduced with permission)

Heart rate variability (HRV) is a technique that has been under investigation for many years though it has not quite broken through into the area of routine clinical application. In part, this may be due to the variety of measures used to quantify HRV. Recently, Sosnowski et al. [157] introduced the heart rate variability fraction which is a much more easily remembered index (cf ejection fraction). This could be one route to greater acceptability (and understanding) of HRV. Further details are to be found in ❷ Chap. 3 of *Specialized Aspects of ECG*.

The use of microprocessor technology has also led to considerable interest in the study of the high-frequency components of the ECG. In particular, much effort has been spent in assessing the prognostic value of so-called late potentials (see ❷ Chap. 7 of *Specialized Aspects of ECG*) where low-amplitude high-frequency waves persist at the end of the QRS complex into the early ST segment. These have been associated with ventricular tachycardia in different groups of susceptible patients. Bedside devices now exist for deriving a plot of the high-frequency averaged ECG with a printout of relevant measurements of area and so on during the last 40 ms of the QRS complex, for example. The high-frequency content of the electrocardiographic signal per se is now enjoying a resurgence of interest almost 50 years after it was first suggested as being of significance in ischemic heart disease [158]. These aspects are also mentioned in ❯ Chap. 7 of *Specialized Aspects of ECG*, where it is concluded that high frequency electrocardiography will be an area of more intensive research in the coming years.

The first artificial cardiac pacemaker was implanted in Stockholm in 1958 [159]. The device was a simple fixed-rate ventricular pacemaker and from this evolved another aspect of electrocardiology. This was followed by rate-responsive pacemakers (possibly dual chamber) that attempt to detect increased activity on the part of the patient and respond by increasing the rate of stimulation in the most appropriate way for the particular condition of the patient. In turn, this has opened up a new area of pacemaker electrocardiography, which is discussed in ❯ Chap. 6 of *Specialized Aspects of ECG*. Instead of simply trying, as in the early days, to decide whether a fixed-rate pacemaker was functioning satisfactorily or not, the problem of assessing whether the modern pacemaker is functioning properly according to its true design performance is a complex task requiring considerable skill on the part of the cardiologist. Many implanted pacemakers now incorporate a so-called "Holter" function, by which is meant a memory facility for recording pacemaker activity.

Cardiac resynchronization therapy involving the use of a catheter electrode to pace the left ventricle via the coronary sinus is a recently introduced technique [160]. This presents challenges to electrocardiographers and automated ECG analysis systems in detecting three pacemaker stimuli, though this is only possible if the so called VV interval (between right and left ventricular stimuli) has a measurable duration of a few milliseconds. Initial work in the author's lab is promising.

The use of animals in medical research must not be forgotten. To this end, an extensive review of the dog electrocardiogram is presented in ❯ Chap. 9 of *Specialized Aspects of ECG*. Interpretation of the canine ECG is an art in itself, requiring a good understanding of the normal appearances in the different breeds. An accompanying ❯ Chap. 10 of *Specialized Aspects of ECG* on comparative electrocardiography provides an exceptionally detailed compendium of appearances in various species of mammals, from certain types of whale to the elephant.

For centuries, the relationship between the electric and magnetic fields has been known. However, it was not until 1963 that the magnetic field of the heart was first detected by Baule and McFee [161]. At that time, as explained in ❯ Chap. 12 of *Specialized Aspects of ECG*, signal averaging had to be used to detect the weak signal from the cardiac magnetic field. In general in the early days, shielded rooms had to be used with equipment which was rather large and immobile. Although the situation has improved in recent years with a reduction in the size of equipment, the technique of magnetocardiography is, as far as is known, still limited to a few research centers in Germany, Italy, Scandinavia and North America. The electric and magnetic vectors of the heart, as of any source, are perpendicular to each other, and as such there has to be a close relationship between the magnetocardiogram and the electrocardiogram. On the other hand, the injury potentials that produce TP depression on the ECG, which is often detected as ST elevation, can be differentiated in the magnetocardiogram. The technique has its proponents, but it still remains to be seen whether any advantages which can be demonstrated outweigh the benefit of the simpler recording equipment required for the electrocardiogram.

The advances in technology have allowed computer databases to contribute to epidemiological investigations as discussed in ❯ Chap. 8 of *Specialized Aspects of ECG* and, to a certain extent, in ❯ Chap. 1 of *Electrocardiology: Comprehensive Clinical ECG*. Although there have been many large-scale studies with electrocardiograms interpreted by conventional means and even coded by hand, it is now the case that computer processing relieves cardiologists and technicians of this chore, though there is a requirement to check the individual results to ensure that technical problems have not interfered with coding. Much can still be gained by diligent, painstaking, methodical collection of ECGs and follow-up of patients over a period of years. Perhaps one of the best known epidemiological studies is that of the population in Framingham in Massachusetts, and many interesting ECG findings have emerged [162, 163]. It was shown that nonspecific ST-T wave changes carried a significantly increased risk of coronary morbidity and mortality and the combination of both seemed most "hazardous." It was concluded that individuals who develop nonspecific ST-T changes without explanation require vigorous preventive management against coronary heart disease. Furthermore, in a separate paper, the same group showed that while ECG data did not contribute to a predictive model for sudden unexpected death, they did improve substantially the predictive model for sudden death in persons with known coronary heart disease. While computer techniques were not used for ECG analysis in these studies, the message is that the use of the ECG in epidemiological studies is invaluable.

Very recently, there has been a rapidly growing interest in utilising ECG measures in genome wide association studies. For example, the long QT interval has been associated with the NOS1AP gene [164]. It can be expected that there will be a growing number of publications in this area in the near future.

1.13   Conclusion

This chapter has presented a necessarily brief review of the history of electrocardiology, and much has had to be omitted. Additional information can be found in many other chapters in the book but it is hoped that if nothing else, the foregoing continues to justify the use of the term "Electrocardiology" rather than "Electrocardiography." Of course, the history of the latter is greater and has received more attention, since most readers will be relatively familiar with the newer aspects of electrocardiology. Perhaps advances over the next few years will be as dramatic as those in the past so that today's techniques will seem so old by comparison that they will merit inclusion in any future historical review.

References

1. Burch, G.E. and N.P. de Pasquale, *A History of Electrocardiography*. Chicago: Year Book Medical, 1964.
2. Burch, G.E., The history of vectorcardiography. *Med. Hist.*, 1985;**5**: 103–131.
3. Cooper, J.K., Electrocardiography 100 years ago. *N. Engl. J. Med.*, 1986;**315**: 461–464.
4. Sykes, A.H., A D Waller and the electrocardiogram, 1887. *Br. Med. J.*, 1987;**294**: 1396–1398.
5. Lamas, G.A., L.R. Koller, E.M. Antman, and T.W. Smith, Electrocardiogram by Einthoven 63 years earlier. *Am. J. Cardiol.*, 1984;**54**: 1163–1165.
6. Burchell, H.B., A centennial note on waller and the first human electrocardiogram. *Am. J. Cardiol.*, 1987;**59**: 979–983.
7. Kossmann, C.E., Unipolar electrocardiography of wilson: A half century later. *Am. Heart J.*, 1985;**110**: 901–904.
8. Barold, S.S., Advanced 12 lead electrocardiography. *Cardiol Clin.*, 2006;**24**: 305–513.
9. Macfarlane, P.W., Renaissance in electrocardiography. *Lancet*, 1999;**353**: 1377–1379.
10. Wellens, H.J.J., The electrocardiogram 80 years after Einthoven. *J. Am. Coll. Cardiol.*, 1986;**7**: 484–491.
11. Fisch, C., The clinical electrocardiogram: A classic. *Circulation*, 1980;**62**(Suppl. III): 1–4.
12. Rijlant, P., The coming of age of electrophysiology and electrocardiography. *NTM-Schriftenr. Gesch. Naturwis,s.Tech.Med.*, 1980;**17**: 108–123.
13. Lempert, G.L., From electrocardiography to electrocardiology. *Adv. Cardiol.*, 1976;**16**: 57–61.
14. Snellen, H.A., A History Of Cardiology. Rotterdam: Donker, 1984.
15. Kölliker, A. and H. Muller, Nachweis der negativen Schwankung des Muskelstroms am naturlich sich contrahirenden Muskel. *Verh. Phys. Med. Ges. Wiirzburg*, 1856;**6**: 528–533.
16. Marey, E.J., Des variations electriques des muscles et du coeur en particulier etudies au moyen de l'electrometer de M Lippmann. *C. R. Acad. Sci.*, 1876;**82**: 975–977.
17. Engelmann, T.W., Ueber das electrische Verhalten des thatigen Herzens. *Pflug. Arch.*, 1878;**17**: 68–99.
18. Burdon Sanderson, J. and F.J.M. Page, Experimental results relating to the rhythmical and excitatory motions of the ventricle of the heart of the frog, and of the electrical phenomena which accompany them. *Proc. R. Soc. London*, 1878;**27**: 410–414.
19. Burdon Sanderson, J. and F.J.M. Page, On the time-relations of the excitatory process in the ventricle of the heart of the frog. *J. Physiol.*, 1879;**2**: 384–435.
20. Waller, A.D., A demonstration on man of electromotive changes accompanying the heart's beat. *J. Physiol.*, 1887;**8**: 229–234.
21. Waller, A.D., On the electromotive changes connected with the beat of the mammalian heart, and of the human heart in particular. *Phil. Trans. R. Soc. London, Ser. B.*, 1889;**180**: 169–194.
22. Besterman, E. and R. Creese, Waller-pioneer of electrocardiography. *Br. Heart J.*, 1979;**42**(1): 61–64.
23. Burch, G.J., On a method of determining the value of rapid variations of a difference of potential by means of the capillary electrometer. *Proc. R. Soc. London (Bioi)*, 1890;**48**: 89–93.
24. Snellen, H.A., *Two Pioneer"s of Electrocardiography. The Correspondence Between Einlhoven and Lewis from 1908–1926*, Rotterdam: Donker, 1983.
25. Einthoven, W., The different forms of the human electrocardiogram and their signification. *Lancet*, 1912;**1**: 853–861.
26. Ader, C., Sur un nouvel appareil enregistreur pour cables sousmarins. *C. R. Acad. Sci. (Paris)*, 1897;**124**: 1440–1442.
27. Einthoven, W., Un nouveau galvanometre. *Arch. Neerl. Sci. Exacles Nal.*, 1901;**6**: 625–633.
28. Bosscha, J., *Dissertatio Physica Inauguralis De Ralvanomelro Differenliali*. Leiden: Menzel, 1854.
29. Burchell, H.B., Did Einthoven invent a string galvanometer? *Br. Heart J.*, 1987;**57**: 190–193.
30. Einthoven, W., Die galvanometrische Registrirung des mensch lichen Elektrokardiogramms, zugleich cine Beurtheilung der Anwendung des Capilar-Elektrometers in der Physiologie. *Plug. Arch.*, 1903;**99**: 472–480.
31. Einthoven, W., Le Telecardiogramme. *Arch. flll. Physiol.*, 1906;**4**: 132–164 (Translation: Matthewson, F.A.L. and Jack, H. *Am. Heart J.*, 1955;**49**: 77–82. Blackburn H.W. *Am. Heart J.*, 1957;**53**: 602–615.)
32. Einthoven, W., Weiteres uber das Elektrokardiogramm. *Plug. Arch.*, 1908;**122**: 517–584.
33. Einthoven, W., G. Fahr, and A. de Waart, Uber die Richtung und die manifeste Grosse der Potentialschwankungen immensch lichen Herzen und uber den Einfluss der Herzlage auf die Form des Elektrokardiogramms. *Pflug. Arch.*, 1913;**150**: 275–315. (Translation: Hoff, H.E., Sekelj, P. *Am. Heart J.*, 1950;**40**: 163–194.)
34. Henson, J.R., Descartes and the ECG lettering series. *J. Hist. Med. Allied Sci.*, 1971;**26**: 181–186.
35. Hurst, J.W., Naming of the waves in the ECG, with a brief account of their Genesis. *Circulation*, 1998;**98**: 1937–1942.
36. Gussak, I., P. Bjerregaard, T.M. Egan, and B.R. Chaitman, ECG phenomenon called the J wave: History, pathophysiology and clinical significance. *J. Electrocardiol.*, 1995;**28**: 49–58.

37. Scherf, D. and A. Schott, *Extrasystoles and Allied Arrhythmias*, 2nd edn, London: Heinemann Medical, 1973.

38. Read, B.E., Gleanings from old Chinese medicine. *Ann. Med. Hist.*, 1926;**8**: 16–19.

39. Hubotter, F., *Die chinesische medizin zu beginn des XX. jahrhunderts und ihr historischer Entwicklungsgang*. Leipzig: Asia Major (Schindler), 1929.

40. Arcieri, J.P., *The Circulation of the Blood And Andrea Cesalpino of Arezzo*, New York: Vanni, 1945.

41. Wenckebach, K.F., *Arhythmia of the Heart: A Physiological and Clinical Study*. Edinburgh: Green, 1904.

42. Mackenzie, J., *The Study of the Pulse, Arterial, Venous, and Hepatic, and of the Movements of the Heart*. Edinburgh: Pentland, 1902.

43. Mackenzie, J., *Diseases of the Heart*. London: Frowde, 1908.

44. Engelmann, T.W., Beobachtungen und Versuche am suspendirten Herzen. 2. Abh. Ueber die Leitung der Bewegungsreize im Herzen. *Pflug. Arch.*, 1894;**56**: 149–202.

45. McWilliam, J.A., Fibrillar contraction of the heart. *J. Physiol.*, 1887;**8**: 296–310.

46. His, W., Ueber die Tiitigkeit des embryonalen Herzens und deren Bedeutung fur die Lehre von der Herzbewegung beim Erwachsenen. *Arb. Med. Klin. Leipzig.*, 1893;**1**: 14–50.

47. His, W., Zur Geschichte des Atrioventrikularbundels nebst Bemerkungen uber die embryonale Herztiitigkeit. *Klin. Wochenschr.*, 1933;**12**: 569–574.

48. Hering, H.E., Ober den Pulsus irregularis perpetuus. *Dtsch. Arch. Klin. Med.*, 1908;**94**: 185–204.

49. Lewis, T., Irregular action of the heart in mitral stenosis: The inception of ventricular rhythm, etc. *Q. J. Med.*, 1909;**2**: 356–367.

50. Samojloff, A., *Eleklrokardiogramme*. Jena: Fischer, 1909.

51. Krikler, D.M., The search for Samojloff: A Russian physiologist in times of change. *Br. Med. J.*, 1987;**295**: 1624–1627.

52. Lepeschkin, E., *Modern Electrocardiography*. Baltimore: Williams and Wilkins, 1951.

53. Lewis, T., *The Mechanism of the Heart Beat,with Special Reference to its Clinical Pathology*, London: Shaw, 1911.

54. Burchell, H., Sir Thomas Lewis: His impact on American cardiology. *Br. Heart J.*, 1981;**46**: 1–4.

55. Snellen, H.A., Thomas Lewis (1881–1945) and cardiology in Europe. *Br. Heart J.*, 1981;**46**: 121–125.

56. Hollman, A., Thomas Lewis the early years. *Br. Heart J.*, 1981;**46**: 233–244.

57. Rosenbaum, M.B., Sir Thomas Lewis: A view from the south. *Br. Heart J.*, 1981;**46**: 349–350.

58. Lewis, T., *The Mechanism and Graphic Registration of the Heart Beat*, 3rd ed. London: Shaw, 1925.

59. Wilson, F.N., A.G. Macleod, and P.S. Barker, The interpretation of the initial deflections of the ventricular complex of the electrocardiogram. *Am. Heart J.*, 1931;**6**: 637–664.

60. Fahr, G., An analysis of the spread of the excitation wave in the human ventricle. *Arch. Intern. Med.*, 1920;**25**: 146–173.

61. Lewis, T., *Research in Medicine and Other Addresses*. London: Lewis, 1939.

62. Wilson, F.N., Report of a case showing premature beats arising in the junctional tissues. *Heart*, 1915;**6**: 17–22.

63. Abildskov, J.A., Prediction of ventricular arrhythmias from ECG waveforms. *J. Electrocardiol.*, 1987;**20**(Suppl.): 97–101.

64. Woolferth, C.C. and F.C. Wood, The Electrocardiographic diagnosis of coronary occlusion by the use of chest leads. *Am. Heart J.*, 1932;**7**: 404 (abstract).

65. Wilson, F.N., A.G. Macleod, and P.S. Barker, Electrocardiographic Leads which record potential variations produced by the heart beat at a single point. *Proc. Soc. Exp. Bioi. Med.*, 1932;**29**: 1011–1012.

66. Wilson, F.N., F.D. Johnston, A.G. Macleod, and P.S. Barker, Electrocardiograms that Represent the potential variations of a single electrode. *Am. Heart J.*, 1934;**9**: 447–471.

67. Kligfield, P., L.S. Gettes, and J.J. Bailley, et al., Recommendations for the standardization and interpretation of the electrocardiogram: Part 1: The electrocardiogram and its technology. *Circulation*, 2007;**115**: 1306–1324.

68. Kossmann, C.E. and F.D. Johnston, The precordial electrocardiogram. I. The potential variations of the precordium and of the extremities in normal subjects. *Am. Heart J.*, 1935;**10**: 925–941.

69. Joint Recommendations of the American Heart Association and the Cardiac Society of Great Britain and Ireland. Standardization of precordial leads. *Am. Heart J.*, 1938;**15**: 107–108.

70. Committee of the American Heart Association for the Standardization of Precordial Leads. Standardization of precordial leads. supplementary report. *Am. Heart J.*, 1938;**15**: 235–239.

71. Committee on Precordial leads of the American Heart Association for the Standardization of Precordial Leads. Standardization of precordial leads. second supplementary report. *J. Am. Med. Assoc.*, 1943;**121**: 1349–1351.

72. Goldberger, E., A simple, indifferent, electrocardiographic electrode of zero potential and a technique of obtaining augmented, unipolar, extremity leads. *Am. Heart J.*, 1942;**23**: 483–492.

73. Pardee, H.E.B., Nomenclature and description of the electrocardiogram. *Am. Heart J.*, 1940;**20**: 655–666.

74. Lewis, T., The spread of the excitatory process in the vertebrate heart. *Phil. Trans. R. Soc. London, Ser. B.*, 1916;**207**: 221–310.

75. Williams, H.B., On the cause of the phase difference frequently observed between homonymous peaks of the electrocardiogram. *Am. J. Physiol.*, 1914;**35**: 292–300.

76. Mann, H., A method of analyzing the electrocardiogram. *Arch. Intern. Med.*, 1920;**25**: 283–294.

77. Mann, H., The monocardiograph. *Am. Heart J.*, 1938;**15**: 681–699.

78. Schellong, F., Elektrographische Diagnostik der Herzmuskelerkrankungen. *Verh. Dtsch. Ges. Inn Med.i* 1936;**48**: 288–310.

79. Wilson, F.N., F.D. Johnston, and P.S. Barker, The use of the cathode-ray oscillograph in the study of the monocardiogram. *J. Clin. Invest.*, 1937;**16**: 664–665.

80. Hollmann, W. and H.E. Hollmann, Neue Elektrokardiographische Untersuchungsmethoden. z. *Kreislaufforsch.*, 1937;**29**: 546–558.

81. Rijlant, P., Introduction a l'etude de la distribution spatiale des variatiolls de potentiel produites par le coeur chez l'homme. *C. R. Seances Soc. Biol.*, 1936;**121**: 1358–1361.

82. Wilson, F.N. and F.D. Johnston, The vectorcardiogram. *Am. Heart J.*, 1938;**16**: 14–28.

83. Burger, H.C. and J.B. Van Milaan, Heart vector and leads. I, II and III. *Br. Heart J.*, 1946;**8**: 157–161, 1947;**9**: 154–160 and 1948;**10**: 229–233.

84. McFee, R., R.M. Stow, and F.D. Johnston, Graphic representation of electrocardiographic leads by means of fluid mappers. *Circulation*, 1952;**6**: 21–29.

85. Brody, D.A., B.D. Erb, and W.E. Romans, The approximate determination of lead vectors and the burger triangle in normal human subjects. *Am. Heart J.*, 1956;**51**: 211–220.

86. McFee, R. and F.D. Johnston, Electrocardiographic leads. I. Introduction. *Circulation*, 1953;8: 554–68. II. Analysis. *Circulation*, 1954;9: 255–266. III. Synthesis. *Circulation*, 1954;**9**:868–880.

87. Frank, E., The image surface of a homogenous torso. *Am. Heart J.*, 1954;**47**: 757–768.

88. Frank, E., An accurate, clinically practical system for spatial vectorcardiography. *Circulation.*, 1956;**13**: 737–749.

89. Wilson, F.N., F.D. Johnston and C.E. Kossmann, The substitution of a tetrahedron for the Einthoven triangle. *Am. Heart J.*, 1947;**33**: 594–603.

90. Rijlant, P., Principe et methode de la vectorcardiographie. *Bull. Acad R. Med. Belg, Ser.*, 1957;**22**: 156–171.

91. Simonson, E., K. Nakagawa, and O.H. Schmitt, Respiratory changes of the spatial vectorcardiogram recorded with different lead systems. *Am. Heart J.*, 1957;**54**: 919–939.

92. Macfarlane, P.W., A hybrid lead system for routine electrocardiography, in *Progress in Electrocardiography*, P W.Macfarlane, Editor, Tunbridge Wells, Pitman Medical, 1979, pp. 1–5.

93. Castillo, H.T., An anatomical orthogonal four-electrode X-Y-Z Lead system for universal ECG recording. *Eur. J. Cardiol.*, 1979;**10**: 395–404.

94. Dower, G., A. Yakush, S.B. Nazzal, R.V. Jutzy, and C.E. Ruiz, Deriving the 12 lead electrocardiogram from four (EASI) electrodes. *J Electrocardiol.*, 1988;**21**(suppl): 182–187.

95. Dower, G.E., H.B. Machado, and J.A. Osborne, On deriving the electrocardiogram from vectorcardiographic leads. *Clin.Cardiol.*, 1980;**3**: 87–95.

96. Edenbrandt, L. and O. Pahlm, Comparison of various methods for synthesizing frank-like vectorcardiograms from the conventional 12-lead ECG, in *Computers in Cardiology IEE Comp Soc*, Baltimore, Maryland, 1987, pp. 71–74.

97. Uijen, G.J.H., A. van Oosterom, and R.T.H. van Dam, The relationship between the 12-lead standard ECG and the XYZ vector leads, in *Proceedings of the 14th International Congress on Electrocardiology*, E.Schubert, Editor, Berlin, Adakemie Verlag, 1988, pp. 301–307.

98. Willems, J., *Common Standards for Quantitative Electrocardiography. 4th Progress Report*. Leuven: Acco, 1984, pp. 199–200.

99. Nelwan, S.,J.A. Kors, S.H. Meij, J.H. van Bemmel, and M. Simoons, Reconstruction of the 12th lead electrocardiogram from reduced lead sets. *J Electrocardiol.*, 2004;**37**: 11–18.

100. Wei, D., T. Kojima, T. Nakayama, and Y. Sakai, US Patent No. 6,721,591: Method of deriving standard 12-lead Electrocardiogram and electrocardiogram monitoring apparatus. *US Patent Office*, 2004.

101. Waller, A.D., Introductory address on the electromotive properties of the human heart. *Br. Med. J.*, 1888;**2**: 751–754.

102. Geselowitz, D.B., Multipole representation for an equivalent cardiac generator. *Proc IRE.*, 1960;**48**: 75.

103. Selvester, R.H., C.R. Collier, and R.B. Pearson, Analog computer model of the vectorcardiogram. *Circulation*, 1965;**31**:45–53.

104. Selvester, R.H., R. Kalaba, C.R.Collier, R. Bellman, and H. Kagiwada, A digital computer model of the vectorcardiogram with distance and boundary effects: Simulated myocardial infarction. *Am. Heart J.*, 1967;**74**: 792–808.

105. Holt, J.H. Jr., A.C.L. Barnard, M.S. Lynn, P. Svendsen, and J.O. Kramer Jr., A study of the human heart as a multiple dipole electrical source. I. normal adult male subjects. *Circulation*, 1969;**40**: 687–696. II. Diagnosis and quantification of left ventricular hypertrophy. *Circulation*, 1969;**40**: 697–710. III.

Diagnosis and quantification of right ventricular hypertrophy. *Circulation*, 1969;**40**: 711–718.

106. Lynn, M.S., A.C.L. Barnard, J.H. Holt, and L.T. Sheffield, A proposed method for the inverse problem in electrocardiography. *Biophys. J.*, 1967;**7**: 925–945.

107. Young, B.D., A Computer Study of the Electrical Activity of the Heart, Ph.D. thesis. Glasgow: University of Glasgow, 1972.

108. Macfarlane, P.W., A.R. Lorimer, R.H. Baxter, and T.D.V. Lawrie, Multiple dipole electrocardiography. *Br. Heart J.*, 1973;**35**:863–864.

109. Intini, A., R.N. Goldstein, P. Jia, et al., Electrocardiographic imaging (ECGI) – A novel diagnostic modality used for mapping of focal ventricular tachycardia in a young athlete. *Heart Rhythm.* 2005;**2**: 1250–1252.

110. Ramanathan, C., R.N. Ghanem, P. Jia, K. Ryu, and Y. Rudy, Noninvasive electrocardiographic imaging for cardiac electrophysiology and arrhythmia. *Nat Med.*, 2004;**10**: 422–428.

111. Boyett, M.R., J. Li, S. Inada, H. Dobrzynski, J.E. Schneider, A.V. Holden, and H. Zhang, Imaging the heart: computer 3-dimensional anatomic models of the heart. *J Electrocardiol.*, 2005;**38**(Suppl): 113–120

112. Nahum, L.H., A. Mauro, H. Chernoff, and R.S. Sikand, Instantaneous equipotential distribution on surface of the human body for various instants in the cardiac cycle. *J. Appl. Physiol.*, 1951;**3**: 454–464.

113. Taccardi, B., B.B. Punske, F. Sachse, X. Tricoche, P. Colli-Franzone, L.F. Pavarino, and C. Zabawa, Intramural activation and repolarization sequences in canine ventricles. Experimental and simulation studies. *J Electrocardiol*, 2005;**38**(Suppl): 131–137.

114. Barr, R.C., M.S. Spach, and G.S. Herman-Giddens, Selection of the number and positions of measuring locations for electrocardiography. *IEEE Trans. Biomed. Eng.*, 1971;**18**: 125–138.

115. Kornreich, F., The missing waveform information in the orthogonal electrocardiogram (Frank leads). I. Where and how can this missing waveform information be retrieved? *Circulation*, 1973;**48**: 984–995.

116. Lux, R.L., M.J. Burgess, R.F. Wyatt, A.K. Evans, G.M. Vincent, and J.A. Abildskov, Clinically practical lead systems for improved electrocardiography: comparison with precordial grids and conventional lead systems. *Circulation*, 1979;**59**: 356–363.

117. Taccardi, B. and Marchetti, G., Distribution of heart potentials on the body surface and in artificial conducting media, in *Int. Symp. Electrophysiology of the Heart*, B. Taccardi, G. Marchetti, Editors. Oxford, Pergamon, 1965, pp. 257–280.

118. Maynard, S.J., I.B.A. Menown, G. Manoharan, J. Allen, J.McC. Anderson, and A.A. J. Adgey, Body surface mapping improves early diagnosis of acute myocardial infarction in patients with chest pain and left bundle branch block. *Heart*, 2003;**89**:998–1002.

119. Burdon Sanderson, J., The mechanical, thermal, and electrical properties of striped muscle, in *Textbook of Physiology*, E.A. Schafer, Editor, Chapter 2, Edinburgh, Pentland, 1900, p. 446.

120. Woodbury, L.A., J.W. Woodbury, and H.H. Hecht, Membrane resting and action potentials of single cardiac muscle fibers. *Circulation*, 1950;**1**: 264–266.

121. Sicouri, S. and C. Antzelevitch, A subpopulation of cells with unique electrophysiological properties in the deep subepicardium of the canine ventricle. The M cell. *Circ. Res*, 1991;**68**: 1729–1741.

122. Antzelevvitch, C., W. Shimuzu, G.X. Yan, S. Sicouri, J. Weissenburger, V.V. Nesterenko, A. Burashnikov, J. Di Diego, J. Saffitz, and G.P. Thomas, The M Cell: its contribution to the ECG and to the normal and abnormal electrical function of the heart. *J Cardiovasc Electrophysiol.*, 1999;**10**: 1124–1152.

123. Rudy, Y., Lessons learned about slow discontinuous conduction from models of impulse propagation. *J Electrocardiol.*, 2005;**38**(Suppl): 52–54.

124. Taccardi, B. and G. Marchetti, Editors, *Int. Symp. Electrophysiology of the Heart*, Oxford, Pergamon, 1965.

125. Hulme, J.T., T. Scheuer, and W.A. Catterall, Regulation of cardiac ion channels by signaling complexes: Role of modified leucine zipper motifs. *J Mol Cell Cardiol.*, 2004;**37**: 625–631.

126. Scher, A.M. and A.C. Young, Ventricular depolarization and the genesis of the QRS. *Ann. N. Y. Acad. Sci.*, 1957;**65**: 768–778.

127. Scher, A.M., Excitation of the heart, in *Handbook of Physiology. Section 2: Circulation*, Vol. 1, W.F. Hamilton, Editor, Washington DC, American Physiological Society, 1962, pp. 287–322.

128. Durrer, D., R.T.H. van Dam, G.E. Freud, M.J. Janse, F.L. Meijler, and R.C. Arzbaecher, Total excitation of the isolated human heart. *Circulation*, 1970;**41**: 899–912.

129. Boineau, J.P., C.B. Miller, R.B. Schuessler, L.J. Autry, A.C. Wylds, and W.R. Roeske, Comparison between activation and potential maps during multicentric atrial impulse origin in dogs, in *Computerized Interpretation of The Electrocardiogram*, R.H.Selvester, and B.D. Geselowitz, Editors, New York, New York Engineering Foundation, 1984, pp. 55–62.

130. Spach, M.S. and R.C. Barr, Origin of epicardial ST-T wave potentials in the intact dog. *Circ. Res.*, 1976;**39**: 475–487.

131. Burgess, M.J., L.S. Green, K. Millar, R. Wyatt, and J.A. Abildskov, The sequence of normal ventricular recovery. *Am. Heart J.*, 1972;**84**: 660–669.

132. Cowan, J.C., Epicardial repolarization sequence and T wave configuration. *Br. Heart J.*, 1988;**59**: 85.

133. Krikler, D.M., Electrocardiography then and now: Where next? *Br Heart J.*, 1987;**57**: 113–117.

134. Watson, H., D. Emslie-Smith, and K.G. Lowe, The intracardiac electrocardiogram of human atrioventricular conducting tissue. *Am. Heart J.*, 1967;**74**: 66–70.

135. Lenegre, J. and P. Maurice, De quelques resultats obtenus par la derivation directe intracavitaire des courants electriques de l'oreillette et du ventricule droits. *Arch. Mal. Coeur Vaiss.*, 1945;**38**: 298–302.

136. Alanis, J., H. Gonzallez, and E. Lopez. The electrical activity of the bundle of his. *J. Physiol.*, 1958;**142**: 127–140.

137. Giraud, G., P. Puech, and H. Latour, Variations de potentiel liees a l'activite du systeme de conduction auriculo ventriculaire chez l'homme (Enregistrement electrocardiographique endocavitaire). *Arch. Mal. Coeur Vaiss.*, 1960;**53**: 757–16.

138. Scherlag, B.J., S.H. Lau, R.H. Helfant, W.D. Berkowitz, E. Stein, and A.H. Damato, Catheter techniques for recording his bundle activity in man. *Circulation*, 1969;**39**: 13–18.

139. Durrer, D., Electrical aspects of human cardiac activity: A clinical-physiological approach to excitation and stimulation. *Cardiovasc. Res.*, 1968;**2**: 1–18.

140. Rosenbaum, M.B., M.V. Elizari, and J.O. Lazzari, *Los Hemibloqueos*. Buenos Aires, Paidos, 1968. (Translation: *The Hemiblocks*. Oldsmar, Florida: Tampa Tracings, 1970.)

141. Grant, R.P., *Clinical Electrocardiography: The Spatial Vector Approach*. New York: Blakiston, 1957.

142. Beattie, J.M., F.A. Gaffney, and C.G. Blomqvist, Transcavitary conduction and the mean frontal QRS axis, in Electrocardiology '87, E. Schubert, and D. Romberg, Editors, Berlin, Akademie Verlag, 1988. pp. 71–74.

143. Brugada, P. and J. Brugada, Right bundle branch block, persistent st elevation and sudden cardiac death: a distinct clinical and electrocardiographic syndrome: A multicenter report. *J Am Coll Cardiol.*, 1993;**20**: 1391–1396.

144. Wilde, A.A.M., C. Antzelevitch, M. Borggrefe, et al., Consensus report. proposed diagnostic criteria for the brugada syndrome. *Eur. Heart J.*, 2004;**23**: 1648–1654.

145. Antzelevitch, A., P. Brugada, M. Borggrefe, et al., Brugada syndrome: report of the second consensus conference. *Circulation*, 2005;**111**: 659–670.

146. Gussak, I., P. Brugada, J. Brugada, et al., Idiopathic short QT interval: A new clinical syndrome? *Cardiology*, 2000;**94**: 99–102.

147. Ott, P. and F.I. Marcus, Electrocardiographic markers of sudden death. *Cardiol. Clin.*, 2006;**24**: 453–469.

148. Stallman, F.W. and H.V. Pipberger, Automatic recognition of electrocardiographic waves by digital computer. *Circ. Res.*, 1961;**9**: 1138–1143.

149. Caceres, C.A., C.A. Steinberg, S. Abrahams, et al., Computer extraction of electrocardiographic parameters. *Circulation*, 1962;**25**: 356–362.

150. Macfarlane, P.W., H. Cawood, T.P. Taylor, and T.D.V. Lawrie, Routine automated electrocardiogram interpretation. *Biomed. Eng.*, 1972;**7**: 176–180.

151. Rosenbaum, D., L.E. Jackson, J.M. Smith, J.N. Ruskin, and R.J. Cohen, Electrical alternans and vulnerability to ventricular arrhythmias. *N. Eng. J. Med.*, 1994;**330**: 235–241.

152. Klingenheben, T., Microvolt T wave alternans for arrhythmia risk stratification in left ventricular dysfunction. *J Am Coll Cardiol.*, 2007;**50**: 174–175.

153. Roberts, W.C. and M.A. Silver, Norman jefferies holter and ambulatory ecg monitoring. *Am. J. Cardiol.*, 1983;**52**: 903–906.

154. MacInnis, H.F., The clinical application of radioelectrocardiography. *Can. Med. Assoc. J.*, 1954;**70**: 574–576.

155. Holter, N.J., New method for heart studies. *Science*, 1961;**134**: 1214–1220.

156. Schmidt, G., M. Malik, P. Barthel, et al., Heart-rate turbulence after ventricular premature beats as a predictor of mortality after acute myocardial infarction. *Lancet*, 1999;**353**: 1390–1396.

157. Sosnowski, M., E. Clark, S. Latif, P.W. Macfarlane, and M. Tendera, Heart rate variability fraction – A new reportable measure of 24-hour R-R interval variation. *Ann of Noninvasive Electrocardiol.*, 2005;**10**: 7–15

158. Langner, P.H. Jr., D.B. Geselowitz, and F.T. Mansure, High-frequency components in the electrocardiograms of normal subjects and of patients with coronary heart disease. *Am. Heart J.*, 1961;**62**: 746–755.

159. Schuller, H. and T. Fahraeus, Pacemaker electrocardiograms: An introduction to practical analysis. *Solna. Siemens-Elema.*, 1983;**1**: 1.

160. Barold, S., M.C. Giudici, B. Herweg, and A.B. Curtis, Diagnostic value of the 12-lead electrocardiogram during conventional and biventricular pacing for cardiac resynchronization. *Cardiol Clin.*, 2006;**24**: 471–490.

161. Baule, G.M. and R. McFee, Detection of the magnetic field of the heart. *Am Heart J.*, 1963;**66**: 95–96.

162. Kannel, W.B., K. Anderson, D.L. McGee, L.S. Degatano, and M.J. Stampfer, Non-specific electrocardiographic abnormality as a predictor of coronary heart disease: The framingham study. *Am. Heart J.*, 1987;**113**: 370–376.

163. Kreger, B.E., L.A. Cupples, and W.B. Kannel, The electrocardiogram in prediction of sudden death. Framingham Study experience. *Am. Heart J.*, 1987;**113**: 377–382.

164. Tobin, M.D., M. Kahonen, P. Braund, T. Nieminen, C. Hajat, M. Tomaszewski, J. Viik, R. Lehtinen, R.A. Ng, P.W. Macfarlane, P.R. Burton, T. Lehtimaki, and N.J. Samani, Gender and effects of a common genetic variant in the NOS1 regulator NOS1AP on cardiac repolarization in 3761 individuals from two independent populations. *Int. J. Epidemiology*, 2008;**37**: 1132–1141.

2 Introductory Physics and Mathematics

R. Plonsey · A. van Oosterom

P. W. Macfarlane et al. (eds.), *Basic Electrocardiology*, DOI 10.1007/978-0-85729-871-3_2,
© Springer-Verlag London Limited 2012

2.1   Introduction

The goal of this chapter is to project an organized presentation of a central core of mathematics and physics that is related to the topics that are discussed elsewhere in this book. Some of the more specialized (and sophisticated) mathematics and physics are not included but, rather, will be found in the particular associated electrocardiographic topic to which they are applied. The reader should also be aware that the choice of material for this chapter is limited to that required for this text; if greater breadth is desired for another purpose, the corresponding reference at the end of this chapter could be consulted.

2.2   Vector Analysis

Mathematical development and application of a variety of electrocardiographic topics presented in this book are greatly facilitated by the use of vector concepts and vector calculus. Some readers may have knowledge of this material, but need a review; a few may have had no formal study of vector analysis, but require that knowledge presently. Presented here are the concepts of gradient, divergence and Laplacian, which play an important role in describing both the heart as a generator of currents and the torso as a site for the flow of these volume-conductor currents.

2.2.1   Scalars and Vectors

All biophysical problems can be described by the behavior of one or more associated variables. For physical quantities, the variables will be either scalars or vectors. If the variable is defined by a simple (single) value (electric potential, conductivity, temperature, etc.), it is designated a scalar. If both magnitude and direction are needed (current density, electric field, force, etc.), then the quantity is described as a *vector*.

In a given preparation, a scalar property might vary as a function of position (the conductivity as a function of position in a body) and this is referred to as a *scalar field*. A vector (blood flow at different points in a major artery) is, similarly, described as a vector field. A scalar is designated by unmodified letters, while vectors in 3D space are denoted with an arrow over the letter. For example, t is used for temperature, $\vec{J}$ for current density, while $\vec{J}(x, y, z)$ denotes a vector field where at each point (x, y, z) a particular vector $\vec{J}$ exists. The magnitude of a vector $\vec{J}$ is written as $|\vec{J}|$, or J.

2.2.2   Vector Addition

The sum (or difference) of two vectors is more complicated than scalar addition (or subtraction) because direction as well as magnitude is involved. If vector $\vec{A}$ is represented by a displacement from 1 to 2 as illustrated in ❷ Fig. 2.1 and vector $\vec{B}$ is represented by a further displacement from 2 to 3, then their sum $\vec{C}$ is clearly the displacement from 1 to 3 as shown. Vector $\vec{C}$ may also be obtained by constructing a parallelogram with $\vec{A}$ and $\vec{B}$ as sides, in which case $\vec{C}$ is the diagonal from the common origin for $\vec{A}$ and $\vec{B}$. This law of vector summation is often referred to as the *parallelogram law*. It can easily be verified geometrically either from ❷ Fig. 2.1 or from the parallelogram construction, that the order of addition of $\vec{A}$ and $\vec{B}$ is immaterial. Vector addition is said to be *commutative, i.e.*

$$\vec{C} = \vec{A} + \vec{B} = \vec{B} + \vec{A} \tag{2.1}$$

The negative of a vector is defined to be a vector of opposite direction but with equal magnitude. The subtraction of vector $\vec{B}$ from $\vec{A}$ can then be expressed as the sum of $\vec{A}$ and $(-\vec{B})$. In ❷ Fig. 2.1, it can be confirmed geometrically that $\vec{B} + (-\vec{C}) = -\vec{A}$, which rearranges to Eqn. (2.1).

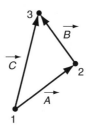

◼ **Fig. 2.1**
Illustration of vector addition

2.2.3 Unit Vectors

The result of multiplying a vector $\vec{A}$ by a scalar m is a new vector with the same orientation but a magnitude m times great. If this is designated by $\vec{B}$, then

$$\vec{B} = m\vec{A} \tag{2.2}$$

$$|\vec{B}| = |m\vec{A}| \text{ or } B = mA \tag{2.3}$$

A unit vector is one which has a magnitude equal to unity. It is sometimes convenient to describe a vector $\vec{A}$ by the product of its magnitude $A = |\vec{A}|$ and a unit vector $\vec{e}_A$ which specifies its direction. Thus, $\vec{A} = A\,\vec{e}_A$. Correspondingly, throughout this chapter $(\vec{e}_x, \vec{e}_y, \vec{e}_z)$ denote (dimensionless) unit vectors along the principal coordinate axes x, y, z of a Cartesian coordinate system. If A_x, A_y and A_z are the projections of vector $\vec{A}$ on the x, y and z axes, respectively, then

$$\vec{A} = A_x\vec{e}_x + A_y\vec{e}_y + A_z\vec{e}_z \tag{2.4}$$

as illustrated in ❷ Fig. 2.2. The magnitude of $\vec{A}$ is related to its rectangular components by

$$A = \left(A_x^2 + A_y^2 + A_z^2\right)^{1/2} \tag{2.5}$$

as is clear from ❷ Fig. 2.2. Equal vectors have the same magnitude and direction and, consequently, equal respective components. For example, (2.1) can be written as

$$\vec{e}_x(A_x + B_x) + \vec{e}_y(A_y + B_y) + \vec{e}_z(A_z + B_z) = \vec{e}_x C_x + \vec{e}_y C_y + \vec{e}_z C_z \tag{2.6}$$

so that

$$A_x + B_x = C_x; \quad A_y + B_y = C_y; \quad A_z + B_z = C_z \tag{2.7}$$

2.2.4 Scalar Product of Two Vectors

The scalar product of two vectors is defined as the scalar representing the product of their magnitudes times the cosine of the angle between them (drawn from a common origin).

From ❷ Fig. 2.3, it can be seen that the scalar product of $\vec{A}$ and $\vec{B}$ is the product of the magnitude of one of them (say B) times the projection of the other on the first (i.e., $A\cos\theta$). For any two vectors that are normal (at right angles) to each other, this means that their scalar product is equal to zero.

The scalar product is denoted as $\vec{A} \bullet \vec{B} = A B \cos\theta$ and correspondingly (usually) referred to as the dot product.

It is clear from the definition that

$$\vec{A} \bullet \vec{B} = \vec{B} \bullet \vec{A} \tag{2.8}$$

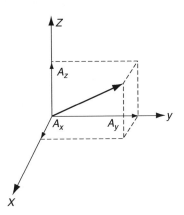

Fig. 2.2
Resolution of a vector into its Cartesian components

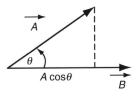

Fig. 2.3
Scalar product of two vectors

so that the *commutative* law of multiplication applies to this type of product. It can also be verified from graphical analysis that

$$(\vec{A} + \vec{B}) \bullet \vec{D} = \vec{A} \bullet \vec{D} + \vec{B} \bullet \vec{D} \tag{2.9}$$

that is, the *distributive* law of multiplication applies to the dot product of two vectors.

Since both the distributive and commutative laws hold, scalar multiplication of vectors follows the familiar rules of algebra. We now apply these rules to the dot product of $\vec{A} = A_x\vec{e}_x + A_y\vec{e}_y + A_z\vec{e}_z$ and $\vec{B} = B_x\vec{e}_x + B_y\vec{e}_y + B_z\vec{e}_z$. The fact that the vectors $\vec{e}_x$, $\vec{e}_y$ and $\vec{e}_z$ have unit lengths and are orthogonal to one another is expressed by the dot products:

$$\vec{e}_x \bullet \vec{e}_x = \vec{e}_y \bullet \vec{e}_y = \vec{e}_z \bullet \vec{e}_z = 1 \text{ and } \vec{e}_x \bullet \vec{e}_y = \vec{e}_y \bullet \vec{e}_z = \vec{e}_z \bullet \vec{e}_x = 0, \tag{2.10}$$

respectively. By using these properties to evaluate $\vec{A} \bullet \vec{B}$ we find that

$$\vec{A} \bullet \vec{B} = A_x B_x + A_y B_y + A_z B_z \tag{2.11}$$

2.2.4.1 Vector Product of Two Vectors

Vector product of two vectors $\vec{A}$ and $\vec{B}$ is defined as vector $\vec{C}$ that is orthogonal to the plane spanned by the two vectors, having as its magnitudes the product of the magnitudes of the two vectors multiplied by sine of the smallest angle needed for rotating $\vec{A}$ to line up with $\vec{B}$ (❷ Fig. 2.3). The vector product is denoted as

$$\vec{C} = \vec{A} \times \vec{B}, \tag{2.12}$$

from which stems the alternative name 'cross-product' for the vector product. For the situation shown in ❷ Fig. 2.3, the vector $\vec{A} \times \vec{B}$ points into the plane of the figure and the vector $\vec{B} \times \vec{A}$ points into the opposite direction, and we have

$$\vec{C} = \vec{A} \times \vec{B} = -\vec{B} \times \vec{A} \tag{2.13}$$

2.2.5   Scalar and Vector Fields

If a fluid-filled container is shaken and swirled, the velocity of the fluid at each point will, in general, be different. The velocity vector is a function of position and this function can be expected to be reasonably well behaved. As noted earlier, a vector function of position constitutes a vector field.

To each point on the surface of the earth, an elevation (above sea level) can be ascertained. Only a single quantity (scalar) is involved and a scalar field is defined in this way. It is convenient to describe such a field by connecting (mapping) points of similar elevation. In this manner, lines on which the field has a constant value are identified, where the constants are chosen from a set of discrete scalar values separated by an interval that is sufficiently large enough for adequate resolution of the field, yet do not have excessive detail.

Isofunction lines, or contour lines, provide valuable graphical information on the topographic field. In a similar way, a representation of an electrical potential field through plotting its isopotential contours depicts, graphically, the behavior of the field.

A vector field may be described in terms of its rectangular (scalar) components so that a vector field would be represented by three scalar fields. A more direct representation is in the construction of flow lines, which are space curves that are tangential to the vector field everywhere. Only a finite number of such lines (they are infinite in number) would be drawn; the number chosen is a trade-off between increasing resolution and excessive complexity. For a two-dimensional map, the total flow between adjoining flow lines is usually chosen to be constant and, consequently, flux density is proportional to the density of the flow lines plotted.

While flow lines are easy to be interpreted when the physical entity constitutes an actual flow (*i.e.*, current), such representation is equally possible for a non-flow type vector field. The direction and density of the flow lines is then simply proportional to the direction and magnitude of the vector field.

2.2.6   Gradient

In this book, there is an interest in situations where an electrical potential field Φ (due to electrical generators in the heart) is established in some region that is electrically conducting (e.g., the torso). A consequence of such an occurrence is a resulting flow of current (which can be described by application of Ohm's law). The direction of current will correspond to the direction of the maximum rate of decrease in potential; the magnitude of the current density will be proportional to the magnitude of this rate of change.

In this section is described the gradient operation which is defined in order to extract, from a scalar potential field, a vector field which is precisely in the direction of the maximum rate of change of potential and with a magnitude equal to that rate of change. Its value (among others) is for evaluating a current flow field from a given potential field.

Let $\Phi(x, y, z)$ be a scalar field (scalar function of position) and assumed that it is a single-valued, continuous and differentiable function of position. Physical fields invariably satisfy these requirements. A surface C of constant value c is defined by

$$\Phi(x, y, z) = c \tag{2.14}$$

In applications of interest, Φ is a potential (electrical or chemical), in which case a surface of constant value is referred to as an equipotential or isopotential surface.

If c takes on a succession of, say, increasing values, a family of nonintersecting equivalued surfaces results. A plot of such equipotential surfaces (or plot of the intersections of these surfaces with principal planes) provides a graphical description of the potential field itself.

Consider two closely spaced points P_1 and P_2, where P_1 lies on the surface C_1 defined by $\Phi(x, y, z) = c_1$ and P_2 may or may not lie on this surface (see ❷ Fig. 2.4). If the coordinates of P_1 are (x, y, z) then the coordinates of P_2 could be described as $[(x + dx), (y + dy), (z + dz)]$. The displacement (a vector) from P_1 to P_2 is simply the vector sum of its rectangular components, namely,

$$d\vec{l} = \vec{e}_x dx + \vec{e}_y dy + \vec{e}_z dz \tag{2.15}$$

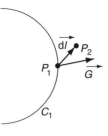

□ Fig. 2.4
Equipotential surface and gradient

Now, the difference in potential from P_1 to P_2 (the total derivative) is

$$d\Phi = \frac{\partial \Phi}{\partial x}dx + \frac{\partial \Phi}{\partial y}dy + \frac{\partial \Phi}{\partial x}dz \tag{2.16}$$

We now define $\vec{G}$ as the vector in 3D space having the above partial derivatives as its rectangular components:

$$\vec{G} = \frac{\partial \Phi}{\partial x}\vec{e}_x + \frac{\partial \Phi}{\partial y}\vec{e}_y + \frac{\partial \Phi}{\partial z}\vec{e}_z \tag{2.17}$$

In view of the definition of the scalar product of two vectors as expressed by (2.11),

$$d\Phi = \vec{G} \bullet d\vec{l} = G\,d\ell\,\cos\theta \tag{2.18}$$

Some of the properties of any nonzero $\vec{G}$ can be deduced from this equation. First, suppose that both P_1 and P_2 lie on C_1 and hence, $d\Phi = 0$. Since P_2 is only an infinitesimal (but nonzero) distance from P_1, $d\vec{l}$ is tangential to C_1 at P_1. Equation (2.18) indicates that in this situation $\cos\theta = 0$ and thus $\vec{G}$ must be normal to C_1. Next, we consider any nonzero $d\vec{l}$ directed from P_1 on C_1 to a field point P_2 on C_2 for which $d\Phi = c_2 - c_1 > 0$. Equation (2.18) also indicates that $d\Phi$ attains a maximum value if $\vec{G}$ and $d\vec{l}$ point in the same direction, and with $d\vec{l}$ directed towards a higher value of Φ, $\vec{G}$ always points toward higher values of Φ.

The magnitude of $\vec{G}$ follows from (2.18). Since

$$d\Phi/dl = G\cos\theta, \tag{2.19}$$

indicating that the derivative of Φ along a line l depends on the local direction, $d\vec{l}$, of the line, the gradient is a *directional derivative*. From (2.19), with $\theta = 0$ and dn a distance directed along the surface normal $\vec{n}$, we have

$$G = d\Phi/dn \tag{2.20}$$

The vector field $\vec{G}$ as defined in (2.17) is called the gradient of a scalar field Φ; if the scalar function is the electric potential, it is called the gradient of the potential.

In summary, a (nonzero) gradient of the potential is a vector field oriented normal to an equipotential surface. It always points towards a region having higher potential values. Its magnitude quantifies the maximum local change in the potential per unit distance.

The gradient of the potential is usually written as $\nabla\Phi$, where

$$\nabla = \vec{e}_x\frac{\partial}{\partial x} + \vec{e}_y\frac{\partial}{\partial y} + \vec{e}_z\frac{\partial}{\partial z} \tag{2.21}$$

is the gradient operator. When applied, each term in (2.21) acts on Φ through the taking of the indicated partial derivatives and appending the corresponding unit vector. It can immediately be verified that this leads, correctly, to the right-hand side of (2.17).

2.2.7   Divergence

A basic vector field required for the analysis of electrophysiology is the electric current density $\vec{J}$ in a volume conductor: the electric current per unit area passing an infinitesimally small area. The structure of the $\vec{J}$ field depends on the presence of sites at which current is either introduced (sources) or withdrawn (sinks). In this respect, the behavior of $\vec{J}(x, y, z)$ is analogous to the vector field that describes fluid flow, which similarly arises from a distribution of sources and sinks. This class of vector field has certain general properties that are exemplified by the current flow field. In the following, the term "sources" is used to include "sinks" (which are, simply, negative sources). It will be shown that a determination of the sources of a field permits that field to be determined everywhere (although, frequently, certain boundary conditions must also be taken into account). For an arbitrary source distribution, $\vec{J}$ will be a complex but well-behaved vector function of position. In particular, for a region that contains no sources, since charge must be conserved the net flow of $\vec{J}$ across the surface bounding any segment of tissue (for example, with inflow taken to be negative while outflow is positive) is required to be zero. This condition is also said to preserve continuity of current. The evaluation of the net flow across a closed surface can then be taken as a measure of the net source (or sink) within the region enclosed by that surface.

For a differential rectangular parallelepiped, an expression that evaluates the net outflow is derived as follows, expressed in rectangular coordinates. Referring to ❷ Fig. 2.5 and assuming a field $\vec{J}(x, y, z)$, the outflow through surface (2) is then $dz\, dy\, (J_x + \frac{1}{2}(\partial J_x/\partial x)\, dx)$+ higher terms, where J_x is the value of $J_x(x, y, z)$ at the center of the parallelepiped (which accounts for the factor of $\frac{1}{2}$ in the expression). For the surface (1), the outflow is $-dz\, dy\, (J_x - \frac{1}{2}(\partial J_x/\partial x)\, dx)-$ dzdy, where the leading minus sign arises because outflow is in the negative x direction. The sum of these contributions is then $dx\, dy\, dz\, \partial J_x/\partial x$. In the same way, the remaining two pairs of faces contribute $dx\, dy\, dz\, \partial J_y/\partial y$ and $dx\, dy\, dz\, \partial J_z/\partial z$. Consequently, their sum is

$$\oint \vec{J} \bullet d\vec{S} = (\partial J_x/\partial x + \partial J_y/\partial y + \partial J_z/\partial z)\, dx\, dy\, dz \qquad (2.22)$$

Note that $\vec{J} \bullet d\vec{S}$ is the outflow of $\vec{J}$ across an arbitrary surface element and that the sign $\oint$ indicates that the integral is over a closed surface. In this case, the differential rectangular parallelepiped described in ❷ Fig. 2.5 is the designated closed surface, which is evaluated in the right-hand side of (2.22).

If both sides of (2.22) are divided by $(dx\, dy\, dz)$, then the ratio $\oint \vec{J} \bullet d\vec{S}/(dx\, dy\, dz)$ is called the divergence of $\vec{J}$. Note that this is evaluated in the limit that the volume $(dx\, dy\, dz)$ approaches zero (the divergence is a differential quantity).

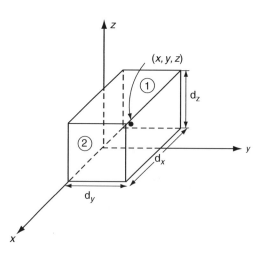

❏ **Fig. 2.5**
Evaluation of divergence

This limit is designated by

$$\mathrm{div}\vec{J} = \lim_{V \to 0} \frac{\oint \vec{J} \bullet \mathrm{d}\vec{S}}{V} = \frac{\partial J_x}{\partial x} + \frac{\partial J_y}{\partial y} + \frac{\partial J_z}{\partial z} \qquad (2.23)$$

This indicates that the divergence of a vector (field) is a scalar (field).

The divergence of $\vec{J}$ equals the net outflow per unit volume of the vector $\vec{J}$ at each point in the space. The definition of the divergence applies to any vector field. The field can be interpreted as a flow and its divergence as a source of the flow field. If the ∇ operator, defined in (2.21), is treated as having vector-like properties, then in view of (2.23) and the properties of the dot product given in (2.11), it follows that

$$\nabla \bullet \vec{J} = \mathrm{div}\vec{J} = \frac{\partial J_x}{\partial x} + \frac{\partial J_y}{\partial y} + \frac{\partial J_z}{\partial z} \qquad (2.24)$$

2.2.8 Gauss' Law

In the previous section, it was pointed out that the net outflow of current from a given volume is a quantity of interest since it is a measure of the net source contained in the volume. For a volume V bounded by a closed surface S, the outflow is given by

$$\mathrm{outflow} = \oint \vec{J} \bullet \mathrm{d}\vec{S}, \qquad (2.25)$$

where $\mathrm{d}\vec{S}$ is a surface element whose direction is along the outward normal. It has just been established that $\nabla \bullet \vec{J}$ evaluates the net outflow per unit volume for an infinitesimally small volume element, so the outflow evaluated in (2.25) can also be found by integrating $\nabla \bullet \vec{J}$ through the volume bounded by S. In fact,

$$\int \nabla \bullet \vec{J} \mathrm{d}V = \oint \vec{J} \bullet \mathrm{d}\vec{S} \qquad (2.26)$$

This relationship holds true for all well-behaved vector fields, such as $\vec{J}$, and is known as Gauss' theorem, or the *divergence theorem*. If the region is source-free, then the net flow across the bounding surface is zero as a consequence. Conversely, if there is a net outflow then within the surface there must be sources with net magnitude equal to the (net) outflow. For a single current dipole (❿ Sect. 2.5.1.2) inside a closed surface, the total current flow passing the surface is zero.

2.2.9 Laplacian

In ❿ Sect. 2.2.6, it has been shown that the gradient operation converts a given scalar field Φ into a vector field $\nabla\Phi$. The divergence operation, on the other hand, converts a vector field into a scalar field. If the vector field is itself the gradient of a scalar function, the result can be expressed through the successive application of the ∇ operator, namely

$$\nabla \bullet \nabla\Phi = \nabla \bullet \left(\vec{e}_x \frac{\partial \Phi}{\partial x} + \vec{e}_y \frac{\partial \Phi}{\partial y} + \vec{e}_z \frac{\partial \Phi}{\partial z} \right)$$
$$= \frac{\partial^2 \Phi}{\partial x^2} + \frac{\partial^2 \Phi}{\partial y^2} + \frac{\partial^2 \Phi}{\partial z^2} \qquad (2.27)$$

The final result can be interpreted as if the original scalar field is operated on by the differential operator:

$$\nabla^2 = \frac{\partial^2}{\partial x^2} + \frac{\partial^2}{\partial y^2} + \frac{\partial^2}{\partial z^2} \qquad (2.28)$$

The operator ∇^2 is called the Laplacian. It converts a scalar potential field into another scalar field (the latter specifying the sources for the first). The properties of the Laplacian are discussed later in this chapter.

2.2.10   Vector Identities

In this section, a short list is presented on the relationships that are known as vector identities. These hold true for all "well-behaved" scalar and vector functions treated in this chapter, with "well-behaved" expressing the fact that taking the various derivatives can be formally justified. Here, and in other chapters, these vector identities will prove useful in deriving biophysical relationships. A proof is included for the first expression; the reader may use this as a model for confirming the others. In the following, Φ and Ψ are taken to be scalar functions, $r = (x^2 + y^2 + z^2)^{1/2}$ and $\vec{A}$ is a vector field.

$$\nabla \bullet (\Phi \vec{A}) = \vec{A} \bullet \nabla \Phi + \Phi \nabla \bullet \vec{A} \tag{2.29}$$

$$\nabla(\Phi \Psi) = \Phi \nabla \Psi + \Psi \nabla \Phi \tag{2.30}$$

$$\nabla \bullet \nabla \Psi = \nabla^2 \Psi = \frac{\partial^2 \Psi}{\partial x^2} + \frac{\partial^2 \Psi}{\partial y^2} + \frac{\partial^2 \Psi}{\partial z^2} \tag{2.31}$$

$$\nabla^2 r = 0 \tag{2.32}$$

For $\vec{R} = (x' - x)\,\vec{e}_x + (y' - y)\,\vec{e}_y + (z' - z)\,\vec{e}_z$, with length $R = \{(x' - x)^2 + (y' - y)^2 + (z' - z)^2\}^{1/2}$, we have

$$\nabla(1/R) = \vec{R}/R^3 = -\nabla'(1/R), \tag{2.33}$$

in which ∇' denotes the differentiation with respect to the primed variables.

    To verify (2.29), replace $\vec{A}$ by its rectangular components $(A_x \vec{e}_x + A_y \vec{e}_y + A_z \vec{e}_z)$ leading to

$$\nabla \bullet (\Phi \vec{A}) = \nabla \bullet (\Phi A_x \vec{e}_x + \Phi A_y \vec{e}_y + \Phi A_z \vec{e}_z) \tag{2.34}$$

Using the definition of the divergence given in (2.24) results in

$$\nabla \bullet (\Phi \vec{A}) = \frac{\partial}{\partial x}(\Phi A_x) + \frac{\partial}{\partial y}(\Phi A_y) + \frac{\partial}{\partial z}(\Phi A_z) \tag{2.35}$$

By the product rule of differentiation, it follows that

$$\nabla \bullet (\Phi \vec{A}) = \Phi \frac{\partial A_x}{\partial x} + A_x \frac{\partial \Phi}{\partial x} + \Phi \frac{\partial A_y}{\partial y} + A_y \frac{\partial \Phi}{\partial y} + \Phi \frac{\partial A_z}{\partial z} + A_z \frac{\partial \Phi}{\partial z} \tag{2.36}$$

Collecting terms gives

$$\nabla \bullet (\Phi \vec{A}) = \Phi \left(\frac{\partial A_x}{\partial x} + \frac{\partial A_y}{\partial y} + \frac{\partial A_z}{\partial z} \right) + A_x \frac{\partial \Phi}{\partial x} + A_y \frac{\partial \Phi}{\partial y} + A_z \frac{\partial \Phi}{\partial z} \tag{2.37}$$

In addition,

$$\vec{A} \bullet \nabla \Phi = \vec{A} \bullet \left(\frac{\partial \Phi}{\partial x} \vec{e}_x + \frac{\partial \Phi}{\partial y} \vec{e}_y + \frac{\partial \Phi}{\partial z} \vec{e}_z \right)$$

$$= A_x \frac{\partial \Phi}{\partial x} + A_y \frac{\partial \Phi}{\partial y} + A_z \frac{\partial \Phi}{\partial z} \tag{2.38}$$

so that substituting (2.38) and (2.24) into (2.37) leads to

$$\nabla \bullet (\Phi \vec{A}) = \vec{A} \bullet \nabla \Phi + \Phi \nabla \bullet \vec{A}, \tag{2.39}$$

which confirms (2.29).

2.2.11   Coordinate Systems

Up to this point, vector fields and vector operations have been expressed in rectangular coordinates, and these are, indeed, the easiest to use as well as being the most frequently used. Often, however, cylindrical or spherical (or other) coordinates are more appropriate. The differential operators of gradient, divergence and Laplacian can be expressed in any of the orthogonal coordinate systems and it is useful to have such expressions available. Their derivation follows their basic definition, taking the coordinate system into account. For example, in ❷ Fig. 2.6(a) the cylindrical coordinate system is illustrated. In this system, an arbitrary point is described by a distance r to the z-axis, an azimuth angle ϕ from the x axis and a distance z along z-axis. ❷ Figure 2.6(b) illustrates the spherical coordinate system. According to the definition and property of $\nabla\Phi$, it is a vector whose component in any direction is the directional derivative of Φ in that direction. Consequently

$$\nabla\Phi = \vec{e}_r \frac{\partial\Phi}{\partial r} + \vec{e}_\phi \frac{\partial\Phi}{\partial\phi} + \vec{e}_z \frac{\partial\Phi}{\partial z} \tag{2.40}$$

Note that in (2.40) the rate of change of Φ per unit length in the ϕ direction requires the limit of $\Delta\Phi/(r\Delta\phi)$ where the denominator is the appropriate element of length and Δ denotes taking of a small difference. The spherical coordinate system is illustrated in ❷ Fig. 2.6(b) where r is the radial distance from the origin, θ is the polar angle and ϕ is the azimuth angle. For this system, the gradient is expressed as

$$\nabla\Phi = \vec{e}_r \frac{\partial\Phi}{\partial r} + \vec{e}_\theta \frac{1}{r}\frac{\partial\Phi}{\partial\theta} + \vec{e}_z \frac{1}{r\sin\phi}\frac{\partial\Phi}{\partial\phi} \tag{2.41}$$

The expressions for the divergence and Laplacian in cylindrical and spherical coordinates are listed below. The reader can verify these using the basic definitions, or by recourse to one of the standard references listed at the end of this chapter.

2.2.11.1   Divergence and Laplacian in Cylindrical Coordinates

$$\nabla \bullet \vec{A} = \frac{1}{r}\frac{\partial}{\partial r}(rA_r) + \frac{1}{r}\frac{\partial A_\phi}{\partial\phi} + \frac{\partial A_z}{\partial z} \tag{2.42}$$

$$\nabla^2\Phi = \frac{1}{r}\frac{\partial}{\partial r}\left(r\frac{\partial\Phi}{\partial r}\right) + \frac{\partial^2\Phi}{\partial\phi^2} + \frac{\partial^2\Phi}{\partial z^2} \tag{2.43}$$

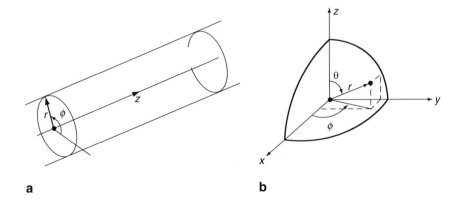

a   b

❏ Fig. 2.6

Coordinate systems: (a) circular cylindrical; (b) spherical

2.2.11.2   Divergence and Laplacian in Spherical Coordinates

$$\nabla \bullet \vec{A} = \frac{1}{r^2} \frac{\partial}{\partial r}(r^2 A_r) + \frac{1}{r \sin \theta} \frac{\partial}{\partial \theta}(A_\theta \sin \theta) + \frac{1}{r \sin \theta} \frac{\partial A_\phi}{\partial \phi} \tag{2.44}$$

$$\nabla^2 \Phi = \frac{1}{r^2} \frac{\partial}{\partial r}\left(r^2 \frac{\partial \Phi}{\partial r}\right) + \frac{1}{r^2 \sin \theta} \frac{\partial \Phi}{\partial \theta}\left(\sin \theta \frac{\partial \Phi}{\partial \theta}\right) + \frac{1}{r^2 \sin^2 \theta} \frac{\partial^2 \Phi}{\partial \phi^2} \tag{2.45}$$

2.2.12   Solid Angle: Definition and Theory

Solid angle is an extension to 3D space of the familiar concept of a 'common' angle in 2D space. For an object in 2D space, the angle of view from some location is defined as the fraction of the circumference of a circle with unit radius, centered at the location of the observer, occupied by the intersections with the circle of the lines connecting all the elements of the object to the center of the circle. In 3D, the analogous definition relates to the similar projection of the object onto the surface of a sphere with unit radius. Being a fraction, the solid angle is unitless. However, to stress its special nature, the solid angle is frequently expressed in the 'unit' star-radian. Observed from an arbitrary point inside a closed surface, this definition results in a total solid angle 4π, as is explained below.

In many of the applications of volume conduction theory, the surface S carries a double layer, which requires assigning a direction to its surface normal. In the sequel, for a closed surface this direction is always taken to be (positive) towards the exterior region: the outward normal.

Consider an observation point $\vec{X}'$ in three-dimensional space in which an arbitrary surface S is situated. Let $d\omega$ be the projection of a small element dS on the surface of a sphere having a unit radius (❷ Fig. 2.7).

Then, the solid angle subtended by dS at $\vec{X}'$ is defined as $d\omega$. The solid angle Ω subtended at $\vec{X}'$ by the entire surface S is found by the addition of all projections $d\omega$ of all elements dS. Mathematically this is expressed as

$$\Omega(S) = \int_S d\omega = \int_S \frac{\cos \alpha \, dS}{R^2}, \tag{2.46}$$

in which R is the length of the vector $\vec{R}$ pointing from surface element dS to observation point $\vec{X}'$, and α the angle between the local surface normal $d\vec{S}$ and $\vec{R}$. If the surface S is decomposed into a set of non-overlapping segments, S1, S2, S3, ... The linearity of integration shows that we have

$$\Omega(S) = \Omega(S_1 \cup S_2 \cup S_3 \cdots) = \Omega(S_1) + \Omega(S_2) + \Omega(S_3) + \cdots \tag{2.47}$$

By defining $d\vec{S}$ as the vector of size dS that is oriented along the outward normal of dS and by using the property of the dot product $\vec{R} \bullet d\vec{S} = R \, dS \cos \alpha$, Eqn. (2.46) can be written as

$$\Omega(S) = \int_S d\omega = \int_S \frac{\vec{R} \bullet d\vec{S}}{R^3} \tag{2.48}$$

The sign of Ω depends on the definition of the direction of both $\vec{R}$ and $d\vec{S}$. Note that the term 'outward' normal relates in a natural manner to closed surfaces only. For a non-closed surface it needs to be defined on the basis of the application involved.

For an observation point $\vec{X}'$ placed at the center of a spherical surface S, the solid angle subtended by S at the $\vec{X}'$ is -4π; its magnitude is equal to the surface area of a unit sphere, the negative sign follows from the definition of the directions of $\vec{R}$ and $d\vec{S}$.

For any arbitrary internal point of non-intersecting closed S, the value of Ω is independent of the actual shape the surface and, moreover, also holds true irrespective of the position of the interior observation point. This most fundamental property can be appreciated by inspecting ❷ Fig. 2.8. In the left panel, a cross section of a closed three-dimensional surface

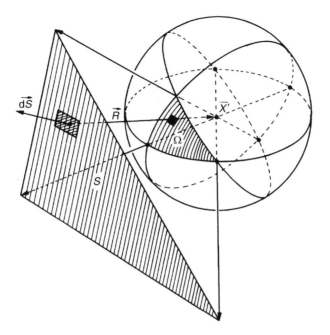

Fig. 2.7
Diagram introducing the solid angle Ω. The outline of a small element dS of an arbitrary surface S is projected on the surface of a sphere with unit radius. The solid angle $d\omega$ subtended by dS at observation point $\vec{X}'$, the center of the sphere, is defined as the area of the projection of dS onto the sphere. The solid angle Ω of S is the sum of the projections $d\omega$ of all elements dS. The surface S may have an arbitrary shape, it is drawn here as triangle for ease of presentation

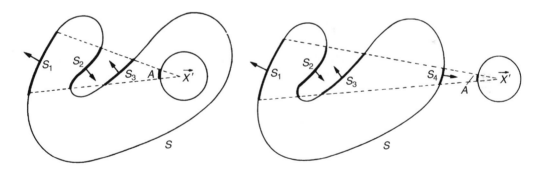

☐ **Fig. 2.8**
Cross-sections of a 3D closed surface S. Observer at $\vec{X}'$. *Left.* Apart from their sign, the solid angles subtended by S_1, S_2, and S_3 are equal to A, the part of a unit sphere around $\vec{X}'$; their sum equals $-A$. *Right*: the situation for an external observation point. Part A of a unit sphere around $\vec{X}'$ has, apart from its sign, the same solid angle as the individual segments S_1, S_2, S_3, and S_4. The sum of the solid angles is zero as a result of the paired sign differences

S is shown in which three segments S_1, S_2 and S_3 are indicated. The observation point lies inside and a unit circle is drawn around it. The area A of the unit sphere represents the solid angle of the segments. Since $\Omega(S_1) = -\Omega(S_2) = \Omega(S_3) = -A$, it follows, by using (2.47), that $\Omega(S_1 \cup S_2 \cup S_3) = \Omega(S_1) + \Omega(S_2) + \Omega(S_3) = -A$. By applying the same type of analysis to the intersections of all possible sectors of the unit sphere with S, it is evident that indeed, for any arbitrary location of an internal point

$$\Omega(S) = -\text{total area of the (unit) sphere} = -4\pi \qquad (2.49)$$

When $\vec{X}'$ is an exterior point of S, we find, by the same type of reasoning (right panel), that

$$\Omega(S) = 0 \tag{2.50}$$

When $\vec{X}'$ lies *on* surface S, the definition of Ω by means of expression cannot be used since $\vec{R}$ = zero. In that situation, $\vec{X}'$ may be taken as having approached S from either the interior or the exterior. Taking this limit from the inside for a locally planar part of the surface, we have

$$\Omega(S) = -2\pi \tag{2.51}$$

An approach from the outside results in

$$\Omega(S) = +2\pi \tag{2.52}$$

For an arbitrarily shaped part of the surface, the limit depends on the local curvature. Whatever the value of the local curvature, the value of the solid angle jumps by a value of 4π when crossing the surface. The sign of the jump is positive if the surface is crossed towards its exterior.

2.3   Static Electric Fields

Electrical activation and recovery of cardiac muscle gives rise to the flow of electric current in the heart and out into the torso. Associated with these currents is the establishment of electrocardiographic potentials within the torso and at the body surface. While the current and potential fields vary with time, at each instant of time they satisfy mathematical expressions which arise in the study of static fields. Accordingly, this section reviews the physical principles associated with the establishment of static electric fields as well as their mathematical description.

2.3.1   Coulomb's Law

Coulomb's famous experiments led to a quantitative description of the force between two point charges. It was established that this force is directed along a line connecting the two point charges (the force is attractive if the charges are of opposite sign and repulsive if the charges are of the same sign) while the force magnitude is proportional to the product of the charge magnitudes and inversely proportional to the square of the distance separating the charges. This description is expressed in the following equation for the force $\vec{F}_{12}$ exerted on charge q_2 by charge q_1, namely,

$$\vec{F}_{12} = \frac{q_1 q_2}{4\pi \varepsilon r_{12}^2} \vec{e}_{12}, \tag{2.53}$$

where e_{12} is a unit vector directed from 1 to 2, r_{12} is the distance between point charges, and ε is the dielectric permittivity of the medium (assumed to be uniform and essentially infinite in extent). Note that the direction and magnitude of the interactive force evaluated by (2.53) correspond to the word description given above. In (2.53), if q_1 and q_2 are expressed in coulombs, r_{12} in meters and ε in farads per meter, then $\vec{F}$ is in newtons. For free space (vacuum), the permittivity $\varepsilon = 8.8542 \cdot 10^{-12}$ Fm^{-1}. Note that $\vec{F}_{12} = -\vec{F}_{21}$ so that "action" is equal and opposite to the "reaction", as required by Newton's laws of mechanics.

❯ Figure 2.9 shows an arrangement of charges for which the force on charge q_o, owing to the presence of several point charges q_1, q_2 and q_3, is to be evaluated. This can be accomplished by the successive application of Coulomb's law (between q_1 and q_o, q_2, and q_o, q_3 and q_o) leading to the component forces $\vec{F}_1$, $\vec{F}_2$ and $\vec{F}_3$, respectively. These are illustrated in ❯ Fig. 2.9 where all the charges are assumed to be of the same sign. The net force exerted on q_o is the vector sum (superposition) of $\vec{F}_1 + \vec{F}_2 + \vec{F}_3 = \vec{F}$. In fact, for any system of point charges, the force exerted on any one of these (designated as q_o) is

$$\vec{F} = \frac{q_o}{4\pi\varepsilon} \sum_i \frac{q_i \vec{e}_{io}}{r_{i0}^2}, \tag{2.54}$$

where r_{i0} is the displacement from the ith charge to the 0th charge.

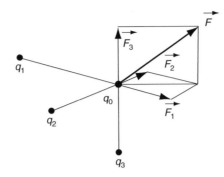

■ Fig. 2.9
Vector sum of electrostatic force components

2.3.2   Electric Field

Force exerted on one charge by another does so across the intervening space, a phenomenon known as "action at a distance". The force can also be viewed as arising from a two-step process whereby one charge is first assumed to establish an electric field, the field then transmits a force to the other charge. For two point charges q_1 and q_2, the first step introduces the concept of the electric field $\vec{E}$ arising from q_1, defined by

$$\vec{E}(r) = \frac{q_1}{4\pi\varepsilon r^2}\vec{e}_r, \tag{2.55}$$

where r is the radial distance from q_1 and $\vec{e}_r$ is the unit vector directed radially away from q_1. Next, the force exerted on the point charge q_2 by this field is given by

$$\vec{F}(r_2) = q\vec{E}(r_2), \tag{2.56}$$

where r_2 is the radial distance to q_2 from q_1. The force on q_2 because of q_1 found by combining (2.55) and (2.56) is precisely that as stated by Coulomb's law and expressed by (2.53).

A more rigorous definition of the electric field, accounting for required point charge nature of charge, with vanishingly small strength, is

$$\vec{E} = \lim_{\Delta q \to 0} (\vec{F}/\Delta q) \tag{2.57}$$

The advantage of the field concept is that it separates the process in which fields are established (by their sources, such as q_1 in (2.55)) from the actions produced by the field (i.e., the force exerted on q_2 in (2.56)). If a number of point charges are present, as in ❷ Fig. 2.9, the electric field at any point in space can be found by superposition, taking into account the contribution from each individual point source and summing vectorially. The net force on a point charge is found from the action of the net field according to (2.56). Where there is a very large number of point charges in a certain region, it is convenient to describe their distribution by means of a charge density function $\rho(x, y, z)$, where

$$\rho = \lim_{\Delta v \to 0} (\Delta q/\Delta v) \tag{2.58}$$

and Δq is the net charge in the volume Δv. The charge density is a function of position. The total charge Q in a volume v is found from (2.58) by integrating through the volume:

$$Q = \int \rho dv \tag{2.59}$$

Since ρdv is an element of charge that is essentially a point source, its electric field $d\vec{E}$ would be given by (2.55), namely

$$d\vec{E} = \frac{\rho dv}{4\pi\varepsilon r^2}\vec{e}_r \tag{2.60}$$

The electric field established by the entire distribution is given by

$$\vec{E}(x',y',z') = \frac{1}{4\pi\varepsilon} \int \frac{\rho(x,y,z)}{r^2}\vec{e}_r dv, \tag{2.61}$$

where r is the length of the vector $\vec{r}$ from an element of charge located at (x, y, z) to the point at which the field is being evaluated: $r = \{(x' - x)^2 + (y' - y)^2 + (z' - z)^2\}^{1/2}$.

Note that the integration in (2.61) is over the unprimed coordinates ($dv = dxdydz$), these being the coordinates in which the source (charge density) is defined. The field point location, given by the primed coordinates, is assumed to be fixed during the integration. In actually performing the integration indicated in (2.61), it must be kept in mind that $\vec{e}_r$ varies according to the location of the source (integration) point and that a vector summation must actually be performed.

2.3.3   Gauss' Flux Theorem

The electric field from a point charge q is given by (2.55). Although $\vec{E}$ does not represent the flow of any substance, it can be treated as if it did; that is, it may be interpreted as an electric flux (flow) density. Then the net flow through an arbitrary, closed surface S surrounding a point charge q can be found from

$$\oint \vec{E} \bullet d\vec{S} = \frac{q}{4\pi\varepsilon} \oint \frac{\vec{e}_r \bullet d\vec{S}}{r^2}, \tag{2.62}$$

with $\vec{e}_r$ a unit vector directed along the vector from the point charge to a point on the surface S. The integrand in (2.62), corresponds to the elementary solid angle $d\omega$ (❷ Sect. 2.2.12) subtended by the elementary surface element dS as observed from the source location:

$$\frac{\vec{e}_r \bullet d\vec{S}}{r^2} = \frac{\vec{r} \bullet d\vec{S}}{r^3} = d\omega \tag{2.63}$$

Consequently,

$$\oint \vec{E} \bullet d\vec{S} = \frac{q}{4\pi\varepsilon} \oint d\omega = \frac{q}{\varepsilon} \tag{2.64}$$

since the total solid angle of any closed surface as viewed from an interior point is 4π. Hence, the total flux emanating from q depends on the magnitude of q. If a number of point charges q_i were enclosed within S, then by superposition the right-hand side of (2.64) becomes, simply, the total charge divided by ε. Thus,

$$\oint \vec{E} \bullet d\vec{S} = \frac{1}{\varepsilon} \sum_i q_i = \frac{Q}{\varepsilon} \tag{2.65}$$

In a similar fashion, if the sources within S were represented by a charge density ρ, then

$$\oint \vec{E} \bullet d\vec{S} = \frac{1}{\varepsilon} \int \rho dv = \int \frac{\rho}{\varepsilon} dv \tag{2.66}$$

Note that since ε is independent of position, it could be moved about freely from across integration or summation signs.

We now combine Gauss' flux theorem ((2.26)) with (2.66), yielding

$$\oint \vec{E} \bullet d\vec{S} = \int \nabla \bullet \vec{E} dv = \int \frac{\rho}{\varepsilon} dv \tag{2.67}$$

which applies to arbitrarily small volume elements and consequently we have

$$\nabla \bullet \vec{E} = \frac{\rho}{\varepsilon} \tag{2.68}$$

2.3.4 Electric Scalar Potential

Equation (2.68) shows that the divergence of the electric field $\vec{E}$ is a scalar function. For all vector fields having this property, it can be shown that they, in turn, are determined uniquely by the negative gradient of another scalar function [1]. In electrostatics, this function is called the electric potential, denoted by Φ, and

$$\vec{E} = -\nabla'\Phi \qquad (2.69)$$

Note that (2.69) defines the electric potential up to a constant only.

The potential difference between two points in space is the work required for moving a unit positive charge from any position A to another position B along a path $\vec{\ell}$ connecting these locations. The work required follows from the line integral along the path:

$$V_{BA} \doteq \Phi_B - \Phi_A = -\int_A^B \vec{E}(\vec{\ell}) \bullet d\vec{\ell} = -\int_A^B \nabla\Phi(\vec{\ell}) \bullet d\vec{\ell}$$

If the work required is positive, the potential at B is higher than in A.

The potential function may thus be found by integration of the scalar function $-\nabla \bullet \vec{E}$. Under static conditions, the outcome of the integration is independent of the path taken.

The property described by (2.69) is demonstrated here in the application to the electric field of a point charge as specified by (2.55). On the basis of the definition of the gradient expressed in spherical coordinates ((2.41)), (2.55) can be written as

$$\vec{E} = \frac{q}{4\pi\varepsilon r^2} = -\nabla'\left(\frac{q}{4\pi\varepsilon r}\right), \qquad (2.70)$$

where ∇' operates at the field point. By using (2.33), (2.70) can also be written as

$$\vec{E} = \nabla\left(\frac{q}{4\pi\varepsilon r}\right) \qquad (2.71)$$

Hence, it is necessary to be particularly careful when designating coordinates.

Examination of (2.70) shows that the electric field $\vec{E}$ is equal to the negative gradient of the scalar function $\Phi = \frac{q}{4\pi\varepsilon r}$. For a collection of point charges, the potential function Φ can be obtained by superposition (in this case, a simple scalar addition) so that

$$\Phi = \frac{1}{4\pi\varepsilon}\sum_i \frac{q_i}{r_i} + c, \qquad (2.72)$$

where r_i is the distance from q_i to the field point and c is an arbitrary constant.

A further generalization considers the potential field from a volume charge density ρ. Since ρdv behaves like a point source, it sets up a field according to (2.72). The entire distribution can be taken into account by superposition (summation) leading to

$$\Phi = \frac{1}{4\pi\varepsilon}\int \frac{\rho}{r}dv + c, \qquad (2.73)$$

which shows the potential to be a weighted volume integral of the (scalar) charge density, the weighting function being $1/r$. The electric field can be found from (2.71) by the gradient operation indicated in (2.69). Note that the field is independent of the choice of the constant c, the value of which is therefore completely arbitrary. This determination of the electric field from multiple sources may be easier to carry out than that indicated in (2.61), which requires vector summation.

Combining (2.68) and (2.69), while dropping the prime, gives

$$\nabla^2\Phi = -\rho/\varepsilon, \qquad (2.74)$$

which is known as Poisson's equation. Dropping the prime is permitted here, in view of the fact that the Laplacian of $1/r$ turns out to be the same for primed and unprimed coordinates (❯ Sect. 2.6.4.1).

Equation (2.73) is an integral form of solution to the partial differential (2.74) as can be verified by direct substitution of (2.74) in (2.73).

2.3.5 Capacitance

Consider two insulated conducting bodies of arbitrary shape. If a voltage V is connected between the two for a period of time, a quantity of charge Q will be transferred from one to the other. The charge will distribute itself on each conducting body in such a way as to result in the electric field tangential to the conductor being reduced to zero (a nonzero tangential field would cause movement and further redistribution of charge). The potential between the two conducting bodies can be found from the steady-state charge distribution by applying (2.72) at each body. If the total charge is doubled, then each charge element ρdv must also double since the system is linear. Consequently, the difference of potential V is proportional to the total charge Q on either body. The constant of proportionality is the capacitance C. That is:

$$C = Q/V, \tag{2.75}$$

where Q is in coulombs, V in volts and C in farads. A conducting pair that holds a greater amount of charge for the same applied voltage will have a higher capacitance.

If the two conducting bodies are parallel, rectangular, conducting plates of area A and separation d (where $d \ll \sqrt{A}$), then the field between the plates will be uniform and

$$V = Ed \tag{2.76}$$

In view of (2.66) and the fact that the field lies solely between the two plates, $EA = Q/\varepsilon$. Consequently,

$$V = \frac{Qd}{\varepsilon A} \tag{2.77}$$

and

$$C = \frac{\varepsilon A}{d} \tag{2.78}$$

This result is strictly correct only for $d \ll \sqrt{A}$, which is a condition for minimum fringing of the field (that is, for a predominantly uniform field). If the medium between the plates is anything other than vacuum, the dielectric permittivity $\varepsilon = \varepsilon_r \varepsilon_0$ is effective where ε_r is the relative permittivity (a dimensionless factor scaling $\varepsilon = \varepsilon_0$ as defined previously (approx. $(1/36\pi)10^{-9}\,\mathrm{F\,m^{-1}}$)).

For biological membranes, which have a high lipid content, $\varepsilon_r = 3$ and $d \cong 3$ nm which is roughly the lipid-layer thickness. The capacitance is then calculated as $0.9\,\mu\mathrm{F\,cm^{-2}}$, a value which is usually measured for nerve tissue and is also applied as the value for the membranes of cardiac myocytes.

2.4 Electric Current Flow in Conductive Media

In the previous section, static electric fields arising from electric charges, where the medium is insulating, were considered. The only property of the medium involved was the specification of the dielectric permittivity ε. Any possible flow of electric current inside the medium was ruled out. While electric fields of cardiac origin also behave (instant by instant) as a static field, such fields generally lie in conducting media. As a consequence, associated with that field is a stationary (steady) current. In a dielectric, no energy is required to maintain a charge configuration and its associated (steady) electric field, but in a conducting body any initial arrangement of charges would quickly dissipate as a result of current flow; the maintenance of a source distribution (and associated electric and current flow field) in a conducting medium requires the continual renewal of such sources. Such steady sources (and associated steady currents) can arise in the presence of physical (electrochemical) batteries. Action currents arising from cellular action potentials (such as those that occur in cardiac muscle) are also based on an electrochemical process. Each cardiac cell, while undergoing activation, can be thought of as an electrochemical cell (battery) and (in effect) a steady current is generated by the (biological) cell. The energy required to maintain the current flow comes, ultimately, from the metabolic processes within the cell.

2.4.1 Ohm's Law of Conductivity

A medium is described as conducting if charged particles are present which are free to move. Electrocardiographic preparations comprise biological tissues (volume conductors) which contain electrolytes. Consequently, they are conducting; their conductivity being caused by the presence of positive and negative ions which can move more or less freely. If an electric field is established in such a medium, each charged particle will experience a force (according to (2.56)) and a flow of charge (i.e., a current) results. The magnitude of current is limited by collisions between the charge carriers and the remaining medium. In fact, if λ is the mean free path (mean distance between collisions), then the time-average drift velocity (for particles with a single electronic charge) is

$$\vec{v} = \frac{q_e \lambda \vec{E}}{2mv_0} = u\vec{E}, \tag{2.79}$$

where $\vec{E}$ is the electric field, q_e is the electronic charge, m is the particle mass, v_0 the average thermal velocity (note that $v \ll v_0$) and u is the mobility. The mobility, mass and mean free path in (2.79) are, of course, specific to the ion species being considered. If the ion concentration is C particles per cubic meter, then the electric current density equals $Cq_e v$ or

$$\vec{J} = \frac{Cq_e^2 \lambda}{2mv_0} \vec{E} \tag{2.80}$$

This expression reflects the convention that positive current is associated with the flow of positive charge.

For an electrolyte, the total current will arise from the movement of several ions, each of which contributes a component given by (2.80). The relative contribution of component ion species to the total current is described by their respective transference numbers. For example, if sodium, potassium and chloride ions constitute the charge carriers and if J is the total current density then

$$J_K = t_K J; \quad J_{Cl} = t_{Cl} J; \quad J_{Na} = t_{Na} J, \tag{2.81}$$

where

$$J = J_K + J_{Cl} + J_{Na} \tag{2.82}$$

The transference numbers t_K, t_{Cl} and t_{Na} for potassium, chloride and sodium depend on their relative ionic concentration and mobility since, for example, using (2.79),

$$J_K = C_K q_e v_K = C_K q_e u_K E \tag{2.83}$$

The linear relationship between $\vec{J}$ and $\vec{E}$, expressed in (2.80), has been verified experimentally under a broad variety of conditions. The coefficient linking these two variables is the electrical conductivity σ, defined through

$$\vec{J} = \sigma \vec{E} \tag{2.84}$$

linking $\vec{E}$, the electric field (V m^{-1}) and $\vec{J}$, the current density (A m^2). As a consequence, the conductivity σ has a dimension (S m^{-1}). Introduced in the way shown above, the conductivity is a scalar constant, a tissue-specific parameter that can be related to molecular quantities through (2.80) or obtained experimentally by the application of (2.84). For some types of tissues, the conductivity has been shown to depend on fiber orientation, which is expressed by calling it *anisotropic*, which demands its specification by means of a tensor.

Equation (2.84) is a differential form of Ohm's law; under dc conditions, it relates to a conduction current arising from the presence of the electric field $\vec{E}$ as a driving force. Under conditions of alternating currents, (2.84) can be generalized if $\vec{J}$ and $\vec{E}$ are interpreted as complex phasors, in which case σ will also, in general, be a complex phasor reflecting reactive properties of the medium. Experimental results, which show that under electrocardiographic conditions σ is essentially real, are described later in this chapter.

2.4.2   Tissue Impedance

An important goal in the biophysical study of electrocardiography is a determination of the currents which flow in the torso owing to the presence of cardiac generators. To accomplish this, it is necessary to describe the electrical conductivity of all torso tissues (along with their geometry). Historically, the following tissues have been thought important enough to require specific inclusion in a rigorous treatment of electrocardiographic current flow: heart muscle, intracavitary blood, lungs, surface fat, surface muscle and the pericardium.

The classical approach to the determination of the conductivity of a material is to incorporate a uniform sample of known size in an electric circuit. A known or measured current is then applied and the resulting voltage is measured. If the voltage is measured at the points at which the current is introduced, the method is called the two-electrode method; if separate voltage lead-off points are used, the method is called the four-electrode method. Since the dimensions of the current-carrying preparation is known, the values of current and voltage are sufficient to determine the conductivity. The four-electrode method, since it avoids electrode interface artifact, is the preferred technique; examples are found in references [2] and [3].

Most biological tissues are not strictly homogeneous, but can be satisfactorily treated as such to a good approximation. The value of conductivity obtained using a typical (macroscopic) sample reflects averaged properties that are normally precise as desired for a simplified, gross, model simulation.

Tissue samples invariably contain biological cells (and cell membranes, of course) so that a determination of conductivity at dc or at different ac frequencies may vary because of the effect of variations in the membrane admittance. For example, in ● Fig. 2.10 the conductivity of a sample (of skeletal muscle) varies with frequency. At a high enough frequency, the membranes become totally "transparent" and no further reduction in conductivity arises. It can also be seen in ● Fig. 2.10 that at low frequencies the conductivity transverse to the fiber axis is lower than that along the axis, a consequence of the greater number of intervening membranes in the former case. At elevated frequencies, when the membrane admittance is negligible, the conductivity becomes isotropic. This example shows that, in fact, the response of a tissue sample to an electric field may not be described by a single scalar conductivity value, but depends on frequency and field orientation (the field displays anisotropy). For muscle, the frequency dependence can be traced to the fact that the current flows both in the intracellular and interstitial space and the mix depends, among other things, on the admittance of the membrane. Anisotropic conductivity can be expected for cardiac as well as for skeletal muscle. However, the range of tissue anisotropy of various tissues as reported in the literature is quite substantial. Moreover, its influence may also affect the appropriate specification of the equivalent primary sources. As a consequence, too detailed analysis of the effect of anisotropy should be carried out with great caution[4]. The effect of anisotropy is an essential element of the

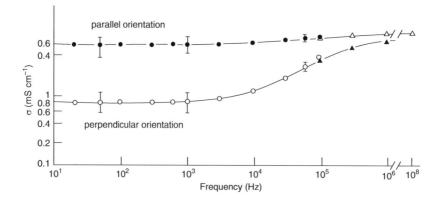

■ Fig. 2.10

Conductivity of canine skeletal muscle at 37°C, in the parallel and perpendicular orientations, measured using a two-electrode (*triangles*), or four-electrode technique (*circles*). Each point represents the average of five separate measurements (four-electrode) or two measurements (two-electrode) in each orientation; typical standard errors are shown (Adapted from Epstein and Foster [3])

■ Table 2.1

Ratio of displacement current to conduction current of tissues at different frequencies [1]

Tissue	Frequency			
	10 Hz	100 Hz	1,000 Hz	10,000 Hz
Lung	0.15	0.025	0.05	0.14
Fatty tissue		0.01	0.03	0.15
Liver	0.20	0.035	0.06	0.20
Heart muscle	0.10	0.04	0.15	0.32

■ Table 2.2

Tissue conductivity (S cm^{-1})

Tissue	Blood	Lung	Liver	Fat	Human trunk
Conductivity	0.67	0.05	0.14	0.04	0.21

bi-domain theory topic addressed in ❷ Chaps. 6 and ❷ 8. Some other aspects are treated in ❷ Chap. 8. The handling of volume conductor effects as presented in this chapter is restricted to the isotropic situations.

Because of the presence of cells and their membranes in tissues, and because the cell membrane has a very high specific capacitance, the macroscopic tissue response to an applied field is both a conduction current and a displacement (capacitive) current. The relative strength of the latter depends on the frequency; for tissue under electrocardiographic conditions, the conductivity (both magnitude and phase) is dispersive (depends on frequency) for this reason.

Measurements on those tissues which are important in electrocardiography show the ratio of displacement to conduction currents to be negligible. Such measurements are summarized in ❷ Table 2.1. It can be concluded that torso tissues may be treated as if they are purely resistive. Mean conductivity values of these tissues are given in ❷ Table 2.2. Additional data may be found in the review papers [5–7].

The validity of conductivity values in ❷ Table 2.2 might possibly be questioned for lung and muscle because for those tissues their cellular structure plays an important role in determining the effective (macroscopic) resistance to current flow. Being complex structures, it may not always be possible or appropriate to describe currents with a simple scalar conductivity parameter. Aside from this proviso, torso tissues are conventionally assumed to be purely resistive, with values of tissue conductivity being essentially those given in ❷ Table 2.2.

2.4.3 Quasistatic Conditions

The conduction current in a physiological preparation with conductivity $\sigma(x, y, z)$ is related to the electric field by (2.84). Since the electric field is conservative, this expression cannot be true at every point of the preparation – that would imply a dissipation of energy (associated with current flow in a resistive medium) with no source of energy. To include the presence of active sources, a nonconservative term is added to (2.84) so that

$$\vec{J} = \sigma \vec{E} + \vec{J}^{\mathrm{i}}, \tag{2.85}$$

where $\vec{J}^{\mathrm{i}}$ is an impressed (applied) current. In (2.85), $\vec{J}^{\mathrm{i}}$ is nonzero only at primary source sites; $\vec{J}^{\mathrm{i}}$ constitutes a nonconservative field. Since the total current in (2.85) is solenoidal (the net flow into or out of any closed region is zero), in order to preserve continuity of current,

$$\nabla \bullet \vec{J} = 0 = \nabla \bullet (\sigma \vec{E}) + \nabla \bullet \vec{J}^{\mathrm{i}} \tag{2.86}$$

If the medium has a homogeneous isotropic conductivity, that is, $\sigma(x, y, z) = \sigma$, then by using (2.29) and (2.86) reduces to

$$\sigma \nabla \bullet \vec{E} + \nabla \bullet \vec{J}^{\mathrm{i}} = 0 \tag{2.87}$$

It is obvious from viewing the electrocardiogram that the potential field arising from sources in the heart varies with time. In fact, for a normal subject at rest, the potential and current flow field is periodic at the heart rate. If the ECG is subjected to a Fourier analysis, it can be determined that the spectral content is from dc to perhaps 100 Hz [8]. The behavior of an ac source in a conducting medium with the size of the human torso and with impedance properties described in ❷ Tables 2.1 and ❷ 2.2 has been studied using Maxwell's equations, which govern such time-varying phenomena [9]. The outcome is that, to a very good approximation, the electric field may be derived as the gradient of a scalar potential, namely

$$\vec{E} = -\nabla \Phi \tag{2.88}$$

If (2.88) is substituted into (2.87), then we obtain

$$\nabla^2 \Phi = \frac{\nabla \bullet \vec{J}^{\,i}}{\sigma} \tag{2.89}$$

The integral solution to Poisson's (2.89) for Φ in the infinite homogeneous medium can be found by comparison with the mathematically equivalent (2.74) and (2.73) of electrostatics. This yields

$$\Phi = \frac{1}{4\pi\sigma} \int \frac{-\nabla \bullet \vec{J}^{\,i}}{r} dv, \tag{2.90}$$

where r is the distance from a point of integration to the fixed point at which the field is being evaluated.

A comparison of (2.88) to (2.90) with (2.69), (2.74) and (2.73) shows that the potential and electric field under electrocardiographic conditions obey the same mathematical relationships as for electrostatics. These are described as quasistatic relationships since, at any instant of time, these potentials appear as if they were static for all time, yet changes in value of potential over time do occur.

Many solutions to problems in electric current flow are equivalent to those of comparable problems in electrostatics. The similarity in the respective fundamental relationships has already been noted. Equation (2.69) and (2.73) can be transformed to (2.88) and (2.73) and vice versa if the following replacements are made:

$$\varepsilon \leftrightarrow \sigma \tag{2.91}$$

$$\rho \leftrightarrow -\nabla \bullet J^{\,i} \tag{2.92}$$

The similarity may be stressed further by introducing the notation $i_v = -\nabla \bullet J^{\,i}$ as an impressed current volume density (A m^{-3}).

2.5   Current Sources

In the previous sections the fundamentals for studying the potential field arising from impressed current sources under quasi-static conditions have been described, as well as the main mathematical tools required for this analysis. We now apply these tools to the description of the main electric current source models that have been found effective.

The analogy between electric current flow in conductive media and electrostatics, the principle of duality, shows up again in the basic expression (2.90), which implies, and permits, the use of the *superposition principle*: the contributions of elementary sources to the potential field simply add up to the (total) potential. The latter is a consequence of the experimentally observed linearity between current strength and resulting potential, which holds true inside the body for natural bioelectric sources.

Bioelectric currents stem from the biochemical processes at the cell membrane. As such, these are not observable. Their presence, nature, and magnitude can only be inferred from the potential field generated; they need to be evaluated from measurements of tissue excitation, with particular reference to the activation of cardiac muscle. The basic expression (2.90) shows that, when interpreting measured potentials, the conductivity of the medium should be included, as well as its distribution throughout the tissue in the case of inhomogeneity.

The discussion begins with a derivation of source–field relationships for the monopole and dipole. It will be seen that these serve as the building blocks of all electrophysiological sources. It should be realized that these source descriptions are models of the actual current generation. They are physical abstractions that serve to describe the observed potentials at some distance from the actual current generating mechanisms only. As such they are referred to as *equivalent sources*. To facilitate the discussion, the medium is assumed to be of infinite extent and have a homogeneous, isotropic conductivity. The potential field generated is referred to as the infinite medium potential. Although this configuration is clearly unrealistic, it facilitates the appreciation of the nature of the source description in isolation of the complexity caused by inhomogeneities. As will be shown in a subsequent section, these complexities can be treated in an "add-on" fashion.

2.5.1 Point Sources

2.5.1.1 Monopole

Consider that a current I_0, emanating from a vanishingly small volume, is impressed into a uniform conducting medium of conductivity σ and infinite in extent. Let the source position be (x, y, z), as illustrated in ❯ Fig. 2.11. This type of current source is analogous to the point charge of electrostatics, and is referred to as a point current source.

The potential field set up inside the medium is evaluated as follows. In view of the symmetry, the current flow is in the radial direction and the current density is uniform on any sphere having the source as its center. Thus if the total current is I_0, then over a concentric spherical surface of radius r the current density $\vec{J}$ is given by

$$\vec{J}(r) = \frac{I_0}{4\pi r^2}\vec{e}_r, \tag{2.93}$$

where $\vec{e}_r$ is a unit vector pointing from the source to the field point (x', y', z') and r denotes their distance: $r = \{(x'-x)^2 + (y'-y)^2 + (z'-z)^2\}^{1/2}$.

Now, according to Ohm's law, the current density $\vec{J}$ and the electric field $\vec{E}$ are related by the conductivity as specified by (2.84). Furthermore, the electric field is obtained as the negative gradient of scalar potential Φ according to (2.88). Consequently,

$$\nabla\Phi = -\frac{I_0}{4\pi\sigma r^2}\vec{e}_r. \tag{2.94}$$

So, using the r component if the gradient operator as listed in (2.41),

$$d\Phi/dr = -\frac{I_0}{4\pi\sigma r^2} \tag{2.95}$$

Integration with respect to r gives an expression for the scalar potential associated with a monopole current source, namely

$$\Phi(r) = \frac{I_0}{4\pi\sigma r} + c \tag{2.96}$$

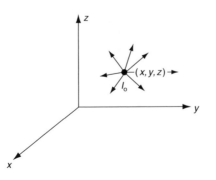

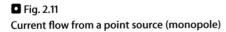

Fig. 2.11
Current flow from a point source (monopole)

The result is directly related to (2.72), by applying duality. The integration constant c may be determined by *choosing* the point in space where the potential is taken to be 0. In the infinite medium configuration, this point is conveniently placed at infinity, which yields: $c = 0$.

2.5.1.2   Dipole

The basic current source of biophysics is the (mathematical) current dipole. It can be introduced by first considering the potential distribution generated by a current (point) source of strength I_0 (expressed in amperes (A)) and a current sink of strength $-I_0$, separated by a (small) distance vector $\vec{\delta}$ (❷ Fig. 2.12), with length δ. This generator configuration is called a "bi-pole," or physical dipole. The magnitudes of the strengths of source and sink are equal. Since no net current can be generated by a biophysical source, the current is merely "pumped around."

For infinitesimally small values of δ, the total field under these conditions can be evaluated by

$$\Phi(\vec{r}') = \frac{I_0}{4\pi\sigma}\frac{\partial(1/R)}{\partial\delta}\delta \tag{2.97}$$

The partial derivative evaluates the rate of change in the field which results from displacing I_0 in the direction of $\vec{\delta}$, and this is multiplied by δ to obtain the actual change in potential. The partial derivative is with respect to the unprimed, source coordinates while the primed, field coordinates are held constant.

In (2.97), the directional derivative of $1/R$ can be recognized, and hence, it can be written as

$$\Phi(\vec{r}') = \frac{I_0}{4\pi\sigma}\nabla(1/R)\bullet\vec{\delta} \tag{2.98}$$

From (2.33) we have

$$\Phi(\vec{r}') = \frac{I_0}{4\pi\sigma}\frac{\vec{R}}{R^3}\bullet\vec{\delta} = \frac{1}{4\pi\sigma}\frac{\vec{R}}{R^3}\bullet\vec{D}, \tag{2.99}$$

which introduces $\vec{D} = I\vec{\delta}$ as the (mathematical) dipole, *defined* as the (hypothetical, equivalent) generator that generates its potentials described by (2.99) throughout the medium, i.e., irrespective of the field point's proximity to the generator. The potential reference at infinity is taken to be zero.

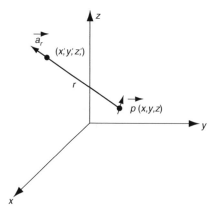

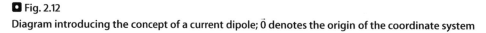

❏ Fig. 2.12

Diagram introducing the concept of a current dipole; $\vec{0}$ denotes the origin of the coordinate system

The dipole is a vector quantity, directed from sink to source. Its physical unit is (A m). As shown, it may be interpreted as the result of a limiting process in which the distance between the two poles of a bi-pole is reduced to zero while keeping the product $I \times \delta$ constant. An alternative expression to (2.99) is

$$\Phi(\vec{r}\,') = \frac{1}{4\pi\sigma} \frac{D\cos\varphi}{R^2},$$ (2.100)

with φ being the angle between $\vec{R}$ and $\vec{\delta}$ (❷ Fig. 2.12).

The current dipole is a useful mathematical concept that may be used to describe (represent, specify) the potential distribution generated by bioelectric sources at a distance. For observation points arbitrarily close to the dipole, the potential prescribed by (2.99) becomes arbitrarily large (infinite), which is clearly physiologically unrealistic. The double layer source model, discussed in ❷ Sect. 2.5.2 as well as in ❷ Chaps. 6–8, does not suffer from this limitation, and has a direct link to the basis of the bioelectric sources, the biochemical phenomena taking place at the cell membrane (❷ Chap. 7).

2.5.1.3 Evaluation

From the way the monopole and the dipole were introduced above, it is evident that they can indeed be classed as *point sources*: their spatial extent is restricted to a single point. They are physical abstractions, valid for describing the potential field at a distance from the source only, as follows from the fact that at close proximity to their position (x, y, z) the potential field as well as the current density that they generate tend to infinite values. This follows from (2.96) and (2.100) for the monopole and the dipole, respectively. This phenomenon is referred to as a point singularity of the potential field.

The single monopole has an additional unrealistic nature when it is applied to a medium that is bounded, as is the human body. In such a medium a single current monopole would keep charging up the tissue continuously (current is the flow of electric charge per unit of time), which is clearly not the case. So it has a value only if accompanied by a sink of equal strength, as was the case while introducing the dipole. Similarly, inside a bounded medium, a collection of current monopoles may be used provided the sum of their strengths equals zero.

In its application to a medium, be it bounded or not, the dipole does not suffer from this lack of realism: no net charge is introduced into the medium. The dipole may be likened to a circulation pump placed in a swimming pool: it "sucks" water at its inlet valve and ejects it at its outlet valve.

The concept of building a dipole from a pair of monopoles can be extended to the inclusion of a larger number of monopoles. Like the mathematical dipole, the total, more complex configuration remains located at a single point in space. A series of current sources of increasing complexity may be conceived in this manner, called *multipoles*. The monopole and the dipole form the first two terms of this series. Conversely, an arbitrary source distribution may be uniquely specified by a weighted sum of the multipoles of increasing order: a so-called multipole expansion [1, 10, 11].

As follows from (2.96), for the monopole, the multipole of order 0, the potential decreases as $1/r$ when moving away from the source. For the dipole, the first-order multipole, the potential decreases as $1/r^2$. For a multipole of order k, the decrease is as fast as $1/r^{k+1}$. This is a highly significant property: with the monopole being absent in a bounded medium, the potential at increasing distances from the source will invariably be dominated by the dipole contributions, the contributions by the higher order terms decreasing more rapidly with distance. This explains the fact that at a distance, the potential field of an arbitrary current source tends to have a dipolar nature. As a rule of thumb, at a distance of, say, 5 times that of the spatial extent of a source, the contributions of the higher order may already be difficult to establish experimentally.

2.5.2 Surface Source Densities

Current monopoles and current dipoles may be used as building blocks for more complex source configurations. To this end, like in electrostatics, these sources may be specified by density functions, specifying their strength per unit of volume. Alternatively, when restricted to some surface, their strength is specified per unit of surface area. The expressions for determining the source–field relationships (in the infinite medium under quasi-static conditions) are (2.85) to (2.90).

These will now be used to describe the properties of two particular variants of distributed surface source densities: the current monopole layer and the current dipole layer. These two source types are the major players in the various applications of volume conduction theory discussed in this book.

2.5.2.1 Monopole Layer; Monolayer

In the case of the current monopole layer, or monolayer, a monopole surface density of strength $J(x, y, z)$ is assumed to be present at a surface S, with $J\,dS$ representing an elementary current source (dimension: A). The dimension of the density function J is A m^{-2}, which is the same as that of the current density $\vec{J}$, but unlike $\vec{J}$ the density is a scalar function.

The potential field for this source is

$$\Phi = \frac{1}{4\pi\sigma} \int \frac{J\,dS}{r} \tag{2.101}$$

To illustrate some of the major properties of the monolayer, the potential along the axis of a disk carrying a uniform monopole current density J is derived. The geometry is shown in ❷ Fig. 2.13, where a cylindrical coordinate system is set up, with the origin at the center of the disk and polar axis normal to the plane of the disk. The disk radius is a. Based on symmetry the contributions of all source points on an annular ring of radius r and width dr, to the potential at a point along the axis at a distance z from the disk are equal:

$$d\Phi(z) = \frac{2\pi r\,dr\,J}{4\pi\sigma(r^2 + z^2)^{1/2}}, \tag{2.102}$$

where the numerator of (2.102) is the total current impressed through the annulus, and $(r^2 + z^2)^{1/2}$ is the distance between source element and observation point.

By adding up the elementary contributions, through the integration of (2.102), we find

$$\Phi(z) = \frac{J}{2\sigma} \int_0^a \frac{r\,dr}{(r^2 + z^2)^{1/2}} = \frac{J}{2\sigma}\left\{(a^2 + z^2)^{1/2} - |z|\right\} + c \tag{2.103}$$

Choosing the potential at infinity to be zero requires setting $c = 0$, which yields

$$\Phi(z) = \frac{J}{2\sigma}\left\{(a^2 + z^2)^{1/2} - |z|\right\} \tag{2.104}$$

From this expression it follows that the potential along the z-axis is continuous at $z = 0$, i.e., when crossing the monolayer. For the electric field along the z-axis the situation is different. Here we have

$$E_z = -\frac{d}{dz}\{\Phi(z)\} = -\frac{J}{2\sigma}\left\{\frac{z}{(a^2 + z^2)^{1/2}} - \frac{z}{|z|}\right\}, \tag{2.105}$$

which is discontinuous at $z = 0$. By denoting the current flow along the z-axis that results from this source configuration as $J_z = \sigma E_z$ it follows that while approaching the disk along the negative z-axis a limiting value of $J_z = -J/2$ is reached, whereas on the other side of the disk we have $J_z = J/2$. This corresponds to an outflow of current away from the monolayer.

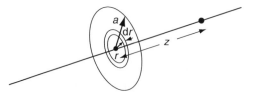

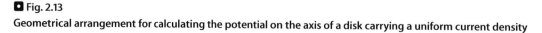

❷ **Fig. 2.13**

Geometrical arrangement for calculating the potential on the axis of a disk carrying a uniform current density

2.5.2.2   Dipole Layer; Double Layer

The distribution of dipole sources confined to a surface S is referred to as a *double layer*. The elements dS of S are taken to carry an elementary current dipole with strength $\vec{M}_S dS$, $\vec{M}_S$ denoting the dipole moment per unit area (dimension: A m/m^2 = A m^{-1}). By using superposition applied to (2.99), the potential field is

$$\Phi = \frac{1}{4\pi\sigma} \int \frac{\vec{M}_S \bullet \vec{r}}{r^3} dS \tag{2.106}$$

If the orientation of the dipole density $\vec{M}_S$ lines up with the normal of the surface S carrying it, then $\vec{M}_S dS = M_S d\vec{S}$ and (2.106) may be written as

$$\Phi = \frac{1}{4\pi\sigma} \int M_S \frac{\vec{r}}{r^3} \bullet d\vec{S} = \frac{1}{4\pi\sigma} \int M_S d\omega, \tag{2.107}$$

where $d\omega$ is an element of solid angle defined earlier (see (2.63)). If, moreover, the double layer strength M_S is uniform (over S), then (2.107) has a simple form, namely

$$\Phi = \frac{M_S}{4\pi\sigma} \Omega, \tag{2.108}$$

where Ω is the solid angle subtended by the entire double layer at the field point (❷ Sect. 2.2.12).

Equation (2.108) has major significance. If S is a closed surface and the double layer is indeed normal to it and has uniform strength, then for any field point external to S we have $\Omega = 0$. For any interior point of S the total solid angle has a magnitude -4π ((2.49) and (2.50)). From this it follows that while crossing the surface S from outside, the solid angle changes by 4π. As a consequence, the potential is discontinuous across the layer, exhibiting a jump of magnitude

$$\Delta\Phi = V_D = M_S/\sigma \tag{2.109}$$

By defining $V_D = M_S/\sigma$, an alternative characterization of the strength of the double layer is obtained and, when applied to (2.107), this yields

$$\Phi = \frac{1}{4\pi} \int V_D \frac{\vec{r}}{r^3} \bullet d\vec{S} = \frac{1}{4\pi} \int V_D d\omega \tag{2.110}$$

For a nonuniform double layer that is oriented along the surface normal, any potential jump observed experimentally reflects the local double layer strength.

The nature of the current dipole layer may be illustrated by taking S once more to be a circular disk of radius a, and computing the potential along the axis of symmetry. This is the same configuration as depicted in ❷ Fig. 2.13, but now the disk carries a uniform dipole density with strength M_S, directed along the z-axis. The potential along the z-axis follows from (2.108). For this axial symmetric configuration the solid angle Ω subtended by the disk at observation point z follows immediately from the definition of the concept *solid angle* as such. For positive values of z the result is

$$\Omega(z) = 2\pi \left\{ \frac{z}{|z|} - \frac{z}{(a^2 + z^2)^{1/2}} \right\} \tag{2.111}$$

The term $z/(a^2 + z^2)^{1/2}$ is equal to the cosine of the top angle α of the cone spanning from z to the disk. When approaching the disk along the negative z-axis, the limiting value for the solid angle is -2π. The negative sign corresponds to the fact that the surface normal is taken to be lined up with the dipole direction, whereas for a negative z the source to field vector points in the opposite direction. When approaching the double layer from the other side, the value of Ω tends to 2π. Recall that total 3D space spans a solid angle of 4π, and close to a plane which remains just one half of that. Thus the solid angle jumps by 4π while crossing the double layer. By writing $V_D = M_S/\sigma$ and substituting (2.111) in (2.108) we find

$$\Phi(z) = \frac{1}{2} V_D \left\{ \frac{z}{|z|} - \frac{z}{(a^2 + z^2)^{1/2}} \right\} = \frac{1}{2} V_D \{ \pm 1 - \cos\alpha \} \tag{2.112}$$

Because of symmetry, the gradient of the potential along the z-axis is directed along this axis. By differentiating (2.112), we find for the component electric field along the z-axis

$$E_z = -\frac{d}{dz}\{\Phi(z)\} = -\frac{1}{2}V_D\left\{XX - \frac{1}{(a^2+z^2)^{1/2}} + \frac{z^2}{(a^2+z^2)^{3/2}}\right\} = \frac{1}{2}V_D\left\{-XX + \frac{a^2}{(a^2+z^2)^{3/2}}\right\} \qquad (2.113)$$

The function $\Phi(z)$ is discontinuous at $z = 0$. This demands some special care while taking its derivative. The term XX expresses the singularity of the derivative at $z = 0$. This has the dipole-like nature of two so-called delta functions with opposite sign that are infinitesimally close at $z = 0$.

Apart from this singularity, the field strength can be seen to be a positive, even function of z. This corresponds to a current flow in one direction: toward the double layer along the negative z-axis, away from it along the positive z-axis. This is in agreement with the circulation pump analogy. Note that close to $z = 0$, the gradient of the potential is proportional to $1/a$, which tends to zero when increasing a, the radius of the disk.

2.5.2.3   Evaluation; Primary and Secondary Sources

The analyses in the previous two sections show that the monolayer and the double layer have a contrasting behavior of the potential at their boundary: for the monolayer the potential is continuous and its gradient is discontinuous. For the double layer it is just the other way round. Although this is demonstrated here for a relatively simple configuration: assuming a uniform strength and a simple shape of S, this type of behavior can be shown to hold true in general (Panofsky & Phillips; p. 20).

Like the monopole, the uniform monolayer has no place by itself in a bounded medium since it does not conserve charge. The nonuniform variant clearly has a place when adding the constraint that the integral of its density over the surface carrying it be zero. Even so, it is rarely used as a model for the true, primary sources that originate from membrane processes. Its natural place is as one of the equivalent sources that are used for treating the relationship between potentials on the heart surface and body surface potentials (❷ Sect. 2.6.4.5).

The double layer source model has a natural place as a primary, equivalent source, as well as a secondary source for treating the effect of inhomogeneities in the electric conductivity of the medium (❷ Sect. 2.6).

2.5.3   Volume Source Densities

A volume distribution of dipole sources can be described by a density function, just as a volume distribution of point charges in electrostatics could be described by a volume charge density function. If $\vec{M}_v$ is a dipole moment per unit volume, with dimension $A\,m^{-2}$, then $\vec{M}_v dv$ is an elementary dipole whose potential field, according to (2.99), is

$$d\Phi = \frac{1}{4\pi\sigma}\frac{\vec{M}_v \bullet \vec{r}}{r^3}dv \qquad (2.114)$$

The total potential field is found by integrating (2.114), giving

$$\Phi = \frac{1}{4\pi\sigma}\int \frac{\vec{M}_v \bullet \vec{r}}{r^3}dv \qquad (2.115)$$

The field of the double layer discussed in the previous section may be viewed as a degenerate case of (2.115), with $\vec{M}_v dv = \vec{M}_S dS$.

More generally, if a conducting region contains an arbitrary impressed current source density $\vec{J}^{\,i}$, then the potential field is

$$\Phi = \frac{1}{4\pi\sigma} \int \frac{-\nabla \bullet \vec{J}^{\,i}}{r} dv \tag{2.116}$$

as was shown in (2.90). The volume of integration expressed in (2.116) relates to any volume that contains all impressed sources; at the surface of such a chosen volume, $\vec{J}^{\,i} = 0$ necessarily. As a consequence, if $\vec{J}^{\,i}/r$ is integrated over such a bounding surface, the result must also be zero. That is

$$\int (\vec{J}^{\,i}/r) \bullet d\vec{S} = 0 \tag{2.117}$$

If the divergence theorem ((2.26)) is applied to (2.117), then

$$\int \nabla \bullet (\vec{J}^{\,i}/r) \, dv = \int \frac{\vec{J}^{\,i}}{r} \bullet d\vec{S} = 0 \tag{2.118}$$

and by application of the vector identity given by (2.29), (2.118) yields

$$\int \vec{J}^{\,i} \bullet \nabla(1/r) dv = - \int (1/r) \nabla \bullet \vec{J}^{\,i} dv \tag{2.119}$$

Consequently (2.116) can be replaced by

$$\Phi = 1/(4\pi\sigma) \int \vec{J}^{\,i} \bullet \nabla(1/r) dv \tag{2.120}$$

from which it follows that

$$\Phi = 1/(4\pi\sigma) \int \vec{J}^{\,i} \bullet \vec{r}/r^3 dv, \tag{2.121}$$

where $\vec{r}$ points from source to field point, as before. A comparison of (2.121) and (2.115) provides an alternative interpretation of the impressed current density $\vec{J}^{\,i}$ $(A\,m^{-2})$ as a dipole moment per unit volume. Note that both interpretations have the same dimensions: $A\,m^{-2} = A\,m/m^3$. The potential field can be found from $\vec{J}^{\,i}$ using either (2.116), where $-\nabla \bullet \vec{J}^{\,i}$ behaves like a current *mono*pole volume density i_v $(A\,m^{-3})$, or (2.121), where $\vec{J}^{\,i}$ behaves like a *di*pole moment volume density $(A\,m^{-2})$.

2.6   Potential Fields in Inhomogeneous Media

Up to this point, all expressions for the potential fields discussed in this chapter have assumed that the sources lie in a volume conductor of infinite extent having a uniform isotropic electric conductivity. When inhomogeneities of the electric conductivity are in fact present, as is always the case in bioelectricity, their effect on the observed potential field must be taken into account. This section describes some of the methods that are used for evaluating these effects. The goal in mind is their application to the determination of electrocardiographic potential fields.

The methods discussed assume the inhomogeneities to be restricted to nonintersecting subregions, each having its individual homogeneous, isotropic electric conductivity.

The most prominent inhomogeneity relates to the fact that the electric conductivity of the region outside the body (air) is zero. As a consequence, in the normal situation, no electric current flow takes place across this surface. Other, major differences in conductivity values with respect to those of the surrounding tissues are those of the lungs (lower conductivity) and the blood inside the cavities of atria and ventricles (higher conductivity).

To introduce the problem, consider a dipole source in a conducting medium of infinite extent. Current flow lines, directed along the local electric field, exists as shown in ❷ Fig. 2.14. Where appropriate, and to distinguish it from the

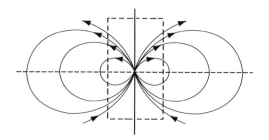

◼ Fig. 2.14
Current flow lines generated by a dipole pointing upward, lying in a uniform, unbounded, conducting medium

inhomogeneous situation, the potential field set up by the electric current generator inside this type of medium will be denoted as the *infinite medium potential* Φ_∞.

Suppose that at some instant the entire region external to the rectangular parallelepiped (shown dotted in ❯ Fig. 2.14) is cut away leaving a nonconducting medium. This constitutes a more realistic model of bioelectrical volume conduction, in a medium of finite extent bounded by air. In this case, since the current cannot enter the nonconducting exterior region, the current flow in the interior region will be diverted such that no current will pass the interface between the conducting and the insulating region.

More generally, if at an instant of time the region external to the parallelepiped in ❯ Fig. 2.14 were to have a different conductivity (not necessarily zero, as just considered), then boundary conditions at the interface between the two regions of different conductivity (labeled by subscripts 1 and 2) need to be satisfied

$$\Phi_1 = \Phi_2 \tag{2.122}$$

$$\sigma_1 \partial \Phi_1 / \partial n = \sigma_2 \partial \Phi_2 / \partial n = J_n, \tag{2.123}$$

where ∂n is taken along the local surface normal to the interface.

Equation (2.123) represents the continuity of the normal component of the current density J_n, which must hold true in the steady state (no accumulation of charge at the interface). This continuity condition and that of potential (2.122) form the basis for finding the potential field set up by an electric current generator inside a piece wise inhomogeneous medium.

If a medium, such as the human torso, can be subdivided into a number of subregions each having a uniform conductivity, a dedicated pair of such conditions will apply at each of the respective interfaces. The total set of these conditions can be shown to be sufficient to uniquely find the current flow pattern [12]. The associated potential field is then, as always, uniquely specified up to a constant only. If the medium is in fact bounded, like the thorax normally is, choosing the location of the reference point for the potential at infinity is no longer possible.

2.6.1   Basic Formulation; Uniqueness Theorem

2.6.1.1   Basic Formulation

The determination of electrocardiographic potential fields arising from bioelectric primary sources is referred to as the Forward Problem of Electrocardiography (❯ Chap. 8). The solution methods discussed here are selected in view of their high conceptual relevance. As introduced above, we consider one or more subregions, each having its own electric conductivity. In one more of these subregions, bioelectric current sources may be situated. The problem of finding the resulting potential field anywhere inside the medium or at its boundary may be handled by finding the potential field resulting from each of these sources separately, followed by adding up their individual contributions (superposition theorem). This is justified by the linearity of the basic source–field relationship:

$$\nabla^2 \Phi = \frac{-i_v}{\sigma_k} = \frac{\nabla \bullet \vec{J}^i}{\sigma_k}, \tag{2.89a}$$

being Poisson's equation.

Inside a homogeneous subregion k with conductivity σ_k, the potential field Φ is found by solving the variant of the differential (2.89a), those without primary bioelectric sources by solving Laplace's equation

$$\nabla^2 \Phi = 0 \tag{2.124}$$

At the boundaries of the subregions the continuity conditions for the potential and the current density normal to the interfaces, (2.122) and (2.123), need to be satisfied

2.6.1.2 Uniqueness Theorem

Once, by whatever means, a solution Φ has been found that satisfies (2.122), (2.123), and (2.124) it can be shown that it is unique up to a constant only. This property is known as the *uniqueness theorem* [12].

2.6.2 Method of Images

The solution method based on images is well known from electrostatics. Because of the analogy between electrostatics and volume conduction theory, cf. (2.91) and (2.92), the same method may also be applied in bioelectricity. However, the number of configurations for which the method can be applied in bioelectric volume conduction problems is rather limited. Here, a discussion on this topic is included to introduce and illustrate some important basic theoretical concepts.

The problem treated is the situation where volume conduction in the semi-infinite space $z \leq 0$ has a conductivity value σ_1. In the remaining (upper) part of space, the conductivity is σ_2. On the z-axis, an electric dipole with strength $\vec{D}$ is situated at $z = -d$, with dipole elements (D_x, D_y, D_z). The problem addressed here is finding the potential field Φ_1 in the lower space, Φ_2 in the upper space and in particular at the interface $z = 0$. Inspired by the image theory of electrostatics, we consider a virtual *infinite* space having a uniform conductivity σ_1, in which we place a (virtual) image source $\vec{V}_2$ at the z-axis at $z = +d$. In the lower semi-space, the dipole potentials generated by both sources clearly satisfy Poisson's equation, irrespective of the strength of $\vec{V}_2$. The potential field in the upper semi-space, Φ_1, is assumed to be generated by a (virtual) image source $\vec{V}_1$ located on the z-axis at $z = -d$; $d > 0$ (with no virtual sources in the upper semi-space). In this upper semi-space the dipole potential generated by $\vec{V}_1$ satisfies Laplace's equation since the upper region is source free. However, without a proper specification of $\vec{V}_1$ and $\vec{V}_2$, it is not guaranteed that the boundary conditions at the interface $z = 0$, (2.122) and (2.123), are met. Without loss of generality, we may put $D_y = 0$, and correspondingly, because of the symmetry involved, $V_{1,y} = 0$ and $V_{2,y} = 0$. In this virtual, infinite space, the potential at, $z = 0$ is continuous if, using the expression for the dipole potential, (2.99),

$$\Phi_1(x,y,0) = \frac{1}{4\pi\sigma_1} \left(\frac{D_x x + D_z d}{R_1^3} + \frac{V_{2,x} x - V_{2,z} d}{R_2^3} \right) = \Phi_2(x,y,0) = \frac{1}{4\pi\sigma_1} \left(\frac{V_{1,x} x + V_{1,z} d}{R_1^3} \right), \tag{2.125}$$

with R_1 the length of $\vec{R}_1 = (x, y, z + d)$ and R_2 the length of $\vec{R}_2 = (x, y, z - d)$, pointing from the respective dipole sources to the field point at $(x, y, z = 0)$. Since $R_1 = R_2$, and the equality is required to hold true independently of x, (2.125) reduces to the conditions

$$V_{1,x} - V_{2,x} = D_x \quad \text{and} \quad V_{1,z} + V_{2,z} = D_z \tag{2.126}$$

Next we demand the virtual sources to be such that the continuity equation for the current density in the original, inhomogeneous situation is also satisfied in the virtual, homogeneous space. To evaluate (2.123), the respective contributions of the dipole sources to the potential in their respective domains are differentiated with respect to z, the z-axis being directed according to the normal of the interface. For $z = 0$, this means that we demand

$$\sigma_1 \frac{\partial \Phi_1}{\partial z}(x,y,0) = \sigma_1 \frac{1}{4\pi\sigma_1}\left(\frac{-3D_x xd + (R_1^2 - 3d^2)D_z}{R_1^5} + \frac{3V_{2,x}xd + (R_2^2 - 3d^2)V_{2,z}}{R_2^5}\right) \tag{2.127}$$

$$\sigma_2 \frac{\partial \Phi_2}{\partial z}(x,y,0) = \sigma_2 \frac{1}{4\pi\sigma_1}\left(\frac{-3V_{1,x}xd + (R_1^2 - 3d^2)V_{1,z}}{R_1^5}\right) \tag{2.128}$$

This equality should hold true, again independently of x, and since $R_1 = R_2$, equating (2.127) to (2.128) yields

$$\kappa V_{1,x} + V_{2,x} = D_x \text{ and } \kappa V_{1,z} - V_{2,z} = D_z, \tag{2.129}$$

with $\kappa = \sigma_2/\sigma_1$. The four equations specified by (2.126) and (2.129) is sufficient to solve the strengths of the components of the virtual sources $\vec{V}_1$ and $\vec{V}_2$. We find

$$\vec{V}_1 = \left(\frac{2}{1+\kappa}D_x, 0, \frac{2}{1+k}D_z\right) \text{ and } \vec{V}_2 = \left(\frac{1-\kappa}{1+\kappa}D_x, 0, -\frac{1-\kappa}{1+\kappa}D_z\right) \tag{2.130}$$

Since the potential fields specified by the combinations of the primary dipole and the virtual dipole sources satisfy the boundary conditions pertaining to the original, inhomogeneous problem formulation, the solutions also apply to the "real world" formulation of the problem. This follows as a direct consequence of the uniqueness theorem, ❯ Sect. 2.6.1.2. Note that, although the medium considered is inhomogeneous, it is still of infinite extent and hence the implied location of the potential reference could be, and was in fact taken, at infinity.

2.6.2.1 Inferences

The relatively simple configuration of ❯ Sect. 2.6.2 provides a suitable entry to introduce and illustrate some basic concepts related to the effect of inhomogeneity of volume conduction.

In combination with the primary dipole source, the virtual source specification implied in (2.130) permits the computation of the field potential everywhere in the medium.

We first consider the potential field $\Phi(x,y)$ at the plane $z = 0$ for the source–volume conductor configuration introduced in ❯ Sect. 2.6.2. By introducing $\vec{V}_2$ as specified by (2.130) in (2.125), we find

$$\Phi(x,y,0) = \frac{1}{4\pi\sigma_1}\frac{D_x x + D_z d}{R^3} + \frac{1}{4\pi\sigma_1}\frac{1-\kappa}{1+\kappa}\frac{D_x x + D_z d}{R^3}, \tag{2.131}$$

with R the length of $\vec{R} = (x,y,\pm d)$. The first term on the right represents the infinite medium potential, the second term the effect of the inhomogeneity. The second term has a source strength that is proportional to that of the primary source term. Correspondingly, $\frac{1-\kappa}{1+\kappa}\vec{V}_2$ constitutes a *secondary* current source; for $\kappa = 1$ (the homogeneous situation), its contribution vanishes. At the plane $z = 0$ we see that (2.131) reduces to

$$\Phi(x,y,0) = \frac{1}{4\pi\sigma_1}\frac{1-\kappa}{1+\kappa}\frac{D_x x + D_z d}{R^3} \tag{2.132}$$

If $\sigma_2 = 0$, corresponding to the medium being nonconductive above $z = 0$, we have $\kappa = 0$ and the potential $\Phi(x,y,0)$ is twice that in the infinite medium:

$$\Phi(x,y,0) = 2\Phi_\infty(x,y,0). \tag{2.133}$$

Next, more generally, we consider the potential field at an arbitrary plane $z = -a$; $a > 0$ in the lower semi-infinite space. Here we have

$$\Phi(x,y,-a) = \frac{1}{4\pi\sigma_1}\frac{D_x x + D_z(-a+d)}{R_1^3} + \frac{1}{4\pi\sigma_1}\frac{1-\kappa}{1+\kappa}\frac{D_x x - D_z(a+d)}{R_2^3}, \tag{2.134}$$

with R_1 the length of $\vec{R}_1 = (x, y, -a + d)$ and R_2 the length of $\vec{R}_2 = (x, y, -a - d)$. Note that $|-a + d|$ is the distance between the location of the primary source and the plane of observation. At this plane R_1 and R_2 are not equal. As a consequence, for $\kappa = 0$ the potential field (2.131) does no longer follow a simple expression of the nature of (2.134).

If the distance d (recall $d > 0$) between primary source and the interface is large compared to $|-a+d|$, the contribution of the secondary source to the potential in (2.134) is small. Consider, for example, the situation where $\kappa = 0$ (bounded medium) and $D_x = 0$ (a primary source dipole pointing toward the interface). By assigning $|-a+d|$ a constant value c, the contribution of the primary source term in (2.134) is proportional to the constant factor $1/c^2$, whereas that of the secondary source is proportional to $1/(2d - c)^2$, which rapidly decreases for increasing values of d.

This indicates that for the interpretation of potential fields observed close to primary sources, the effect of *distal* inhomogeneities may, to a first-order approximation, be neglected.

2.6.2.2 Alternative Secondary Sources

The secondary source description stemming from the method of images is by no means unique. Alternative variants are the introduction of monolayers or double layers at the interfaces between the inhomogeneous subregions. The potential field set up by the virtual sources satisfies Laplace's equation, that of the primary sources (the infinite medium solution) satisfies the associated Poisson's equation. The strength of such virtual sources may be computed such that all boundary conditions are satisfied, and thus (unicity theorem) the sum of both fields in the virtual, infinite space into which the primary and secondary sources are introduced is also the solution for the "real world" problem.

2.6.3 Spherically Shaped Interfaces

Although including inhomogeneity, the volume conductor treated in ❯ Sect. 2.6.2 is still insufficient for the analysis of the bioelectric potentials, since the semi-space is of infinite extent. The method of images may be applied to treating bounded media, but here the bounding geometry needs to be restricted, e.g., to be box-like.

For some types of geometric alternative, analytical methods are available for solving the involved volume conduction problem. A particular class is formed by spherical interfaces. In this section, the method of handling such interfaces is discussed, and is illustrated with respect to their application to a single bounded sphere, the earliest bounded volume conductor model considered in electrocardiography.

2.6.3.1 General Solution of Laplace's Equation; Spherical Harmonics

As shown in ❯ Sect. 2.6.2.2, the potential field generated by the secondary sources should satisfy Laplace's equation, and for treating spherical boundaries the expression of Laplace's equation in spherical coordinates (r, θ, ϕ), (2.45), is the natural starting point. It can be shown that the general *solution* to (2.45) can be formulated as a sum of basic analytical functions, involving, in general, an infinite member of terms [1, 10]. This expression reads

$$\Phi(r, \theta, \phi) = \sum_{n=0}^{\infty} \sum_{m=0}^{n} (a_{n,m} \cos m\phi + b_{n,m} \sin m\phi)(c_{n,m} r^n + d_{n,m} r^{-(n+1)}) P_n^m(\mu), \qquad (2.135)$$

with $\mu = \cos \theta$. The function $P_n^m(\mu)$ is the associated Legendre function of degree n and order m [13, p. 332]. In combination with the sine and cosine functions involved, these functions form the set of the so-called spherical harmonics. For $m = 0$ these are referred to as the Legendre polynomials $P_n(\mu) = P_n^0(\mu)$. The factors $a_{n,m}$, $b_{n,m}$, $c_{n,m}$, and $d_{n,m}$ are the expansion coefficients that specify the solution $\Phi(r, \theta, \phi)$. The great significance of the expansion (2.135) stems from the fact that the spherical harmonics form an orthogonal set. This means that the integral over a product of two such functions of the same order and degree is nonzero, whereas it will be zero if any of the two orders or degrees differs. As a

2

consequence, a unique set of expansion coefficients may be computed for any potential field $\Phi(r, \theta, \phi)$. The derivatives of $P_n(\mu)$ are related to the associated Legendre function, in fact we have:

$$\frac{\mathrm{d}^m}{\mathrm{d}\mu^m} P_n(\mu) = (-1)^m (1 - \mu^2)^{-m/2} P_n^m(\mu), \tag{2.136}$$

[13 p. 334]. For $n = 0, 1, 2, 3$ the Legendre polynomials are

$$P_0(\mu) = 1, \quad P_1(\mu) = \mu, \quad P_2(\mu) = \frac{1}{2}(3\mu^2 - 1) \text{ and } P_3(\mu) = \frac{1}{2}(5\mu^3 - 3\mu), \tag{2.137}$$

those for higher degrees follow from the recurrence expression

$$(k + 1)P_{k+1}(\mu) = (2k + 1)\mu P_k(\mu) - kP_{k-1}(\mu) \tag{2.138}$$

These polynomials are orthogonal over the interval $-1 < \mu < 1$. The integral of $(P_n(\mu))^2$ over this interval, called the squared norm of $P_n(\mu)$, is

$$\int_{-1}^{1} (P_n(\mu))^2 \mathrm{d}\mu = \frac{2}{2n + 1} \tag{2.139}$$

2.6.3.2   Application: Current Dipole Inside a Bounded Sphere

As an example of the use of spherical harmonics, we compute the potential field generated by a current dipole placed inside a bounded sphere with radius a, centered around the origin. Other applications of this method are worked out in other chapters of this volume.

The internal homogeneous conductivity of the sphere is taken to be σ. Without loss of generality, the dipole is placed on the z-axis at $z = d, 0 \leq d < a$, and its strength taken to be $\vec{D} = (D_x, 0, D_z)$. The infinite medium potential, expressed in Cartesian coordinates is

$$\Phi_\infty(x, y, z) = \frac{1}{4\pi\sigma} \frac{D_x x + D_z(z - d)}{R^3} = \frac{1}{4\pi\sigma} \frac{D_x x}{R^3} + \frac{1}{4\pi\sigma} \frac{D_z(z - d)}{R^3} \tag{2.140}$$

The first term on the right represents the contribution to the potential field of the component of the dipole vector that is tangential to the surface of the sphere, the second term that of the radial component. The expression of the same function in spherical coordinates reads

$$\Phi_\infty(r, \theta, \phi) = \frac{1}{4\pi\sigma} \frac{D_x r \sin\theta \cos\phi}{(\sqrt{r^2 + d^2 - 2dr\cos\theta})^3} + \frac{1}{4\pi\sigma} \frac{D_z(r\cos\theta - d)}{(\sqrt{r^2 + d^2 - 2dr\cos\theta})^3} \tag{2.141}$$

After introducing $\mu = \cos\theta$, in the second term on the right the function

$$\frac{r\cos\theta - d}{(\sqrt{r^2 + d^2 - 2dr\mu})^3} = \frac{\partial}{\partial d}\left(\frac{1}{\sqrt{r^2 + d^2 - 2dr\mu}}\right) = \frac{\partial}{\partial d}\left(\frac{1}{R}\right), \tag{2.142}$$

as can be verified by differentiation. Similarly, in the first term on the right of (2.141), the function

$$\frac{r}{(\sqrt{r^2 + d^2 - 2dr\mu})^3} = \frac{1}{d}\frac{\partial}{\partial\mu}\left(\frac{1}{R}\right) \tag{2.143}$$

The function $1/R$ may be expanded in a Taylor series. For $r > d$ the result is

$$\frac{1}{R} = \frac{1}{r}\sum_{\ell=0}^{\infty}\left(\frac{d}{r}\right)^\ell P_\ell(\mu)$$

and for $r < d$ we have

$$\frac{1}{R} = \frac{1}{d} \sum_{\ell=0}^{\infty} \left(\frac{r}{d}\right)^{\ell} P_{\ell}(\mu) \tag{2.144}$$

The appearance of the Legendre polynomials in this Taylor series expansion is not accidental: in fact the Legendre polynomials have been defined on the basis of this expansion. These properties allow the two terms in the right hand side of (2.141) to be expanded as a series of Legendre polynomials, thus opening the way for solving the bounded medium potential. This is demonstrated here by computing the potential field generated by the radial dipole component. The treatment of the contribution of the tangential dipole component may be carried out in a similar way.

For $r > d$ the infinite medium potential generated by radial dipole is

$$\Phi_{\infty}(r,\theta,\phi) = \frac{D_z}{4\pi\sigma} \frac{r\mu - d}{(\sqrt{r^2 + d^2 - 2d\mu})^3} = \frac{D_z}{4\pi\sigma} \frac{\partial}{\partial d}\left(\frac{1}{R}\right)$$

and by using (2.144) we find

$$\Phi_{\infty}(r,\theta,\phi) = \frac{D_z}{4\pi\sigma} \frac{1}{r^2} \sum_{\ell=1}^{\infty} \ell \left(\frac{d}{r}\right)^{\ell-1} P_{\ell}(\mu) \tag{2.145}$$

Note that the summation starts at $\ell = 1$, as the term for $\ell = 0$ is wiped out by the factor ℓ that results from the applied differentiation. Also note that the expression on the right does not depend on ϕ, in agreement with the axial-symmetric nature of this part of the problem.

To this infinite medium potential we now add the general solution of Laplace's Equation (2.135) and demand that the potential field expressed by the sum satisfies the boundary condition at the surface of the sphere. For a bounded medium this means that the normal derivative of the field is zero. The nature of the problem is such that a relatively simple form of (2.135) is involved. First, because of the axial-symmetric nature of both the infinite medium potential and the volume conductor, no terms involving ϕ should play a role. Second, since the contribution to the potential field at the origin is desired to be finite, all terms involving negative powers of r should be absent. This leaves as the possible contribution satisfying Laplace's equation

$$\Phi(r,\theta,\phi) = \sum_{n=0}^{\infty} c_n r^n P_n(\mu), \tag{2.146}$$

and, for $r > d$ the general nature of the total potential field is

$$\Phi(r,\theta,\phi) = \frac{D_z}{4\pi\sigma} \frac{1}{r^2} \sum_{\ell=1}^{\infty} \ell \left(\frac{d}{r}\right)^{\ell-1} P_{\ell}(\mu) + \sum_{n=0}^{\infty} c_n r^n P_n(\mu) \tag{2.147}$$

The expansion coefficients c_n remain to be determined from the boundary condition. Because of the radial symmetry of the volume conductor, the normal derivative of the interface is found by differentiation with respect to r and the boundary condition is satisfied if this derivative is zero for $r = a$.

Carrying out the differentiation, followed by substituting $r = a$, leads to the equation

$$-\frac{D_z}{4\pi\sigma} \frac{1}{a^3} \sum_{\ell=1}^{\infty} \ell(\ell+1) \left(\frac{d}{a}\right)^{\ell-1} P_{\ell}(\mu) + \sum_{n=0}^{\infty} (n c_n a^{n-1}) P_n(\mu) = 0 \tag{2.148}$$

The determination of the expansion coefficients from this expression may seem to be difficult. However, as demonstrated in the sequel, it is a straightforward, standard procedure based on the application of the orthogonality properties of the Legendre polynomials (❯ Sect. 2.6.3.1). The procedure is as follows. For all integer values of k, $k \geq 0$, multiply both sides of (2.148) by $P_k(\mu)$ followed by the integration of the result with respect to μ over the interval $-1 < \mu < 1$. Because of the orthogonality properties of the Legendre polynomials, for any given k the terms in the first summation yield nonzero terms only for $\ell = k$, and those of the second summation only for $n = k$. Moreover, by using the expression for the norms of the Legendre polynomials, (2.139), we find

$$-\frac{D_z}{4\pi\sigma} \frac{1}{a^3} k(k+1) \left(\frac{d}{a}\right)^{k-1} \frac{2}{2k+1} - + c_k k a^{k-1} \frac{2}{2k+1} = 0 \tag{2.149}$$

From this expression the expansion coefficients c_k can be computed easily. Note that, for didactic reasons, the norms of the Legendre polynomials are included in (2.149), but in fact drop out of the equation. Moreover, for $k = 0$ the equation does not yield a value for c_k. For other values of k we find

$$c_k = \frac{D_z}{4\pi\sigma}(k+1)\frac{d^{k-1}}{a^{2a+1}}.\tag{2.150}$$

Substitution of this result in (2.147) then yields as the final solution for the potential field for $d < r \le a$:

$$\Phi(r,\theta) = \frac{D_z}{4\pi\sigma r^2}\sum_{k=1}^{\infty}k\left(\frac{d}{r}\right)^{k-1}P_k(\mu) + \frac{D_z}{4\pi\sigma r^2}\sum_{k=1}^{\infty}(k+1)\left(\frac{d}{r}\right)^{k-1}\left(\frac{r}{a}\right)^{k+2}P_k(\mu)\tag{2.151}$$

2.6.3.3 Discussion

The relatively simple configuration of ❷ Sect. 2.6.3.2 provides a suitable means for illustrating some basic consequences of the bounded nature of a volume conductor, as is worked out in the sequel. As indicated, (2.151) holds true in the domain $d < r \le a$. For the remaining part of the sphere, $r < d$, the potential field may be found using the same procedure as in ❷ Sect. 2.6.3.2, but now using the Taylor expansion valid for this region as shown in the second part of (2.144). The computation of the complete potential field generated by the tangential dipole component may be carried out in a similar way.

Notes:

1. In (2.151), the first expression on the right represents the infinite medium potential, while the second represents the effect of the sphere being bounded. This second term may be interpreted as the field arising from a virtual, secondary source placed in an infinite medium. Its magnitude depends linearly on that of the primary source. The nature of the secondary source may be diverse. A potential field inside the sphere having the required nature may be generated by a virtual dipole having an appropriate position and strength, a monolayer at the interface or a double layer at the interface.

2. The contribution of the secondary source tends to zero if the boundary is distal, i.e., if $a \gg r$, due to the factor $(r/a)^{k+2}$. As a consequence, the potential field observed at a distance to the source that is small relative to the distance to the boundary tends to the infinite medium potential; for the interpretation of observed potentials at this field point, the boundary effects may be neglected.

3. For observation points on the spherical boundary, $r = a$, (2.151) reduces to

$$\Phi(r,\theta) = \frac{D_z}{4\pi\sigma a^2}\sum_{k=1}^{\infty}(2k+1)\left(\frac{d}{a}\right)^{k-1}P_k(\mu)\tag{2.152}$$

For a dipole located at the center of the sphere $(d \to 0)$, the only remaining term in the summation is the one for $k = 1$. This leaves

$$\Phi(r,\theta) = 3\frac{D_z}{4\pi\sigma a^2}\cos\theta,\tag{2.153}$$

since, (2.137), $P_1(\mu) = \mu = \cos\theta$. This demonstrates that for a dipolar source placed at the center of a spherical surface, the effect of bounding the sphere produces a potential field on the spherical boundary that is threefold that of the infinite medium potential. For source locations close to the spherical surface, the effect of bounding the medium is less, tending to the factor 2 (2.133) for a planar boundary. For an arbitrary bound, the factor may be expected to lie within these two limits, 2 and 3.

4. While evaluating the expansion coefficients c_k, (2.150) no value could be identified for $k = 0$. The Legendre polynomial for $k = 0$, (2.137), $P_0(\mu) = 1$. This leaves the mean value of the potential field undetermined. The potential field (2.151) has an implicit zero mean of the potential over the boundary, as a consequence of excluding a term for $k = 0$ and the orthogonality of the Legendre polynomials.

5. The mean level of the potential is unrelated to the impressed current density, as was discussed in ❯ Sect. 2.5.1.1. For a bounded medium the location in space as a reference for measured potential difference cannot be chosen at infinity, but must be selected somewhere on, or inside, the boundary. The selection of this location may be guided by practical considerations. However, contrary to a frequently encountered belief, no universal, theoretical optimum exists [14, 15].

2.6.4 Realistically Shaped Interfaces; The Boundary Element Method

Although the inclusion of spherical bounds or interfaces, like the basic version treated in ❯ Sect. 2.6.3, are more realistic than the one treated in ❯ Sect. 2.6.2, they still only poorly resemble the shapes of the interfaces of the most prominent inhomogeneities, such as the torso boundary, the high conductivity of blood, or the low conductivity of lung tissue.

For the treatment of volume conduction effects involving such shapes, analytical methods of the type described in the previous section are not available. Instead, several numerical methods have been developed over the past few decades. The most prominent are the finite difference method (FDM), the finite element method (FEM), the finite volume method (FVM), and the boundary element method (BEM). The BEM lacks the possibility of treating situations involving anisotropic electric conductivity that some of the other methods have but its conceptual relevance is higher. It is for this reason that this topic is treated in this chapter. The other methods (FDM, FEM, and FVM) are discussed in ❯ Chap. 8. The BEM is based on formulations described by in 1939 by Smythe [10].

2.6.4.1 Mathematical Preliminaries

The mathematics involved in the theory of the BEM uses some specific results from the field of vector calculus. To make this section self-contained, these results are listed here. As in ❯ Sect. 2.2.2, all specific conditions required are assumed to be satisfied. Dedicated proofs can be found in the standard references listed at the end of this chapter. Throughout, in the scalar function 1/R, R denotes the length of the vector $\vec{R} = \vec{r}' - \vec{r}$ pointing from (source) point $\vec{r}$ to (field) point $\vec{r}'$ (compare ❯ Sect. 2.2.10), $\vec{A}$ is a vector field, Ψ and Φ are arbitrary scalar functions.

- For vector field $\vec{A}$ within a volume closed by a boundary S

$$\int_V \nabla \bullet \vec{A} dV = \int_S \vec{A} \bullet d\vec{S} \quad \text{(Gauss' divergence theorem; (2.26))} \tag{2.154}$$

$$\nabla^2 \frac{1}{R} = -4\pi\delta(\vec{r}',\vec{r}) = \nabla'^2 \frac{1}{R} \tag{2.155}$$

This is the result that is most specific for this section. The function $\delta(\vec{r}',\vec{r})$ is the 3D Dirac delta function. It is a so-called distribution function, defined through the properties of a volume integral over a volume V of its product with a scalar function $f(\vec{r})$. The defining equations are

$$\int_V \delta(\vec{r}',\vec{r})f(\vec{r})dV = 0 \quad \text{if V does not encompass } \vec{r}', \tag{2.156}$$

$$\text{else,} \quad \int_V \delta(\vec{r}',\vec{r})f(\vec{r})dV = f(\vec{r}') \tag{2.157}$$

Note that this definition implies that $\int_V \delta(\vec{r}',\vec{r})dV = 1$ and, hence, its unit is m^{-3}.

- Application of Gauss' theorem to $\vec{A} = \Psi\nabla\Phi$ yields

$$\int_V \nabla \bullet \Psi\nabla\Phi dV = \int_V \nabla\Psi \bullet \nabla\Phi dV + \int_V \Psi\nabla^2\Phi dV = \int_S \Psi\nabla\Phi \bullet d\vec{S} \tag{2.158}$$

This result is known as Green's first theorem.

- Correspondingly, by exchanging Ψ and Φ, we have

$$\int_V \nabla \bullet \Phi \nabla \Psi \, dV = \int_V \nabla \Phi \bullet \nabla \Psi \, dV + \int_V \Phi \nabla^2 \Psi \, dV = \int_S \Phi \nabla \Psi \bullet d\vec{S} \qquad (2.159)$$

- Finally, by subtracting second equation in (2.158) from the corresponding part of (2.159), we see that

$$\int_V \Phi \nabla^2 \Psi \, dV - \int_V \Psi \nabla^2 \Phi \, dV = \int_S \Phi \nabla \Psi \bullet d\vec{S} - \int_S \Psi \nabla \Phi \bullet d\vec{S} \qquad (2.160)$$

This result is known as Green's second theorem.

2.6.4.2 Equivalent Surface Sources

The BEM is based on the use of equivalent surface sources [10, 16–18]. To introduce this, we first consider the source–volume–conductor configuration shown in ❷ Fig. 2.15. It depicts a volume segment bounded by a closed surface S. Its interior has uniform conductivity σ and contains a primary, impressed current source (dotted region). Its exterior is left unspecified: it may or may not contain primary sources and may or may not have the same conductivity.

Starting point for the theory described here is Green's second theorem, (2.160), in which we substitute $\Psi = \frac{1}{R}, \vec{R} = \vec{r}' - \vec{r}$ pointing from (source) point $\vec{r}$ to (field) point $\vec{r}'$ as before, and take for Φ the potential field inside S, which leads to

$$\int_V \Phi \nabla^2 \frac{1}{R} \, dV - \int_V \frac{1}{R} \nabla^2 \Phi \, dV = \int_S \Phi \nabla \frac{1}{R} \bullet d\vec{S} - \int_S \frac{1}{R} \nabla \Phi \bullet d\vec{S} \qquad (2.161)$$

All integrations are carried out with respect to the unprimed variable $\vec{r}$, and $d\vec{S}$ is the local outward normal of S. The four integrals shown are worked out as follows.

Based on (2.155) and (2.157), the first one is found to be equal to $-4\pi \Phi(\vec{r}')$. The second integral equals $-4\pi \Phi_\infty(\vec{r}')$, the potential field generated by the primary sources inside S when placed in an infinite medium having a conductivity σ. This follows from (2.116). The third integral may be written as $\int_S \Phi(\vec{r}) \, d\omega$, with $d\omega$ the solid angle subtended by $d\vec{S}$ at $\vec{r}'$ (combine (2.63) and (2.33)). Note that for $\vec{r}$ on S, as is the case for this integral and $\vec{r}'$ an interior point of surface S, $\vec{R}$ is pointing inward and consequently the sign of $d\omega$ is negative. Finally, in the fourth integral $\nabla \Phi \bullet d\vec{S}$ is equal to $-E_n dS$, with E_n the normal component of the electric field at $\vec{r}$ on S. For the latter, by using (2.84), we may write $E_n(\vec{r}) = J_n(\vec{r})/\sigma$, with $J_n(\vec{r})$ the normal component of the current density passing the surface S at $\vec{r}$.

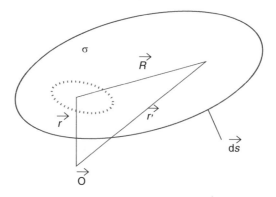

❏ Fig. 2.15
A part of space, delineated by a surface S, with uniform conductivity σ. Primary current sources are located in the region surrounding $\vec{r}$. The field point is $\vec{r}'$, $\vec{R} = \vec{r}' - \vec{r}$

Substitution of the above expressions for the four integrals of (2.161), followed by a reordering of the terms, results in the following, fundamental expression

$$\Phi(\vec{r}') = \Phi_\infty(\vec{r}') - \frac{1}{4\pi} \int_S \Phi(\vec{r}) d\omega(\vec{r}', \vec{r}) - \frac{1}{4\pi\sigma} \int_S \frac{J_n(\vec{r})}{R(\vec{r}', \vec{r})} dS(\vec{r}) \tag{2.162}$$

It signifies that at any point inside any volume V with homogeneous conductivity σ, bounded by a surface S, the potential field can be expressed as the sum of the local infinite medium potential, a weighted sum (integral) of the potentials $\Phi(\vec{r})$ at S, and a weighted sum (integral) of the normal component of the current density $J_n(\vec{r})$ passing surface S.

The two additions represent the effect of the conditions in the external domain: the effects of any primary sources present in that domain and/or differences of the electric conductivity with respect to the internal, homogeneous value σ. Based on the results from ❷ Sect. 2.5.2, the first of these contributions may be interpreted as arising from a virtual double layer source, (2.107), the second one as a virtual mono layer source, (2.101), both located at S.

2.6.4.3 Application to Homogeneous, Bounded Volume Conductors

The results of the previous subsection facilitate the introduction of the BEM for evaluating the effect of bounds on the electric conductivity having an arbitrary shape. To this end, we reconsider the same situation as depicted in ❷ Fig. 2.15, now taking the part of space exterior of S to be nonconducting. This being the case, no current will pass S and (2.162) reduces to

$$\Phi(\vec{r}') = \Phi_\infty(\vec{r}') - \frac{1}{4\pi} \int_S \Phi(\vec{r}) d\omega(\vec{r}', \vec{r}) \tag{2.163}$$

In this expression, $\Phi(\vec{r})$ represents the potential field at S in the bounded state, which needs to be known before the potential at an arbitrary internal point can be computed. To find $\Phi(\vec{r})$, the field point $\vec{r}'$ is moved toward S. While assuming no primary current sources close to S, the potential field $\Phi(\vec{r}')$ is continuous, and in the limit of approaching S we have $\Phi(\vec{r}) = \Phi(\vec{r}')$. Expression $d\omega(\vec{r}', \vec{r}) = \vec{R} \cdot d\vec{S}/R^3$ requires special attention, since both numerator and denominator approach zero when $\vec{r}'$ approaches $\vec{r}$. Its value may be found by taking an appropriate limit L. For a (locally) planar surface its value is $L = -2\pi$, in which 2π is the solid angle subtended by a planar semi-space and the minus sign stems from the fact that locally, $\vec{R}$ and $d\vec{S}$ point in opposite directions. In numerical computations based on (2.163), the surface S is approximated by a large number of small triangles. In early applications, the field points $\vec{r}'$ were situated at the centers of gravity of these triangles, in which case $L = -2\pi$ for all field points (on S). In this case (2.163) may be formulated as

$$\Phi(\vec{r}') = \Phi_\infty(\vec{r}') - \frac{1}{4\pi} \oint_S \Phi(\vec{r}) d\omega(\vec{r}', \vec{r}) - \frac{-2\pi}{4\pi} \Phi(\vec{r}'), \tag{2.164}$$

in which the integration excludes the small region dS around $\vec{r}' = \vec{r}$, yielding

$$\Phi(\vec{r}') = 2\Phi_\infty(\vec{r}') - \frac{1}{2\pi} \oint_S \Phi(\vec{r}) d\omega(\vec{r}', \vec{r}) \tag{2.165}$$

In numerical implementations in which the field points are formed by the triangle vertices, the absolute value of $L = L(\vec{r})$ depends on the local curvature of S. For locally convex surface patches (as seen from the outside) it is less than 2π, while for concave surface patches it is greater than 2π.

Numerical Implementation

For each of N observation points on S, the numerical handling of (2.165) leads to a linear equation in the unknown values $\varphi_n = \Phi(\vec{r}_n')$, $n = 1, 2 \ldots N$. The total set of N equations in the N unknown φ_n values can be solved by computer implementations of the appropriate methods of linear algebra. The solution found is unique only up to a constant, corresponding to the physics of the problem. It requires the specification of a point of the medium acting as a potential reference to make the solution unique, just like when measuring bioelectric potentials. This point may be chosen at will. The outcome of the entire procedure for determining all elements φ_n of a N-dimensional numerical vector φ may be formulated as a matrix multiplication of the (numerical) vector φ_∞ by a transfer matrix, say $\mathbf{A}$, constituting a numerically determined set of weighting coefficients, representing the effect of all volume conductor effects (inhomogeneities and bounds of the volume conductor) [19]

$$\varphi = \mathbf{A}\varphi_\infty \tag{2.166}$$

The matrix $\mathbf{A}$ is a linear operator acting on the infinite medium potentials.

The computation of the involved elementary solid angles $d\omega(\vec{r}',\vec{r})$ can be approximated using a discretized representation of the surfaces involved, based on small triangular elements. Analytical expressions for the basic, required computations are available in [20, 21].

Discussion

The method described above constitutes the essence of the BEM. Frequently, the interest lies in determining the potentials on the bounding surface only. The determination of the elements of the transfer matrix constitutes the most elaborate part of the BEM. However, once the potential $\Phi(\vec{r})$ on S has been determined, the potential field at any interior point can be found by means of (2.163).

For several applications, it is of particular significance, and a pronounced advantage of the BEM over some of the other methods such as the FEM, that the transfer matrix $\mathbf{A}$ depends on the geometry of S only. Hence, when considering a set of different locations of the source points, the most elaborate part of the procedure, the computation of $\mathbf{A}$, needs to be carried out only once, which greatly facilitates inverse procedures [22].

As discussed in ❯ Sect. 2.6.4.3, based on the results from ❯ Sect. 2.5.2, the integral in (2.163) may be interpreted as representing the contribution from a virtual double layer source at S. This is specific for the variant of the BEM described here. An alternative BEM approach has been formulated in which the virtual source of S is a monolayer. This was in fact the case in the very first application of the BEM in electrocardiography [18].

2.6.4.4 Application of the BEM to Inhomogeneous Volume Conductors

The BEM can be extended to the handling of the effect of internal regions of the volume conductor having a different, homogenous conductivity. This is worked out here in some detail for an application to a single inhomogeneous region inside a bounded volume conductor. The generalization for multiple inhomogeneous regions is straightforward.

The starting point for the theory described here is once more Green's second theorem, (2.160).

We apply it separately to the subregions I and II illustrated in ❯ Fig. 2.16. Subregion I has conductivity σ_1 and is bounded by surfaces S_1 and S_2. It is assumed to contain primary sources. Subregion II is bounded by S_2, has conductivity σ_2 and is assumed to be source free.

For subregion I, with both the integration variable $\vec{r}$ and the field point lying within subregion I, (2.161),

$$\Phi_I(\vec{r}') = \Phi_{I,\infty}(\vec{r}') - \frac{1}{4\pi}\int_{S_1}\Phi(\vec{r})d\omega(\vec{r}',\vec{r}) + \frac{1}{4\pi}\int_{S_2}\Phi(\vec{r})d\omega(\vec{r}',\vec{r}) + \frac{1}{4\pi\sigma_1}\int_{S_2}\frac{J_n(\vec{r})}{R(\vec{r}',\vec{r})}dS(\vec{r}) \tag{2.167}$$

The first term on the right represents the potential generated by the primary sources in an infinite medium having the conductivity of the source region, which will be referred to as σ_s. In the case illustrated, this conductivity is $\sigma_s = \sigma_1$. The third term on the right stems from the fact that the subregion is bounded by both S_1 and S_2. The difference in sign compared with the corresponding term for S_1 stems from the fact that the outward normal of region I at S_2 is the reverse of the outward normal of region II at S_2. The latter also explains the sign of the final term involving the current density across S_2. This term is clearly nonzero, since the conductivity of region II is nonzero.

Next, we leave the field point within subregion I, while applying Green's second theorem to region II.

$$\int_{V_{II}}\Phi\nabla^2\frac{1}{R}dV - \int_{V_{II}}\frac{1}{R}\nabla^2\Phi dV = \int_{S_2}\Phi\nabla\frac{1}{R}\bullet d\vec{S} - \int_{S_2}\frac{1}{R}\nabla\Phi\bullet d\vec{S} \tag{2.168}$$

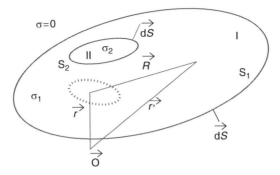

◻ Fig. 2.16

Volume conductor. Region I is bounded by surfaces S_1 and S_2, with uniform conductivity σ_1. Internal region II is bounded by S_2, with uniform conductivity σ_2. Primary current sources are located within region I, around arbitrary point $\vec{r}$ of region I. Field point $\vec{r}'$ is also shown in region I, with $\vec{R} = \vec{r}' - \vec{r}$

The first integral on the left is zero since $\vec{r}'$ is exterior to subregion I ((2.156) and (2.155)). The second integral is also zero since there are no primary sources within subregion II: $\nabla^2 \Phi = 0$. Hence, as was the case when deriving (2.162), we now have

$$0 = -\frac{1}{4\pi} \int_{S_2} \Phi(\vec{r}) d\omega(\vec{r}', \vec{r}) - \frac{1}{4\pi\sigma_2} \int_{S_2} \frac{J_n(\vec{r})}{R(\vec{r}', \vec{r})} dS(\vec{r}) \tag{2.169}$$

By comparing (2.167) and (2.169) it can be seen that the integrals involving $J_n(\vec{r})$ are identical: both represent the current density across S_2. As a consequence these integrals will be eliminated by multiplying (2.167) by σ_1, and multiplying (2.169) by σ_2, followed by the addition of both equations. After rearranging the terms of this addition and dividing the result by σ_1, the following expression is found for $\Phi_I(\vec{r}')$, the potential field inside subregion I.

$$\Phi_I(\vec{r}') = \frac{\sigma_s}{\sigma_1} \Phi_{I,\infty}(\vec{r}') - \frac{1}{4\pi} \int_{S_1} \Phi(\vec{r}) d\omega(\vec{r}', \vec{r}) - \frac{1}{4\pi} \frac{\sigma_2 - \sigma_1}{\sigma_1} \int_{S_2} \Phi(\vec{r}) d\omega(\vec{r}', \vec{r}) \tag{2.170}$$

Besides the infinite medium contribution of the primary sources, the expression shows two virtual double layer sources, one for each of the surfaces that form the border of subregion I. Note that for $\sigma_1 = \sigma_2$, the contribution of the final term is zero, as required. The factor σ_s/σ_1 in the first term on the right, a factor equal to one in the current example, arises when the primary sources are present in a subregion different to the one where the potential field is evaluated.

When the field point $\vec{r}'$ is located in subregion II, the same method as shown above may be used to find the potential field. The result is

$$\Phi_{II}(\vec{r}') = \frac{\sigma_s}{\sigma_2} \Phi_{II,\infty}(\vec{r}') - \frac{1}{4\pi} \int_{S_1} \Phi(\vec{r}) d\omega(\vec{r}', \vec{r}) - \frac{1}{4\pi} \frac{\sigma_2 - \sigma_1}{\sigma_2} \int_{S_2} \Phi(\vec{r}) d\omega(\vec{r}', \vec{r}), \tag{2.171}$$

which, apart from a different scaling factor, is the same as (2.170). However, note that all solid angle terms, the factors weighting the equivalent double layer strengths, are different because of the different location of field point $\vec{r}'$.

If K, possibly nested, subregions are present within the bounded volume conductor, the potential field within any subregion k, a generalization of (2.170) and (2.171) can be formulated as

$$\Phi_k(\vec{r}') = \frac{\sigma_s}{\sigma_k^-} \Phi_{k,\infty}(\vec{r}') - \frac{1}{4\pi} \sum_{\ell=1}^{K} \frac{\sigma_\ell^- - \sigma_\ell^+}{\sigma_k^-} \int_{S_\ell} \Phi_\ell(\vec{r}) d\omega(\vec{r}', \vec{r}), \tag{2.172}$$

in which subregion k is defined by the label of its outermost interface, where σ_ℓ^+ is the conductivity just outside the interface ℓ and σ_ℓ^- is the conductivity just inside. If $k = 1$ is the surface encompassing the entire medium, and if its exterior is nonconducting, then $\sigma_1^+ = 0$.

Discussion

Equation (2.172) constitutes the essence of the BEM. It expresses the potential field in any number of inhomogeneous subregions as the sum of the contributions to the potential inside a virtual infinite medium of (a scaled version of) the impressed primary sources and those of virtual double layer sources at each of the interfaces bounding the subregions. The strength of these secondary sources is small if the differences between conductivity values at both sides of an interface are small.

In a practical application (2.172) can only be used if the potentials $\Phi_\ell(\vec{r})$ at the interfaces are known. These may be computed numerically in the same manner as discussed in the previous subsection for the single interface problem.

2.6.4.5   The BEM Used To Compute Potentials On The Heart Surface

The final demonstration of the use of the BEM discussed here is its application to the computation of the transfer between potentials on the heart surface and the potentials on the body surface. The inverse of this transfer function is the key element for the computation of potentials on the heart surface from observed body surface potentials. This topic is discussed in ❯ Chap. 9. The methods are based on the fact that if no primary sources are present within a volume conductor bounded by a surface S_1 and an internal *closed* region S_1 the potential fields on these surfaces are linked in a unique manner. The medium in between may contain different subregions having a different conductivity. The treatment presented here considers just S_1 representing the body surface, and the surface S_2, representing a surface closely encompassing the heart. This surface is usually referred to as the epicardium, but its identification with the pericardium is more appropriate.

The volume conductor of the problem addressed is shown in ❯ Fig. 2.17. The transfer can be computed on the basis of (2.167), which describes the field in subregion I. Since there are no primary sources in this subregion, this equation reduces to

$$\Phi(\vec{r}') = -\frac{1}{4\pi}\int_{S_1}\Phi_1(\vec{r})d\omega(\vec{r}',\vec{r}) + \frac{1}{4\pi}\int_{S_2}\Phi_2(\vec{r})d\omega(\vec{r}',\vec{r}) + \frac{1}{4\pi\sigma_1}\int_{S_2}\frac{J_n(\vec{r})}{R(\vec{r}',\vec{r})}dS(\vec{r}) \qquad (2.173)$$

In the computation of the forward transfer, the potential field $\Phi_2(\vec{r})$ on S_2 is assumed to be known. This leaves $\Phi_1(\vec{r})$, the potential on S_1, as well as the current density $J_n(\vec{r})$ at S_2, to be determined. As in the preceding subsections the numerical approximation of these functions is carried out by placing field points on S_1 and S_2. For N_1 points placed on S_1 and M_2 points placed on S_2 this results in a system of $N_1 + M_2$ linear equations in the unknown variables φ_n and J_m. The system has a unique solution for any set of assumed values φ_m on S_2. The indeterminacy of the potential that needed to be addressed in the ❯ Sect. 2.6.3.3 is not present here, since the specified φ_m values implicitly define the mean level of the potential [23]. The application of these types of numerical methods is discussed in ❯ Chap. 8 (❯ Sect. 8.5.4).

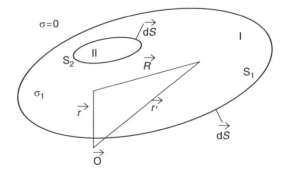

◘ Fig. 2.17

Volume conductor. Region I is bounded by surfaces S_1 and S_2, with uniform conductivity σ_1 Internal region II, bounded by S_2, contains primary sources, conductivity unspecified. No primary current sources are present within region I; $\vec{r}$ is an arbitrary point of region I. Field point $\vec{r}'$ is restricted to region I, with $\vec{R} = \vec{r}' - \vec{r}$

Appendix A   Tools from Linear Algebra and Their Notation

A.1   Introduction

In some chapters of this book, notations and methods are used that are taken from linear algebra. These are the basic tools involved in the numerical computation of potential fields (❯ Chap. 2): the forward problem (❯ Chap. 8) and in particular for solving various variants of the inverse problem (❯ Chap. 9). This appendix introduces some of the basic concepts. For a formal, more complete treatment the reader is referred to the general literature on linear algebra and its numerical implementation. Highly valuable examples are: [24–27]. Specific variants of vectors and matrices, as well as of various definitions and notations used are listed in ❯ Sect. A.5.

A.1.1   Vectors

In ❯ Sect. 2.2, the vector concept is introduced in its application to 3D space. Any vector $\vec{A}$ can be seen to be characterized by three elements, A_x, A_y, and A_z (❯ Sect. 2.2.3). Addition and multiplication rules are treated in ❯ Sects. 2.2.3–2.2.4. In linear algebra these concepts have been generalized by introducing variables that are specified by the values of an arbitrary number of elements. Different types of notations for such "numerical" vectors can be found in the literature. Here introduced are the notations used throughout this book.

In the sequel, the term "vector" will refer to a variable that is specified by a set of numbers being its elements. These elements may either be listed in a single row or in a single column. In the latter situation, a vector is referred to as a column vector, which is denoted by a bold lower case symbol. For vector **a** with m elements we have

$$\mathbf{a} = \begin{bmatrix} a_1 \\ a_2 \\ \cdot \\ \cdot \\ a_m \end{bmatrix} \tag{A.1}$$

The listing of the values of the complete set of elements of a column vector may demand much space. A more economical way is to listing the same values in a row. Accordingly, **a** may also be defined by its "transpose": $\mathbf{a}^T$, defined as

$$\mathbf{a}^T = \begin{bmatrix} a_1 & a_2 & \cdot & \cdot & a_m \end{bmatrix}, \tag{A.2}$$

which is called a row vector. The notation ^{T}, signifies "transpose", a term that is clarified in ❯ Sect. A.1.3.

In analogy with vectors in 3D space, a numerical vector having m elements is called an m-dimensional vector. Note that for $m = 1$ the vector reduces to a scalar.

There is a particular role for vectors comprising zero elements only. Such vectors are called zero vectors (❯ Sect. A.5).

A.1.2   Basic Vector Algebra

A.1.2.1   Vector Addition

The familiar rules of addition that apply to "ordinary," i.e., scalar, variables can be extended to vectors by defining that these rules be applied to all corresponding elements. Applied to vectors **a** and **b** demands that both vectors have the same number of elements, and that the elements s_i, $i = 1, \cdots, m$ of the sum vector **s**:

$$\mathbf{s} = \mathbf{a} + \mathbf{b} \tag{A.3}$$

be $s_i = a_i + b_i$.

A.1.2.2 Vector Multiplication

The most elementary version of multiplication involving vectors is the one in which a vector is multiplied by a scalar. The elements of vector $\mathbf{a}$ after multiplication by a scalar c is carried out by multiplying all elements a_i of $\mathbf{a}$ by the scalar, which implies a uniform scaling of the elements by c. As a consequence we have

$$c\,\mathbf{a} = \mathbf{a}\,c. \tag{A.4}$$

Note that a combination of the definition of vector addition and scalar multiplication with $c = -1$ also defines the subtraction of vectors:

$$\mathbf{v} = \mathbf{a} - \mathbf{b} = \mathbf{a} + (-1)\mathbf{b}. \tag{A.5}$$

All these properties can be seen to be straightforward generalizations of those defined in ❷ Sect. 2.2.2 for the vectors in 3D space. In a similar fashion to what is shown in ❷ Sect. 2.2.4, the scalar product of two vectors $\mathbf{a}$ and $\mathbf{b}$ is the scalar d that is the outcome of the pair-wise multiplication of their elements, followed by the summation of the resulting products:

$$d = \sum_{i=1}^{m} a_i b_i = \mathbf{a}^T\,\mathbf{b} = \mathbf{b}^T\,\mathbf{a}. \tag{A.6}$$

The significance of the notation $\mathbf{a}^T\mathbf{b}$ is explained in the next section.

If the product of two vectors is zero the vectors are said to be orthogonal, analogous to the definition in ❷ Sect. 2.2.4. The generalization of the magnitude of a 3D vector (❷ Sect. 2.2.3) leads to the definition of the "norm" of a vector as:

$$|\mathbf{a}| = \sqrt{\mathbf{a}^T\mathbf{a}}. \tag{A.7}$$

It is interesting to note that even the concept of the angle between two vectors in 3D space (❷ Sect. 2.2.2) can be carried over to two vectors in n-dimensional space, an angle that is computed as

$$\alpha = \mathrm{acos}\left(\frac{\mathbf{a}^T\mathbf{b}}{|\mathbf{a}|\,|\mathbf{b}|}\right). \tag{A.8}$$

A.1.3 Matrices

Many numerical methods lead to a problem formulation involving a collection of several, say n, column vectors of dimension m. This collection is called a matrix. In the sequel, bold face capitals are used to denote matrices. Matrix $\mathbf{A}$, with elements $a_{i,j}$, $i = 1, \cdots, m; j = 1, \cdots, n$, can be visualized as

$$\mathbf{A} = \begin{bmatrix} a_{1,1} & a_{1,2} & \cdots & a_{1,j} & \cdots & a_{1,n} \\ . & . & \cdots & . & \cdots & . \\ a_{i,1} & a_{i,2} & \cdots & a_{i,j} & \cdots & a_{i,n} \\ . & \cdots & \cdots & . & \cdots & . \\ a_{m,1} & a_{m,2} & \cdots & a_{m,j} & \cdots & a_{m,n} \end{bmatrix} \tag{A.9}$$

There are $m \times n$ elements in the above matrix; its size is defined as (m, n). If $m = n$ the matrix is called "square."

Next to any matrix $\mathbf{A}$ of size (m, n) there is a corresponding one, the transposed matrix $\mathbf{A}^T$ of size (n, m). Its elements are the elements $a_{j,i}$ of $\mathbf{A}$.

If, in matrix $\mathbf{A}$, $n = 1$, the matrix reduces to a single column. Thus, an m-dimensional column vector may be viewed as a matrix of size $(m, 1)$. Similarly, a row vector having n elements may be viewed as a matrix of size $(1, n)$. The notation $\mathbf{a}^T$ introduced for a row vector paves the way for a unified formalism for multiplications involving matrices, vectors, or both.

Definitions of specific matrices and their properties are listed in ❷ Sect. A.5.

A.1.3.1   Matrix Addition

As explained for vectors, the familiar rules of addition that apply to "ordinary," i.e., scalar, variables can be extended to matrices by demanding that these rules be applied to all corresponding elements. Applied to vectors $\mathbf{A}$ and $\mathbf{B}$ this requires that both matrices be of the same size and that the elements $s_{i,j}$, $i = 1, \cdots, m$; $j = 1 \cdots, n$, of the sum $\mathbf{S}$:

$$\mathbf{S} = \mathbf{A} + \mathbf{B} \qquad (A.10)$$

be $s_{i,j} = a_{i,j} + b_{i,j}$.

A.1.3.2   Multiplication and Matrices

The most elementary version of multiplication involving matrices is the one in which a matrix is multiplied by a scalar. As worked out for the vector, multiplication by a scalar c is carried out by multiplying all elements $a_{i,j}$ of $\mathbf{A}$ by c. This also defines the difference of two matrices, as shown for the vector.

The most important, basic multiplication of two matrices is defined as follows. Let $\mathbf{A}$ be a matrix of size (m, n) and $\mathbf{B}$ a matrix of size (n, p), then their product is defined as the matrix $\mathbf{C}$ of size(m, p):

$$\mathbf{C} = \mathbf{AB} \qquad (A.11)$$

having elements

$$c_{i,\ell} = \sum_{j=1}^{n} a_{i,j} b_{j,\ell}. \qquad (A.12)$$

Note that this definition demands that the number of columns of $\mathbf{A}$ be the same as the number of rows of $\mathbf{B}$. It is only if this condition is satisfied that this type of matrix multiplication is meaningful.

Contrary to the multiplication rules for scalars, this matrix multiplication does not have the property of commutativity, i.e., generally,

$$\mathbf{AB} \neq \mathbf{BA}. \qquad (A.13)$$

This can be seen most easily by comparing the multiplication of $\mathbf{A}$ specified by row vector [1 2 3] and $\mathbf{B}$ a column vector specified by its transpose: [1 0 −2]. By applying the rules of matrix multiplication (A.12) we see that

$$\mathbf{AB} = \begin{bmatrix} 1 & 2 & 3 \end{bmatrix} \begin{bmatrix} 1 \\ 0 \\ -2 \end{bmatrix} = -5. \qquad (A.14)$$

In contrast,

$$\mathbf{BA} = \begin{bmatrix} 1 \\ 0 \\ -2 \end{bmatrix} \begin{bmatrix} 1 & 2 & 3 \end{bmatrix} = \begin{bmatrix} 1 & 2 & 3 \\ 0 & 0 & 0 \\ -2 & -4 & -6 \end{bmatrix}. \qquad (A.15)$$

Another basic property of matrix multiplication is

$$(\mathbf{AB})^T = \mathbf{B}^T \mathbf{A}^T, \qquad (A.16)$$

as can be verified from the definition of "transpose" and the rule of matrix multiplication (A.12).

linearity

By combining the properties of matrix addition and multiplication it follows that

$$\mathbf{A}(\mathbf{B} + \mathbf{C}) = \mathbf{AB} + \mathbf{AC}, \tag{A.17}$$

expressing the associatative law of matrix multiplication. The full set of definitions given identifies matrix multiplication as a so-called linear operation.

The rank of a matrix, denoted as $rank(\mathbf{A}) = r \le \min(m, n)$, is the maximum number of independent columns or rows it comprises. For the product of two matrices $\mathbf{A}$ and $\mathbf{B}$ we have [24]

$$rank(\mathbf{AB}) = \min(rank(\mathbf{A}), rank(\mathbf{B})). \tag{A.18}$$

A.2   Solving Linear Equations: the Problem Definition

The basic problems that require the use of linear algebra for their solution can be formulated as: find $\mathbf{x}$ that satisfies the matrix equation

$$\mathbf{y} = \mathbf{Ax} + \mathbf{n}. \tag{A.19}$$

The symbols denote

$\mathbf{y}$, a column vector, of size $(m, 1)$ representing known or observed variables

$\mathbf{A}$, a matrix, of size (m, n) usually representing a model based transfer

$\mathbf{x}$, a column vector, either directly representing a signal or its parameters

$\mathbf{n}$, a column vector, size$(m, 1)$, usually referred to as noise. It represents any   In some applications, a set of t column
   uncertainties in the problem formulation or measurement errors.

As a consequence, it is an unknown vector, but its statistical properties may be known.

Vectors (multiple realizations) $\mathbf{y}$ and $\mathbf{n}$ are available and the problem to be solved is: find matrix $\mathbf{X}$ that satisfies the equation

$$\mathbf{Y} = \mathbf{AX} + \mathbf{N} \tag{A.20}$$

involving matrices with

$size(\mathbf{Y}) = (m, t)$

$size(\mathbf{X}) = (n, t)$

$size(\mathbf{N}) = (m, t)$, and

$size(\mathbf{A}) = (m, n)$ as in (A.19)

In the practice of analyzing observed data there is generally no exact solution to the so-called linear systems (A.19) or (A.20). Instead, the true solutions are replaced by estimates, $\widehat{\mathbf{x}}$ for (A.19), computed such that the difference between both sides of the equation is as small as possible. The next section introduces this approach.

A.3   Solution Types

The problem formulation as outlined in ❷ Sect. A.2 leads to two essentially different types of solutions. These are discussed here for the basic variant of the problem formulation (A.19) with $\mathbf{n} = \mathbf{0}$.

A.3.1   True Solutions

The basic variant of the problem formulation (A.19) reads as

$$\mathbf{y} = \mathbf{Ax}, \tag{A.21}$$

with $\mathbf{A}$ a matrix of size (m, n) and rank r. This system of equations may, or may not have a solution. Three different situations can be distinguished.

- There is no solution. This is the case when the vector products of all possible vectors $\mathbf{Ax}$ and $\mathbf{y}$ are nonzero. An equivalent statement of this condition is $rank([\mathbf{y}\,\mathbf{A}]) > rank(\mathbf{A})$.
- There is a single, unique solution. This is the case when $rank([\mathbf{y}\,\mathbf{A}]) = rank(\mathbf{A})$ and $rank(\mathbf{A}) = r = n$.
- A multitude of different solutions exists. This is the case when $rank([\mathbf{y}\,\mathbf{A}]) = rank(\mathbf{A})$ and $r < n$. This follows from the definition of the rank of a matrix: $r < n$ signifies that there exist nonzero vectors $\mathbf{z}$ such that $\mathbf{Az} = \mathbf{0}$. Thus, if $\mathbf{x}$ is a solution to $\mathbf{Ax} = \mathbf{y}$ then $\mathbf{A}(\mathbf{x} + \mathbf{z}) = \mathbf{y}$, which indicates that $\mathbf{x} + \mathbf{z}$ is also a solution. A matrix for which $r < n$ is called a rank-deficient matrix.

If the system has a solution it is called consistent, otherwise it is called inconsistent.

In linear algebra the treatment of (A.21) is usually restricted to square versions of $\mathbf{A}$. If $r = n$, a unique solution exists, but for this situation only, which can be denoted as

$$\mathbf{x} = \mathbf{A}^{-1}\mathbf{y}, \tag{A.22}$$

with $\mathbf{A}^{-1}$ denoting the inverse of matrix $\mathbf{A}$. Note that under these conditions the existence of a unique solution $\mathbf{x}$ depends on the properties of $\mathbf{A}$ only and not on the involved $\mathbf{y}$. With $rank(\mathbf{A}) = n$, matrix $\mathbf{A}$ is called non-singular, otherwise: singular.

This document is directed towards solving (A.21) in the more general situation where $\mathbf{A}$ is not square.

A.3.2 Least Squares Solutions

The linear systems that arise in several applications of numerical analysis are often inconsistent and, or rank deficient. It is for the handling of these situations that the methods used in this chapter have been developed. Such methods are based on the minimization of the squared Euclidean norm of $\mathbf{y} - \mathbf{Ax}$. As such they are called "least squares methods."

If no further information is available on the nature of the problem (A.21) the so-called ordinary least squares (OLS) solution $\widehat{\mathbf{x}}$, [28], can be computed. This is the solution resulting from minimizing with respect to $\mathbf{x}$ of RES^2, the squared (Euclidean) norm of the difference vector $\mathbf{r} = \mathbf{y} - \mathbf{Ax}$, i.e., $\|\mathbf{y} - \mathbf{Ax}\|_2^2$. Accordingly, the solution $\widehat{\mathbf{x}}$ is taken from

$$\min_{\mathbf{x}} \|\mathbf{y} - \mathbf{Ax}\|_2^2. \tag{A.23}$$

The minimization is carried out by equating all partial derivatives of the squared norm in (A.23) with respect to the elements of $\mathbf{x}$ to zero. The result of this procedure leads to the following condition, which needs to be satisfied by any least square solution $\widehat{\mathbf{x}}$,

$$\mathbf{A}^T \mathbf{A}\widehat{\mathbf{x}} = \mathbf{A}^T \mathbf{y}. \tag{A.24}$$

An important property of (A.24) is that it has at least one solution [27], irrespective of whether the system $\mathbf{Ax} = \mathbf{y}$ is consistent. How these are found is treated below.

A.3.2.1 Specific Notations

After minimization, the following variables can be distinguished:
$\widehat{\mathbf{x}}$ $\equiv$ the OLS solution
$\mathbf{y}$ $\approx \mathbf{A}\widehat{\mathbf{x}}$ $\widehat{\mathbf{x}}$ solves the system in the least squares sense
$\widehat{\mathbf{y}}$ $= \mathbf{A}\widehat{\mathbf{x}}$
$\widehat{\mathbf{r}}$ $= \mathbf{y} - \mathbf{A}\widehat{\mathbf{x}}$, the residual difference $(=\mathbf{y} - \widehat{\mathbf{y}})$
RES $=$ the norm of $\widehat{\mathbf{r}}$

A.3.2.2   The Over Determined Situation: $m \geq n$

1. *full-rank case*: $r = rank(\mathbf{A}) = n$
   In this situation a unique solution to (A.24)

$$\widehat{\mathbf{x}} = (\mathbf{A}^T\mathbf{A})^{-1}\mathbf{A}^T\mathbf{y} \tag{A.25}$$

   exists, as follows immediately from (A.24). It requires $\mathbf{A}^T\mathbf{A}$ to be non-singular, which is the case in this full-rank situation.

2. *rank-deficient case*: $r < n$
   If $r < n$ matrix $\mathbf{A}^T\mathbf{A}$ is singular and (A.25) cannot be used, and so (A.25) does not have a non-unique solution. The solution can be made unique by imposing additional constraints on the solutions. A frequently used constraint is to demand that the norm of the solution vector $\mathbf{x}$ be minimal. Other types of constraints as well as their implementations are discussed in ❷ Chap. 9.

A.3.2.3   The Underdetermined Situation: $m < n$.

1. *full-rank case*: $m = r < n$
   Here a multitude of solutions to (A.21) exist. A unique solution

$$\widehat{\mathbf{x}} = \mathbf{A}^T(\mathbf{A}\mathbf{A}^T)^{-1}\mathbf{y} \tag{A.26}$$

   is found by requiring it to be the one that minimizes the norm of $\mathbf{x}$, subject to the constraint $\mathbf{y} = \mathbf{A}\mathbf{x}$. The fact that $m = r$ guarantees that $\mathbf{A}\mathbf{A}^T$ is non-singular, and thus the solution is indeed unique.

2. *rank-deficient case*: $r < m < n$
   Here, again, a multitude of solutions exist, all having the same value of RES, and can be made unique only by imposing appropriate constraints.

A.3.3   General Methods

Several different methods have been described in the literature for solving the basic equations (A.19) or (A.20). All of these require the inversion of a matrix, either one included in the basic equations, or the one resulting from the least squares approach (A.25). Usually, the solution is made unique by imposing a constraint that minimizes the norm of the solution.

Algorithm HFTI [26] as well as SVD [25] produce LS solutions for all cases, yielding minimum norm solutions in the underdetermined situations.

Algorithm HFTI produces the solution only, algorithm SVD yields a decomposition into three matrices from which the solution $\mathbf{x}$ can be found easily, as is shown below. The SVD is summarized in ❷ Sect. A.4. Both algorithms can also be used to find (to estimate) the covariance of the solution (the estimate) for the general situation involving noise.

For the SVD-based approach involving any matrix of rank r, the least squares solution having minimum norm is

$$\widehat{\mathbf{x}} = \mathbf{V}_r\mathbf{\Sigma}_r^{-1}\mathbf{U}_r^T\mathbf{y}, \tag{A.27}$$

with $\mathbf{\Sigma}_k^{-1}$ a square diagonal matrix having elements $1/\sigma_i$ for $i = 1, r$.
For the notation used, see ❷ Sect. A.4.1.

A.4   The Singular Value Decomposition

One of the major tools of linear algebra is the singular value decomposition of a matrix. It has a great value in theoretical derivations as well as for practical computations. The treatment in this section is mainly descriptive. Proofs of the various statements can be found in Refs. [24–26]. However, they also follow directly from the way in which the various matrices are constructed by the SVD algorithm.

A.4.1 The Basic Statement

For any real matrix $\mathbf{A}$ of size (m, n) there exist matrices $\mathbf{U}$ of size (m, m) and $\mathbf{V}$ (n, n), and a matrix $\mathbf{\Sigma}$ of size (m, n) having non-negative elements $\sigma_i = \sigma_{i,i}$ for $1 \leq i \leq k \leq \min(m, n)$, all remaining elements being zero, such that

$$\mathbf{A} = \mathbf{U\Sigma V}^T. \tag{A.28}$$

This so-called factorization of $\mathbf{A}$ is referred to as its singular value decomposition (SVD).

The elements σ_i, $i = 1, k$, are called the singular values of $\mathbf{A}$. They are usually ordered such that $\sigma_i \geq \sigma_{i+1}$, accompanied by a reordering of the corresponding columns of $\mathbf{U}$ and $\mathbf{V}$, $\mathbf{u}_i$ and $\mathbf{v}_i$, $i = 1, k$, respectively.

The matrices $\mathbf{U}$ and $\mathbf{V}$ have the following properties:

- $\mathbf{U}$ (size(m, m)) is orthogonal: $\mathbf{U}^T\mathbf{U} = \mathbf{I}$, hence $\mathbf{U}^T = \mathbf{U}^{-1}$.
- $\mathbf{V}$ (size(n, n)) is orthogonal: $\mathbf{V}^T\mathbf{V} = \mathbf{I}$, hence $\mathbf{V}^T = \mathbf{V}^{-1}$.

The integer variable k can be shown to be equal to the rank r of the matrix.

Based on the rank r of $\mathbf{A}$, the ordered variant of the decomposition can be partitioned as

$$\mathbf{A} = \begin{bmatrix} \mathbf{U}_r & \mathbf{U}_{m-r} \end{bmatrix} \begin{bmatrix} \mathbf{\Sigma}_r & \mathbf{0} \\ \mathbf{0} & \mathbf{0} \end{bmatrix} \begin{bmatrix} \mathbf{V}_r^T \\ \mathbf{V}_{n-r}^T \end{bmatrix},$$

where the matrix subscripts denote the number of columns of the respective matrices.

By excluding the entries for $\sigma_i = 0$ this partitioning indicates that a different factorization of $\mathbf{A}$ is

$$\mathbf{A} = \mathbf{U}_r \mathbf{\Sigma}_r \mathbf{V}_r^T, \tag{A.29}$$

the so-called "lean" variant of the decomposition. It expresses the essence of the decomposition in its application to solving the linear system. Some computer codes generate $\mathbf{U}_r$ and $\mathbf{V}_r$ only. It involves the first r columns of matrices $\mathbf{U}$ and $\mathbf{V}$. Matrix $\mathbf{\Sigma}_r$ is a diagonal matrix of size (r, r) comprising positive diagonal elements.

For the submatrices involved one has

- The columns of $\mathbf{U}_r$ are orthogonal: $\mathbf{U}_r^T\mathbf{U}_r = \mathbf{I}_r$.
- The columns of $\mathbf{U}_{m-r}$ are orthogonal: $\mathbf{U}_{m-r}^T\mathbf{U}_{m-r} = \mathbf{I}_{m-r}$.
- The columns of $\mathbf{V}_r$ are orthogonal: $\mathbf{V}_r^T\mathbf{V}_r = \mathbf{I}_r$.
- The columns of $\mathbf{V}_{n-r}$ are orthogonal: $\mathbf{V}_{n-r}^T\mathbf{V}_{n-r} = \mathbf{I}_{n-r}$.

Note that, since $\mathbf{U}_r$ and $\mathbf{V}_r$ need not be square, their transposed versions generally do not represent their inverses.

Yet another form of the basic expression (A.28) is

$$\mathbf{A} = \sum_{i=1}^{r} \sigma_i \mathbf{u}_i \mathbf{v}_i^T, \tag{A.30}$$

expressing $\mathbf{A}$ as a sum of the matrix products of corresponding column vectors $\mathbf{u}_i$ and $\mathbf{v}_i$: $\mathbf{u}_i \mathbf{v}_i^T$, each being a so-called rank-one matrix.

2

A.4.2 Applications of the Decomposition

For square, non-singular matrices ($m = n = r$) the inverse of matrix $\mathbf{A}$ as required in (A.21) can be computed from the three matrices (factors) resulting from the SVD algorithm: equation (A.28). Since all three factors involved are non-singular and have the same size we immediately find, by applying the properties listed in ❷ Sect. A.5, as well as the orthogonality of $\mathbf{U}$ and $\mathbf{V}$,

$$\mathbf{A}^{-1} = (\mathbf{U\Sigma V}^T)^{-1} = (\mathbf{V}^T)^{-1}\mathbf{\Sigma}^{-1}\mathbf{U}^{-1} = \mathbf{V\Sigma}^{-1}\mathbf{U}^T. \tag{A.31}$$

Because of the diagonal nature of $\mathbf{\Sigma}$ and the fact that all its elements σ_i are positive, matrix $\mathbf{\Sigma}^{-1}$ is also diagonal, having elements $1/\sigma_i$.

If matrix $\mathbf{A}$ is singular or non-square, it does not have an inverse. As discussed in ❷ Sect. A.3.2, one then reverts to least squares methods. At one stage or another, of these methods require solving expressions like (A.21). Below it is shown that the least squares solution to this problem having a minimal norm is

$$\widehat{\mathbf{x}} = \mathbf{V}_r\mathbf{\Sigma}_r^{-1}\mathbf{U}_r^T\mathbf{y}, \tag{A.32}$$

with all matrices shown as defined in (A.29).

We start by demonstrating that this solution is a least squares solution, which requires that it satisfies condition (A.24). To this end, we multiply the left side of (A.32) by $\mathbf{A}^T\mathbf{A}$ and the right side by the same factor, now expressed by in terms of the equivalent variant (A.29). This is permitted since $\mathbf{A}$ and $\mathbf{A}_r$ have the same rank. We then find, by using the properties of the matrices $\mathbf{V}_r$, $\mathbf{\Sigma}_r$ and $\mathbf{U}_r$ as specified above, that

$$\begin{aligned} \mathbf{A}^T\mathbf{A}\widehat{\mathbf{x}} &= \mathbf{V}_r\mathbf{\Sigma}_r\mathbf{U}_r^T \ \mathbf{U}_r\mathbf{\Sigma}_r\mathbf{V}_r^T\mathbf{V}_r\mathbf{\Sigma}_r^{-1}\mathbf{U}_r^T\mathbf{y}, \\ &= \mathbf{V}_r\mathbf{\Sigma}_r\mathbf{\Sigma}_r\mathbf{\Sigma}_r^{-1}\mathbf{U}_r^T\mathbf{y} \\ &= \mathbf{V}_r\mathbf{\Sigma}_r\mathbf{U}_r^T\mathbf{y} \\ &= \mathbf{A}^T\mathbf{y}. \end{aligned} \tag{A.33}$$

Finally, we show that solution $\widehat{\mathbf{x}}$ as found from (A.32) has a minimum norm. Let $\widehat{\mathbf{x}} + \mathbf{z}$ be any other vector resulting in the same (minimal) residual. Equation (A.32) shows that $\widehat{\mathbf{x}}$ is a linear combination of the first r columns of $\mathbf{V}$ appearing in the full SVD of $\mathbf{A}$. The weighting coefficients are the r-dimensional row vector $\mathbf{\Sigma}_r^{-1}\mathbf{U}_r^T\mathbf{y}$. Adding an arbitrary linear combination of the $n - r$ columns of matrix $\mathbf{V}_{n-r}$, with weighting coefficients $\mathbf{w}$ to the least squares solution $\widehat{\mathbf{x}}$ will result in the same residual since

$$\mathbf{A}\mathbf{V}_{n-r}\mathbf{w}^T \ = \ \begin{bmatrix} \mathbf{U}_r & \mathbf{U}_{m-r} \end{bmatrix} \begin{bmatrix} \mathbf{\Sigma}_r & \mathbf{0} \\ \mathbf{0} & \mathbf{0} \end{bmatrix} \begin{bmatrix} \mathbf{V}_r^T \\ \mathbf{V}_{n-r}^T \end{bmatrix} \mathbf{V}_{n-r}\mathbf{w}^T,$$

and so

$$\mathbf{A}\mathbf{V}_{n-r}\mathbf{w}^T = \mathbf{U}_{m-r}\mathbf{0}\mathbf{w}^T = \mathbf{0}. \tag{A.34}$$

This proves that the vector $\widehat{\mathbf{x}} + \mathbf{V}_{n-r}\mathbf{w}^T$ is also a least squares solution. However, its norm is necessarily higher because of the fact that the basis vectors, the columns of $\mathbf{V}_r$ and $\mathbf{V}_{n-r}$, are orthogonal.

The matrix $\mathbf{A}^+ \stackrel{\Delta}{=} \mathbf{V}_r\mathbf{\Sigma}_r^{-1}\mathbf{U}_r^T$ is called the natural pseudo-inverse of matrix $\mathbf{A}$.

A.5   Definitions and Notations

The following notations are used throughout.

General

$\triangleq$	is defined as
iff	if and only if
$\approx$	equals in the least squares sense
T	the transpose of a vector or a matrix
$\perp$	is orthogonal to

Vectors

Column vectors are denoted by bold-face lower-case characters
e.g., $\mathbf{x}$, their elements as x_i, $i = 1, \cdots, n$

$\mathbf{0}$	a vector having all elements = 0
$\mathbf{x} = \mathbf{0}$	a vector having all elements $x_i = 0$
$\mathbf{x} > \mathbf{0}$	a vector having all elements $x_i \geq 0$ with at least one element $x_i > 0$
$\|\mathbf{x}\|$	norm of a vector (Euclidean norm): $\|\mathbf{x}\| \triangleq (\sum_i x_i^2)^{1/2}$
dependent	k vectors are called dependent if set of numbers $\alpha(i), i = 1, \cdots, k$ exist, not all zero, such that $\mathbf{x}_1\alpha_1 + \mathbf{x}_2\alpha_2 + \cdots + \mathbf{x}_k\alpha_k = \mathbf{0}$, else they are called independent

Matrices
General

Matrices are denoted by bold-face upper-case characters, e.g., $\mathbf{A}$,
Matrix $\mathbf{A}$ of size (m, n) has elements $a_{i,j}$, $i = 1, \cdots, m; j = 1, \cdots, n$

$r = rank(\mathbf{A})$	rank r, of a matrix is the maximum number of independent columns or rows it contains; $r <= \max(m, n)$
$\mathbf{A}^+$	denotes a pseudo-inverse of matrix $\mathbf{A}$
$\mathbf{A}^{\circ}$	alternative notation of a pseudo-inverse of matrix $\mathbf{A}$
$\mathbf{0}$	a matrix having zero elements only
$\mathbf{A} \neq \mathbf{0}$	a matrix having at least one element $a_{i,j} \neq 0$
$\mathbf{U}$	is an orthogonal matrix if $\mathbf{U}^T\mathbf{U} = \mathbf{I}$, i.e., if all its columns, treated as vectors, are mutually orthogonal and their scalar products equal one
$\|\mathbf{A}\|_F$	Freebies norm (also Euclidean norm): $\|\mathbf{A}\|_F \triangleq (\sum_i \sum_j a_{i,j}^2)^{1/2}$

Square matrices

$\mathbf{D}$	a diagonal matrix. All off-diagonal elements are zero
$\mathbf{D}=\mathbf{D}^T$	$\mathbf{D}$ diagonal
$\mathbf{I}$	the identity matrix: a diagonal matrix having unit diagonal elements
$\mathbf{A}^{-1}$	denotes the inverse of matrix $\mathbf{A}$: a matrix such that $\mathbf{A}^{-1}\mathbf{A} = \mathbf{A}\mathbf{A}^{-1} = \mathbf{I}$
$(\mathbf{AB})^{-1} = \mathbf{B}^{-1}\mathbf{A}^{-1}$	(non-singular square matrices of the same size)
$\mathbf{AA} = \mathbf{A}^2$	notation valid for square matrices only
$\kappa(\mathbf{A})$	condition number of matrix $\mathbf{A}$ with respect to inversion: $\kappa(\mathbf{A}) \triangleq \|\mathbf{A}\|. \|\mathbf{A}^{-1}\|$
$tr(\mathbf{A})$	the trace of $\mathbf{A}$: $tr(\mathbf{A}) \triangleq \sum_i a_{i,i}$

Statistics

$E(\mathbf{x})$ the mathematical expectation of $\mathbf{x}$ if its elements are stochastic

i.i.d.   "independent and identically distributed" elements of a stochastic vector

$Cov(\mathbf{x})$ $\overset{\Delta}{=} E\{(\mathbf{x} - E(\mathbf{x}))(\mathbf{x} - E(\mathbf{x}))^T\}$, the covariance of $\mathbf{x}$; in matrix notation: $\boldsymbol{\Gamma}_{\mathbf{x}}$

$Var(\mathbf{x})$ $\overset{\Delta}{=} diag(\boldsymbol{\Gamma}_{\mathbf{x}})$, the variance of $\mathbf{x}$

white noise   independent samples drawn from a zero-mean Gaussian distribution

References

1. Panofski, W.K.H. and M. Phillips, Classical Electricity and Magnetism. 1962. Addison-Wesley: London.
2. Schwan, W.H.K. and C.F. Kay, The conductivity of living tissues. Ann N.Y. Acad Sci., 1957;65: p. 1007–1013.
3. Epstein, B.R. and K.R. Foster, Anisotropy in the dielectric properties of skeletal muscle. Med. Biol. Eng. Comp., 1983;21: p. 51–56.
4. Plonsey, R. and A. van Oosterom, Implications of Macroscopic Source Strength on Cardiac Cellular Activation Models. J. Electrocardiol., 1991;24/2: p. 99–112.
5. Rush, S., J.A. Abildskov, and R.S. McFee, Resistivity of body tissues at low frequencies. Circulation Res., 1963;7: p. 262–267.
6. Geddes, L.A. and L.E. Baker, The Specific Resistance of Biological Material, a Compendium of Data for the Biomedical Engineer and Physiologist. Med. Biol. Eng. Comput., 1967;5: p. 271–293.
7. Gabriel, C., S. Gabriel, and E. Corthout, The dielectric properties of biological tissues, (I): Literature Survey. Phys. Med. Biol., 1996;41: p. 2231–2249.
8. Thomas, C.W., Electrocardiographic measurement system response, in Pediatric Electrocardiography, J. Liebman, R. Plonsey, and P.C. Gilette, Editors. Williams and Wilkins: Baltimore. 1982. pp. 40–59.
9. Plonsey, R. and D. Heppner, Considerations of Quasistationarity in Electrophysiological Systems. Bull. Math. Biophys., 1967;29: 657–664.
10. Smythe, W.R., Static and Dynamic Electricity. 1968. McGraw-Hill: New York.
11. Geselowitz, D.B., Multipole Representation for an Equivalent Cardiac Generator. Proc. IRE, 1960: pp. 75–79.
12. Jackson, J.D., Classical Electrodynamics, 2 edn., 1975. New York: John Wiley & Sons.
13. Abramowitz, M. and I.E. Stegun, Handbook of mathematical functions, 1970; New York: Dover.
14. Burger, H.C., The Zero of Potential: A Persistent Error. Am. Heart J., 1955;49: 581–586.
15. Geselowitz, D.B., The Zero of Potential. IEEE Eng. Med. Biol. Mag., 1998;17(1): 128–132.
16. Geselowitz, D.B., Bioelectric potentials in an inhomogeneous volume conductor, in QPR. 1960, MIT, p. 218–226.
17. Plonsey, R., The formulation of bioelectric source-field relationships in terms of surface discontinuities, J. Franklin Inst., 1974; 317–324.
18. Gelernter, H.L. and J.C. Swihart, A Mathematical-physical Model of the Genesis of the Electrocardiogram. Biophys. J., 1964;4: p. 285–301.
19. Oostendorp, T.F. and A. van Oosterom, Source parameter estimation in inhomogeneous volume conductors of arbitrary shape. IEEE Trans. Biomed. Eng., 1989;BME 36(3): 382–391.
20. van Oosterom, A. and J. Strackee, The Solid Angle of a Plane Triangle. IEEE Trans. Biomed. Eng., 1983;BME 30: 125–126.
21. Munck, J.C.D., A Linear Discretization of the Volume Conductor Boundary Integral Equation using Analytically Integrated Elements. IEEE Trans. Biomed. Eng., 1992;BME 39: 986–990.
22. Oostendorp, T.F. and A. van Oosterom, Source parameter estimation in inhomogeneous volume conductors of arbitrary shape. IEEE Trans. Biomed. Eng., 1989;BME 36: 382–391.
23. van Oosterom, A. and T.F. Oostendorp, On Computing Pericardial Potentials and Current Densities. J. Electrocardiol., 1992; 25(Suppl): 102–106.
24. Golub, G.H. and C.F. Van Loan, Matrix Computations, The Johns Hopkins University Press, Baltimore, 1996. 3rd edition.
25. Forsythe, G.E., M.A. Malcolm, and C.B. Moler, Computer Methods for Mathematical Computations, Prentice-Hall, Englewood Cliffs, N.J., 1977.
26. Lawson, C.L. and R.J. Hanson, Solving Least Squares Problems, Prentice-Hall, Englewood Cliffs, N.J., 1974.
27. Steward G.W., Introduction to Matrix Computations, Academic Press, New York, 1973.
28. Beck J.V. and K.J. Arnold, Parameter Estimation in Engineering and Science, Wiley, New York, 1977.

General References

Smythe, W.R., Static and Dynamic Electricity. New York: McGraw-Hill, 1968; first published in 1939.
Stratton, J.A., Electromagnetic Theory. New York: McGraw-Hill, 1941.
Jackson J.D. Classical Electrodynamics. New York: Wiley, 1962.
Panofsky W.K.H, Phillips M. Classical Electricity and Magnetism, 2nd ed. Reading, MA: Addison-Wesley, 1962.
Plonsey R, Collin R. Principles and Applications of Electromagnetic Fields. New York: McGraw-Hill, 1961.

Plonsey R. *Bioelectric Phenomena*. New York: McGraw-Hill, 1969.

Gulrajani, R.M. *Bioelectricity and Biomagnetism*. New York: Wiley, 1998.

Plonsey R., Barr R.C., *Bioelectricity: A Quantitative Approach*, third edition. New York: Springer, 2007.

Appendix Bibliography

1. Golub GH and Van Loan CF. *Matrix Computations*. The Johns Hopkins University Press, Baltimore, 1996. 3rd edition.
2. Forsythe GE, Malcolm MA, and Moler CB. *Computer Methods for Mathematical Computations*. Prentice-Hall, Englewood Cliffs, N.J., 1977.
3. Lawson CL and Hanson RJ. *Solving Least Squares Problems*. Prentice-Hall, Englewood Cliffs, N.J., 1974.
4. Steward GW. *Introduction to Matrix Computations*. Academic Press, New York, 1973.
5. Beck JV and Arnold KJ. *Parameter Estimation in Engineering and Science*. Wiley, New York, 1977.

Part II

Cardiac Electrophysiology

3 Cellular Electrophysiology

A. Zaza · R. Wilders · T. Opthof

P. W. Macfarlane et al. (eds.), *Basic Electrocardiology*, DOI 10.1007/978-0-85729-871-3_3,

3.1   Introduction

The beginning of the era of cardiac electrophysiology can be attributed to the end of the nineteenth century, when Einthoven discovered the ECG and described its configuration [1], defining it more quantitatively in a later study [2]. While the ECG remains an essential clinical tool and a symbol of cardiac electrophysiology, the discipline has evolved to address the function of single myocytes, or even of specific processes within myocytes.

Myocytes represent the functional unit of the cardiac muscle; nonetheless, the heart behaves more or less like an electrical syncytium, whose global activity depends on low resistance coupling between the myocytes. The phrase "more or less" is used here intentionally to imply that, while the activity intrinsic to individual myocytes is affected by coupling, its features remain recognizable within the context of the whole heart and are important to determine its function.

The ECG signal represents the electrical activity of the whole organ and its relation with the activity of individual myocytes is quite complex. Indeed, the potentials recorded by body surface electrodes are affected by spatial and temporal summation of myocyte activity at different locations in the heart. This results in so many electrical signals being cancelled, especially during the repolarization phase [3], that the same ECG pattern may be compatible with different activation and repolarization sequences. This implies that it would be theoretically possible to construct the ECG from the action potentials of all underlying myocytes, but we cannot deduce individual myocyte behavior from the ECG, a condition recognized by biophysicists as the "inverse problem" [4]. In the same way, analysis of the mechanisms and modulation of the electrical activity of single myocytes provides information relevant to the function of the whole heart, which cannot be obtained from the ECG.

This chapter deals with the basic mechanisms of myocyte functioning such as excitation, repolarization, and automaticity, which are relevant to the initiation and orderly propagation of electrical activity in the whole heart. The aim is to provide a link between phenomena at the molecular level, potential targets of drug therapy or genetic manipulation, and macroscopic electrical behavior. We have focused on issues essential to pursue this aim, sacrificing for the sake of clarity, some of the overwhelming complexity of cardiac cell physiology. Reviews have been quoted to cover settled topics, and references reserved for original papers and more recent or controversial issues.

3.1.1   Annotation Conventions

Knowledge of a few conventions on the annotation of physical parameters is useful for understanding the following discussion.

1. Following commonly used annotation, we have used E to denote electrochemical equilibrium potentials (e.g., E_K for potassium equilibrium potential) and V to denote membrane potential (V_m, V_{rest}). For the sake of clarity, it should be stressed that both E and V denote an electrical potential difference across the cell membrane and thus have identical units (mV).
2. The symbol I_m refers to *net current across the cell membrane*. I_m may reflect the algebraic summation of currents carried by different ion channels, possibly with different signs. Thus, $I_m = 0$ does not necessarily imply that individual currents are also null. Individual currents are appropriately annotated (e.g., I_{Na} for Na^+ current).
3. In defining the sign of potentials and currents, the extracellular electrode is used as reference (i.e., at 0 mV by convention). Thus: (1) $V_m = -80$ mV means that the intracellular side is 80 mV negative to the extracellular one; (2) membrane current has a positive sign whenever positive charges leave the cell (outward current); inward current has a negative sign.
4. The term "mole" refers to a quantity of substance (containing a number of molecules equal to Avogadro's number), whereas the term "molar" (M) refers to a concentration (1 M = 1 mol/L).

3

3.2   Outline of Structure and Function

3.2.1   Myocyte Structure and Relation to Excitation–Contraction Coupling

Each myocyte is surrounded by a plasma membrane named sarcolemma. Its basic structure is a lipid bilayer, a few nanometers thick, impermeable to ions and with a high dielectric constant. Ions can cross the sarcolemmal membrane only via specialized embedded proteins, named ion channels. The sarcolemma forms multiple invaginations perpendicular to the long cell axis, named T-tubules (❷ Fig. 3.1). They serve as extensions of the cell surface and host a large density of ion channels and transporters important for excitation-contraction coupling. Myocytes contain a specialized cisternal system, the sarcoplasmic reticulum (SR), in which Ca^{2+} is actively accumulated by ATP-driven transport (SR Ca-ATPase or SERCA). The SR is in close vicinity (about 10 nm) to the T-tubule sarcolemma on one side and to the contractile apparatus on the other, but is not in contact with them. This kind of structural arrangement is essential for the coupling between electrical excitation of the sarcolemma and massive release of Ca^{2+} from the SR. Indeed, coupling is mediated by a relatively small influx of Ca^{2+} through voltage-gated sarcolemmal Ca^{2+} channels (L-type channels, carrying I_{CaL}), which open Ca^{2+}-activated Ca^{2+} channels in the SR membrane (ryanodine receptor (RyR) channels), a process named Ca^{2+}-induced Ca^{2+}-release (CICR) [5] (❷ Fig. 3.1c). Each L-type Ca^{2+}-channel on the sarcolemma corresponds to a cluster of RyR channels on the SR membrane, forming a sort of Ca^{2+} release unit. RyR channels within a unit open and close in a "cooperative" fashion, so as to make Ca^{2+} release of the cluster a quantal (all-or-none) process. Such unitary Ca^{2+}

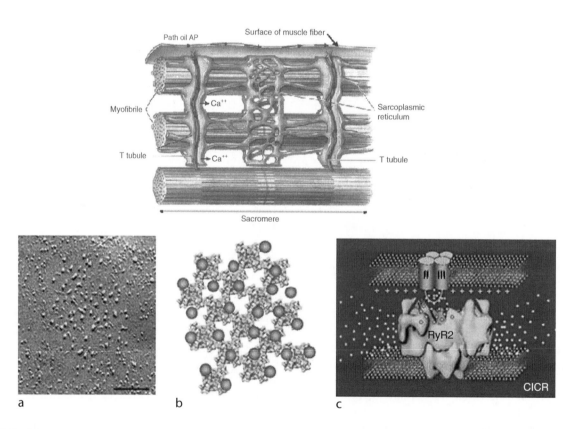

❏ Fig. 3.1

Myocyte structure. *Upper panel*: arrangement of T-tubules, sarcoplasmic reticulum (SR) and sarcomeres within a cardiac myocyte. *Bottom panels*: (**a**) clustering of Ryanodine receptors (RyR) on SR membrane, (**b**) spatial relationship between dihydropyridine receptor (*yellow*) in sarcolemma and underlying RyR clusters (*green*); (**c**) Ca^{2+} release by RyR, induced by Ca^{2+} entry through dihydropyridine receptor (CICR: Ca^{2+} induced Ca^{2+} release) releases have been named "Ca^{2+} sparks" [6]; physiological contraction is triggered by the fusion of multiple sparks into a "Ca^{2+} transient," supported by synchronous activation of all release units by Ca^{2+} entry through L-type Ca^{2+}-channels during the action potential.

The transmission of action potentials from cell to cell occurs via non-selective, large-conductance ion channels, closely packed in large arrays named gap junctions. These are primarily located within the intercalated disks connecting myocytes along their longitudinal axis, but are also present on lateral margins, to provide side-to-side connections. Each cardiac gap junction channel is made of 12 connexin molecules. Six of these form a hemichannel (connexon) in one myocyte, which faces another hemichannel in the adjacent myocyte. Together they form a full channel providing electrical continuity between myocytes. There are several isoforms of these connexins, but the most important one, abundantly present in working atrial and ventricular muscle, is connexin43 (Cx43; see for review [7]). Intercalated disks also provide the physical structure where mechanical force can be transmitted.

3.2.2   Tissue Structure and Relation to Global Heart Excitation

There are five functionally and anatomically separate types of heart muscle: sinoatrial (SA) node, atrioventricular (AV) node, His-Purkinje system, atrial muscle and ventricular muscle. To date there is no convincing evidence for the existence of "internodal pathways". Under normal circumstances only the first three are capable of pacemaker function. The SA node generates the cardiac impulse, whereas the AV node and His-Purkinje system have a prominent role in its conduction. The primary function of the remaining atrial and ventricular muscle tissues is force development, as expressed by the comprehensive definition of "working myocardium." The bundle of His and Purkinje fibers were anatomically described in the nineteenth century, and the SA and AV nodes were discovered during the first decade of the twentieth century [8, 9]. Indeed, an impressive, comprehensive review of the origin and conduction of the heartbeat appeared as the opening paper in the very first issue of *Physiological Reviews* in 1921 [10]. At that time the principal structural components of the heart were known, but the study of function had to await a number of important technical breakthroughs. First, in 1949, Ling and Gerard introduced the microelectrode, which permitted the measurement of transmembrane potentials [11]. Thirty years later, two important techniques were developed. Cell isolation techniques permitted the study of the characteristics of single myocytes [12]. The patch clamp technique paved the path for the study of membrane currents at the level of individual membrane channels [13].

The SA node is composed of a heterogeneous population of cells with some common features. The myocytes are small and generally spindle-shaped. They have little contractile material, which is not organized in myofibrils with a clearly periodical structure. Compared to their relatively low myofilament density, they have a remarkably high mitochondrial density. They do not have a significant T-tubular system, but they do possess many caveolae [14]: cholesterol-rich membrane domains containing a high density of receptor and channel proteins. In the SA node, myocytes form clusters and bundles surrounded by abundant collagen. The SA node border is deeply interdigitated with the surrounding atrial myocardium, forming structures in which relatively thin atrial bundles penetrate a larger mass of nodal myocytes.

Whether propagation from the SA node to the AV node occurs through specialized conduction tissue is an unresolved issue. Internodal pathways have not been conclusively demonstrated and the dominating opinion is that the conduction pattern results from the longitudinally oriented tissue architecture of the crista terminalis at the junction between the intercaval area and the right atrium.

AV nodal cells are similar in both shape and function to those of the SA node [14, 15]. In contrast to the SA node with its central origin of the cardiac impulse and radial propagation, the AV node has two functional inputs and one functional output communicating with the bundle of His. Under pathological conditions, this morphological and functional triangular make-up provides the substrate for AV nodal reentrant arrhythmias. Even in structurally normal hearts, isolated echobeats can be provoked by appropriate stimulation protocols, not only in animal studies [15], but also in humans [16].

The specialized conduction system distal to the AV node (His bundle, bundle branches, fascicles and Purkinje network) is composed of Purkinje myocytes, longitudinally oriented in bundles, packed by dense connective tissue. Purkinje myocytes are of similar shape but larger than working myocytes, have less contractile material and contain large amounts of glycogen. Connexins are abundantly expressed, particularly in terminal gap-junctional connections. Myocytes at the transition between Purkinje fibers and working ventricular muscle have an intermediate morphology [17].

Atrial and ventricular myocytes are rod-shaped and about 100 μm long. Ventricular myocytes are about 20 μm wide, atrial ones are slightly thinner. Both cell types contain a large amount of contractile proteins, organized in clearly periodic myofibrils, a large number of mitochondria and glycogen deposits. T-tubules are well developed in ventricular myocytes, but almost missing in atrial myocytes. The latter contain secretory granules, related to their endocrine activity (atrial natriuretic peptide (ANP) secretion).

The morphological and functional differences between cardiac tissues account for orderly impulse propagation, providing the coordinated contraction required for pump efficiency. After the initiation of the cardiac impulse in the sinus node (invisible in the surface ECG) the impulse travels rapidly over the atria, giving rise to the P wave in the ECG, followed by atrial contraction. The impulse conducts through the AV node for a considerable time (between 120 and 200 ms; invisible in the ECG, leading to the PR interval), during which period the ventricles fill passively and are assisted by atrial contraction. Once the impulse has passed the AV node, the His-Purkinje system is activated. Again this system has not enough mass to show up on the ECG. The function of the His-Purkinje system is to warrant rapid ventricular activation (visible in the ECG as the QRS complex with a duration of about 100 ms). Moreover the site of earliest (septal) activation is closer to the apex than to the base (in the human heart, not in the murine heart, for example), which is relevant for hemodynamic reasons. Finally, after a long plateau phase of the ventricular action potentials (invisible in the ECG, leading to the ST segment), the ventricles repolarize, leading to the T wave in the ECG. In the next sections we describe the basic active and passive membrane properties at the cellular and organ level.

3.3 Biological Membranes

3.3.1 Bilayer Structure and Physical Properties

The basic structural component of biological membranes is a phospholipid bilayer, formed by molecules containing a hydrophylic head and a hydrophobic tail (amphiphilic molecules). When put in water, pairs of such molecules turn their tails to each other and their heads to face the water. Many such pairs form a sort of carpet, with a hydrophobic core and hydrophylic shell, whose energy of interaction with water (hydration energy) provides a strong stabilizing mechanism. In spite of its structural stability, the phospholipid bilayer is fluid. Its constituent molecules are in continuous random motion, which occasionally generates small gaps in the hydrophobic core, through which water molecules can pass. Thus, in spite of its lipidic nature, the bilayer is significantly permeable to water by simple diffusion [18]. In biological membranes, additional water permeability can be provided by water channel proteins, named "aquaporins," which are variably expressed in different cell types [19]. While uncharged molecules dissolve in the bilayer and freely permeate it by diffusion, charged molecules, such as ions, do not.

Due to its impermeability to ions and thinness, the phospholipid bilayer is able to separate charges at a very close distance (20–30 nm) and favors their electrostatic interaction (high dielectric constant); thus, the bilayer is an electrical condenser (or capacitor). The *capacity* of a condenser (charge accumulated per unit voltage, $C = \Delta Q / \Delta V$) (Electrical capacity is expressed in farad (F), $1\,F = 1\,C/V$. It should be noted that $1\,F$ is a large capacity, e.g., found in heavy-duty industrial condensers.) is proportional to its surface area. The presence of membrane invaginations (T-tubules, caveolae etc.) increases the ratio between membrane surface and cell volume. Capacity per unit area (specific capacitance) is rather constant among biological membranes and amounts to about $1\,\mu F/cm^2$.

3.3.2 Special Routes for Ion Permeation: Ion Channels

To allow ion permeation, a hydrophilic pathway must be created through the phospholipid bilayer. This is provided by "ion channels," protein molecules inserted in the bilayer and connected to the cytoskeleton [20].

Ion channels allow permeation of ions by generating a water-filled pore or, more often, by providing a path of charged amino acidic residues which temporarily bind the ion, freeing it from its hydration shell. Since each permeation path may bind different ions with different affinities, permeation is selective. Selectivity of ion channels is very important functionally and may range among different channels from loose (e.g., cations vs. anions, monovalents vs. divalents) to very strict (e.g., K^+ vs. Na^+, Ca^{2+} vs. Mg^{2+}).

3.3.3   Ion Movements Require Energy: Electrochemical Potentials

Energy is required to move ions along the channel (i.e., to make them jump from one binding site to the next). This energy (also named "driving force") is provided by the electrochemical gradient, generated across the membrane by (1) the presence in the cytosol of non-diffusible anions (mainly negatively charged proteins, to which the membrane is totally impermeable); (2) active redistribution of ions, operated mainly by the Na^+/K^+ pump through consumption of metabolic energy (ATP). The direction of current flow in an ion channel is always along the electrochemical gradient of the ion which permeates the channel. Only active transporters (different from channels) can move ions against their gradient, by using metabolic energy.

The "electrochemical" gradient is a potential energy generated simultaneously by a difference in concentration (generating chemical energy) and in charge (generating electrical energy). When chemical and electrical energies are equal in magnitude and of opposite sign they cancel each other and the net ion flow is null. This condition is named "electrochemical equilibrium" and the membrane potential at which it occurs, is called "equilibrium potential." To exemplify, given the physiological distribution of K^+ ions across the membrane, with a high intracellular concentration (≈ 150 mM) and a low extracellular concentration (≈ 4 mM), the equilibrium potential of K^+ (E_K) is about -94 mV (negative toward the cytosol). This implies that if the membrane potential is equal to -94 mV the net K^+ flow across the membrane is null. When the membrane potential (V_m) differs from E_K, K^+ flows through the membrane, carrying a current proportional to the difference between V_m and E_K, also known as the "driving force" for the ion. The current is outward if V_m is more positive than E_K and vice versa. The V_m value at which the current reverses its direction is also named "reversal potential" of the current. If the channel is selectively permeable to a single ion species (e.g., K^+) the current reversal potential and the ion equilibrium potential coincide. If the channel is permeable to different ions, the current reversal potential is in between the equilibrium potentials of the individual ions, and its precise value is determined by the ratio of the respective permeabilities. For instance, if the channel is permeable to both K^+ ($E_K \approx -94$ mV) and Na^+ ($E_{Na} \approx +70$ mV), the current reversal potential will be positive to -94 mV and will approach $+70$ mV as the Na^+/K^+ permeability ratio increases.

3.3.4   Changes in Membrane Selective Permeability: Ion Channel Gating

Changes in membrane selective permeability are caused by the opening and closing of selective ion channels. Opening and closing correspond to changes in the conformation of the channel protein (or "state" of the channel). The energy required for such transitions (gating energy) can be of a different kind for different channels. For most cardiac channels, gating energy is provided by the transmembrane electrical potential field (voltage–gated channels), which acts by orienting charged amino acid residues in the channel protein. However, some channels in the heart respond to the binding of a specific molecule (ligand-gated channels), to membrane stretch (stretch-activated channels) etc.

Each specific current (e.g., I_{Na}) is actually carried by a large number of individual channel proteins of the same kind (e.g., single Na^+ channels) which can either be closed or open. The sum of such single channel currents generates an ensemble (or "macroscopic") current, whose magnitude can vary in an apparently "continuous" fashion. The historical interpretation of channel gating (Hodgkin-Huxley model, see ❷ Sect. 3.14.1) considers "ensemble" currents, carried by "ensemble" channels. Conductance of the ensemble channel (g) is given by

$$g = x \times g_{max}, \tag{3.1}$$

in which g_{max} is maximal conductance and x (gating variable, ranging from 0 to 1) is the fraction of g_{max} actually expressed in a given condition. Channel "gating" (activation, deactivation etc.) is modeled by varying the value of x.

In the following discussion, we will always refer to *ensemble* "channel," "current," "conductance," etc. Nonetheless, the relation between single channel and ensemble behavior can be easily understood by considering g_{max} as the g value observed when all single channels are open ($x = 1$) and x as the fraction of all single channels which are open in a given condition (also named the "open probability" of the single channel). Channel "gating" corresponds to changes in the open probability.

To summarize, the amount of current flowing through an ion channel is proportional to the product of (1) the driving force for the permeating ion(s) and (2) the channel conductance:

$$I = x \times g_{max} \times (V_m - E_{rev}),$$ (3.2)

where g_{max} represents the maximal conductance (all channels open), x the proportion of g_{max} actually available (activation variable) and the term in parenthesis corresponds to the driving force. Notably, in voltage-gated channels, x and the driving force are both affected by V_m. Moreover, in some of them (e.g., I_{Na} and I_{CaL}), the same V_m change (e.g., depolarization) leads to two subsequent transitions: the channel is first activated (x approaches 1) and then "inactivated" (made non-conductive). This is expressed by adding an "inactivation variable" y, with a dependency on V_m opposite to that of x:

$$I = x \times y \times g_{max} \times (V_m - E_{rev}).$$ (3.3)

In this case, the current is present when both x and y are not null; thus, upon depolarization, the current flows only for a very short time (a few ms), i.e., when x is already greater than 0 and y is not yet 0. Subsequent return of y to 1 (allowing current to pass) is referred to as "recovery from inactivation" and it is the cause of excitation "refractoriness." For further discussion on modeling of ion channel gating, the reader is referred to ❷ Sect. 3.14.1.

By convention (see ❷ Sect. 3.1.1), outward current makes V_m more negative (repolarization or hyperpolarization). Similarly, inward current makes V_m more positive (depolarization). For cations (e.g., Na^+, Ca^{2+}, K^+) the direction of ion movement and current coincide. Anions (e.g., Cl^-) leaving the cell cause membrane depolarization and are said to generate an "inward current."

3.4 How Membrane Current Affects Membrane Potential

Thus far, we have addressed the dependency of ionic currents on membrane potential (voltage dependent gating). Now it is time to ask the opposite question: how does membrane current change membrane potential? We will start considering the case of net membrane current (I_m). If the membrane would behave as a simple resistance (R_m), the change in membrane potential (ΔV_m) would be given by Ohm's law ($\Delta V_m = I_m \times R_m$). However, a membrane is also a condenser, which needs to be charged by I_m before V_m develops to the value predicted by Ohm's law; thus, the change in V_m always follows I_m with a lag proportional to membrane capacity (C_m). This can be expressed by the following relation:

$$-dV_m/dt = I_m/C_m$$ (3.4)

which states that I_m magnitude determines the *velocity* ($-dV_m/dt$) by which the V_m change takes place (This relation is valid only if I_m is used entirely to charge C_m, i.e., in the absence of current flow along the cytoplasm (axial current = 0). This is generally true in a single myocyte, but not during propagation between electrically coupled myocytes. In the latter case, part of I_m is used as axial current, thus leading to a smaller dV_m/dt.) (the minus sign implies that inward I_m moves V_m in the positive direction). A larger C_m makes the relationship between *velocity* and current shallower. C_m is constant in a given cell; thus, in practice it is safe to state that, at least in a single myocyte, the velocity of depolarization (or repolarization) linearly depends on the absolute magnitude of net transmembrane current. Such a simple relation is pivotal to the understanding of action potential complexity.

To predict the effect of a specific ionic current (e.g., I_{Na}) on membrane potential the following should be considered. At each instant V_m tends to a value equal to the reversal potential of I_m (E_m), whose composition changes over time. (Before V_m achieves the reversal potential of I_m, membrane capacity needs to be filled up with charge (saturated). When a channel opens (membrane permeability changes), charge flows through it and charges capacity; the larger the current, the faster the charging process. The reversal potential (at which current is null) is truly achieved only at steady state, i.e., when the capacitor is charged to saturation.) During rest, the prevailing permeability is that for K^+. Accordingly V_m is close to E_K (e.g., -90 mV); during excitation Na^+ permeability prevails (Na^+ channels open and K^+ channels close), thus V_m quickly approaches $+70$ mV (fast depolarization). Thereafter, K^+ permeability increases again over Na^+ and V_m returns toward E_K (repolarization).

3.5   Maintaining Electrochemical Gradients: Membrane Transports

An alternative path for the movement of molecules through biological membranes is provided by membrane transporters. Similar to ion channels, transporters are protein molecules embedded in the phospholipid bilayer that undergoes conformational changes when exposed to energy. However, they show notable functional differences with respect to channels. These consist mainly of (1) lower and more sharply saturable transport rates, and (2) the capability, at least for "active transporters," of transporting molecules against their electrochemical gradient by using other energy sources.

The lower transport rates and complete saturability depend on the fact that the conformational change corresponds to translocation of one or few bound molecules at a time, rather than to opening of a continuous permeation path. Thus, translocation is slow and, once all the binding sites on the protein are occupied, flow cannot increase further (saturation). Flow through channels may also saturate to some extent and recent observations suggest that, under specific conditions, transporters can actually behave as ion channels. This has led us to question the ground for a sharp distinction between the two types of mechanism; nonetheless, such a distinction remains meaningful for most applications.

Active transporters can (1) directly hydrolyze ATP to ADP and use its energy to propel the transport; (primary active transport, e.g., the Na^+/K^+ pump), or (2) simultaneously transport one substance against its gradient and a different one along its gradient, with the latter providing the propulsion energy (secondary active transport, e.g., the Na^+/Ca^{2+} exchanger). In the case of secondary transport, the propelling gradient must be maintained by another active transport. For instance, by extruding Na^+, the Na^+/K^+ pump generates the inward Na^+ gradient necessary to actively extrude Ca^{2+} through the Na^+/Ca^{2+} exchanger and to actively extrude protons through the Na^+/H^+ exchanger.

If the number of charges carried in the two directions is not the same, the transport will also generate an electrical current and is said to be "electrogenic." If a transport is electrogenic it is also sensitive to V_m; in this case, as for ion channels, an electrochemical "equilibrium potential" of the transport can be measured, at which transport is null and current flow reverses. Under physiological conditions, the Na^+/K^+ pump carries outward current (I_{NaK}) throughout the electrical cycle (i.e., its equilibrium is more negative than physiological values of V_m). The Na^+/Ca^{2+} exchanger current (I_{NaCa}) is inward during diastole (corresponding to Ca^{2+} extrusion) but, due to the attending changes in cytosolic Ca^{2+} concentration, tends to reverse during systole (Ca^{2+} may enter through the exchanger, which then acts in "reverse mode"). More details on membrane transport can be found in [21].

3.6   Resting Membrane Potential

Most nerve and muscle cells and also epithelial cells have a negative resting membrane potential (V_{rest}) between −60 and −90 mV. This potential difference exists over a membrane only 5 nm thick and therefore the electrical field is very strong, in the order of 10^5 V/cm. Such a powerful electrical field will influence the behavior of single ions strongly. A constant and stable V_{rest} is needed in the working atrial and ventricular muscles that are supposed to follow a stimulus generated elsewhere.

As mentioned above, the value of V_{rest} in the working myocardium is mainly determined by the presence of an overwhelming K^+ conductance, based on the membrane current named "inward rectifier" (I_{K1}), which is open at negative potentials. High permeability to K^+ brings V_{rest} close to the K^+ equilibrium potential and effectively prevents its oscillations. Smaller contributions to V_{rest} are also made by currents generated by Na^+/K^+ and Na^+/Ca^{2+} transports. Since V_{rest} is based on the K^+ electrochemical gradient, even small increases in extracellular concentration of this ion may cause membrane depolarization (e.g., in acute ischemia). The effect of a decrease in extracellular K^+ is more complex: while it would tend to make V_{rest} more negative, it also causes a marked decrease in I_{K1} conductance, resulting in loss of polarization. The two effects balance off at a K^+ concentration of about 3 mM and V_{rest} may become very unstable at lower concentrations. This is one of the mechanisms underlying the adverse effect of hypokalemia on cardiac electrical stability and explains why severe hypokalemia (as severe hyperkalemia) is incompatible with life.

3

3.7   Excitability

Excitability concerns conversion of a small triggering stimulus to a large, stereotypical response (the action potential). Such a conversion implies the existence of a voltage "threshold," below which the triggering stimulus is ineffective (subliminal). Thus, membrane excitation occurs in two phases: (1) achievement of the threshold, in which the membrane passively responds to the triggering current (*electrotonic* phase); (2) autoregenerative excitation, which involves active membrane properties (i.e., voltage dependent channel gating) and becomes independent of the triggering stimulus.

Two autoregenerative processes cooperate to determine the threshold: (1) activation of an inward current (I_{Na}) and (2) removal of the outward current responsible for stabilizing diastolic potential (I_{K1}). The former is due to the positive feed-back interaction between I_{Na} and V_m. The latter depends on the peculiar voltage dependency of I_{K1}, whose conductance is dramatically decreased if V_m is depolarized to a certain extent above its resting value. This I_{K1} property, named "inward rectification," is caused by intracellular cations (polyamines, Mg^{2+} and Ca^{2+}) plugging the channel when attracted into its pore by the favorable potential gradient provided by depolarization [22–24]. I_{Na} activation and I_{K1} depression are simultaneously a cause and consequence of depolarization, as required by an autoregenerative process.

Achievement of the activation threshold (electrotonic phase) depends on both amplitude and duration of the triggering stimulus. We can understand this by realizing that the sarcolemma has both electrical resistance (R_m) and capacity (C_m). A current (I_m) injected into the membrane charges C_m along an exponential time course, to produce a steady-state voltage (V_{mSS}) given by $V_{mSS} = I_m \times R_m$. If V_{mSS} is equal to the activation threshold (liminal stimulus), excitation may require the whole charging time (several ms); on the other hand, if V_{mSS} exceeds the threshold (supraliminal stimulus), excitation may be achieved before V_{mSS} is fully developed, that is in a shorter time.

There is a relationship between the amplitude and the duration of the stimulus required to achieve excitation. This relation is named "strength-duration" curve and its steepness depends on tissue properties. The minimum stimulus amplitude which, irrespective of duration (made very long), is required for excitation is named "rheobase." The term "chronaxy" refers to the minimum effective duration of a stimulus of an amplitude twice the rheobase. Such parameters are also useful in defining the energies required to stimulate the myocardium by external sources (e.g., artificial pacemakers). At the functional level the basic concept of rheobase can be regarded as the diastolic threshold for activation. Refractory periods are normally assessed by short stimuli (e.g. 2 ms) with an amplitude twice the threshold one.

3.8   Action Potential

The ability to generate action potentials (AP) is the distinctive feature of excitable cells, for which conserved propagation of the electrical signal is a functional requirement. The AP is essentially an electrical transient, which can propagate over long distances preserving its amplitude. Such a "constancy" of the AP is achieved by basing its initiation (excitation followed by depolarization) and termination (repolarization) on autoregenerative phenomena which, once initiated, become independent of the triggering stimulus. To initiate the autoregenerative process, the triggering stimulus must achieve a "threshold" of amplitude and duration.

3.8.1   The Cardiac Action Potential Contour

The cardiac electrical cycle has been schematically divided in five "phases," four of them describing the AP contour and one the diastolic interval (❯ Fig. 3.2).

Phase 0 refers to the autoregenerative depolarization, which occurs when the excitation threshold is exceeded. Phase 0 is supported by activation of two inward (depolarizing) currents, I_{Na} and I_{CaL}. Membrane depolarization quickly activates these channels and, with a delay of several milliseconds for I_{Na} and of tens of ms for I_{CaL}, inactivates them. Thus, membrane depolarization provides both the triggering and breaking mechanism for the autoregenerative depolarization. Although short-lived, I_{Na} is large and provides most of the charge influx required for propagation (see below). I_{CaL} has a small component with fast activation/inactivation (I_{CaT}) and a larger one with slower kinetics (I_{CaL}). I_{CaL} mediates most of Ca^{2+} influx required to trigger myocyte contraction and may support propagation under conditions in which I_{Na} is not expressed or functional (e.g., in the nodes). Phase 0 depolarization also activates K^+ currents, which contribute to

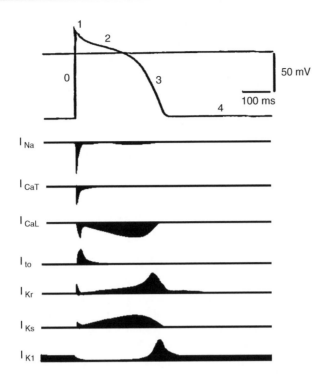

◘ Fig. 3.2
Phases of a prototypical ventricular action potential (AP) and underlying currents. The numbers refer to the 5 phases of the action potential. In each current profile the horizontal line represents the zero current level; inward currents are below the line and outward ones are above it. See text for abbreviations of the membrane currents

its termination and to subsequent repolarization. Among these, the transient outward current (I_{to}) is sufficiently fast to limit depolarization rate during phase 0.

Phase 1 is the initial phase of repolarization, mainly supported by I_{to}. The latter is a K^+ current that, similarly to I_{Na}, is activated and quickly inactivated by depolarization. Thus, I_{to} supports fast repolarization. Recovery of I_{to} from inactivation occurs during the diastole and is slow enough to make this current poorly available at high heart rates. I_{to} is unequally expressed across the ventricular wall (see below), thus phase 1 is more prominent in subepicardial layers than in subendocardial ones [25].

Phase 2, also named AP "plateau," is the slow repolarization phase, which accounts for the peculiar configuration of the cardiac AP. The net transmembrane current flowing during phase 2 is small and it results from the algebraic summation of inward and outward components. The outward one (promoting repolarization) mainly consists of depolarization-activated K^+ currents collectively named "delayed rectifiers" (I_K). I_K is actually the sum of rapid (I_{Kr}) and slow (I_{Ks}) components, carried by separate channels with different properties and pharmacology [26]. The interplay and roles of I_{Kr} and I_{Ks} in determining repolarization rate will be discussed in more detail below. The inward phase 2 currents (opposing repolarization) are mostly carried by "window" components of I_{Na} and I_{CaL}, which flow when V_m is such that the activated state of these channels is not yet completely offset by the inactivation process. Thus, very small proportions of I_{Na} and I_{CaL} can contribute to the whole duration of phase 2 [27, 28]. Small Na^+ currents with slow inactivation gating also exist in Purkinje fibers [29]. The current generated by the operation of the Na^+/Ca^{2+} exchanger (I_{NCX}) can variably contribute to phase 2, according to the magnitude and course of the cytosolic Ca^{2+} transient and to the subsarcolemmal Na^+ levels [30].

Phase 3 is the terminal phase of repolarization, and differs from phase 2 for its faster repolarization rate. Phase 3 is dominated by I_{Kr} and I_{K1}, both characterized by a kinetic property, named "inward rectification" [23, 31, 32], suitable to support autoregenerative processes [33]. Initiation of phase 3 is probably supported by I_{Kr}, with a threshold determined

3

by the balance between its onset and waning of phase 2 inward currents. I_{K1} takes over during the final part of phase 3 [33, 34] and effectively "clamps" membrane potential back to its diastolic value.

Phase 4 describes membrane potential during diastole. In myocytes expressing a robust I_{K1} (e.g., atrial and ventricular myocytes), V_m is stabilized at a value close to the current reversal and a significant current source is required to re-excite the cell. On the other hand, if I_{K1} is poorly expressed (Purkinje myocytes) or absent (nodal cells) [35, 36], phase 4 becomes more positive and unstable. Under such conditions even small inward currents may cause progressive depolarization, eventually leading to re-excitation (automatic behavior) [37]. Besides the time-dependent currents, specific for each AP phase, time-independent (or "background") currents may also contribute to the whole AP course. These mainly include the Na^+/K^+ pump current (I_{NaK}) and the Na^+/Ca^{2+} exchanger current (I_{NCX}). Direction and magnitude of these currents during the various AP phases will be determined essentially by their electromotive force, which may vary according to the distribution of the transported ions across the cell membrane.

3.8.2 The Repolarization Process

3.8.2.1 Large Hearts have Long APs

❯ Figures 3.3 (from [38]) shows that action potentials are longer at low heart rate and that their duration is somewhat proportional to heart size (short in rat and mouse, longer in rabbit, guinea-pig, dog etc.). This may be dictated by functional needs. In an electrical syncytium, such as myocardium, the direction of propagation is indifferent; thus, any point along a propagation path, unless refractory, can be re-excited by activity occurring distal to it [39]. Thus, extinction of excitation during each cycle requires that cells at any point of the propagation path remain refractory until all cells downstream

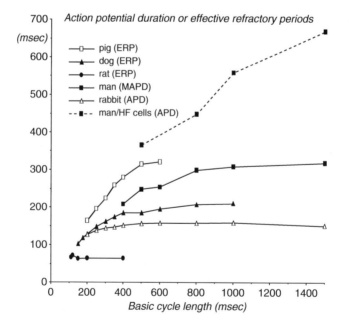

◻ Fig. 3.3

Cycle length and action potential duration (*APD*) or effective refractory period (*ERP*). Only in the rat, ERP seems independent of cycle length. In man, two relations are shown. The solid line with filled squares represents monophasic action potential duration in the normal human heart (*MAPD*). The dashed line with filled squares shows APD measured in single myocytes obtained from explanted hearts from patients with heart failure (*HF*). In heart failure, action potentials are prolonged compared to those in non-failing hearts. This is due to the combined effect of heart failure and to cell isolation which causes per se prolongation of the action potential by loss of electrotonic interaction (See also [43]) (Modified from [38])

have been activated. In accordance with the seminal theoretical work of Wiener and Rosenblueth [40] and Moe [41], the "leading circle" theory [42] predicts that the minimum length of the propagation path at which re-excitation can occur, named wavelength (WL in cm), equals the product of refractory period (RP in s) and conduction velocity (CV in cm/s)

$$WL = RP \times CV.$$

Thus, in a large heart with a large mass, re-excitation can be prevented only by a large RP × CV product. This requirement is fulfilled in larger animals by prolonged RP, resulting from long AP duration (APD). (Since I_{Na} quickly recovers from inactivation once V_m has repolarized, the refractory period is largely determined by APD under normal conditions.) The same functional requirement justifies the observation that APD is generally longer at proximal than at distal sites along a physiological propagation path. Therefore, it is understandable that preservation of correct temporal and spatial repolarization patterns is essential for maintenance of cardiac electrical stability [43].

In addition to the fact that APD is longer in species with larger hearts, ❷ Fig. 3.3 also shows the pivotal effect of electrotonic interaction on APD. Thus, APD in *isolated* human ventricular myocytes is substantially longer than in *intact* heart. This effect is probably much stronger than the APD prolongation caused by myocardial remodeling during the development of hypertrophy and heart failure (see also [43]).

3.8.2.2 Where Stability and Flexibility Meet

The need for repolarization stability and optimization of its synchrony contrasts with that of adapting APD to changes in heart rate, and with the existence, even during normal functioning, of numerous factors potentially perturbing the repolarization profile. (Notably those linking AP profile to mechanical activity, through Ca^{2+}-sensitivity of many among currents active during repolarization (I_{CaL}, I_{NCX}, I_{Ks}, I_{K1})) Thus, mechanisms to buffer perturbations and to allow flexible rate-adaptation must coexist in repolarization; understanding these might help us in predicting conditions at risk of cardiac electrical instability. Some clues may be provided by considering how the properties of I_{Kr} and I_{Ks} might be suited to afford repolarization stability at different heart rates.

I_{Ks} is a repolarizing current, which when increased, tends to shorten APD; it has slow systolic activation and slow diastolic deactivation [26]. Only a small proportion of total I_{Ks} is activated during an AP and its deactivation may be incomplete during short diastolic intervals (DI). Thus, an increment in the APD/DI ratio, as the one occurring as rate is increased, allows more I_{Ks} to be activated and less to be deactivated during each cycle. This makes I_{Ks} a good tool for APD rate-adaptation, particularly in the high heart-rate range, when incomplete diastolic deactivation becomes significant [33]. However, recent reports indicate that I_{Ks} deactivation may be distinctly faster in dog [44] and man [45] than in the guinea pig [46]; therefore, the role of I_{Ks} in human rate-dependency of repolarization is controversial. I_{Ks}'s contribution to rate-adaptation is also mediated by the sensitivity of this current to ß-adrenergic stimulation [26, 47] and to increases in cytosolic Ca^{2+} [48], both conditions physiologically associated with tachycardia. APD prolongation allows for more I_{Ks} activation which, in turn, shortens APD again; thus, APD and I_{Ks} are tied in a negative feed-back loop. This points to a potential role of I_{Ks} in stabilizing APD at each cycle length and in limiting its maximal duration at long ones [49]. At the same time, this negative feed-back loop may also set a limit to the maximum amount of shortening of APD at extreme high heart rates, when the reduction of relaxation time (diastole) may exceed that of activation time (systole). Under these circumstances I_{Ks} would tend to become a steady-state current. However, it should be considered that negative feed-back loops are paradoxically prone to oscillate whenever the conditions change quickly as compared to their response time. This may result in specific forms of APD instability, such as APD alternans, facilitated by abrupt changes in heart rate [50].

As shown in recent experiments, I_{Kr} kinetic features and response to heart rate are entirely different from those described above for I_{Ks} [33]; I_{Kr} deficiency also leads to major repolarization instability [51], suggesting a complementary role for the two K^+ currents. At variance with what has initially been hypothesized [52], at high heart rates I_{Kr} conductance may increase similarly to that of I_{Ks} [33]. However, the mechanism underlying the rate-dependent enhancement is fundamentally different between the two currents. ❷ Figure 3.4 (modified from [33]) shows that the extent of I_{Kr} activation is in fact independent of the diastolic interval. APs recorded at paced cycle length of 250 ms and 1,000 ms were applied to drive the membrane as I_{Kr} was recorded under voltage clamp conditions (❷ Fig. 3.4). In one case (left panels) APs were applied as originally recorded (i.e., with both AP profile and diastolic interval variable), in the other (right panels)

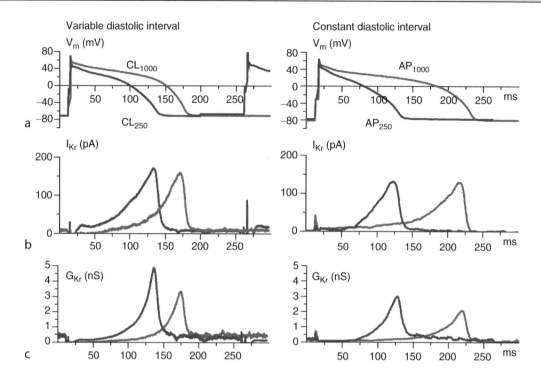

Fig. 3.4

Rate-dependency of I_{Kr}. (**a**) each panel shows action potential waveforms recorded at cycle lengths (*CL*) of 250 (*blue*) and 1,000 (*red*) ms. (**b**) I_{Kr} recorded during repetitive application, at the appropriate CL, of the action potentials shown in A. (**c**) I_{Kr} conductance (G_{Kr}), obtained by dividing the traces in B by the K^+ driving force (calculated from the traces in (**a**)). In the *right side panels*, the experiment was repeated by applying the waveforms in A after adjusting the CL to keep the diastolic interval constant. A remarkable increase in I_{Kr} amplitude and speed is observed at the shorter CL, irrespective of whether the diastolic interval is changing or not. This indicates that I_{Kr} increase at shorter CL is secondary to the change in action potential shape, rather than depending on CL itself (Modified from [33])

the cycle length was adjusted to keep the diastolic interval constant. In both cases, I_{Kr} conductance (G_{Kr}) was larger and faster at the shorter cycle length. This suggests that AP profile, rather than diastolic interval, determined I_{Kr} magnitude and course. As shown in ❷ Fig. 3.5 (modified from [33]), the feature of AP profile responsible for I_{Kr} rate-dependency is actually the repolarization rate. Modeling studies suggest that dependency of I_{Kr} conductance on repolarization rate can be explained by the interplay between the processes of deactivation and recovery from inactivation [33]. Since larger I_{Kr} results in faster repolarization, I_{Kr} and APD may be tied in a positive feed-back loop, acting as an "autoregenerative" repolarization mechanism. On the other hand, as I_{Kr} increase at high rates was the consequence of APD shortening; the latter must have been initiated by other mechanisms, probably including I_{Ks}. These findings suggest complementary roles for I_{Ks} and I_{Kr} and may explain why the effects of their simultaneous inhibition are more than additive [53].

Repolarization results from a balance between outward and inward currents. Thus, the properties of inward current components are equally important in determining repolarization course. Besides their role in sustaining the AP plateau, ion movements through I_{CaL}, I_{Na} and I_{NCX} determine the Ca^{2+} flux balance across the sarcolemma. Thus, unlike outward ones, inward currents are directly involved in contractile function and in its modulation.

The feature of I_{Na} and I_{CaL} most relevant to the course of repolarization is probably the rate and extent of their inactivation during the AP plateau. Normally I_{Na} is quickly inactivated by voltage and only a *small* "window" component persists during repolarization. Since such a component is a minor proportion of activated I_{Na}, even apparently small deviations from normal inactivation properties may lead to significant increments in plateau current [54–56]. I_{CaL} inactivation is partly voltage-dependent and partly induced by subsarcolemmal Ca^{2+}, through a Ca^{2+}-binding protein (Ca-calmodulin)

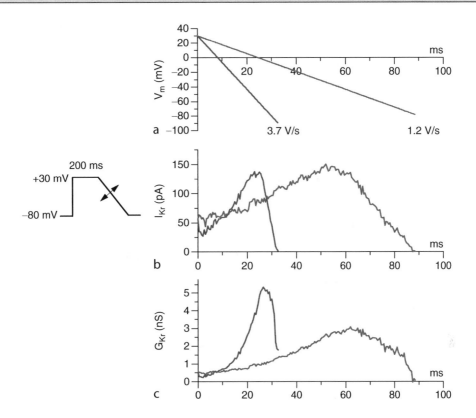

☐ Fig. 3.5

I_{Kr} dependency on repolarization rate. (a) I_{Kr} was recorded during repolarizing ramps of different velocity (voltage protocol shown in the *inset*). (b) I_{Kr} recorded during the two ramps. (c) I_{Kr} conductance (G_{Kr}) obtained by dividing the traces in **b** by the K$^+$ driving force (calculated from the traces in (**a**)) (Modified from [33])

[57, 58]. Ca^{2+}-induced I_{CaL} inactivation provides feedback regulation of Ca^{2+} influx and is part of a set of mechanisms adjusting APD to intracellular Ca^{2+} content. Changes in subsarcolemmal Ca^{2+} profile may cause major APD changes [59]. The availability of I_{CaL} during AP plateau strictly depends on the time course of membrane potential within the "window" range. Plateau prolongation may cause autoregenerative oscillatory depolarization (EADs) based on undue I_{CaL} reactivation [60]. Thus, even if intrinsically normal, I_{CaL} may amplify repolarization abnormality secondary to other causes. Finally, the direction and magnitude of I_{NCX} are sensitive to the Ca^{2+} transient profile, which may be altered in response to the needs of contractility modulation. With this in mind, inward currents seem to serve contractility requirements better than repolarization stability. Thus, for the repolarization process per se, inward currents might be viewed as a source of perturbation which, under normal conditions, is buffered by sufficiently strong outward currents.

3.9 Pacemaker Function

The high right atrium had been recognized as the "primum movens" as well as the "ultimum moriens" for over centuries. Doubt, however, has existed on the question of whether automaticity was an intrinsic property of the heart, or whether, alternatively, the heart depended on the brain for its rhythmic activity. This controversy was still not completely settled when Eyster and Meek published their famous review in the very first issue of *Physiological Reviews* [10]. The discovery of the sinus node [8] in the mole's heart by Martin Flack in the late summer of 1906, as described by Sir Arthur Keith in a historical paper dating back to 1942 [61], provided an anatomical base for the natural pacemaker of the heart. The relation between function and ultrastructure was reported in 1963 by Trautwein and Uchizono [62], although it took until 1978

3

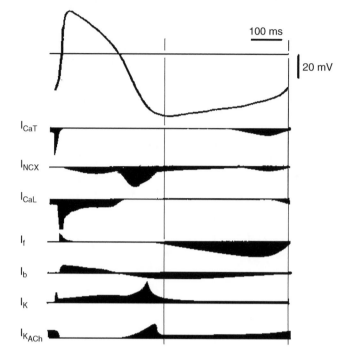

◘ Fig. 3.6

Outline of membrane currents of sinus node cells: current profiles (drawn by hand) are time aligned with the action potential. *Vertical lines* delimit diastolic depolarization. While the time course of currents approximates the real one, their relative magnitude may not be accurate

before the anatomical location of myocytes, from which sinus node action potentials had been recorded, was identified by tagging through the recording electrode [63].

Cardiac cells express currents of opposite sign and different time courses (e.g., I_{CaL} and I_K), linked by a common dependency on V_m (❷ Fig. 3.6). In such a situation the genesis of spontaneous V_m oscillations is very likely, unless there is a specific mechanism to prevent them (e.g., I_{K1} expression in non-pacemaker cells). Thus, multiple mechanisms may contribute to automaticity, and the absence of this function, rather than its presence, may be viewed as a functional specificity. This view is supported by the observation that, at early stages of maturation, all cardiac cells are spontaneously active and electrophysiological differentiation into working myocytes corresponds to the onset of I_{K1} expression [64]. This provides the theoretical ground for localized I_{K1} knock-out, obtained through genetic manipulation, as a means to artificially generate biological pacemakers in the ventricle [37].

A distinguishing feature of nodal tissues is indeed the lack of I_{K1} expression [35], which is responsible for many of the functional peculiarities of pacemaker cells. These include (1) the presence of diastolic depolarization, and (2) maximum (most negative) diastolic potentials of −60 to −40 mV, i.e., positive to those generated by a constantly high K^+ permeability. Such depolarized potentials would, per se, functionally inactivate I_{Na}; moreover, this current is also transcriptionally downregulated in the nodes, making the upstroke of their action potentials dependent on I_{CaL} (Ca^{2+}-dependent action potentials).

In light of this, it is not surprising that the attempt to identify the mechanism for the initiation of the heartbeat with a specific current has been a matter of scientific controversy in recent years [65, 66]. Nonetheless, in spite of the aspecific nature potentially underlying automaticity, pacemaker tissues (nodal and Purkinje cells) are equipped with a current, named I_f, with properties suitable to support pacemaker function and its modulation by autonomic transmitters [65]. I_f is only scantily expressed in non-pacemaker tissues and has properties which make its functional role negligible under physiological conditions in those tissues [67, 68]. The specific role of I_f will be discussed below, along with that of other currents contributing to diastolic depolarization.

3.9.1 Currents Underlying Diastolic Depolarization and its Autonomic Modulation

The membrane currents of sinus node cells have been reviewed in detail [14, 66, 69] and are summarized in ❷ Fig. 3.6.

Diastolic depolarization occurs at a low rate, thus requiring only a small amount of net inward transmembrane current (several pA in a single SA myocyte). However, such small net inward current results from the balance of larger inward and outward components; the direct effect of an increase in inward components is acceleration of depolarization (increased sinus rate), the opposite is true in case of an increase in outward ones.

Three voltage- and time-dependent currents, I_f and I_{CaL} (inward) and I_K (outward), are active during diastolic depolarization and are modulated by autonomic transmitters. (Other currents of smaller magnitude, or not directly modulated by neurotransmitters (I_{CaT}, I_{NCX}) are present during diastolic depolarization. Their role in pacemaking is discussed in ❷ Sect. 3.9.2.) These are superimposed on time-independent (background) currents, including inward (I_b) (Several different inward background currents, potentially contributing to I_b, have been described. Dissection of I_b in its components is not essential to the understanding of pacemaking and will not be discussed further) and outward (I_{KACh}) ones.

I_f is an inward current (carried by Na^+ at diastolic potentials); when increased it accelerates diastolic depolarization. Contrary to most cardiac currents, I_f is activated by membrane hyperpolarization [65]; the more negative the diastolic potential, the larger the I_f activation. Being triggered by the preceding repolarization, I_f may contribute to initiation of diastolic depolarization [70]. Due to its peculiar voltage-dependency and kinetics, I_f may provide an efficient buffer mechanism preventing excessive slowing of sinus rate by other mechanisms (see below). I_f is directly stimulated by binding of cytosolic cAMP [71]; thus, it is reciprocally regulated by membrane receptors increasing adenylate cyclase activity (ß-adrenergic, glucagone) and decreasing it (M2-muscarinic, A1-adenosine etc.) [72, 73]. I_{CaL} plays a role both in diastolic depolarization and in the generation of the upstroke of the SA nodal AP. Thus, its inhibition may cause pacemaker slowing and arrest in central nodal cells. However, I_{CaL} activates only in the terminal portion of diastolic depolarization [70] and it is probably not involved in its initiation (but see [74]). I_{CaL} is stimulated by cAMP-dependent protein kinase (PKA) [75]. Its receptor modulation is slower (channel phosphorylation requires extra time) but is consensual to that of I_f.

At first glance, it may be surprising that I_K (an outward current) is important to support pacemaking. Indeed, its main role is to repolarize the membrane to its maximum diastolic potential. However, I_K-mediated repolarization is essential for I_f activation (see above); this accounts for the apparently paradoxical observation that I_K inhibition leads to pacemaker slowing [76]. I_K deactivation is slow, causing a decay of outward current during the whole diastolic depolarization. If summed to adequately large background inward current (I_b), such a decay would result in a progressive increase of net inward current, which might alone sustain diastolic depolarization. Such a mechanism, although not specific to pacemaker tissues, might serve a backup function in the SA node [77]. I_K is stimulated by PKA and by cytosolic Ca^{2+} [48] therefore it is enhanced by the same receptors stimulating I_{CaL}. I_K stimulation should theoretically slow the rate; however, a larger I_K leads to more I_f activation, and the net effect is hardly predictable.

I_{KACh} is an inward rectifier K^+ current, structurally and functionally similar to I_{K1} [78]. However, different from I_{K1}, I_{KACh} channels are active only in the presence of acetylcholine (or adenosine). I_{KACh} activation adds outward current during diastolic depolarization, brings it to more negative potentials and, if sufficiently large, may cause pacemaker arrest. However, I_{KACh}-induced hyperpolarization activates I_f to a larger extent, which may limit the direct depressant effect [77]. A physiological amount of vagal stimulation is accompanied by an increase in membrane conductance [79]. When a decrease of I_f would be the predominant effect of vagal stimulation, a decrease in membrane conductance, *not an increase* would be expected. This might suggest that $I_{K,Ach}$ activation constitutes the most relevant mediator of cholinergic pacemaker modulation [79]. Nonetheless, acetylcholine concentrations required to activate I_{KACh} in sinoatrial myocytes also inhibit I_f [80]. Therefore, physiological pacemaker regulation may be based on simultaneous modulation of both currents. This view is supported by model simulations. ❷ Figure 3.7 suggests that modulation of both currents may provide more efficient rate control than separate modulation of either I_{KACh} or I_f. Functional

3

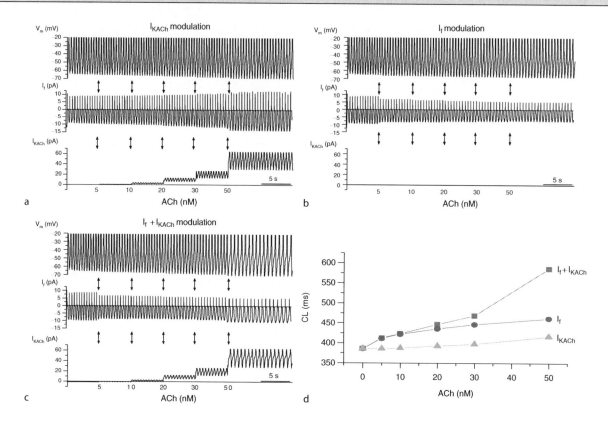

◘ Fig. 3.7

Interaction between I_{KACh} and I_f modulation by acetylcholine (*ACh*) in the control of pacemaker rate. Model simulations of sinoatrial pacemaking (Oxsoft Heart model [Noble D. *Oxsoft Heart 4.8 Program Manual*. Oxford, UK: Oxsoft Ltd. 1997]) considering the action of ACh as I_{KACh} activation only (**a**), I_f inhibition only (**b**) and combined I_{KACh} and I_f modulation (**c**). In each panel the *top trace* shows membrane potential (shown only negative to −20 mV to illustrate changes in maximum diastolic potential), the *middle trace* I_f and the *bottom trace* I_{KACh}. *Vertical arrows* mark the change in ACh concentration. (**d**) Pacemaker cycle length is plotted vs. ACh concentration for the three simulations. ACh effect on I_{KACh} and I_f was simulated according to the quantitative data in [80]. The simulation shows that coupled modulation of the two currents is required to modulate CL on a wide range of ACh concentrations. In particular, the effect of I_{KACh} modulation alone is very small because it is offset by the increase in I_f, secondary to membrane hyperpolarization (A. Zaza, unpublished data)

coupling between the two currents is probably instrumental in a wide-range and fail-safe regulation of sinus rate by vagal activation.

Controversy on the role of each of the above currents in SA pacemaking (I_f and I_{CaL}) largely stems from the observation that pharmacological blockade of either of them may fail to suppress diastolic depolarization. This is not only true for I_f [81], but under conditions of Ca^{2+}-independent excitability, true also for I_{CaL} [14]. On the one hand this may reflect the existence, within SA myocytes, of multiple pacemaker mechanisms, possibly taking over when one is abolished. On the other hand, this might also be the consequence of fail-safe mechanisms, determined by the kinetic properties of pacemaker currents. ❷ Figure 3.8 shows model simulations in which I_f was deliberately made essential for diastolic depolarization. The model predicts that even after 80% I_f blockade, pacemaker activity and its cholinergic modulation would still be preserved. While the mechanisms underlying this surprising observation are discussed elsewhere [82], this demonstrates that the interpretation of the effects of current blockade on cellular electrical activity may be quite complex.

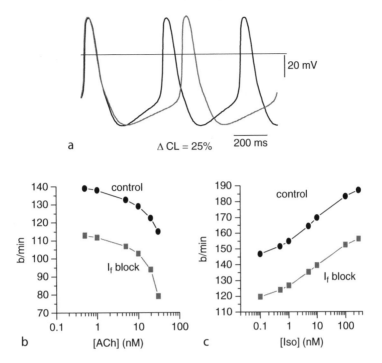

❏ Fig. 3.8

Effect of I_f blockade on pacemaker rate and its modulation in an I_f–dependent pacemaker model. Model (Oxsoft Heart [Noble D. *Oxsoft Heart 4.8 Program Manual*. Oxford, UK: Oxsoft Ltd. 1997]) parameters were set to obtain complete pacemaker arrest in the presence of 100% I_f inhibition (I_f-dependent pacemaking). (**a**) I_f inhibition by 80% (red trace, e.g., by 2 mM Cs$^+$) caused only 25% prolongation of cycle length (similar to the change experimentally observed with 2 mM Cs$^+$). (**b**) Pacemaker rate changes induced by ACh under control conditions and in the presence of 80% I_f blockade. ACh effects simulated by I_f and I_{KACh} modulation as in ❷ Fig. 3.7. (**c**) Pacemaker rate changes induced by ß-receptor stimulation with isoprenaline (*Iso*) under control conditions and in the presence of 80% I_f blockade. Iso effects simulated by I_f and I_{CaL} modulation according to the quantitative data in [72]. The simulation shows that such a large amount of I_f blockade results in only a moderate decrease in pacemaker rate, and preservation of its autonomic modulation, although full blockade of I_f causes quiescence (A. Zaza, unpublished data)

3.9.2   Intracellular Ca^{2+}-Dynamics may Contribute to Pacemaking

Pacemaker function of various cardiac tissues, including SA myocytes, is inhibited by ryanodine, an alkaloid which blocks Ca^{2+} release from the sarcoplasmic reticulum. This observation has raised interest in the role of intracellular Ca^{2+} dynamics in the genesis and modulation of SA pacemaking. Earlier reports of ryanodine effects have been followed by confocal microscopy studies establishing temporal and causal relationship between (1) voltage-dependent activation of sarcolemmal I_{CaT} during diastole, (2) a small "pre-systolic" Ca^{2+} release from the sarcoplasmic reticulum, and (3) the genesis of a slow inward current transient, crucially contributing to achievement of the SA activation threshold [83]. As for other Ca^{2+}-dependent membrane potential oscillations, in this case the Na$^+$/Ca^{2+} exchanger may also be primarily involved in coupling the pre-systolic SR Ca^{2+} release to the genesis of inward current transient [84, 85]. The contribution of the SR to SA pacemaker activity has been further extended by more recent studies suggesting that pre-systolic SR Ca^{2+} release may even occur as part of an oscillatory phenomenon, intrinsic to SR and independent of voltage-gated activation of sarcolemmal Ca^{2+} channels. A direct role of the "SR Ca^{2+} oscillator" in the pacemaker activity is suggested by correlation between the intrinsic frequencies of the two phenomena [86]. While SR-based pacemakers are common in smooth muscle cells, this represents the first example of such a mechanism in cardiac muscle.

Inhibition of SR Ca^{2+} release by ryanodine has also been reported to abolish ß-adrenergic receptor (ß-AR) modulation of pacemaker rate [87]. Although this finding is consistent with the important effect of ß-AR on SR function, it does not imply that adrenergic modulation of pacemaker rate may entirely occur through SR modulation. Indeed, sarcolemmal currents involved in pacemaker control (I_f, I_{CaL}) are altered by the change in cytosolic Ca^{2+} caused by ryanodine by beta AR.

The finding of a role for SR in pacemaking has potentially important pathophysiological implications because SR dysfunction is common in cardiac disease and possibly part of the maladaptive response associated with myocardial hypertrophy/failure. Nonetheless, the emphasis recently put on this novel pacemaker mechanism should not lead to the conclusion that SR-mediated phenomena are the only relevant mechanism in the genesis and modulation of sinoatrial automaticity.

3.9.3   Redundancy and Safety Factor in Pacemaking

As described above, redundancy in pacemaking mechanisms may be intrinsic to each myocyte. Nonetheless, a further factor in pacemaker safety is probably how the sinus node cells communicate with each other and with the surrounding atrium. The interest in the specificity in SA intercellular coupling stems from the apparent disproportion between the small excitation source, provided by the SA node, and the large current sink (electrical load) imposed on it by the surrounding atrial tissue, to which the impulse must propagate. Moreover, in the presence of low resistance coupling, quiescent and more polarized atrial myocytes would tend to "clamp" SA myocyte potential, thus preventing diastolic depolarization. This makes the coexistence of pacemaking and sinoatrial synchronization and conduction towards the atrium an apparent mystery.

As in the whole heart, gap junctions are a prerequisite for conduction in the SA node. Still, it has been argued that the spread of activation within the sinus node should be regarded as synchronization rather than as conduction [88]. Semantics or not, the resistance for intercellular current spread is high in the sinus node centre, mainly due to low density of gap junctions [89]. Moreover, at variance with working myocardium, smaller sinus node cells from the (putative) primary pacemaker area virtually lack connexin43. Their gap junctions are made of connexin40 and connexin45 proteins only [90]. Honjo et al. [90] have found, however, that larger sinoatrial cells from the (putative) more peripheral area – relevant for communication with the surrounding atrial muscle- express connexin45 and connexin43. Connexin45 has a lower unitary conductance than connexin43 [7]. As a consequence the "space constant" in the sinus node is around 300–500 µm, as compared to several mm in Purkinje fibers. This implies that pacemaker cells within the sinus node centre do not "see" much of their surroundings. From the central, primary pacemaker region, towards the periphery, the density of gap junction increases [91], thus establishing the lower resistance connection required for effective sinoatrial propagation. Centrifugal changes in the densities of intrinsic membrane currents [14] and gap junctions [91] predict that the "space constant" might be different according to the direction of propagation (node to atrium vs atrium to node); this prediction awaits experimental confirmation. This special feature is, however, functionally exemplified by the fact that the centre of the sinus node is "blind" to the effects of atrial fibrillation. Indeed, during this arrhythmia, central nodal cells continue their regular spontaneous discharge, unaffected by neighboring chaotic activity occurring at cycle lengths as short as 100 ms [92]. Thus, the delicate requirement to reconcile pacemaking with sinoatrial propagation is solved by a suitable arrangement of intercellular coupling, still adequate for pacemaker synchronization, but limiting the influence of atrial tissue. Nonetheless, coupling of the sinus node to the right atrium does slow pacemaker rate, as demonstrated experimentally [93, 94] and in computer simulations [95]. I_f response to membrane hyperpolarization (see above) contributes to the limiting of such an effect.

3.9.4   Functional Inhomogeneity in the Sinus Node

One of the most intriguing features of the sinus node is that its intrinsic cycle length is remarkably constant, although this is not the case with respect to its individual myocytes. Thus, isolated sinus node cells show substantial beat-to-beat

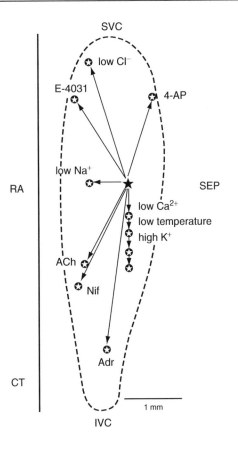

◘ Fig. 3.9

Shifts in pacemaker location within the sinus node. Scheme of (rabbit) sinus node with primary pacemaker location (*asterisk*).
Arrows indicate shift of the site of pacemaker dominance under various conditions: *SVC* superior vena cava, *SEP* interatrial
septum, *IVC* inferior vena cava, *CT* crista terminalis, *RA* right atrium, *E-4031* blocker of the rapid component of delayed rectifier
current (I_{Kr}), *4-AP* 4-aminopyridine (blocker of transient outward current (I_{to})), *Adr* adrenaline, *Nif*, nifedipine (blocker of L-type
Ca^{2+} current), *Ach* acetylcholine (Based on [14] and [97]. Reproduced from [14] with permission from Elsevier Science)

variability [93, 96] but this irregularity already disappears in clusters of sinus node cells of less than 1 mm × 1 mm [93, 94].
Sinus node cells in small clusters have shorter action potentials than in the intact node [93]. The intact sinus node is
in fact an inhomogeneous mixture of cells with different responses to environmental changes. A larger number of sinus
nodal myocytes is not only required to obtain beat-to-beat regularity, but also to expand the frequency range of beating.
Changes in the ionic composition of the extracellular fluid, drugs and autonomic stimulation induce pacemaker shifts
between different areas within the sinus node [14, 97] with different pacemaker rates (❷ Fig. 3.9, from [14]). This probably
reflects not only the presence, within the node, of cell populations with different channel expression and receptor density,
but also the presence of inhomogeneity in innervation. The functional implication is that, the whole sinus node is capable
of producing a larger range of cycle lengths than individual sinus node cell. Also, an intact heterogeneous sinus node
may produce a larger cycle length range than an homogeneous one. Positive chronotropy results from myocytes with
the highest sensitivity to the applied agent, f.e. noradrenalin. Negative chronotropy by vagal activation results from shift
of pacemaking from the area with highest intrinsic rate to another one with lower intrinsic rate, but less sensitive to the
depressant effect of acetylcholine [98, 99] (see also ❷ Fig. 3.9). The chronotropic response of the intact sinus node cannot
be deduced from the chronotropic responses of its constituent cells [97–99].

3.9.5 Abnormal Automaticity

Abnormal automaticity is defined as the occurrence of spontaneous firing in cardiac cells which are normally quiescent (e.g., working atrial and ventricular myocytes). Since such cells lack the mechanisms underlying physiological pacemaker function, abnormal automaticity is based on different mechanisms, put into action by pathological conditions. A common cause of abnormal automaticity is partial membrane depolarization, to a range of potentials at which I_{K1} conductance is reduced. Under such conditions, diastolic potential becomes unstable and is likely to be driven by mechanisms which are normally silenced. Such mechanisms may be based on the interplay between time- and voltage-dependent currents with opposite signs, such as I_{CaL} and I_K and on Ca^{2+}-activated currents. The intrinsic rate of an abnormal focus based on such mechanisms is generally proportional to the degree of membrane depolarization [100]. It has been recently observed that in hypertrophic ventricular myocytes I_f may be expressed at an abnormally high density and with kinetic properties [101] favoring its role in pacemaker activity. Thus it is possible that, under specific pathological conditions, I_f may contribute to abnormal automaticity.

Action potentials resulting from abnormal automaticity generally arise in partially depolarized membranes, in which I_{Na} is partially or completely inactivated. Thus, depending on the extent of I_{Na} inactivation, their upstroke may be partially or completely dependent on I_{CaL} [102]. Accordingly, abnormal automaticity is often suppressed by Ca^{2+} channel inhibition.

If abnormal automaticity occurs at a rate exceeding the sinoatrial one, the automatic focus becomes the dominant pacemaker and its activity may be propagated to the whole heart. If the abnormal automatic rate is lower than the sinoatrial one, its discharge can become manifest only if the automatic focus is protected from resetting by the dominant activity. This may occur through a unidirectional "entry block," which prevents propagation of sinoatrial activity to the abnormal focus, but allows propagation of abnormal activity to the surrounding myocardium. Even if reset by sinoatrial activity (i.e., in the absence of entry block), abnormal foci are less sensitive to overdrive suppression than normal pacemaker tissue [103]. They may therefore become active during slow heart rate and are not easily overdriven when the sinus node resumes its activity. Low rate abnormal automaticity is a common mechanism of "parasystolic" arrhythmias and "escape" ventricular beats. Due to its dependency on Ca^{2+} current, abnormal automaticity is strongly enhanced by ß-adrenergic stimulation.

Subacute and chronic myocardial infarction are probably the conditions in which abnormal automaticity is most common and a frequent cause of arrhythmia [39]. Tissue at the junction between the pulmonary veins and the left atrium is particularly prone to abnormal automaticity [104]. Its role in triggering atrial fibrillation has been recently identified with a major impact on the therapeutic approach to this arrhythmia [105].

3.10   Ionic Homeostasis and Electrical Activity

Bioelectricity constitutes by far the fastest communication system of the body. Action potentials come with a price. They disturb the ionic homeostasis, which has ultimately to be corrected by the Na^+/K^+ pump at the dispense of metabolic energy. The disturbance of the homeostasis is surprisingly small. If we consider a cylindrical myocyte with a length of $100\,\mu m$ and a diameter of $20\,\mu m$, we arrive at a cellular surface of $6,912\,\mu m^2$ and a cellular volume of $31,416\,\mu m^3$. The surface is necessary for the calculation of the number of ions that pass the membrane during the action potential upstroke, which can be considered as a depolarizing step of $100\,mV$. We need the volume in order to calculate the disturbance of the cellular Na^+ concentration under the assumption that all depolarizing current is carried by Na^+ ions. The amount of charge related to an upstroke of the action potential can be calculated with

$$Q = C \times V$$

in which Q is charge in coulomb (C), C is cell capacitance in farad (F) and V is voltage in volt (V). The typical capacitance of cellular membranes is $1\,\mu F/cm^2$. Thus, with the above cellular surface of $6,912\,\mu m^2$, the capacitance of one myocyte is 6.9×10^{-11} F. Here we have neglected the effect of caveolae on the cell surface, which might double it. Because the amplitude of the action potential ($100\,mV$) equals $0.1\,V$, we obtain a total charge (see formula) of 6.9×10^{-12} C. Because the passage of the membrane by 1 mol equals a charge of $96,500$ C (Faraday constant), the amount of 6.9×10^{-12} C is carried by 7.2×10^{-17} mol of Na^+ ions. Multiplying by the number of Avogadro (6.022×10^{23}, i.e., the number of ions or molecules in 1 mol) then yields the number of Na^+ ions that passes the sarcolemma of a myocyte with a length of 100 μm and a width of 20 μm during the upstroke of an action potential with an amplitude of 100 mV. This number amounts to 43 million. The number may seem impressive, but in a cellular volume of 31,416 μm^3 (see above), which equals 3.14×10^{-11} L, these 43 million Na^+ ions only increase the intracellular Na^+ concentration by 2.3 μM. Given the intracellular Na^+ concentration of 10 mM, one action potential results in an increase of 0.02% in the intracellular Na^+ concentration. Thus, assuming for the sake of simplicity that the action potential configuration does not change over time, the intracellular Na^+ concentration would double after 5,000 action potentials, that is, after more than 1 h at normal heart rate, if this "extra" Na^+ were not pumped back by the Na^+/K^+ pump.

Although the concentration increase of Na^+ (2.3 μM) per action potential is small compared with the normal Na^+ concentration (10 mM), this concentration step is substantial compared with both the systolic and diastolic intracellular Ca^{2+} concentrations, which are at and below the micromolar level.

3.11 Region-Specific Currents

While the nodes represent the most striking case of functional specificity within the heart, relevant differences in action potential shape and underlying currents also characterize other cardiac tissues. Rather than providing a systematic description of regional variations in electrical activity, the aim of this section is to illustrate some examples of major pathophysiological relevance.

3.11.1 Receptor-Activated Current (I_{KACh}) Replaces I_{K1} in the Nodes and is Highly Expressed in the Atria

As discussed above, I_{K1} is responsible for diastolic membrane potential stability in working myocardium and its absence from nodal tissues is instrumental to pacemaker function. Nonetheless, all atrial tissues (including the nodes) express at high density I_{KACh}, an inward-rectifier current strictly related to I_{K1} in terms of channel structure and function [78]. However, unlike I_{K1} constitutive activation, I_{KACh} is turned on by the binding of acetylcholine or adenosine to M2 and A1 receptors respectively. Activation occurs through direct channel interaction with beta-gamma subunits of receptor coupled G-proteins (G_i or G_o) [106]. I_{KACh} activation leads to substantial hyperpolarization of the diastolic potential and decreased membrane input resistance, both contributing to lower excitability, and APD shortening. This translates into negative chronotropic and dromotropic effects in nodal myocytes and reduced refractoriness in the atria. Recent reports suggest that I_{KACh} channels are also present in ventricular myocytes, but their functional expression is limited by competition with other K^+ currents (e.g., I_{K1}) for a common pool of subsarcolemmal K^+ [107]. I_{KACh} function also depends on PKA-mediated phosphorylation [108] and on the availability of a membrane phospholipid component (PIP2), which is a substrate of phospholipase C (PLC). Accordingly, I_{KACh} availability is limited by PLC activating receptors (endothelin, angiotensin, α-adrenergic, etc.) that consume PIP2 [109].

3.11.2 Different Delayed Rectifier Currents Underlie Repolarization in the Atria

Atrial repolarization, characterized by a prominent phase 1, is distinctly faster than ventricular repolarization. This suggests differences in the expression of repolarizing currents. I_{to} and two components of delayed-rectifier current, with properties similar to I_{Ks} and I_{Kr} in the ventricle, have been described in canine [110] and human atrial myocytes [111]. However, atrial myocytes also express an additional depolarization activated K^+ current characterized by (1) fast activation and deactivation; (2) slow and only partial inactivation; (3) sensitivity to low (μM) 4-aminopyridine concentrations. Currents with such properties have been identified in animal and human atrial myocyte by different groups and named I_{sus} [112], I_{Kur} [113], and I_{so} [114]. Despite slightly different properties, possibly due to different recording conditions, all these currents are probably carried by the same channel protein $K_v1.5$. Due to its kinetic properties I_{Kur} may contribute to the whole repolarization process. Since its amplitude is reduced at high stimulation rates [115], I_{Kur} probably does not play a role in rate-dependent APD shortening. In terms of molecular nature, I_{Kur} is closer to I_{to}, with which it shares pharmacological properties, than to ventricular delayed rectifiers. This provides the rationale for targeting I_{Kur} as a tool for selective prolongation of atrial repolarization.

3.11.3 Differential Expression of K$^+$ Currents Generates a Gradient of Electrophysiological Properties Across the Ventricular Wall

In subepicardial layers phase 1 is prominent and results in a "spike and dome" AP morphology, which is at variance with subendocardial layers, in which the repolarization course is more monotonic [25]. As a consequence, a significant gradient of action potential morphologies exists across the ventricular wall [116]. Different phase 1 amplitude is the consequence of a gradient in functional I_{to} expression, resulting from non-uniform distribution of a functionally essential channel subunit [117]. Electrical heterogeneity across the ventricular wall is also contributed by lower expression of I_{Ks} in midmyocardial layers [118], albeit established at non-physiological conditions. Myocytes isolated from these layers (M cells) are characterized by a particularly steep rate-dependency of repolarization, with marked APD prolongation at long CLs [119]. Lack of I_{Ks} also makes isolated M cells susceptible to develop early afterdepolarizations during sympathetic activation. The functional significance of these transmural inhomogeneities has been subject to vigorous debate even in the dog, the species in which M cells have been extensively investigated [120, 121]. Recently, Janse and coworkers, in a study performed with high density recording over and within the wall, showed that transmural repolarization is remarkably synchronous in the canine left ventricle [122]. The role of M cells in the human heart has only been assessed in a very limited number of studies. M cells have been identified in the human wedge preparation [123], but not in whole human hearts [124, 125], and also not in a larger wedge preparation obtained from the human heart [125]. A midmural zenith in action potential duration cannot be demonstrated in the left human ventricle [124], let alone a midmural zenith in repolarization time [125]. Although the electrical peculiarity of M cells may be less apparent within the myocardial syncytium, they may become functionally important in the presence of I_{Kr} blockers, when they have been suggested to lead to repolarization abnormalities [121]. However, even under such challenging conditions the role of M cells has been questioned [126]. While methodological differences might contribute to the discrepancy between these studies, the contribution of M cells to overall cardiac repolarization remains controversial. Overall, intercellular coupling (electrotonic interaction) seems to substantially blunt repolarization heterogeneity within the ventricular wall. This may be particularly true in larger species, including man, with long action potential duration and relatively high membrane resistance during repolarization, which in turn, is likely to increase intercellular communication (see below) [43, 125].

3.12 Cardiac Channel Proteins

The molecular identity of most cardiac ion channels has been identified; the corresponding proteins have been cloned and can be expressed by heterologous transfection in various cell types [127]. Many functional studies are nowadays performed on heterologously expressed channel clones, whose nomenclature is often unrelated to that of the native current. ❷ Table 3.1 summarizes the correspondence between each native current and its molecular counterpart (see also [128]).

    Each functional channel results from the interaction between several proteins (subunits): an α-subunit, usually including permeation and gating structures, and one or more β-subunits, which confer to the channel specific kinetic and pharmacological properties. Within the cell membrane, α-subunits are generally clustered in tetramers. The latter may be composed by a single (homeotetramers) or different (heterotetramers) isoforms of the protein, often resulting in different functional properties [129]. In many instances, expression of the cloned proteins does not precisely reproduce the functional properties of the native current. This is true even if all the α- and β-subunits known to contribute to the channel are coexpressed. Moreover, function of a channel clone can change according to the cell type in which it is expressed [130], to reflect the multiplicity of factors contributing to the function of the native channel. Nonetheless, functional changes induced by drugs or structural abnormalities (mutations) in cloned channels expressed in mammalian cell lines have been thus far reasonably predictive of those occurring in native ones [131]. Thus, as long as its intrinsic limitations are duly considered, heterologous expression of channel clones is a useful tool for electrophysiological studies.

◼ **Table 3.1**
Correspondence between cardiac ionic currents and channel proteins

Current	α-subunit(s)	β-subunits	Notes
I_{Na}	$Na_V1.5$ (SC5NA)	$\beta1$, $\beta2$, $\beta3$	TTX-sensitive type
I_{CaT}	$Ca_V3.1$ (α_{1G})	$\gamma6$	Mainly in nodes
I_{CaL}	$Ca_V1.2$ (α_{1C}), $Ca_V1.3$ (α_{1D})	β, γ, δ	$Ca_V1.3$ in nodes
I_f	HCN1 + HCN4	MiRP1 (KCNE2)	Specific for pacemaker tissues
I_{K1}	$K_{ir}2.1$ (IRK1)	$K_{ir}2.2$	"Inward rectifier"
I_{KATP}	$K_{ir}6.2$	SUR	Inactive at physiological [ATP]
I_{KACh} (I_{Kado})	$K_{ir}3.4$ (GIRK4) + $K_{ir}3.1$ (GIRK1)		Activated by ACh or adenosine; mostly atrial and nodal
I_{to}	$K_V4.2$ + $K_V4.3$	KChIP2	Mainly subepicardial
I_{Kur} (I_{Ksus})	$K_V1.5$	KChAP, $K_V\beta_1$, $K_V\beta_2$	Specific for atrium
I_{Kr}	$K_V11.1$(HERG)	MiRP1 (KCNE2)	Rapid "delayed rectifier"
I_{Ks}	$K_V 7.1$(KVLQT1)	minK (KCNE1)	Slow "delayed rectifier"
I_{NCX} (I_{TI})	NCX1		Na^+/Ca^{2+} exchanger current
I_{NaK}	NaK α 1,2,3	$\beta1$, $\beta2$	Na^+/K^+ pump current
I_{GJ}	Cx43 (ventricle), Cx40, Cx45 (nodes)		Gap-junctional current

Denomination of α-subunits according to the IUPHAR compendium of voltage-gated ion channels [128]. Other frequently used denominations in parentheses

3.13 Propagation

3.13.1 General Mechanism of Propagation

If considered in detail, propagation of excitation through the heart is very complex, as described in some excellent reviews by Kléber, Janse and Fast [132], and Kléber and Rudy [133]. Nonetheless, a relatively simple description of its basic principles is possible and very useful for the understanding of cardiac pathophysiology.

During propagation there is a difference in membrane potential between the excited myocytes (i.e., the site of an action potential) and the still unexcited neighboring one. This difference defines the "activation front." Let us suppose that an activation front moves from left to right through a strand of myocytes. At the left the inside of the myocytes is positively charged (due to inward current of Na^+ ions from the extracellular space into the intracellular space), whereas the inside of the not yet excited myocytes is still at the resting membrane potential of about −90 mV. This potential difference causes an intracellular current flow along the cell axis and through gap junctions, i.e., the positive charge moves from the excited cell to the unexcited one. At the same time, in the extracellular space a current flows in the opposite direction; this is because the extracellular side of the excitation site is made negative by the movement of Na^+ ions into the cell. To summarize, during propagation, local current moves forward through the intracellular space and backward in the extracellular space, forming a complete "propagation circuit." As a result of intracellular current positive charge accumulates under the membrane of the cell to be excited and depolarizes it to the excitation threshold; this triggers a new autoregenerative I_{Na} activation (action potential). The latter, in turn, serves as the "source" of charge for excitation of the next cell and the process is repeated. In this process, the cell(s) to be excited can be viewed as the electrical "load" to be imposed on the charge "source." The relevant parameter is actually the amount of membrane capacity to be charged, which directly depends on the area of membrane electrically coupled to the source. For propagation to occur, the charge supplied by the source must at least match the charge required by the load. Under physiological conditions, the former largely exceeds the latter; such a redundancy of the system is important in establishing a "safety factor" for propagation, which may prevent the occurrence of conduction block in a wide range of conditions.

Propagation is characterized by its "conduction velocity" (in cm/s) and the "safety factor," which we consider in more detail in the next two subsections.

3.13.2   Conduction Velocity

The speed at which the activation front travels essentially depends on how many cells along the propagation path can be simultaneously excited by the charge supplied by the "source." This, in turn depends on (1) the amount of source charge (I_{Na} density in working myocardium and I_{CaL} density in the nodes), and (2) how far along the cell axis charge can travel without being dissipated to the extracellular space. According to cable theory, the latter can be characterized by the ratio between specific membrane resistance (R_m, in $\Omega \cdot m^2$) and specific axial resistance (R_i, in $\Omega \cdot m$) (R_m and R_i are expressed here with the conventional units of "specific resistance". The term a/2 is omitted if R_m is specific resistance per circumference unit ($\Omega \cdot m$) and R_i is specific resistance per cross-sectional area (Ω/m)) and is defined by a parameter named "space constant" (λ):

$$\lambda \sim \sqrt{\{(R_m/R_i) \times (a/2)\}}$$

where a is the radius of the cable and λ is the distance over which the amplitude of a small voltage deflection has decayed to 37% of its original value. R_m essentially depends on how many membrane ion channels are open, whereas R_i is determined by the sum of cytoplasmic, gap junctional, and extracellular resistances.

In the sinus node, R_m is high due to the absence of I_{K1}; however this is off-set by a high R_i due to the low density and conductance of gap junctions, thus resulting in a small λ (≤ 0.5 mm). In the Purkinje system, in which I_{K1} is small compared with the working ventricular myocardium, but large compared with the sinus node, and in which the gap junctional density is high, λ can be in the order of several mm, substantially larger than in the working myocardium. It should be noted that, for technical and theoretical reasons, λ is measured only at the resting membrane potential [134], at which R_m is substantially different than during an action potential. For instance, during the upstroke of the action potential R_m is smaller, due to the massive opening of Na^+ channels; during the plateau phase and early repolarization R_m is higher (no I_{K1}, small currents). This predicts that λ may be maximal, thus supporting optimal electrotonic interaction, during the action potential plateau and the early phase of repolarization. The fact that electrotonic interaction may be lower in smaller animals (e.g., rodents) due to their shorter action potential duration, caused by larger repolarizing currents and leading to a smaller R_m during repolarization, is starting to be recognized [43, 135].

An important consequence of the role of gap junctional resistance is that it creates a physiologically relevant difference in velocity between propagation parallel to cell orientation (longitudinal propagation) or perpendicular to it (transverse propagation). This difference is named "electrical anisotropy" and can be explained as follows. Cardiac myocytes are elongated (about 70–100 µm long and 10–20 µm wide); when packed in the tissue they can establish side-to-side and end-to-end connections. Thus axial current will travel in both directions. However, to travel the same tissue distance (e.g., 1 cm), current must cross about fivefold more cell borders (i.e., gap junctions) in the transverse than in the longitudinal direction. Gap junctions are "in series" with respect to axial current flow, which implies that their individual resistances are summed. Thus as far as the contribution of gap junctions in R_i (specific axial resistance; sum of cytoplasmic, gap junctional, and extracellular resistances) is involved, it can be expected that conduction velocity is lower in transversal than in longitudinal direction. Variation in the density of gap junction expression and more complex arrangement of cells (e.g., end-to-side connections) may also contribute to determine the anisotropy ratio. Measured anisotropy ratio is about 2.7 in dog [132], but it might be substantially less in human ventricle, where these simple measurements are surprisingly scarce [136]. An anisotropy ratio even larger than predicted by tissue geometry may reflect propagation "discontinuity" [137], resulting in junctional delays larger than predicted for continuous propagation.

These considerations have an interesting bearing on conduction velocity in hypertrophy and heart failure. Both are in general associated with delayed conduction [138], which is often considered to be the result of decreased conduction velocity. However, hypertrophy per se (increase in cell size), results in a smaller number of junctions per unit length of the propagation path. Thus, as long as no factors other than cellular dimensions change during hypertrophy, an increase and *not* a decrease, in tissue conduction velocity is expected, as was recently confirmed experimentally [139]. Under such circumstances an observed conduction delay is explained by increased cardiac mass, which is insufficiently compensated for by *increased* conduction velocity. On the other hand, at more severe stages of hypertrophy, concomitant interstitial fibrosis and changes in gap junction expression may cause a decrease in conduction velocity itself. Further pathological changes in the density of membrane channels, also known as remodeling, may exacerbate this process.

Besides electrotonic interaction, conduction velocity is also affected by the magnitude of the current source, which is substantially larger for I_{Na} than for I_{CaL}. Thus, differential expression of these currents contributes to the large difference in conduction velocity among cardiac tissues. Longitudinal conduction velocities are in the order of 2 and 5 cm/s in SA and AV nodes respectively, and around 60 cm/s in atrial and ventricular working myocardium. In specialized conducting tissues conduction velocity is higher; values of 100 and 130 cm/s can be measured in crista terminalis and Bachman's bundle respectively and 200–300 cm/s in Purkinje fibers [132].

3.13.3   Safety Factor of Propagation

As introduced above, the propagation safety factor is determined by the ratio between the electrical charge supplied by the "source" and that required by the "load" [132, 133, 140]. The former is primarily determined by the magnitude of depolarizing current (I_{Na} in the working myocardium and Purkinje, I_{CaL} in the nodes) available at a given time. The latter is determined by the electrical capacity to be charged, physically represented by the membrane area electrically coupled to the source. Under physiological conditions, the current size available in a single cell is large enough to charge the membrane capacity of the cell itself plus a number of connected cells.

Source/load mismatch can result from (1) depression of I_{Na} (or I_{CaL} in the nodes), by incomplete recovery from inactivation (partial membrane depolarization, extrasystoles falling in the relative refractory period etc.), drugs or genetic defects with loss of function (e.g., the LQT3 syndrome), and (2) tissue geometry such as to impose a large load on a small source. Illustrative examples of the latter are discrete Purkinje-myocardial junctions, at which a small number of Purkinje cells are coupled to a relatively large mass of underlying myocardium (i.e., a large membrane capacity). Under such circumstances the safety factor is low for orthodromic and high for antidromic propagation, setting the stage for the occurrence of unidirectional conduction block. In the case of the Purkinje-myocardial junction the potential source/load mismatch is compensated by a very high expression of Na^+ channels and long action potential duration in Purkinje cells. However, under pathological conditions, a similar tissue geometry may be generated by patchy fibrosis, producing expanses of myocardium connected by relatively thin bundles of excitable tissue. In this case compensatory mechanisms are absent and arrhythmias resulting from unidirectional block (reentry) are greatly facilitated.

Although safety factor and conduction velocity are affected in the same direction by several factors (e.g., I_{Na} magnitude), their changes are not always consensual. Indeed, an increase in gap junctional resistance decreases conduction velocity (smaller λ), but may simultaneously increase the safety factor [141]. This is because the effective membrane capacity "seen" by the source decreases when coupling resistance increases [142]. This is the mechanism underlying the observation that, although longitudinal propagation is faster, depression of I_{Na} may lead to blocking of longitudinal propagation with persistence of the transverse one [143]. The relation between safety factor, conduction velocity and coupling resistance is illustrated in ❷ Fig. 3.10.

Under source/load mismatch conditions, I_{CaL} may become necessary to support propagation even if I_{Na} is intact [144, 145]. This unexpected observation has been interpreted as follows. Due to discrete distribution of axial resistance (at gap junctions), a small delay occurs whenever excitation crosses a cell border. Thus, even if apparently continuous at macroscopic level, propagation is "discontinuous" at the microscopic one [146]. Under source/load mismatch conditions such delays may be increased and outlast the duration of I_{Na} flow. In this case the smaller, but longer lasting I_{CaL} may become pivotal to provide the sustained generator current required for excitation of the downstream cell. Thus, not only the magnitude, but also the duration of the generator current may be important in determining the safety factor of propagation.

3.14   Mathematical Models

Over the past decades patch-clamp experiments have provided us with detailed information on the different types of ion channels that are present in the cardiac cell membrane. The sophisticated cardiac cell models that are available today can help us understand how the different types of ion channels act together to produce the cardiac action potential (cf. ❷ Figs. 3.6 and ❷ 3.8). Moreover, such models have become essential instruments for the assessment of the functional

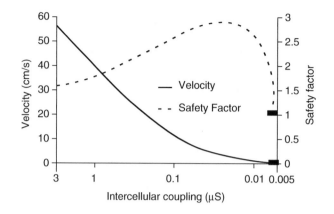

◘ Fig. 3.10

Influence of junctional coupling conductance on conduction velocity and safety factor. Conduction velocity (*left* ordinate) and safety factor for conduction (*right* ordinate) as a function of intercellular coupling (*abscissa*). At first glance, against intuition, a decrease in intercellular coupling leads to a transient increase in safety of conduction, before conduction blocks (Reproduced from [128] with permission from Physiological Reviews. This figure is adapted from Fig. 3.5a in Shaw RM, Rudy Y. Circ Res 1997; 81: 727–741)

implications of changes in density or kinetics of ion channels, e.g., changes due to ion channel mutations underlying the congenital long-QT syndrome.

Back in 1928, van der Pol and van der Mark presented the first mathematical description of the heartbeat, which is in terms of a relaxation oscillator [147]. Their work has given rise to a family of models of nerve and heart "cells" (excitable elements) in terms of their key properties, i.e., excitability, stimulus threshold, and refractoriness. These models are relatively simple with a minimum number of equations and variables [148, 149]. Because they are compact, these models have been widely used in studies of the spread of excitation in tissue models consisting of large numbers of interconnected "cells" (e.g., [149]).

A major drawback of this family of models is the absence of explicit links between the electrical activity and the underlying physiological processes like the openings and closures of specific ion channels. Today's sophisticated cardiac cell models provide such links and are all built on the framework defined by the seminal work of Hodgkin and Huxley [150], for which they received the Nobel Prize in Physiology or Medicine in 1963.

3.14.1 The Seminal Hodgkin-Huxley Model

Hodgkin and Huxley investigated the electrical activity of the squid giant axon, on which they published a series of five (now classical) papers in 1952. In their concluding paper they summarized their experimental findings and presented "a quantitative description of membrane current and its application to conduction and excitation in nerve" [150]. This "quantitative description" included a mathematical model derived from an electrical equivalent of the nerve cell membrane. They identified sodium and potassium currents flowing across the giant axon membrane and represented these in terms of the sum of conductive components that we now identify as ion channels, and membrane capacitance. In the electrical equivalent, the cell membrane was represented by a capacitor (cf. ❷ Sect. 3.3.1) in parallel with three resistors representing the sodium conductance, the potassium conductance and a leakage conductance. The associated sodium and potassium currents were described using the mathematical formulation introduced in ❷ Sect. 3.3.4.

In their series of papers, Hodgkin and Huxley demonstrated that g_m can be separated into sodium and potassium components (g_{Na} and g_K, respectively), which are both functions of V_m and time. In their analysis they introduced the

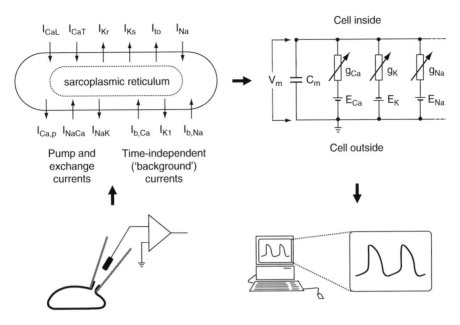

◻ Fig. 3.11
Common layout of cardiac cell models. Data from patch-clamp experiments (*bottom left*) provide quantitative information on each of the individual membrane current components (*top left*). This information is turned into an electrical equivalent (*top right*). The resulting equations, together with equations describing intracellular processes, e.g., the calcium uptake and release by the sarcoplasmic reticulum, are then compiled into a computer model of the cardiac cell, e.g., an SA nodal cell model (*bottom right*)

concept of activation and inactivation "gates" and provided equations governing the time and voltage dependence of these gates. Upon a change in V_m, x (the gating variable introduced in ❷ Sect. 3.3.4) changes with time as:

$$dx/dt = \alpha \times (1 - x) - \beta \times x, \qquad (3.5)$$

where α and β are "rate constants," which are both functions of V_m. In this concept, α is the rate at which x gates change from the closed to the open state, whereas β is the rate at which x gates change from the open to the closed state.

As illustrated in ❷ Fig. 3.11, today's ionic cardiac cell models still follow the concept of Hodgkin and Huxley. The ionic currents that have been identified in patch-clamp experiments are described in terms of "activation" and "inactivation" and turned into components of an electrical circuit, which underlies the set of model equations. The only extension to the concept of Hodgkin and Huxley is the inclusion of an additional set of equations governing the changes in intracellular ion concentrations (sodium, potassium, and calcium) and the intracellular calcium uptake and release processes ("second-generation models," see ❷ Sect. 3.14.4).

3.14.2 Early Cardiac Cell Models (1960–1989)

The Hodgkin and Huxley concept was first applied to cardiac cells by Noble [151, 152]. His model of cardiac Purkinje fibers was relatively simple and had five variables. With more experimental data becoming available, the model was updated twice, in the seventies by McAllister et al. [153] and in the eighties by DiFrancesco and Noble [154]. The latter two models formed the basis for the development of ventricular, atrial, and sinoatrial cell models (❷ Table 3.2; [151–162]).

■ Table 3.2

Early ionic models of mammalian cardiac cells (1960–1989)

Model	Parent model
Purkinje fibre models	
Noble [151, 152]	–
McAllister et al. [153]	Noble [151, 152]
DiFrancesco and Noble [154]	McAllister et al. [153]
Ventricular cell models	
Beeler and Reuter [155]	McAllister et al. [153]
Drouhard and Roberge [156]	Beeler and Reuter [155]
Atrial cell models	
Hilgemann and Noble [157]	DiFrancesco and Noble [154]
Sinoatrial cell models (rabbit)	
Yanagihara et al. [158]	–
Irisawa and Noma [159]	Yanagihara et al. [158]
Bristow and Clark [160]	McAllister et al. [153]
Noble and Noble [161]	DiFrancesco and Noble [154]
Noble et al. [162]	Noble and Noble [161]

3.14.3　Detailed Cardiac Cell Models (1990–2005)

According to current standards, the models that were developed during the first three decades of cardiac cell modeling (❷ Table 3.2; [151–162]) were simple, with a small number of variables and equations, and of a generic nature, with limited specificity regarding species or location within the tissue. This changed rapidly during the subsequent period. Starting in the early nineties, a large number of cardiac cell models of increasing complexity have been developed, profiting from the immense progress made in cardiac cellular electrophysiology and the powerful computer resources that have become available (❷ Table 3.3; [153, 163–194]). Among these models, the "Luo-Rudy II" ventricular cell model [167], also known as "phase-2 Luo-Rudy" or "LR2" model, has become a classical one. Several more recent ventricular and atrial cell models have been built upon the Luo-Rudy equations. After the Luo-Rudy II model was published in 1994, it has been updated several times, keeping track with experimental data appearing in literature. The source code of the current version of the model ("LRd model"), as well as that of several other models, is available on the Internet (see ❷ Sect. 3.14.8).

3.14.4　First-Generation and Second-Generation Models

In the early ionic models of cardiac cells, all the concentrations of the various ionic species were held fixed, so that no provision had to be made for pumps and exchangers to regulate these concentrations. We refer to models that incorporate variable ion concentrations as well as pumps and exchangers as "second-generation" models, in contrast to the earlier "first-generation" models [195]. There are two major problems with the more physiologically realistic second-generation models, in which, besides membrane potential and gating variables, ion concentrations vary in time: (1) drift, with very slow long-term trends in some of the variables, particularly some ionic concentrations, and (2) degeneracy, with non-uniqueness of equilibrium solutions such as steady states and limit cycles (see [195] and primary references cited therein). Drift has been managed in several ways, including stimulus current assignment to a specific ionic species [196]. The other major problem noted with second-generation models is degeneracy. Essentially, second-generation models form a system of $N-1$ equations in N unknowns. As a result, there is a continuum of equilibrium points ("steady-state solutions"), rather than isolated equilibrium points, so that, e.g., the resting potential of a quiescent system depends on the initial conditions.

■ Table 3.3

Detailed ionic models of mammalian cardiac cells (1990–2005)

Model	Species	Parent model
Ventricular cell models		
Noble et al. [163]	Guinea pig	Earm and Noble [164]
Luo and Rudy [165]	Guinea pig	Beeler and Reuter [155]
Nordin [166]	Guinea pig	–
Luo and Rudy [167]	Guinea pig	Luo and Rudy [165]
Jafri et al. [168]	Guinea pig	Luo and Rudy [167]
Noble et al. [169]	Guinea pig	Noble et al. [163]
Priebe and Beuckelmann [170]	Human	Luo and Rudy [167]
Winslow et al. [171]	Canine	Jafri et al. [168]
Pandit et al. [172]	Rat	Demir et al. [173]
Puglisi and Bers [174]	Rabbit	Luo and Rudy [167]
Bernus et al. [175]	Human	Priebe and Beuckelmann [170]
Matsuoka et al. [176]	Guinea pig	–
Bondarenko et al. [177]	Mouse	–
Shannon et al. [178]	Rabbit	Puglisi and Bers [174]
Ten Tusscher et al. [179]	Human	–
Iyer et al. [180]	Human	–
Hund and Rudy [181]	Canine	Luo and Rudy [167]
Atrial cell models		
Earm and Noble [164]	Rabbit	Hilgemann and Noble [167]
Lindblad et al. [182]	Rabbit	–
Courtemanche et al. [183]	Human	Luo and Rudy [167]
Nygren et al. [184]	Human	Lindblad et al. [182]
Ramirez et al. [185]	Canine	Courtemanche et al. [183]
Sinoatrial cell models		
Wilders et al. [186]	Rabbit	–
Demir et al. [173]	Rabbit	–
Dokos et al. [187]	Rabbit	Wilders et al. [186]
Demir et al. [188]	Rabbit	Demir et al. [173]
Zhang et al. [189]	Rabbit	–
Zhang et al. [190]	Rabbit	Zhang et al. [189]
Zhang et al. [191]	Rabbit	Zhang et al. [189]
Kurata et al. [192]	Rabbit	–
Sarai et al. [193]	Rabbit	–
Lovell et al. [194]	Rabbit	–

*Model has Markov type channel gating

This can be overcome through a "chemical" approach using an explicit formula for the membrane potential of cells in terms of the intracellular and extracellular ionic concentrations [197].

When using cardiac cell models, one should realize that first-generation models tend to reach a steady state within only a few beats, whereas second-generation models should be run for a much longer time to reach steady state. For example, in the canine atrial cell model by Kneller et al. [196] action potential duration reached steady state after approximately 40 min of pacing, which limits its suitability for performing large-scale (whole-heart) simulations, where simulating a single beat may take several hours on a state-of-the-art computer. Furthermore, it should be emphasized that the equations representing the calcium subsystem of the second-generation models are still evolving and even the latest comprehensive models fail to adequately represent fundamental properties of calcium handling and inactivation of L-type calcium current by intracellular Ca^{2+} (see, e.g., [180, 198] and primary references cited therein).

3.14.5 Deterministic, Stochastic and Markov Models

Until a few years ago, cardiac cell models all employed the traditional Hodgkin-Huxley formulation of ion channel gating. In this concept, the state of an ion channel is defined by one or more independent gates that can each flip between their open and closed state, with the channel being open if and only if all of its gates are in their open position. Accordingly a channel with n different gates, can reside in any of 2^n different states (❯ Fig. 3.12a). It had been noted that many ionic currents can more accurately be described using state diagrams that are not limited to the Hodgkin-Huxley concept of one or a few independent gates. The generic Markov type models, named after the mathematician Andrei Markov (1856–1922), are used instead. Markov models allow for more complex interactions between open, closed or inactivated states, as illustrated in ❯ Fig. 3.12b, and thus have the advantage of being more closely related to the underlying structure and conformation of the ion channel proteins. A disadvantage is that Markov models often introduce additional differential equations to the model that must be solved, thus slowing the computation time. In the recent comprehensive model of a rabbit ventricular myocyte by Shannon et al. [178], Markov channel models were therefore generally avoided unless considered necessary.

Markov models should not be confused with stochastic models. Cardiac cell models employing Markov type channel gating are as deterministic as models employing the Hodgkin-Huxley channel gating. The number of ion channels occupying a certain channel state is represented as a fraction (between 0 and 1) that changes with time as a continuous number. The changes with time are described by a set of differential equations governing the *average* behavior of the thousands of individual ion channels. Stochastic models are non-deterministic (probabilistic) models in which the stochastic "random" openings and closures of each individual ion channel are taken into account. The number of ion channels occupying a certain channel state is then represented as a discrete number that changes "randomly" with time: the computation of changes in these numbers with time involves drawing of random numbers instead of solving differential equations. As a consequence, action potential parameters may show beat-to-beat fluctuations, like experimental recordings [199, 200]. Stochastic ionic models of cardiac pacemaker cells have been developed by Wilders et al. [199] and Guevara and Lewis [201]. Recently, Greenstein and Winslow [202] have developed an ionic model of the canine ventricular myocyte incorporating stochastic gating of L-type calcium channels and ryanodine-sensitive calcium release channels.

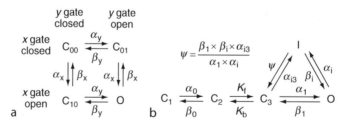

◩ Fig. 3.12

Hodgkin-Huxley and Markov type models of I_{Kr} (HERG, *KCNH2*) channel gating. (a) State diagram of classical Hodgkin-Huxley type model. The conductive state of the channel is controlled by two independent activation and inactivation gates (*x* and *y*, respectively), resulting in four different channel states. (b) State diagram of Markov type scheme (after [207]). C_1, C_2, and C_3 are closed states, O is the open state, and I the inactivated state. All transition rates, except K_f and K_b, are a function of membrane potential. Ψ is defined as a function of other transition rates to satisfy the microscopic reversibility condition

3.14.6   Computational Aspects

The original computations by Hodgkin and Huxley [150] were done by hand. As memorized by Huxley in his Nobel lecture, "this was a laborious business: a membrane action took a matter of days to compute, and a propagated action potential took a matter of weeks." For his initial Purkinje fiber action potential simulations, Noble [151, 152] could make use of the university computer for which he had to write a program in machine code. It took 2 h of CPU time to simulate a single action potential of the 5-variable model. In the seventies, Beeler and Reuter used a mainframe computer to solve the differential equations of their 8-variable ventricular cell model. A single action potential could be computed in about 40 s [155]. In subsequent decades, computational power has grown exponentially. Simulating a single Noble or Beeler-Reuter action potential now takes no more than one or a few milliseconds on a moderate personal computer. Nevertheless, computational efficiency is still an important issue when modeling cardiac cells. Models have not only become much more complex, but also require much longer time to reach steady state (see ❷ Sect. 3.14.4). Computational efficiency is of course, of particular importance in large-scale tissue or whole-heart simulations.

The ongoing demand for computational power is illustrated by the development of human ventricular cell models. The models by Priebe and Beuckelmann [170] and ten Tusscher et al. [198], with 15 and 16 variables, respectively, are of a similar complexity. Both use Hodgkin and Huxley type equations for the ionic currents and they model intracellular sodium, potassium, and calcium dynamics. The Iyer et al. [180] human ventricular cell model uses Markov type models rather than Hodgkin-Huxley type equations to describe the dynamics of the major ionic currents. As set out above, this allows one to fit single channel experimental data and to incorporate knowledge on ion channel structure, but this comes at the cost of a much higher number of variables; as many as 67 in the case of the Iyer et al. model [180].

Apart from the number of variables, the computational efficiency of a model is also determined by the "stiffness" of its equations: a model with "stiff" equations requires a small integration time step for a stable and precise solution of its differential equations. Ten Tusscher et al. [198] compared the computational efficiency of the above human ventricular cell models under standardized conditions, using simple Euler forward integration, which is the most widely used integration method for large-scale spatial simulations in electrophysiology. They observed that the Priebe & Beuckelmann and the ten Tusscher et al. models allowed for a much larger integration time step (20 μs) than the Iyer et al. model (0.02 μs). Together, the differences in the number of variables and the integration time step cause simulations with the Priebe and Beuckelmann and the tenTusscher et al. models to be approximately equally fast, whereas the Iyer et al. model is almost 1,000 times "slower."

3.14.7   Multicellular Simulations

The "bidomain" model has been widely accepted as the major approach for theoretical and numerical investigation of macroscopic electric phenomena in cardiac tissue. It is based on the representation of the tissue as two interpenetrating extra- and intracellular domains each of them having different conductivities along and across the direction of the fibers [203]. The state variables describing the system are the local intracellular and extracellular potentials (φ_i and φ_e, respectively), with the transmembrane potential defined as $V_m = \varphi_i - \varphi_e$. Although the bidomain model gives the most accurate approximation of heart tissue, it requires considerable computational power for calculations, both in terms of CPU speed and computer memory. The bidomain model of the human heart developed by Potse et al. [204], for example, requires > 20 GB of computer memory and takes 2 days on a 32-processor parallel computer to simulate a complete cardiac cycle. This explains why large-scale simulations are often "monodomain," i.e., φ_e is ignored and set to zero. Differences between monodomain and bidomain simulation results are small enough to permit the use of a monodomain model for propagation studies, even when extracellular potentials are required. However, bidomain models should be used if external currents are applied (pacing, defibrillation) [204].

Ionic models of single cardiac cells are also "monodomain": as in experiments on isolated cardiac cells, the extracellular space is grounded to earth (cf. ❷ Fig. 3.11). Given the required computational power, only simple first-generation cardiac cell models, with few variables and equations, can be used in large-scale bidomain simulations. Thus, bidomain simulations do not permit highly detailed studies of the effects of individual ionic currents on cardiac activation. This also holds, to a lesser extent, for monodomain simulations. Cardiac cell models that are typically used in large-scale simulations include the simplified ionic models by Fenton and Karma [205] and Bernus et al. [175].

3

◻ Table 3.4

Cardiac cell models available on the Internet

Source code
Source code of numerous models in CellML format Web address: http://www.cellml.org/
Source code of cardiac cell models from the Rudy group (C++, Matlab) Web address: http://rudylab.wustl.edu/
Source code of cardiac cell models from the Winslow group (C++, Fortran) Web address: http://www.ccbm.jhu.edu/
Source code of the "Kyoto model" (several formats) Web address: http://www.card.med.kyoto-u.ac.jp/Simulation/
C++ source code of the Bernus et al. [175] human ventricular cell model Web address: http://www.physiol.med.uu.nl/wilders/
C++ source code of the ten Tusscher et al. [179] human ventricular cell model Web address: http://www-binf.bio.uu.nl/khwjtuss/
Fortran source code of the Zhang et al. [189, 190] rabbit sinoatrial cell models Web address: http://personalpages.umist.ac.uk/staff/H.Zhang-3/
Ready-to-use Java applets
Applets of numerous ionic models from the Centre for Arrhythmia Research at Hofstra University Web address: http://arrhythmia.hofstra.edu/
iCell: Java-based interactive cell modeling resource Web address: http://ssd1.bme.memphis.edu/icell/
Ready-to-use Windows program
LabHEART: Windows version of Puglisi & Bers rabbit ventricular cell model [174] Web address: http://www.meddean.luc.edu/templates/ssom/depts/physio/labheart.cfm

See Table 1 of [206] for a comprehensive list of tools for cardiac cell modeling

3.14.8   Cardiac Cell Models on the World Wide Web

The source code of various cardiac cell models is available through the Internet. This code can be compiled into a computer program using the appropriate "compiler," which requires basic computer programming skills. ❷ Table 3.4 lists some of the sites at which source code is made available. A few "ready-to-use" programs are also available. These include Java applets of several ionic models as well as a Windows version of the rabbit ventricular cell model by Puglisi and Bers [174].

Several efforts have been made to set a language standard for cardiac cell modeling. One example is the "CellML" language, which is an open standard based on the XML markup language, being developed by the Bioengineering Institute at the University of Auckland and affiliated research groups. The purpose of CellML is to store and exchange computer-based mathematical models. A large number of models are already available on the CellML website (❷ Table 3.4). To run simulations, a simulation environment that imports CellML files is required.

References

1. Einthoven, W., Über die Form des menschlichen Electrocardio-gramms. *Pflug. Arch. Ges. Phys.*, 1895;**60**: 101–123.
2. Einthoven, W., The different forms of the human electrocardio-gram and their signification. *Lancet*, 1912;**1**: 853–861.
3. Burgess, M.J., K. Millar, and J.A. Abildskov, Cancellation of electrocardiographic effects during ventricular recovery. *J. Electrocardiol.*, 1969;**2**: 101–107.
4. Van Oosterom, A., Genesis of the T wave as based on an equiv-alent surface source model. *J. Electrocardiol.*, 2001;**34**(Suppl.): 217–226.
5. Fabiato, A. and F. Fabiato, Contractions induced by a calcium-triggered release of calcium from the sarcoplasmic reticu-lum of single skinned cardiac cells. *J. Physiol.*, 1975;**249**:469–495.

6. Cheng, H., W.J. Lederer, and M.B. Cannell, Calcium sparks: elementary events underlying excitation-contraction coupling in heart muscle. *Science*, 1993;**262**: 740–744.

7. Van Veen, A.A.B., H.V.M. Van Rijen, and T. Opthof, Cardiac gap junction channels: modulation of expression and channel properties. *Cardiovasc. Res.*, 2001;**51**: 217–229.

8. Keith, A. and M. Flack, The form and nature of the muscular connection between the primary divisions of the vertebrate heart. *J. Anat. Physiol.*, 1907;**41**: 172–189.

9. Tawara, S., *Das Reizleitungssystem des Säugetierherzen*. Jena, 1906.

10. Eyster, J.A.E. and W.J. Meek, The origin and conduction of the heart beat. *Physiol. Rev.*, 1921;**1**: 1–43.

11. Ling, G. and R.W. Gerard, The normal membrane potential of frog sartorius muscle. *J. Cell. Compar. Physiol.*, 1949;**34**: 383–396.

12. Powell, T. and V.W. Twist, A rapid technique for the isolation and purification of adult cardiac muscle cells having respiratory control and a tolerance to calcium. *Biochem. Biophys. Res. Commun.*, 1976;**72**: 327–333.

13. Neher, E., B. Sakmann, and J.H. Steinbach, The extracellular patch-clamp: a method for resolving currents through individual open channels in biological membranes. *Pflug. Arch.*, 1978;**375**: 219–228.

14. Boyett, M.R., H. Honjo, and I. Kodama, The sinoatrial node, a heterogeneous pacemaker structure. *Cardiovasc. Res.*, 2000;**47**: 658–687.

15. Meijler, F.L. and M.J. Janse, Morphology and electrophysiology of the mammalian atriventricular node. *Physiol. Rev.*, 1988;**68**: 608–647.

16. Schuilenburg, R.M. and D. Durrer, Atrial echo beats in the human heart elicited by induced atrial premature beats. *Circulation*, 1968;**37**: 680–693.

17. Tranum-Jensen J., A.A.M. Wilde, J.T. Vermeulen, and M.J. Janse, Morphology of electrophysiologically identified junctions between Purkinje fibers and ventricular muscle in rabbit and pig hearts. *Circ. Res.*, 1991;**69**: 429–437.

18. Harris, H.W., Jr., Molecular aspects of water transport. *Pediatr. Nephrol.*, 1992;**6**: 304–310.

19. Benga, G., Birth of water channel proteins-the aquaporins. *Cell. Biol. Int.*, 2003;**27**: 701–709.

20. Calaghan, S.C., J.Y. Le Guennec, and E. White, Cytoskeletal modulation of electrical and mechanical activity in cardiac myocytes. *Prog. Biophys. Mol. Biol.*, 2004;**84**: 29–59.

21. Fozzard, H.A. and R.B. Gunn, Membrane transport, in *The Heart*, 2nd ed., H.A. Fozzard, E. Haber, R.B. Jennings, A.M.J. Katz, and H.E. Morgan, Editors. New York: Raven Press, 1991, pp. 99–110.

22. Matsuda, H. and J.D.S. Cruz, Voltage-dependent block by internal Ca^{++} ions of inwardly rectifying K^+ channels in guinea-pig ventricular cells. *J. Physiol.*, 1993;**470**: 295–311.

23. Lopatin, A.N., E.N. Makhina, and C.G. Nichols, Potassium channel block by cytoplasmic polyamines as the mechanism of intrinsic rectification. *Nature*, 1994;**372**: 366–369.

24. Zaza, A., M. Rocchetti, A. Brioschi, A. Cantadori, and A. Ferroni, Dynamic Ca^{2+}-induced inward rectification of K^+ current during the ventricular action potential. *Circ. Res.*, 1998;**82**: 947–956.

25. Litovsky, S.H. and C. Antzelevitch, Transient outward current prominent in canine ventricular epicardium but not endocardium. *Circ. Res.*, 1988;**62**: 116–126.

26. Sanguinetti, M.C. and N.K. Jurkiewicz, Two components of cardiac delayed rectifier K^+ current. Differential sensitivity to block by class III antiarrhythmic agents. *J. Gen. Physiol.*, 1990;**96**: 195–215.

27. Attwell, D., I.S. Cohen, D.A. Eisner, M. Ohba, and C. Ojeda, The steady state TTX-sensitive ("window") sodium current in cardiac Purkinje fibres. *Pflug. Arch.*, 1979;**379**: 137–142.

28. Hirano, Y., A. Moscucci, and C.T. January, Direct measurement of L-type Ca^{++} window current in heart cells. *Circ. Res.*, 1992;**70**: 445–455.

29. Gintant, G.A., N.B. Datyner, and I.S. Cohen, Slow inactivation of a tetrodotoxin-sensitive current in canine Purkinje fibers. *Biophys. J.*, 1984;**45**: 509–512.

30. Bers, D.M., Sarcolemmal Na/Ca exchange and Ca-pump, in *Excitation-Contraction Coupling and Cardiac Contractile Force*, D.M. Bers, Editor. Boston: Kluwer Academic Publishers, 2002, pp. 133–160.

31. Ishihara, K., T. Mitsuiye, A. Noma, and M. Takano, The Mg^{2+} block and intrinsic gating underlying inward rectification of the K^+ current in guinea-pig cardiac myocytes. *J. Physiol.*, 1989;**419**: 297–320.

32. Smith, P.L., T. Baukrowitz, and G. Yellen, The inward rectification mechanism of the HERG cardiac potassium channel. *Nature*, 1996;**37**: 833–836.

33. Rocchetti, M, A. Besana, G.B. Gurrola, L.D. Possani, and A. Zaza, Rate-dependency of delayed rectifier currents during the guinea-pig ventricular action potential. *J. Physiol.*, 2001;**534**: 721–732.

34. Shimoni, Y., R.B. Clark, and W.R. Giles, Role of inwardly rectifying potassium current in rabbit ventricular action potential. *J. Physiol.*, 1992;**448**: 709–727.

35. Noma, A., T. Nakayama, Y. Kurachi, and H. Irisawa, Resting K conductances in pacemaker and non-pacemaker heart cells of the rabbit. *Jpn. J. Physiol.*, 1984;**34**: 245–254.

36. Cordeiro, J.M., K.W. Spitzer, and W.R. Giles, Repolarizing K^+ currents in rabbit heart Purkinje cells. *J. Physiol.*, 1998;**508**: 811–823.

37. Miake, J., E. Marbán, and H.B. Nuss, Biological pacemaker created by gene transfer. *Nature*, 2002;**419**: 132–133.

38. Janse, M.J., T. Opthof, and A.G. Kléber, Animal models of cardiac arrhythmias. *Cardiovasc. Res.*, 1998;**39**: 165–177.

39. Janse, M.J. and A.L. Wit, Electrophysiological mechanisms of ventricular arrhythmias resulting from myocardial ischemia and infarction. *Physiol. Rev.*, 1989;**69**: 1049–1169.

40. Wiener, N. and A. Rosenblueth, The mathematical formulation of the problem of conduction of impulses in a network of connected excitable elements, specifically in cardiac muscle. *Arch. Inst. Cardiol. Mex.*, 1946;**16**: 205–265.

41. Moe, G.K. and C. Mendez, Basis of pharmacotherapy of cardiac arrhythmias. *Mod. Conc. Cardiov. Dis.*, 1962;**31**:739–744.

42. Allessie, M.A., F.I.M. Bonke, and F.J.G. Schopman, Circus movement in rabbit atrial muscle as a mechanism of tachycardia. The "leading circle" concept: a new model of circus movement in cardiac tissue without the involvement of an anatomical obstacle. *Circ. Res.*, 1977;**41**: 9–18.

43. Conrath, C.E. and T. Opthof, Ventricular repolarization. An overview of (patho)physiology, sympathetic effects, and

genetic aspects. *Prog. Biophys. Mol. Biol.*, 2005;**92**(3): 269–307. doi:10.1016/jpbiomolbio.2005.05.009.

44. Stengl, M., P.G. Volders, M.B. Thomsen, R.L. Spätjens, K.R. Sipido, and M.A. Vos, Accumulation of slowly activating delayed rectifier potassium current (I_{Ks}) in canine ventricular myocytes. *J. Physiol.*, 2003;**551**: 777–786.

45. Virág, L., N. Iost, M. Opincariu, J. Szolnoky, J. Szécsi, G. Bogáts, P. Szenohradszky, A. Varró, and J.G. Papp, The slow component of the delayed rectifier potassium current in undiseased human ventricular myocytes. *Cardiovasc. Res.*, 2001;**49**: 790–797.

46. Lu, Z., K. Kamiya, T. Opthof, K. Yasui, and I. Kodama, Density and kinetics of I_{Kr} and I_{Ks} in guinea pi45d r rabbit ventricular myocytes explain different efficacy of I_{Ks} blockade at high heart rate in guinea pig and rabbit. *Circulation*, 2001;**104**:951–956.

47. Volders, P.G., M. Stengl, J.M. van Opstal, U. Gerlach, R.L. Spätjens, J.D. Beekman, K.R. Sipido, and M.A. Vos, Probing the contribution of I_{Ks} to canine ventricular repolarization: key role for ß-adrenergic receptor stimulation. *Circulation*, 2003;**107**: 2753–2760.

48. Nitta, J.-I., T. Furukawa, F. Marumo, T. Sawanobori, and M. Hiraoka, Subcellular mechanism for Ca^{2+} -dependent enhancement of delayed rectifier K^+ current in isolated membrane patches of guinea pig ventricular myocytes. *Circ. Res.*, 1994;**74**: 96–104.

49. Jost, N., L. Virág, M. Bitay, J. Takács, C. Lengyel, P. Biliczki, Z. Nagy, G. Bogáts, D.A. Lathrop, J.G. Papp, and A. Varró, Restricting excessive cardiac action potential and QT prolongation: a vital role for I_{Ks} in human ventricular muscle. *Circulation*, 2005;**112**: 1392–1399.

50. Saitoh, H, J.C. Bailey, and B. Surawicz, Alternans of action potential duration after abrupt shortening of cycle length: differences between dog Purkinje and ventricular muscle fibers. *Circ. Res.*, 1988;**62**: 1027–1040.

51. Curran, M.E., I. Splawski, K.W. Timothy, M.G. Vincent, E.D. Green, and M.T. Keating, A molecular basis for cardiac arrhythmia: HERG mutations cause long QT syndrome. *Cell*, 1995;**80**: 795–803.

52. Jurkiewicz, N.K. and M.C. Sanguinetti, Rate-dependent prolongation of cardiac action potentials by a methanesulfonanilide class III antiarrhythmic agent. Specific block of rapidly activating delayed rectifier current by dofetilide. *Circ. Res.*, 1993;**72**:75–83.

53. Biliczki, P., L. Virág, N. Iost, J.G. Papp, and A. Varró, Interaction of different potassium channels in cardiac repolarization in dog ventricular preparations: role of repolarization reserve. *Br. J. Pharmacol.*, 2002;**137**: 361–368.

54. Bennett, P.B., K. Yazawa, N. Makita, and A.L. George, Jr., Molecular mechanism for an inherited cardiac arrhythmia. *Nature*, 1995;**376**: 683–685.

55. Clancy, C.E., M. Tateyama, H. Liu, X.H. Wehrens, and R.S. Kass, Non-equilibrium gating in cardiac Na^+ channels: an original mechanism of arrhythmia. *Circulation*, 2003;**107**: 2233–2237.

56. Berecki, N.G., J.G. Zegers, Z.A. Bhuiyan, A.O. Verkerk, R. Wilders, and A.C.G. van Ginneken, Long-QT syndrome related sodium channel mutations probed ny dynamic action potential clamp technique. *J. Physiol.*, 2006;**570**: 237–250.

57. Lee, K.S., E. Marbán, and R.W. Tsien, Inactivation of calcium channels in mammalian heart cells: joint dependence on membrane potential and intracellular calcium. *J. Physiol.*, 1985;**364**: 395–411.

58. Zuhlke, R.D., G.S. Pitt, K. Deisseroth, R.W. Tsien, and H. Reuter, Calmodulin supports both inactivation and facilitation of L-type calcium channels. *Nature*, 1999;**399**: 159–162.

59. Goldhaber, J.I., L.H. Xie, T. Duong, C. Motter, K. Khuu, and J.N. Weiss, Action potential duration restitution and alternans in rabbit ventricular myocytes: the key role of intracellular calcium cycling. *Circ. Res.*, 2005;**96**: 459–466.

60. January, C.T. and J.M. Riddle, Early after depolarizations: mechanism of induction and block A role for L-type Ca^{2+} current. *Circ. Res.*, 1989;**64**: 977–990.

61. Keith, A., The sino-auricular node: a historical note. *Br. Heart J.*, 1942;**4**: 77–79.

62. Trautwein, W. and K. Uchizono, Electron microscopic and electrophysiologic study of the pacemaker in the sinoatrial node of the rabbit heart. *Z. Zellforsch. Mikrosk. Anat.*, 1963;**61**: 96–109.

63. Taylor, J.J., L.S. d'Agrosa, and E.M. Berns, The pacemaker cell of the sinoatrial node of the rabbit. *Am. J. Physiol.*, 1978;**235**: H407–H412.

64. Maltsev, V.A., A.M. Wobus, J. Rohwedel, M. Bader, and J. Hescheler, Cardiomyocytes differentiated in vitro from embryonic stem cells developmentally express cardiac-specific genes and ionic currents. *Circ. Res.*, 1994;**75**: 233–244.

65. DiFrancesco, D., Pacemaker mechanisms in cardiac tissue. *Annu. Rev. Physiol.*, 1993;**55**: 451–467.

66. Irisawa, H., H.F. Brown, and W. Giles, Cardiac pacemaking in the sinoatrial node. *Physiol. Rev.*, 1993;**73**: 197–227.

67. Yu, H., F. Chang, and I.S. Cohen, Pacemaker current i_f in adult canine cardiac ventricular myocytes. *J. Physiol.*, 1995;**485**: 469–483.

68. Robinson, R.B., H. Yu, F. Chang, and I.S. Cohen, Developmental change in the voltage-dependence of the pacemaker current, i_f, in rat ventricle cells. *Pflug. Arch.*, 1997;**433**: 533–535.

69. DiFrancesco, D., The cardiac hyperpolarizing-activated current I_f. *Prog. Biophys. Mol. Biol.*, 1985;**46**: 163–183.

70. Zaza, A., M. Micheletti, A. Brioschi, and M. Rocchetti, Ionic currents during sustained pacemaker activity in rabbit sino-atrial myocytes. *J. Physiol.*, 1997;**505**: 677–688.

71. DiFrancesco, D. and M. Mangoni, Modulation of single hyperpolarization-activated channels (I_f) by cAMP in the rabbit sino-atrial node. *J. Physiol.*, 1994;**474**: 473–482.

72. Zaza, A., R.B. Robinson, and D. DiFrancesco, Basal responses of the L-type Ca^{2+} and hyperpolarization-activated currents to autonomic agonists in the rabbit sinoatrial node. *J. Physiol.*, 1996;**491**: 347–355.

73. Zaza, A., M. Rocchetti, and D. DiFrancesco, Modulation of the hyperpolarization activated current (I_f) by adenosine in rabbit sinoatrial myocytes. *Circulation*, 1996;**94**: 734–741.

74. Verheijck, E.E., A.C.G. van Ginneken, R. Wilders, and L.N. Bouman, Contribution of L-type Ca^{2+} current to electrical activity in sinoatrial nodal myocytes of rabbits. *Am. J. Physiol.*, 1999;**276**: H1064–H1077.

75. Reuter, H., Calcium channel modulation by neurotransmitters, enzymes and drugs. *Nature*, 1983;**301**: 569–574.

76. Verheijck, E.E., A.C.G. van Ginneken, J. Bourier, and L.N. Bouman, Effects of delayed rectifier current blockade by E-4031 on impulse generation in single sinoatrial nodal myocytes of the rabbit. *Circ. Res.*, 1995;**76**: 607–615.

77. Noble, D., J.C. Denyer, H.F. Brown, and D. DiFrancesco, Reciprocal role of the inward currents $I_{b,Na}$ and I_f in controlling and stabilizing pacemaker frequency of rabbit sino-atrial node cells. *Proc. R. Soc. Lond. B Biol. Sci.*, 1992;**250**:199–207.

78. Nishida, M. and R. MacKinnon, Structural basis of inward rectification: cytoplasmic pore of the G protein-gated inward rectifier GIRK1 at 1.8 Å resolution. *Cell*, 2002;**111**:957–965.

79. Duivenvoorden, J.J., L.N. Bouman, T. Opthof, F.F. Bukauskas, and H.J. Jongsma, Effect of transmural vagal stimulation on electrotonic current spread in the rabbit sinoatrial node. *Cardiovasc. Res.*, 1992;**26**: 678–686.

80. DiFrancesco, D., P. Ducouret, and R.B. Robinson, Muscarinic modulation of cardiac rate at low acetylcholine concentrations. *Science*, 1989;**243**: 669–671.

81. Boyett, M.R., I. Kodama, H. Honjo, A. Arai, R. Suzuki, and J. Toyama, Ionic basis of the chronotropic effect of acetylcholine on the rabbit sinoatrial node. *Cardiovasc. Res.*, 1995;**29**:867–878.

82. Zaza, A. and M. Rocchetti, Regulation of the sinoatrial pacemaker: selective I_f inhibition by ivaradine, in *Heart Rate Management in Stable Angina*, K. Fox and R. Ferrari, Editors. London: Taylor & Francis, 2005, pp. 51–67.

83. Huser, J., L.A. Blatter, and S.L. Lipsius, Intracellular Ca^{2+} release contributes to automaticity in cat atrial pacemaker cells. *J. Physiol.*, 2000;**524**: 415–422.

84. Bogdanov, K.Y., T.M. Vinogradova, and E.G. Lakatta, Sinoatrial nodal cell ryanodine receptor and Na^+-Ca^{2+} exchanger: molecular partners in pacemaker regulation. *Circ. Res.*, 2001;**88**: 1254–1258.

85. Lakatta, E.G., V.A. Maltsev, K.Y. Bogdanov, M.D. Stern, and T.M. Vinogradova, Cyclic variation of intracellular calcium: a critical factor for cardiac pacemaker cell dominance. *Circ. Res.*, 2003;**92**: e45–e50.

86. Vinogradova, T.M., Y.Y. Zhou, V. Maltsev, A. Lyashkov, M. Stern, and E.G. Lakatta, Rhythmic ryanodine receptor Ca^{2+} releases during diastolic depolarization of sinoatrial pacemaker cells do not require membrane depolarization. *Circ. Res.*, 2004;**94**: 802–809.

87. Vinogradova, T.M., K.Y. Bogdanov, and E.G. Lakatta, Beta-adrenergic stimulation modulates ryanodine receptor Ca^{2+} release during diastolic depolarization to accelerate pacemaker activity in rabbit sinoatrial nodal cells. *Circ. Res.*, 2002;**90**: 73–79.

88. Michaels, D.C., E.P. Matyas, and J. Jalife, Mechanisms of sinoatrial pacemaker synchronization: a new hypothesis. *Circ. Res.*, 1987;**61**: 704–714.

89. Masson-Pévet, M.A., W.K. Bleeker, and D. Gros, The plasma membrane of leading pacemaker cells in the rabbit sinus node. A quantitative structural analysis. *Circ. Res.*, 1979;**45**: 621–629.

90. Honjo, H., M.R. Boyett, S.R. Coppen, Y. Takagishi, T. Opthof, N.J. Severs, and I. Kodama, Heterogeneous expression of connexins in rabbit sinoatrial node cells: correlation between connexin isoform and cell size. *Cardiovasc. Res.*, 2002;**53**: 89–96.

91. Masson-Pévet, M.A., W.K. Bleeker, E. Besselsen, B.W. Treytel, H.J. Jongsma, and L.N. Bouman, Pacemaker cell types in the rabbit sinus node: a correlative ultrastructural and electrophysiological study. *J. Mol. Cell. Cardiol.*, 1984;**16**: 53–63.

92. Kirchhof, C.J. and M.A. Allessie, Sinus node automaticity during atrial fibrillation in isolated rabbit hearts. *Circulation*, 1992;**86**: 263–271.

93. Opthof, T., A.C.G. VanGinneken, L.N. Bouman, and H.J. Jongsma, The intrinsic cycle length in small pieces isolated from the rabbit sinoatrial node. *J. Mol. Cell. Cardiol.*, 1987;**19**: 923–934.

94. Kodama, I. and M.R. Boyett, Regional differences in the electrical activity of the rabbit sinus node. *Pflug. Arch.*, 1985;**404**: 214–226.

95. Joyner, R.W. and F.J.L. van Capelle, Propagation through electrically coupled cells: how a small SA node drives a large atrium. *Biophys. J.*, 1986;**50**: 1157–1164.

96. Wilders, R. and H.J. Jongsma, Beating irregularity of single pacemaker cells isolated from the rabbit sinoatrial node. *Biophys. J.*, 1993;**65**: 2601–2613.

97. Opthof, T., The mammalian sinoatrial node. *Cardiovasc. Drugs Ther.*, 1988;**1**: 573–597.

98. Mackaay, A.J.C., T. Opthof, W.K. Bleeker, H.J. Jongsma, and L.N. Bouman, Interaction of adrenaline and acetylcholine on cardiac pacemaker function. *J. Pharmacol. Exp. Ther.*, 1980;**214**: 417–422.

99. Mackaay, A.J.C., T. Opthof, W.K. Bleeker, H.J. Jongsma, and L.N. Bouman, Interaction of adrenaline and acetylcholine on sinus node function, in *Cardiac Rate and Rhythm*, L.N. Bouman and H.J. Jongsma, Editors. The Hague: Nijhoff, 1982, pp. 507–523.

100. Katzung, G.B. and H.A. Morgenstern, Effects of extracellular potassium on ventricular automaticity and evidence of a pacemaker current in mammalian ventricular myocardium. *Circ. Res.*, 1977;**40**: 105–111.

101. Cerbai, E, R. Pino, F. Porciatti, G. Sani, M. Toscano, M. Maccherini, G. Giunti, and A. Mugelli, Characterization of the hyperpolarization-activated current, I_f, in ventricular myocytes from human failing heart. *Circulation*, 1997;**95**: 568–571.

102. Imanishi, S., Calcium-sensitive discharges in canine Purkinje fibers. *Jpn. J. Physiol.*, 1971;**21**: 443–463.

103. Dangman, K.H. and B.F. Hoffman, Studies on overdrive stimulation of canine cardiac Purkinje fibers: maximal diastolic potential as a determinant of the response. *J. Am. Coll. Cardiol.*, 1983;**2**: 1183–1190.

104. Cheung, D.W., Electrical activity of the pulmonary vein and its interaction with the right atrium in the guinea-pig. *J. Physiol.*, 1981;**314**: 445–456.

105. Haissaguerre, M., P. Jais, D.C. Shah, A. Takahashi, M. Hocini, G. Quiniou, S. Garrigue, A. Le Mouroux, P. Le Metayer, and J. Clementy, Spontaneous initiation of atrial fibrillation by ectopic beats originating in the pulmonary veins. *New Engl. J. Med.*, 1998;**339**: 659–666.

106. Logothetis, D.E., Y. Kurachi, J. Galper, E.J. Neer, and D.E. Clapham, The beta-gamma subunits of GTP-binding proteins activate the muscarinic K^+ channel in heart. *Nature*, 1987;**325**: 321–326.

107. Bender, K., M.C. Wellner-Kienitz, L.I. Bosche, A. Rinne, C. Beckmann, and L. Pott, Acute desensitization of GIRK current in rat atrial myocytes is related to K^+ current flow. *J. Physiol.*, 2004;**561**: 471–483.

108. Müllner, C., D. Vorobiov, A.K. Bera, Y. Uezono, D. Yakubovich, B. Frohnwieser-Steinecker, N. Dascal, and W. Schreibmayer, Heterologous facilitation of G protein-activated K^+ channels by beta-adrenergic stimulation via cAMP-dependent protein kinase. *J. Gen. Physiol.*, 2000;**115**: 547–558.

109. Cho, H., D. Lee, S.H. Lee, and W.K. Ho, Receptor-induced depletion of phosphatidylinositol 4,5-bisphosphate inhibits inwardly rectifying K^+ channels in a receptor-specific manner. *Proc. Natl. Acad. Sci. USA*, 2005;**102**: 4643–4648.

110. Gintant, G.A., Two components of delayed rectifier current in canine atrium and ventricle. Does I_{Ks} play a role in the reverse rate dependence of class III agents? *Circ. Res.*, 1996;**78**: 26–37.

111. Wang, Z., B. Fermini, and S. Nattel, Rapid and slow components of delayed rectifier current in human atrial myocytes. *Cardiovasc. Res.*, 1994;**28**: 1540–1546.

112. Wang, Z., B. Fermini, and S. Nattel, Sustained depolarization-induced outward current in human atrial myocytes. Evidence for a novel delayed rectifier K$^+$ current similar to Kv1.5 cloned channel currents. *Circ. Res.*, 1993;**73**: 1061–1076.

113. Crumb, W.J., Jr., B. Wible, D.J. Arnold, J.P. Payne, and A.M. Brown, Blockade of multiple human cardiac potassium currents by the antihistamine terfenadine: possible mechanism for terfenadine-associated cardiotoxicity. *Mol. Pharmacol.*, 1995;**47**: 181–190.

114. Amos, G.J., E. Wettwer, F. Metzger, Q. Li, H.M. Himmel, and U. Ravens, Differences between outward currents of human atrial and subepicardial ventricular myocytes. *J. Physiol.*, 1996;**491**: 31–50.

115. Koidl, B., P. Flaschberger, P. Schaffer, B. Pelzmann, E. Bernhart, H. Machler, and B. Rigler, Effects of the class III antiarrhythmic drug ambasilide on outward currents in human atrial myocytes. *Naunyn Schmiedebergs Arch. Pharmacol.*, 1996;**353**: 226–232.

116. Antzelevitch, C., S. Sicouri, S.H. Litovsky, A. Lukas, S.C. Krishnan, J.M. Di Diego, G.A. Gintant, and D.W. Liu. Heterogeneity within the ventricular wall. Electrophysiology and pharmacology of epicardial, endocardial, and M cells. *Circ. Res.*, 1991;**69**: 1427–1449.

117. Rosati, B., F. Grau, S. Rodriguez, H. Li, J.M. Nerbonne, and D. McKinnon, Concordant expression of KChIP2 mRNA, protein and transient outward current throughout the canine ventricle. *J. Physiol.*, 2003;**548**: 815–822.

118. Liu, D.W. and C. Antzelevitch, Characteristics of the delayed rectifier current (I_{Kr} and I_{Ks}) in canine ventricular epicardial, midmyocardial, and endocardial myocytes. A weaker I_{Ks} contributes to the longer action potential in the M cell. *Circ. Res.*, 1995;**76**: 351–365.

119. Sicouri, S. and C. Antzelevitch, A subpopulation of cells with unique electrophysiological properties in the deep subepicardium of the canine ventricle. The M cell. *Circ. Res.*, 1991;**68**: 1729–1741.

120. Anyukhovsky, E.P., E.A. Sosunov, R.Z. Gainullin, and M.R. Rosen, The controversial M cell. *J. Cardiovasc. Electrophysiol.*, 1999;**10**: 244–260.

121. Antzelevitch, C., W. Shimuzu, G.-X. Yan, S. Sicouri, J. Weissenburger, V.V. Nesterenko, A. Burashnikov, J. Di Diego, J. Saffitz, and G.P. Thomas, The M cell: its contribution to the ECG and to normal and abnormal electrical function of the heart. *J. Cardiovasc. Electrophysiol.*, 1999;**10**: 1124–1152.

122. Janse, M.J., E.A. Sosunov, R. Coronel, T. Opthof, E.P. Anyukhovsky, J.M.T. de Bakker, A.N. Plotnikov, I.N. Shlapakova, P. Danilo, Jr., J.G.P. Tijssen, and M.R. Rosen, Repolarization gradients in the canine left ventricle before and after induction of short-term cardiac memory. *Circulation*, 2005;**112**: 1711–1718.

123. Drouin, E., F. Charpentier, C. Gauthier, K. Laurent, and H. Le Marec, Electrophysiological characteristics of cells spanning the left ventricular wall of human heart: evidence for the presence of M cells. *J. Am. Coll. Cardiol.*, 1995;**26**: 185–192.

124. Taggart, P., P.M.I. Sutton, T. Optof, R. Coronel, R. Trimlett, W. Pugsley, and P. Kallis, Transmural repolarisation in the left ventricle in humans during normoxia and ischaemia. *Cardiovasc. Res.*, 2001;**50**: 454–462.

125. Conrath, C.E., R. Wilders, R. Coronel, J.M.T. De Bakker, P. Taggart, J.R. De Groot, and T. Opthof, Intercellular coupling through gap junctions masks M cells in the human heart. *Cardiovasc. Res.*, 2004;**62**: 407–414.

126. Bauer, A., R. Becker, K.D. Freigang, J.C. Senges, F. Voss, A. Hansen, M. Müller, H.J. Lang, U. Gerlach, A. Busch, P. Kraft, W. Kubler, and W. Schols, Rate- and site-dependent effects of Propafenone, Dofetilide and the new I_{Ks}-blocking agent Chromanol 293b on individual muscle layers of the intact canine heart. *Circulation*, 1999;**100**: 2184–2190.

127. Roden, D.M., J.R. Balser, A.L. George, Jr., and M.E. Anderson, Cardiac ion channels. *Annu. Rev. Physiol.*, 2002;**64**: 431–475.

128. Catterall, W.A. and G. Gutman, Introduction to the IUPHAR compendium of voltage-gated ion channels. *Pharmacol. Rev.*, 2005;**57**: 385.

129. Hanlon, M.R. and B.A. Wallace, Structure and function of voltage-dependent ion channel regulatory β subunits. *Biochemistry*, 2002;**41**: 2886–2894.

130. Qu, J., C. Altomare, A. Bucchi, D. DiFrancesco, and R.B. Robinson, Functional comparison of HCN isoforms expressed in ventricular and HEK 293 cells. *Pflug. Arch.*, 2002;**444**: 597–601.

131. Yang, T., D. Snyders, and D.M. Roden, Drug block of I_{Kr}: model systems and relevance to human arrhythmias. *J. Cardiovasc. Pharm.*, 2001;**38**: 737–744.

132. Kléber, A.G., M.J. Janse, and V.G. Fast, Normal and abnormal conduction in the heart, in *Handbook of Physiology. Section 2 The Cardiovascular System, vol. 1 The Heart*. Oxford: Oxford University Press, 2001, pp. 455–530.

133. Kléber, A.G. and Y. Rudy, Basic mechanisms of cardiac impulse propagation and associated arrhythmias. *Physiol. Rev.*, 2004;**84**: 431–488.

134. Weidmann, S., Electrical constants of trabecular muscle from mammalian heart. *J. Physiol.*, 1952;**118**: 348–360.

135. Sampson, K.J. and C.S. Henriquez, Electrotonic influences on action potential duration dispersion in small hearts: a simulation study. *Am. J. Physiol. Heart Circ. Physiol.*, 2005;**289**: H350–H360.

136. Taggart, P., P.M.I. Sutton, T. Opthof, R. Coronel, R. Trimlett, W. Pugsley, and P. Kallis, Inhomogeneous transmural conduction during early ischaemia in patients with coronary artery disease. *J. Mol. Cell. Cardiol.*, 2000;**32**: 621–630.

137. Spach, M.S., Transition from continuous to discontinuous understanding of cardiac conduction. *Circ. Res.*, 2003;**92**:125–126.

138. Winterton, S.J., M.A. Turner, D.J. O'Gorman, N.A. Flores, and D.J. Sheridan. Hypertrophy causes delayed conduction in human and guinea pig myocardium: accentuation during ischaemic perfusion. *Cardiovasc. Res.*, 1994;**28**: 47–54.

139. Wiegerinck, R.F., A.O. Verkerk, C.N. Belterman, T.A.B. van Veen, A. Baartscheer, T. Opthof, R. Wilders, J. de Bakker, and R. Coronel, Larger cell size in rabbits with heart failure increases myocardial conduction velocity and QRS duration. *Circulation*, 2006;**113**: 806–813.

140. Wang, Y. and Y. Rudy, Action potential propagation in inhomogeneous cardiac tissue: safety factor considerations and ionic mechanism. *Am. J. Physiol. Heart Circ. Physiol.*, 2000;**278**: H1019–H1029.

141. Shaw, R.M. and Y. Rudy, Ionic mechanisms of propagation in cardiac tissue. Roles of the sodium and L-type calcium currents during reduced excitability and decreased gap junction coupling. *Circ. Res.*, 1997;**81**: 727–741.

142. Spach, M.S., W.T. Miller, III, D.B. Geselowitz, R.C. Barr, J.M. Kootsey, and E.A. Johnson, The discontinuous nature of propagation in normal canine cardiac muscle. Evidence for recurrent discontinuities of intracellular resistance that affect the membrane currents. *Circ. Res.*, 1981;**48**: 39–54.

143. Spach, M.S., P.C. Dolber, and J.F. Heidlage, Influence of the passive anisotropic properties on directional differences in propagation following modification of the sodium conductance in human atrial muscle. A model of reentry based on anisotropic discontinuous propagation. *Circ. Res.*, 1988;**62**: 811–832.

144. Sugiura, H. and R.W. Joyner, Action potential conduction between guinea pig ventricular cells can be modulated by calcium current. *Am. J. Physiol.*, 1992;**263**: H1591–H1604.

145. Rohr, S. and J.P. Kucera, Involvement of the calcium inward current in cardiac impulse propagation: induction of unidirectional conduction block by nifedipine and reversal by Bay K 8644. *Biophys. J.*, 1997;**72**: 754–766.

146. Spach, M.S., Transition from a continuous to discontinuous understanding of cardiac conduction. *Circ. Res.*, 2003;**92**: 125–126.

147. van der Pol, B. and J. van der Mark, The heartbeat considered as a relaxation oscillation and an electrical model of the heart. *Philos. Mag.*, 1928;**6**: 763–775.

148. FitzHugh, R., Impulses and physiological states in theoretical models of nerve membrane. *Biophys. J.*, 1961;**1**: 445–466.

149. van Capelle, F.J.L. and D. Durrer, Computer simulation of arrhythmias in a network of coupled excitable elements. *Circ. Res.*, 1980;**47**: 454–466.

150. Hodgkin, A.L. and A.F. Huxley, A quantitative description of membrane current and its application to conduction and excitation in nerve. *J. Physiol.*, 1952;**117**: 500–544.

151. Noble, D., Cardiac action and pacemaker potentials based on the Hodgkin-Huxley equations. *Nature*, 1960;**188**: 495–497.

152. Noble, D., A modification of the Hodgkin-Huxley equations applicable to Purkinje fibre action and pace-maker potentials. *J. Physiol.*, 1962;**160**: 317–352.

153. McAllister, R.E., D. Noble, and R.W. Tsien, Reconstruction of the electrical activity of cardiac Purkinje fibres. *J. Physiol.*, 1975;**251**: 1–59.

154. DiFrancesco, D. and D. Noble, A model of cardiac electrical activity incorporating ionic pumps and concentration changes. *Philos. Trans. R. Soc. Lond. B Biol. Sci.*, 1985;**307**: 353–398.

155. Beeler, G.W. and H. Reuter, Reconstruction of the action potential of ventricular myocardial fibres. *J. Physiol.*, 1977;**268**: 177–210.

156. Drouhard, J.P. and F.A. Roberge, Revised formulation of the Hodgkin-Huxley representation of the sodium current in cardiac cells. *Comput. Biomed. Res.*, 1987;**20**: 333–350.

157. Hilgemann, D.W. and D. Noble, Excitation-contraction coupling and extracellular calcium transients in rabbit atrium: reconstruction of the basic cellular mechanisms. *Proc. R. Soc. Lond. B Biol. Sci.*, 1987;**230**: 163–205.

158. Yanagihara, K., A. Noma, and H. Irisawa, Reconstruction of sino-atrial node pacemaker potential based on the voltage clamp experiments. *Jpn. J. Physiol.*, 1980;**30**: 841–857.

159. Irisawa, H. and A. Noma, Pacemaker mechanisms of rabbit sinoatrial node cells, in *Cardiac Rate and Rhythm*, L.N. Bouman and H.J. Jongsma, Editors. The Hague: Nijhoff, 1982, pp. 35–51.

160. Bristow, D.G. and J.W. Clark, A mathematical model of primary pacemaking cell in SA node of the heart. *Am. J. Physiol.*, 1982;**243**: H207–H218.

161. Noble, D. and S.J. Noble, A model of sino-atrial node electrical activity based on a modification of the DiFrancesco-Noble (1984) equations. *Proc. R. Soc. Lond. B Biol. Sci.*, 1984;**222**: 295–304.

162. Noble, D., D. DiFrancesco, and J.C. Denyer, Ionic mechanisms in normal and abnormal cardiac pacemaker activity, in *Neuronal and Cellular Oscillators*, J.W. Jacklet, Editor. New York: Marcel Dekker, 1989, pp. 59–85.

163. Noble, D., S.J. Noble, G.C. Bett, Y.E. Earm, W.K. Ho, and I.K. So, The role of sodium-calcium exchange during the cardiac action potential. *Ann. NY Acad. Sci.*, 1991;**639**: 334–353.

164. Earm, Y.E. and D. Noble, A model of the single atrial cell: relation between calcium current and calcium release. *Proc. R. Soc. Lond. B Biol. Sci.*, 1990;**240**: 83–96.

165. Luo, C.-H. and Y. Rudy, A model of the ventricular cardiac action potential: depolarization, repolarization and their interaction. *Circ. Res.*, 1991;**68**: 1501–1526.

166. Nordin, C., Computer model of membrane current and intracellular Ca^{2+} flux in the isolated guinea pig ventricular myocyte. *Am. J. Physiol.*, 1993;**265**: H2117–H2136.

167. Luo, C.-H. and Y. Rudy, A dynamic model of the cardiac ventricular action potential, I: simulations of ionic currents and concentration changes. *Circ. Res.*, 1994;**74**: 1071–1096.

168. Jafri, S., J.R. Rice, and R.L. Winslow, Cardiac Ca^{2+} dynamics: the roles of ryanodine receptor adaptation and sarcoplasmic reticulum load. *Biophys. J.*, 1998;**74**: 1149–1168.

169. Noble, D., A. Varghese, P. Kohl, and P. Noble, Improved guinea-pig ventricular cell model incorporating a diadic space, i_{Kr} and i_{Ks}, and length- and tension-dependent processes. *Can. J. Cardiol.*, 1998;**14**: 123–134.

170. Priebe, L. and D.J. Beuckelmann, Simulation study of cellular electric properties in heart failure. *Circ. Res.*, 1998;**82**: 1206–1223.

171. Winslow, R.L., J. Rice, S. Jafri, E. Marbán, and B. O'Rourke, Mechanisms of altered excitation-contraction coupling in canine tachycardia-induced heart failure, II: model studies. *Circ. Res.*, 1999;**84**: 571–586.

172. Pandit, S.V., R.B. Clark, W.R. Giles, and S.S. Demir, A mathematical model of action potential heterogeneity in adult rat left ventricular myocytes. *Biophys. J.*, 2001;**81**: 3029–3051.

173. Demir, S.S., J.W. Clark, C.R. Murphey, and W.R. Giles, A mathematical model of a rabbit sinoatrial node cell. *Am. J. Physiol.*, 1994;**266**: C832–C852.

174. Puglisi, J.L. and D.M. Bers, LabHEART: an interactive computer model of rabbit ventricular myocyte ion channels and Ca transport. *Am. J. Physiol. Cell Physiol.* 2001;**281**: C2049–C2060.

175. Bernus, O., R. Wilders, C.W. Zemlin, H. Verschelde, and A.V. Panfilov, A computationally efficient electrophysiological model of human ventricular cells. *Am. J. Physiol. Heart Circ. Physiol.*, 2002;**282**: H2296–H2308.

176. Matsuoka, S., N. Sarai, S. Kuratomi, K. Ono, and A. Noma, Role of individual ionic current systems in ventricular cells hypothesized by a model study. *Jpn. J. Physiol.*, 2003;**53**:105–123.

177. Bondarenko, V.E., G.P. Szigeti, G.C. Bett, S.J. Kim, and R.L. Rasmusson, Computer model of action potential of mouse ventricular myocytes. *Am. J. Physiol. Heart Circ. Physiol.*, 2004;**287**: H1378–H1403.

178. Shannon, T.R., F. Wang, J. Puglisi, C. Weber, and D.M. Bers, A mathematical treatment of integrated Ca dynamics within the ventricular myocyte. *Biophys. J.*, 2004;**87**: 3351–3371.

179. ten Tusscher, K.H., D. Noble, P.J. Noble, and A.V. Panfilov, A model for human ventricular tissue. *Am. J. Physiol. Heart Circ. Physiol.*, 2004;**286**: H1573–H1589.

180. Iyer, V., R. Mazhari, and R.L. Winslow, A computational model of the human left-ventricular epicardial myocyte. *Biophys. J.*, 2004;**87**: 1507–1525.

181. Hund, T.J. and Y. Rudy, Rate dependence and regulation of action potential and calcium transient in a canine cardiac ventricular cell model. *Circulation*, 2004;**110**: 3168–3174.

182. Lindblad, D.S., C.R. Murphey, J.W. Clark, and W.R. Giles, A model of the action potential and underlying membrane currents in a rabbit atrial cell. *Am. J. Physiol.*, 1996;**271**: H1666–H1691.

183. Courtemanche, M., R.J. Ramirez, and S. Nattel, Ionic mechanisms underlying human atrial action potential properties: insights from a mathematical model. *Am. J. Physiol.*, 1998;**275**: H301–H321.

184. Nygren, A., C. Fiset, L. Firek, J.W. Clark, D.S. Lindblad, R.B. Clark, and W.R. Giles, Mathematical model of an adult human atrial cell: the role of K$^+$ currents in repolarization. *Circ. Res.*, 1998;**82**: 63–81.

185. Ramirez, R.J., S. Nattel, and M. Courtemanche, Mathematical analysis of canine atrial action potentials: rate, regional factors, and electrical remodeling. *Am. J. Physiol. Heart Circ. Physiol.*, 2000;**279**: H1767–H1785.

186. Wilders, R., H.J. Jongsma, and A.C.G. van Ginneken, Pacemaker activity of the rabbit sinoatrial node: a comparison of mathematical models. *Biophys. J.*, 1991;**60**: 1202–1216.

187. Dokos, S., B. Celler, and N. Lovell, Ion currents underlying sinoatrial node pacemaker activity: a new single cell mathematical model. *J. Theor. Biol.*, 1996;**181**: 245–272.

188. Demir, S.S., J.W. Clark, and W.R. Giles, Parasympathetic modulation of sinoatrial node pacemaker activity in rabbit heart: a unifying model. *Am. J. Physiol.*, 1999;**276**: H2221–H2244.

189. Zhang, H., A.V. Holden, I. Kodama, H. Honjo, M. Lei, T. Varghese, and M.R. Boyett, Mathematical models of action potentials in the periphery and center of the rabbit sinoatrial node. *Am. J. Physiol. Heart Circ. Physiol.*, 2000;**279**: H397–H421.

190. Zhang, H., A.V. Holden, D. Noble, and M.R. Boyett, Analysis of the chronotropic effect of acetylcholine on sinoatrial node cells. *J. Cardiovasc. Electrophysiol.*, 2002;**13**: 465–474.

191. Zhang, H., A.V. Holden, and M.R. Boyett, Sustained inward current and pacemaker activity of mammalian sinoatrial node. *J. Cardiovasc. Electrophysiol.*, 2002;**13**: 809–812.

192. Kurata, Y., I. Hisatome, S. Imanishi, and T. Shibamoto, Dynamical description of sinoatrial node pacemaking: improved mathematical model for primary pacemaker cell. *Am. J. Physiol. Heart Circ. Physiol.*, 2002;**283**: H2074–H2101.

193. Sarai, N., S. Matsuoka, S. Kuratomi, K. Ono, and A. Noma, Role of individual ionic current systems in the SA node hypothesized by a model study. *Jpn. J. Physiol.*, 2003;**53**:125–134.

194. Lovell, N.H., S.L. Cloherty, B.G. Celler, and S. Dokos, A gradient model of cardiac pacemaker myocytes. *Prog. Biophys. Mol. Biol.*, 2004;**85**: 301–323.

195. Krogh-Madsen, T., P. Schaffer, A.D. Skriver, L.K. Taylor, B. Pelzmann, B. Koidl, and M.R. Guevara, An ionic model for rhythmic activity in small clusters of embryonic chick ventricular cells. *Am. J. Physiol. Heart Circ. Physiol.*, 2005;**289**: H398–H413.

196. Kneller, J., R.J. Ramirez, D. Chartier, M. Courtemanche, and S. Nattel, Time-dependent transients in an ionically based mathematical model of the canine atrial action potential. *Am. J. Physiol. Heart Circ. Physiol.*, 2002;**282**: H1437–H1451.

197. Endresen, L.P., K. Hall, J.S. Hoye, and J. Myrheim, A theory for the membrane potential of living cells. *Eur. Biophys. J.*, 2000;**29**: 90–103.

198. ten Tusscher, K.H., O. Bernus, R. Hren, and A.V. Panfilov, Comparison of electrophysiological models for human ventricular cells and tissues. *Prog. Biophys. Mol. Biol.*, 2006;**90**: 326–345.

199. Wilders, R. and H.J. Jongsma, Beating irregularity of single pacemaker cells isolated from the rabbit sinoatrial node. *Biophys. J.*, 1993;**65**: 2601–2613.

200. Zaniboni, M., A.E. Pollard, L. Yang, and K.W. Spitzer, Beat-to-beat repolarization variability in ventricular myocytes and its suppression by electrical coupling. *Am. J. Physiol. Heart Circ. Physiol.*, 2000;**278**: H677–H687.

201. Guevara, M.R. and T.J. Lewis, A minimal single-channel model for the regularity of beating in the sinoatrial node. *Chaos*, 1995;**5**: 174–83.

202. Greenstein, J.L. and R.L. Winslow, An integrative model of the cardiac ventricular myocyte incorporating local control of Ca^{2+} release. *Biophys. J.*, 2002;**83**: 2918–2945.

203. Henriquez, C.S., Simulating the electrical behavior of cardiac tissue using the bidomain model. *Crit. Rev. Biomed. Eng.*, 1993;**21**: 1–77.

204. Potse, M., B. Dubé, J. Richer, A. Vinet, and R.M. Gulrajani, A comparison of monodomain and bidomain reaction-diffusion models for action potential propagation in the human heart. *IEEE Trans. Biomed. Eng.*, 2006;**53**(12): 2425–2435.

205. Fenton, F. and A. Karma, Vortex dynamics in three-dimensional continuous myocardium with fiber rotation: filament instability and fibrillation. *Chaos*, 1998;**8**: 20–47.

206. Sarai, N., S. Matsuoka, and A. Noma, SimBio: a Java package for the development of detailed cell models. *Prog. Biophys. Mol. Biol.*, 2006;**90**: 360–377.

207. Mazhari, R., J.L. Greenstein, R.L. Winslow, E. Marbán, and H.B. Nuss, Molecular interactions between two long-QT syndrome gene products, HERG and KCNE2, rationalized by in vitro and in silico analysis. *Circ. Res.*, 2001;**89**: 33–38.

4 Activation of the Heart

M.J. Janse

P. W. Macfarlane et al. (eds.), *Basic Electrocardiology*, DOI 10.1007/978-0-85729-871-3_4,
© Springer-Verlag London Limited 2012

4.1   Introduction

The cardiac electrical impulse is initiated in the sinoatrial node and spreads rapidly over the atria, slowly through the atrioventricular node, and rapidly over the specific ventricular conduction system and myocardium of both ventricles [1]. These excitable tissues are able to generate an action potential in response to a suprathreshold current stimulus. The voltage difference between excited and resting tissue drives local current circuits that excite the resting tissue thereby causing spread of excitation in a wave-like manner. The main factors that determine propagation are (1) the properties of the ionic channels in the cell membrane, (2) the passive electrical properties of the tissue, and (3) in two- or three-dimensional media the curvature of the excitation wave . In atrial and ventricular myocardium, and in the specific ventricular conduction system, the current responsible for the action potential upstroke and for delivering local current for propagation is carried by Na^+ ions. In the cells of the sinoatrial node and the atrioventricular node a major contribution is made by the Ca^{2+} current. In tissue with a high degree of electrical cell-to-cell uncoupling and in tissue with geometrical discontinuity, flow of inward Ca^{2+} current becomes necessary to maintain propagation [2, 3]. The various regions of the heart differ with respect to distribution of ionic channels, and with respect to passive electrical properties, which depend on cell morphology, type and distribution of gap junctions, and the arrangement of cells in strands and layers. Therefore values of conduction velocity vary from about 0.05 m/s, the lowest value found in the atrioventricular node, to about 3.5 m/s, the highest value in the His-Purkinje system [4].

4.2   The Sinoatrial Node

The morphological sinoatrial, or sinus node, first described by Keith and Flack in 1907 [5], lies at the junction of the superior vena cava and the right atrium close to the crest of the atrial appendage. Its boundaries are not sharply defined in all species [6, 7]. The node consists of two types of myocytes [6–9]. The central nodal cells are arranged in a complex interdigitating manner interspersed with connective tissue. They contain very few myofilaments. The intracellular organized structures (myofilaments, mitochondria, nuclei and sarcoplasmic reticulum tubules) occupy only 50% of the cell volume, whereas in atrial cells these structures comprise 90% of cell volume. The second type of myocytes is transitional in that it changes gradually from the typical central nodal cell to an ordinary atrial cell. In some species, such as the rabbit, the zone of transitional cells is large, in others, such as the dog or the pig, it is narrow. The boundary between transitional and atrial cells is morphologically often poorly defined. Studies using immunohistochemical staining techniques did show a sharp boundary between nodal and atrial cells [10]. Nodal cells reacted with a monoclonal antibody against bovine Purkinje fibers and did not react to an antibody against connexion 43. Atrial cells on the other hand did not react to the antibody against Purkinje fibers but did react with the connexion 43 antibody. Since no electrophysiologic measurements were made, and no morphological studies were performed to quantify the number of intracellular organelles and filaments, no certainty exists whether some cells defined as atrial by immunohistochemical criteria might not be transitional according to other criteria. In a study combining immunohistochemistry, electrophysiology and electronmicroscopy [11], it was found, in contrast to previous studies, that atrial cells could be found in the very center of the node. Furthermore, the sinus node comprised three morphologically distinct cells that had the same electrophysiological characteristics. In contrast to the traditional concept of a transitional zone in which the transition from nodal cells to atrial cells occurred gradually, the situation in human, feline, and canine nodes is such that typical nodal cells are intermingled with atrial cells, and the transition is formed by a zone in which the density of atrial cells gradually increases from the central node to the crista terminalis [7, 11, 12].

A striking feature of the sinus node, including that in the human, is the presence of abundant connective tissue surrounding the nodal cells [13–17]. There are marked species differences regarding the amount of collagen. In cats 75–95% of the volume of the sinus node may consist of collagen; in pigs 75%, and in guinea-pigs 50% [14–16]. Attempts to correlate the amount of connective tissue with age yielded variable results. Thus, in humans approximately 50% of the sinus node in young individuals has been reported to be occupied by myocytes, while at the age of 70 years the proportion of the node occupied by myocytes may be as low as 10% [17]. In another study, the relative volume of collagen in the sinus node was found to remain constant once adulthood was reached in both cats and humans. No consistent relationship between the amount of collagen and sino-atrial conduction time could be established [18]. An increase in the amount of adipose tissue between the transitional cells has been reported to be age related [19].

The first combined electrophysiological and morphological studies on the pacemaker of the heart were performed in 1910 [20, 21]. The site of origin of the heartbeat was determined by searching for the site of primary extracellular negativity, which was found on the epicardial surface of the canine right atrium in the sulcus terminalis near the vena cava superior. This site of "primary negativity" coincided with the site of the histological sinus node. Transmembrane potentials from pacemaker cells were first recorded from the sinus venosus of the frog heart in 1952 [22] and in 1955 from the sinus node of mammalian hearts [23]. These studies revealed the most characteristic electrophysiological feature of pacemaking cells: spontaneous diastolic depolarization of the membrane potential. A number of ionic currents are involved in normal pacemaking in the sinus node: a decay in outward current carried by potassium ions following repolarization, an inward current carried by sodium ions, called If, which is activated after repolarization, and finally the slow inward current carried by calcium ions, which is activated as the membrane depolarizes [24–28].

In 1963 Trautwein and Uchizono [29] determined the ultrastructure of cells very close to cells from which typical pacemaker potentials were recorded, and in 1978 direct identification of the cell from which the pacemaker potential had been recorded was made [30]. Not unexpectedly, pacemaker potentials originated from nodal cells. Microelectrode recording in isolated, superfused rabbit heart preparations [8, 9, 31–34] resulted in maps depicting the spread of excitation during spontaneous sinus beats (see ❷ Fig. 4.1). Dominant pacemaker cells, i.e., those with the earliest action potential upstrokes, the fastest rate of diastolic depolarization, the slowest rate of rise of the action potential, and a gradual transition from diastolic to systolic depolarization, comprise a small area of about 0.3 mm square, containing about 5,000 cells that fire synchronously. Gap junctions, although less frequent than in transitional or atrial cells, were found in every cell contour in ultrathin sections. It was estimated that every cell in the pacemaker center was coupled to other cells via at least 100 gap junctions [8]. This is far in excess of what is needed to ensure synchronisation of diastolic depolarization [35, 36].

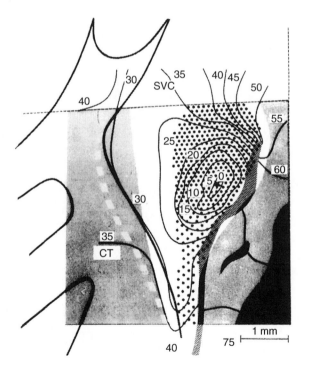

❑ Fig. 4.1
Isochronal map of spread of excitation from the sinus node of an isolated rabbit heart preparation. Numbers correspond to activation times in ms. Configuration of action potentials is shown along the pathway of conduction from central node towards the atrium. The dashed line indicates the beginning of the atrial electrogram used as a time reference. Towards the periphery the action potentials show an increase in amplitude and dV/dtmax and a decrease in the rate of diastolic depolarization. The hatched area is an area of conduction block (© Reproduced with permission from Bleeker et al. [9])

This is in apparent contrast with a study in which the sinus node failed to react with antibodies against connexion 43 [10], although in another study nodal cells did show a reaction [37].

Electrotonic interaction between atrial and nodal cells plays a crucial role in the functioning of the sinus node. Pacemaker activity in the peripheral transitional cells is suppressed because they are coupled to atrial cells, which do not have the capacity for spontaneous diastolic depolarization. Because the constant resting potential of atrial cells is more negative than the maximum diastolic potential of transitional cells, an electrotonic current flows from atrial to transitional cells, hyperpolarizing the latter and thus suppressing diastolic depolarization. When transitional cells are isolated from the surrounding atrium, their intrinsic pacemaking rate is actually higher than that from the centrally located "dominant" pacemaker [16, 38, 39]. Computer simulations have shown that a critical degree of coupling between atrial and transitional cells, as well as a gradual decrease in coupling resistance from central nodal cells towards the atrium, are necessary for the small group of nodal cells to activate the atrium. When coupling resistance is too low, electrotonic current from the large mass of surrounding atrial tissue will suppress diastolic depolarization. When coupling resistance is too high, the current provided by the small group of dominant pacemaker cells will not be sufficient to depolarize atrial cells to threshold [40].

As shown in ❷ Fig. 4.1 conduction from the central node towards the crista terminalis in the isolated rabbit heart preparation occurs preferentially in an oblique cranial direction. This can be explained by the tissue architecture, conduction being faster in areas where fibers are arranged in parallel. Conduction block occurs towards the interatrial septum, due to a reduced excitability of cells in this region [41]. In intact hearts, the excitation process is more complicated. First of all, alterations in the activity of the autonomic nervous system not only cause changes in sinus rate, they also produce pacemaker shifts. Under the influence of acetylcholine, the dominant pacemaker shifts away from the central area of the node towards transitional cells in the cauda; adrenalin induces a pacemaker shift towards a more inferior site [42–44]. Extracellular recordings form intact canine and human hearts [45, 46] showed that in the area of the sinus node two deflections of low amplitude and frequency precede the large high-frequency deflection caused by activity of atrial tissue: a "diastolic slope" corresponding to diastolic depolarization and an "upstroke slope" corresponding to systolic depolarization. Asynchronous activity of several pacemaking groups was recorded, suggesting that, despite strong coupling within one group of pacemaking cells, intergroup coupling may not be strong. Earliest right atrial activation could result from impulses arising from more than one automatic group within the sinus node. Studies by Boineau and co-workers in the canine heart showed that impulses were simultaneously initiated from up to three atrial sites separated by more than 1 cm [47–49]. Multiple depolarization waves originating from these sites, merged into a common wavefront after 10–15 ms. Changes in heart rate were associated with changes in the sites of origin. It was argued that these findings should be explained by a multicenter pacemaker model, and that the system of atrial pacemakers is much larger than the sinus node, extending both craniocaudally and mediolaterally. At extreme heart rates, extranodal pacemakers could dominate the pacemakers in the sinus node. Thus, whereas in isolated preparations the site of the dominant pacemaker is constant, in the heart in vivo, considerable pacemaker shifts may occur and the earliest activated atrial areas may shift as well. ❷ Fig. 4.2 shows that in the human heart, simultaneous atrial activation may occur at multiple sites [50]. To quote Cosio et al.: "The expression 'sinus node area' is commonly used as a reference for the diagnosis of ectopic atrial tachycardia; however, our data show that the origin of activation can be so wide as to make this expression almost meaningless" [50].

4.3 Subsidiary Pacemakers with Normal Automaticity

Cells with the capacity of spontaneous diastolic depolarization can be found in other areas of the heart besides the sinus node, particularly along the crista terminalis and in the inter-atrial septum, in the atrioventricular junction and in the specialized ventricular conduction system [51–53]. The intrinsic rate of impulse formation is highest in the sinus node and decreases progressively in pacemakers in the atrium, atrioventricular junction and His-Purkinje system. Normally, the sinus node is the dominant pacemaker over a wide range of heart rates because diastolic depolarization of latent pacemakers is inhibited by repeated excitation by impulses from the sinus node. This inhibition is called overdrive suppression [54]. Overdrive suppression is mediated by enhanced activity of the Na^+/K^+ pump. This pump, depending on energy derived from a membrane-bound ATPase, is responsible for maintaining ionic homeostase by pumping Na^+ ions

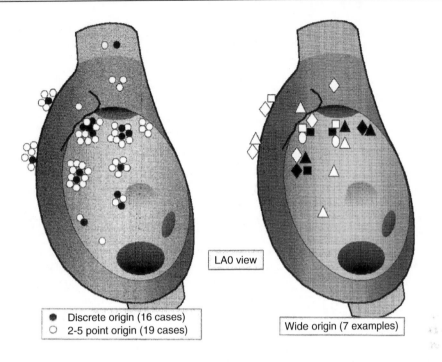

LA0 view

● Discrete origin (16 cases)
○ 2-5 point origin (19 cases)

Wide origin (7 examples)

⬛ Fig. 4.2
Schematic representation of the right human atrium in a left anterior oblique view displaying points of earliest activation. The orifices of the superior vena cava, inferior vena cava, coronary sinus, and the ring of the oval fossa are shown for orientation. *Left*: Points of onset of activation in all patients are represented in black for cases with single endocardial zero points and in white for cases with multiple points of onset. *Right*: Seven examples of onset of activation simultaneously in multiple points are represented. Each shape and tone (black or white) identifies multiple sites in each patient (© Reproduced with permission from Cosio et al. [50])

that entered the cell during the action potential upstroke out of the cell, and pumping K^+ ions that left the cell during repolarization back into the cell. When a latent pacemaker is driven by the sinus node at a faster rate than its normal intrinsic rate more Na^+ ions enter the cell than would have been the case if the pacemaker were firing at its own intrinsic rate. The activity of the Na^+/K^+ pump is largely determined by the level of intracellular Na^+ concentration [55], so that pump activity is enhanced during high rates of stimulation. Since the pump drives three Na^+ ions out of the cell against two K^+ ions into the cell, it generates a net outward current that hyperpolarizes the cell membrane and counteracts inward currents responsible for spontaneous diastolic depolarization. If the dominant pacemaker is stopped, for example by strong vagal stimulation, the overdrive suppression is responsible for a period of quiescence which lasts until the intracellular Na^+ concentration, and hence pump current, becomes small enough to allow subsidiary pacemakers to depolarize spontaneously to threshold. Impulse generation by latent pacemakers begins at a low rate and gradually speeds up to a final steady state. When sudden atrioventricular block occurs and pacemaker cells in the distal atrioventricular node or His-Purkinje cells need a long time to recover from overdrive suppression, the period of cardiac standstill may be long enough to cause loss of consciousness (Adams-Stokes attack).

Another mechanism that may suppress subsidiary pacemakers is electrotonic interaction between pacemaker cell and non-pacemaker cells. This mechanism is particularly important in preventing overt pacemaker activity in the central part of the atrioventricular node. In these cells the action potential upstroke is, like that of the central sinus node, largely dependent on the slow inward calcium current. Therefore, in those cells far less Na^+ ions enter the cell than in cells of the atrium and His-Purkinje system. As a result there is far less stimulation of the Na^+/K^+ pump during overdrive and less overdrive suppression. Isolated small preparations of atrioventricular nodal cells have intrinsic pacemaker activity that is as rapid as that in the sinus node and is not easily overdrive suppressed [53]. Because of electrotonic inhibition, ectopic pacemaker activity seldom occurs in the central atrioventricular node. Normally, the atrioventricular nodal pacemakers that drive the heart during complete atrioventricular block are located in the distal node [51]. These cells are overdrive suppressible.

4.4   Atrial Activation

Lewis, who was the first to map the spread of excitation in the atria, described this process as follows: "the excitation wave in the auricle may be likened to the spread of fluid poured upon a flat surface, its edges advancing as an ever widening circle, until the whole surface is covered; such variation as exists in the rate of travel along various lines in the auricle is fully accounted for by the simple anatomical arrangement of the tissue" [56]. In the accompanying figure the isochrones deviate over the crista terminalis, indicating preferential conduction over that bundle. The right atrium is a "bag full of holes." The orifices of the superior and inferior vena cava, the ostium of the coronary sinus, and the fossa ovalis divide the atrial myocardium into various muscular bands. Owing to this architecture, there are only a limited number of routes available for conduction of the impulse from sinus node to atrioventricular node. From the many studies in which atrial activation was mapped [31, 57–66], it emerged that internodal conduction follows routes indicated by gross anatomical landmarks. The crista terminalis and the anterior limb of the fossa ovalis are the main routes for preferential conduction between the sinus node and the atrioventricular node, and these prominent muscle bands provide a dual input to the atrioventricular node. A similar activation sequence as that found in isolated rabbit heart was found in the human heart during surgery [66]. Here also, the AV node received a dual input. In most patients, the anterior septum was activated some 10 ms prior to the posterior input via the crista terminalis. In patients with a low crista terminalis pacemaker the AV node was activated via the crista terminalis 15–20 ms before activation of the anterior input (NB: in the older literature the terms anterior and posterior are used. Given the position of the heart in the body, it is better to use "superior" instead of "anterior," and "inferior" instead of "posterior").

There are two main routes for the sinus impulse towards the left atrium: an anterior one corresponding to Bachmann's bundle, and a posterior one via interatrial posteromedial connections inserting around the orifices of the right pulmonary veins [67, 68]. Some authors consider Bachmann's bundle as the most important connection [67], others find the posterior interatrial connection as important as Bachmann's bundle for activation from right to left, whereas activation from left to right occurs predominantly via Bachmann's bundle [68].

Irrespective of the site of earliest breakthrough, the pattern of left atrial activation is determined by a line of conduction block related to an abrupt change in left atrial endocardial fiber orientation and wall thickness at the lateral margin of the septal pulmonary bundle as this traverses the posterior left atrium between the pulmonary veins towards the septal mitral annulus [69]. A third interatrial connection exists through the coronary sinus [70–74]. This muscular connection has a variable anatomy in the human heart [74], and is particularly important during pacing from the coronary sinus [68].

A typical feature of left atrial activation is that different wavefronts simultaneously proceed in different directions and that wavefronts frequently collide [50, 61]. In a study on atrial activation of the horse, it was said that the explanation for the "chaotic pattern of left atrial activation may be that the two great pulmonary veins break the left atrial surface into discontinuous islets in which no general front of depolarization can develop" [62]. The major portion of the left atrium depolarizes after right atrial activation has been completed. In the canine heart, atrial activation is completed in approximately 60 ms, in the isolated human heart after 90–100 ms [59, 61, 63].

During retrograde atrial activation, studied while pacing the ventricles at a rate higher than the sinus rate, the pattern of left atrial activation is similar to that during sinus rhythm [63, 64, 75–77]. The retrograde wavefront quickly spreads up the interatrial septum to emerge very early at Bachmann's bundle. Activation then proceeds over this bundle to activate the left atrium in much the same way as during sinus rhythm. When the atrium is paced from the posteroinferior left atrium or from a site just posterior (or rather inferior) to the ostium of the coronary sinus, Bachmann's bundle is activated late, and P waves in leads I, III, and avF are negative. When Bachmann's bundle was activated early, as during ventricular pacing or from an atrial site anterior (superior) to the coronary sinus, P waves are positive [75, 77]. The time of arrival of a retrograde wavefront at Bachmann's bundle is therefore critical in determining the polarity of a "retrograde" P wave.

4.5   Specialized Internodal Pathways?

Controversy regarding the spread of activation of the sinus impulse has existed since the discovery of the sinus node and the atrioventricular node. In 1909 Thorel [78] claimed to have demonstrated continuity between both nodes via a tract of "Purkinje-like" cells. This possibility was debated during a meeting of the Deutschen pathologischen Gesellschaft in 1910 [79] and the consensus of this meeting was that both nodes were connected by simple atrial myocardium. In the 1960s and 1970s, the concept of specialized internodal tracts was again promoted, notably by James [70]. This promotion was so successful that the tracts are denoted in the well-known atlas of Netter [80] in a fashion analogous to that used to delineate the ventricular specialized conduction system. In the 1960s and 1970s pediatric cardiac surgeons took care not to damage these tracts. The specialized tracts were considered to play a role in the genesis of atrial flutter [81]. A review of the early literature, together with own experimental and histological data was presented by Janse and Anderson in 1974 [82]. It was concluded that there was no well-defined specialized conduction system connecting the sinus node to the atrioventricular node. The definitive proof that specialized internodal tracts do not exist was given by Spach and co-workers [83]. They argued that preferential conduction in atrial bundles could either be due to the anisotropic properties of the tissue or to the presence of a specialized tract. If the point of stimulation would be shifted to various sites of the bundle, isochrones of similar shape would result from stimulating multiple sites if the anisotropic properties primarily influenced local conduction velocities. On the other hand, isochrones of different shapes would be obtained if there was a fixed position specialized tract in the bundle. Their experimental results clearly provided evidence that preferential conduction in the atria is due to the anisotropic properties of cardiac muscle.

4.6   The Atrioventricular Junction

The atrial part of the atrioventricular (AV) junction is contained within the triangle of Koch, as depicted for the human heart in ❷ Fig. 4.3. The triangle is delineated by the tendon of Todaro, the attachment of the septal leaflet of the tricuspid valve, and by the ostium of the coronary sinus. In 1906, Tawara [85] described a spindle-shaped compact network of small cells in the superior part of Koch's triangle. These cells were connected via *Knotenpunkte* in which four or five fibers were joined together. It was this characteristic that prompted him "for simplicity's sake" to call this compact network *Knoten* (node). Nowadays, this part of the AV junction is usually called the compact node. The compact node is surrounded by transitional cells. Although Tawara did not use the term transitional cells, he wrote that between the compact node and the atrial musculature "the cells are very small. They do not form a complicated network, but course more or less parallel. They are joined into several small bundles, separated by strands of connective tissue, which in this area is abundant" (p. 136). "These bundles are connected to atrial muscle...these connections are so gradual that no sharp boundary can be detected. ... Either single cells become gradually larger and change inconspicuously into atrial fibers, or several small bundles gradually join into a broader bundle which then merges with atrial muscle" (p. 137). There is room for confusion when speaking of the atrioventricular (AV) node, because some authors mean by this the compact node only, others the whole area occupied by compact node and transitional cells. Tawara was unable to determine precisely where the atrium ended and the specialized AV nodal region begins, because of the gradual change from atrial to transitional cells, as were subsequent investigators [86–88]. When traced superiorly, the compact node, without any perceptible change in cellular configuration, enters the central fibrous body. This point marks the transition from compact node to the penetrating atrioventricular bundle, or bundle of His. Tawara noted that at the point of entry in the central fibrous body, typical nodal cells were interspersed with larger His bundle cells. Again, on a histological basis, he could not tell where the AV node ended and the His bundle began. "I set the boundary at the site where this system penetrates into the membranous septum" (p. 127; all quotations from Tawara are in my translation).

4.7   Activation of the Atrioventricular Nodal Area

In 1960, Paes de Carvalho and de Almeida studied the activation pattern of the AV node in isolated rabbit heart preparations [87]. Based on activation times and transmembrane action potential characteristics, they described three cell

4

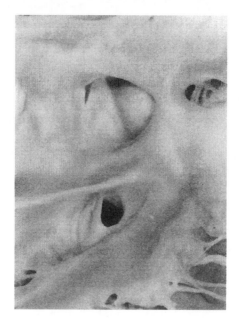

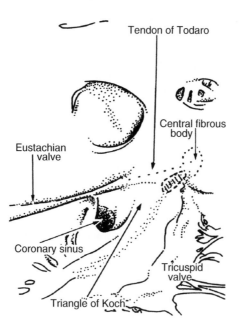

◘ Fig. 4.3

Anatomy of the AV junction. Photograph and sketch of a normal human heart showing the anatomical landmarks of the triangle of Koch. The approximate site of the compact AV node is indicated by the stippled area adjacent to the central fibrous body (© Reproduced with permission from Janse et al. [84])

types arranged in different layers and classified them into atrionodal (AN), nodal (N), and nodo-His (NH). N cells had action potentials with low amplitudes and upstroke velocities, the AN zone was a transitional zone between fast conducting atrial tissue and the slowly conducting N zone, and the NH zone was a transitional zone between the N zone and the His bundle, where conduction became rapid and action potential upstroke velocity became high. AN potentials were found to be generated by transitional cells, N potentials by the compact node, and NH potentials by the distal AV node [89]. However, N potentials could also be recorded from transitional cells and from cells in the tract of lower nodal cells in continuity with the His bundle. This raises the question whether there is a strict correlation between cellular electrophysiology and histology. In a study on isolated, arterially perfused canine and porcine hearts, it was found that cells with N type action potentials were not confined to the triangle of Koch, but extended along both AV orifices. These cells had low resting membrane potentials between −55 and −65 mV, a maximum upstroke velocity lower than 5 V/s, a low action potential amplitude between 45 and 65 mV, and they responded to the administration of adenosine by a further reduction of action potential amplitude and upstroke velocity. Histologically, these cells were similar to atrial cells, but they lacked the gap-junctional protein connexin 43 (Cx43) [90]. It is possible that immunohistochemistry is a more discriminating tool than light microscopy in delineating various cell types in the AV junction. Thus, Petrecca and co-workers [91] showed a paucity of sodium channel immunofluorescence in the central compact node. A gradual increase of expression was detected when moving to the peripherally located circumferential transitional cells. In the transitional zone, and in the lower nodal cell tract, levels of sodium channel immunoreactivity were comparable to that found in atrial and ventricular myocardium. The pattern of distribution of Cx43 was similar to that of the sodium channel, with a paucity of Cx43 immunoreactivity central mid-nodal cells. Both factors contribute to the slow conduction in the N zone.

There are only two studies in which mapping of Koch's triangle have been performed by both extra- and intracellular electrodes simultaneously [92, 93]. Mapping with extracellular electrodes is difficult because the rate of change in extracellular deflections may be very slow, because extracellular potentials may have multiple deflections, and because activation of the central node is a three-dimensional event where slow, low-amplitude action potentials in deep layers may not generate extracellular potentials of sufficient amplitude to be recorded by surface electrodes. The two studies mentioned above differ with respect to the cause of extracellular potentials with double components. In a study on superfused rabbit and canine preparations [92], where extracellular waveforms with multiple deflections were found at the posterior (inferior) approach to the node, the initial rapid deflection corresponded to the action potential upstroke of superficial atrial cells, the second, usually slower deflection originated from underlying nodal cells. In a study on arterially, blood-perfused canine and porcine hearts, the initial rapid deflection originated from deep atrial cells, the second slow deflection from more superficial nodal cells [93].

In shows an activation map of the superfused rabbit heart preparation, where sites transmembrane potential were recorded, the activation sequence is depicted in 20 ms intervals, with time zero being the activation time of a site close to the sinus node. The main features of the activation sequence are (1) there is a dual input into the AV nodal region, a posterior (inferior) one via the crista terminalis and an anterior (superior) one in front of the ostium of the coronary sinus; (2) in the central part of Koch's triangle, the activation pattern is complex and isochronal lines cannot be drawn. This is so in part because at one location superficial cells may be excited up to 40 ms earlier than deeper cells. The speed of propagation is very slow; it takes some 60 ms to cover a distance of about 1 mm, which corresponds to a conduction velocity in the order of 1.7 cm/s; (3) in the last part to be activated (at 90–110 ms), activation is rapid and synchronous. There is a sharp demarcation between cells activated early and cells activated late. The anterior (superior) input does not bypass the central node but curves posteriorly (inferiorly) to merge with the posterior (inferior) input. One feature is not apparent is this case is the existence of "dead-end pathways." These consist of cells that do not participate in transmitting the impulse from atrium to His bundle and vice versa. They can be identified by expressing their moment of excitation as a percent of the atrium-His bundle and His bundle-atrium conduction time during anterograde and retrograde conduction, respectively. The sum of these times for cells in the mainstream is around 100%. For dead end pathway cells, this sum far exceeds 100%, indicating that they activated too late in both modes of conduction. One dead-end pathway consists of atrial overlay fibers terminating in the base of the septal leaflet of the tricuspid valve, another one branches off the central node and extends posteriorly (inferiorly) along the tricuspid orifice [89, 95].

4.8   Dual Atrioventricular Nodal Pathways and Reentry

The two atrial inputs into the AV nodal area have different properties. When pacing the atria at a relatively fast rate, stimulation on the crista terminalis (inferior input) still results in 1:1 conduction to the His bundle, while pacing at the same rate on the superior input causes 2:1 block [96]. It is now customary to call these inputs "slow" and "fast" pathways, which are thought to underlie AV nodal reentry.

As early as 1913, Mines [97] described what he called a reciprocating rhythm after electrical stimulation of the auricle-ventricle preparation of the electric ray, a species which does not have a real atrioventricular node as described by Tawara. He reasoned that the atrioventricular connection had two divisions with a slight difference in the rate of recovery. A premature stimulus delivered to the ventricle "should spread up to the auricle by that part of the A-V connection having the quicker recovery process and not by the other part. In such a case, when the auricle would be excited by this impulse. The other portion of the A-V connection would be ready to take up transmission again back to the ventricle. Provided the transmission in each direction was slow, the chamber at either end would be ready to respond (its refractory phase being short) and thus the condition once established would tend to continue, unless upset by the interpolation of a premature systole" [97]. A similar explanation was given 2 years later by White, who described a clinical case where, during AV dissociation, idioventricular beats were sometimes conducted back to the atria, and the retrograde inverted P wave was followed by a narrow QRS complex [98]. In 1926, Scherf and Shookhoff studied reciprocating rhythms in dogs and introduced the term "longitudinal dissociation" [99], Moe et al. in 1956 suggested "dual AV transmission" [100], and Rosenblueth in 1958 coined the phrase "ventricular echoes" [101]. Reciprocation in the other direction, where an atrial premature impulse turns back in the AV node to reexcite the atria as an echo was also described [102].

When catheters were used for intracardiac recording and stimulation in patients, many studies reported on the induction of both atrial and ventricular echoes in hearts without apparent conduction abnormalities and without arrhythmias, so that functional longitudinal dissociation was considered to be a property of the normal AV node [102–106]. Animal studies supported this conclusion [100, 107, 108]. In some animal studies, it was possible, if only occasionally, to induce repetitive reciprocation leading to sustained AV nodal reentrant tachycardia [109–112], but in humans with normal AV nodal function this was not observed. In patients with spontaneous AV nodal reentrant tachycardias, this arrhythmia could easily be induced by premature stimulation [103, 106, 113].

A key factor thought to indicate the presence of dual AV pathways is the so-called discontinuity in the AV conduction curve during premature stimulation, which can be demonstrated both in individuals with and without spontaneous tachycardia [103, 106]. During atrial premature stimulation the interval between the premature atrial response and the subsequent His bundle deflection (the A2–H2 interval) gradually prolongs with increasing prematurity until at certain coupling interval it abruptly increases ("jumps") and then continues to increase gradually. The explanation is that with moderate prematurity AV conduction proceeds over a fast pathway that has a long refractory period. When at a certain coupling interval the fast pathway is refractory, conduction now occurs over the slow pathway having a shorter refractory period. During ventricular premature stimulation, the exits of slow and fast pathways correspond the posterior (inferior) and anterior (superior) inputs found in animal experiments [96, 114, 115]. These findings form the basis for successful surgical or catheter ablation of either fast or slow pathway to cure AV nodal reentrant tachycardia [116, 117]. No anatomical abnormalities have been detected in the AV nodal region in patients with proven dual AV nodal pathways [118], but it has been shown that fast and slow pathways are formed by connexin 43-expressing bundles, surrounded by tissue without connexin 43 [119].

There is a long standing debate on the precise location of the reentrant circuit, and on the question whether atrial tissue forms a substantial part of the circuit. Josephson and Miller [120] introduced premature atrial stimuli during the tachycardia prior to the time the atria would have been retrogradely activated by the reentrant wave. Even when perinodal atrial myocardium was depolarized 10–130 ms before the expected arrival of the retrograde wavefront, the tachycardia was not interrupted, nor was its cycle length changed. Mignone and Wallace [108] came to the same conclusion by showing that perinodal atrial tissue could be made refractory by pre-excitation without abolishing ventricular echoes. However, other investigators [121–123] suggested that atrial tissue, including the sinus septum above the ostium of the coronary sinus, is involved in the circuit. The fact that AV nodal reentrant tachycardia can successfully be terminated by catheter ablation of sites far from the compact node was also seen as evidence that atrial tissue is involved in the circuit. However, in isolated, blood-perfused canine hearts, it was demonstrated that the reentrant pathway during ventricular and atrial echo beats was confined to the compact node [124, 125]. Interestingly, in these hearts there was no "jump" in the AV or VA conduction curve during premature stimulation of atria or right bundle branch. It is of course possible that in sustained AV nodal reentrant tachycardia, the circuit is different from that during single echo beats.

4.9   Factors That Cause AV Nodal Delay

There is no single factor responsible for the slowing of the impulse as it traverses the AV nodal area. Various geometrical factors, such as the small size of AV nodal cells, the paucity of intercellular connections, and the complex network of small bundles separated by connective tissue where summation and collision of impulses occur, play a role in addition to the role of the slow calcium inward current, which is the dominant current depolarizing AV nodal cells.

Conduction velocity in a linear cable is proportional to the square root of the fiber diameter. Given a diameter of Purkinje fibers of 50 µm, and of 7 µ for AV nodal cells, the ratio of conduction velocity of both tissues would be 2.7, if fiber diameter would be the only factor. In fact, the ratio is much higher, conduction velocity in the Purkinje system being in the order of meters per second, that in the N zone being less than 5 cm/s.

Several studies have measured space constants in the AV node [126–129]. The reported values are much lower than those for other cardiac tissue, with the lowest value in the N zone in the order of 170 µm. All measurements were made in superfused tissue, where the large volume of extracellular fluid acts as an extracellular shunt resistance. In densely packed tissue, extracellular resistance has a value similar to the intracellular resistance, and the space constant of arterially perfused papillary muscle is 357 µm, as compared to 528 µm in superfused tissue [130]. Thus, in the intact heart, the space constant of the densely packed compact node may be much smaller than that of isolated, superfused tissue. Assuming that the extracellular resistance would be the same as in an arterially perfused papillary muscle, and that intracellular resistance is a higher by a factor ten, conduction velocity in the node would be about three times less than in ventricular tissue, in the order of 20 cm/s, which still is about ten times that of the lowest values found in the N zone.

Summation of impulses, arriving more or less simultaneously over converging pathways, appears to play an important role in AV conduction [96, 131–133]. As already mentioned, AV nodal conduction is much less effective when the site of initial activation is switched from crista terminalis to the interatrial septum [96]. Zipes et al. [133] separated both nodal inputs by making a cut through the roof and floor of the coronary sinus. Premature stimulation of each input separately gave rise to a local response in an n cell, while simultaneous stimulation of both inputs resulted in a fully developed action potential that was propagated to the His bundle.

There is no doubt that the calcium current plays a dominant role in depolarizing nodal cells. However, the question whether central AV nodal cells have no sodium channels at all, or are merely inactivated by the low resting potential, has not been settled.

Recovery from inactivation of the slow calcium current is slow, and may lag behind completion of repolarization [134]. This may be an important factor in causing cycle length-dependent conduction delay. ❷ Figure 4.4 shows selected action potentials from the AV nodal area during application of five successive atrial premature stimuli at progressively shorter coupling intervals. The key feature is that with prolongation of the atrium-His bundle conduction time, the action potential upstroke of cells in the N region separate into two components. The first component coincides with the upstroke of the last activated AN cells, the second component with the upstroke of the earliest activated NH cells. No action potential were recorded with upstrokes occurring in between these two components. The cycle length-dependent conduction delay appears to be caused by a local discontinuity of conduction, rather than by a progressive slowing of continuous propagation. One may also speak of "saltatory" conduction. The explanation given by Billette et al. [135] is that the excitability of the N cells progressively diminished at short cycle lengths, so that at very short cycles the N cells acted as a purely passive barrier between late AN cells and early NH cells, capable only of transmitting electrotonic currents that would slowly bring NH cells to threshold.

4.10   Ventricular Activation

In the mammalian heart, the impulse that has passed through the AV node reaches the ventricular myocardium by way of the specialized conduction system, consisting of the His bundle, the main right and left bundle branches, and the peripheral Purkinje network, which at discrete sites – the Purkinje-ventricular muscle junctions – is in contact with

HANDBOOK OF PHYSIOLOGY ~ THE HEART

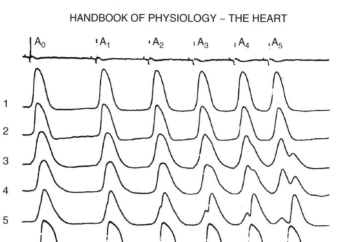

□ Fig. 4.4

Cycle length-dependence of AV nodal conduction. Action potentials show dependency of first and second component of the upstroke of N cells on late AN cells and early NH cells. Signals 1 and 2 were recorded from AN cells, signals 3, 4 and 5 from N cells, and signal 6 from an NH cell. *Inset* shows position of cells. First component is largest in N cells close to AN cells, second component is largest in cells close to NH cells (© Reproduced with permission from Billette et al. [135])

ventricular myocardium. Proximal to the Purkinje-muscle junctions the specialized conduction system has no functional contact with the myocardium because it is isolated from it by a thin collagenous sheet [136]. Conduction velocity in the bundle branches is high, in the order of 2 m/s [4].

It is often assumed that the main left bundle in its course below the membranous part of the interventricular septum splits into two divisions: the anterior and posterior fascicles. As shown in ❷ Fig. 4.5, in a number of hearts there is a more or less separate middle fascicle occupying the left midseptal area [137]. This was already described by Tawara in 1906 [85]. In isolated, Langendorff-perfused human hearts, three distinct areas of initial myocardial activation have been found that correspond to the transition of these three fascicles into the peripheral Purkinje network (6, see ❷ Fig. 4.6).

Because of the many connections between the main branches of the left sided conduction system, only extensive lesions result in complete block in the left bundle branch system. In clinical electrocardiography, a distinction is made between incomplete bundle branch block, anterior and posterior fascicular block, and complete bundle branch block [138].

After activation of the subendocardial myocardium by the specialized conduction system, at anterior, midseptal and posterior sites on the septum, excitation of the left ventricular wall in the human and canine heart occurs by myocardial conduction in an endocardial to epicardial direction with a more or less concentric arrangement of the isochrones [63, 139]. Epicardial breakthrough in the human left ventricle occurs almost simultaneously in anterior and posterior paraseptal areas located halfway between apex and base, after about 30 ms following onset of ventricular activation.

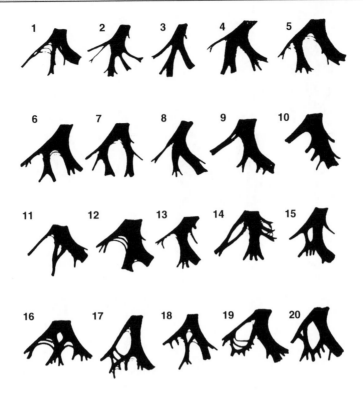

🔲 Fig. 4.5
Division of the left bundle branch. An illustration of the variation of the structure of the divisions of the left bundle in 20 different human hearts (© Reproduced with permission from Demoulin and Kulbertus [137])

The septum is largely activated in a left-to-right direction, although a small part of this structure is activated in the opposite direction by a wavefront originating in the lower right septal surface. The basal portions of the septum, particularly the posterior parts, are devoid of Purkinje fibers and are the last to be depolarized.

The papillary muscles are activated via false tendons, consisting mainly of Purkinje fibers, that run through the ventricular cavity from the septal surface to the apex of the anterior and posterior papillary muscles. From there, activation proceeds over the sheet of Purkinje fibers to excite the muscles via the Purkinje-muscle junctions (see later) at their base, nearly synchronously with the onset of depolarization of the initially activated left septal areas.

The myocardium of the left ventricular wall consists of discrete muscle layers that follow a curving radial path from the subendocardium to the subepicardium [140]. To which extent the laminar organization of the ventricular wall affects propagation is unclear. Intramural recordings, utilizing needles with multiple electrodes at 1 mm distance have not revealed discontinuities in the spread of excitation from endocardium to epicardium [63]. On a microscopic scale, one might suppose that the pathway of activation is convoluted, if the muscle layers are electrically insulated and make contact only via direct muscle branches. It is possible that the structural anisotropy may lead to irregular pattern of activation when coupling between muscle layers becomes impaired, but direct evidence for this is lacking.

The right bundle branch in its course over the right endocardial surface of the septum ends at the base of the anterior papillary muscle, where it gives off branches to the lower right anterior surface of the septum, to the free right ventricular wall at the pretrabecular area, and to the subendocardial Purkinje network of the right ventricular free wall [140, 141]. Initial right ventricular activation occurs near the base of the papillary muscle and the overlying free wall (see ❷ Fig. 4.6). From there, activation proceeds in a right-to-left direction in the septum, and tangentially towards the epicardium of the right ventricular free wall. Right ventricular epicardial breakthrough occurs about 25 ms after onset of left septal activation. The last parts of the right ventricle to be activated are the outer layers of the outflow tract and the crista supraventricularis.

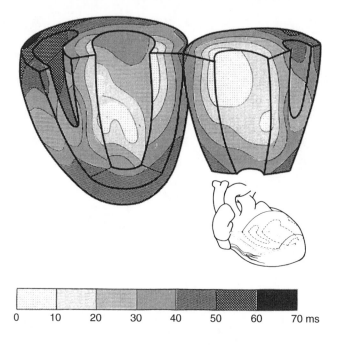

0   10   20   30   40   50   60   70 ms

◨ Fig. 4.6

Activation sequence of ventricular myocardium in an isolated, Langendorff-perfused normal human heart, as determined from intramural electrodes. The ventricles are shown opened, according to the *inset* in the *lower right*. Note initial activation at three sites of the inside of the left ventricle and terminal activation in the right ventricular conus. Activation of the interventricular septum begins at the left endocardial surface and meets between 30 and 40 ms with an excitation front that has started at 20–25 ms in the right ventricle. Activation times are in milliseconds after the onset of left ventricular activation (© Reproduced with permission from Durrer et al. [63])

4.11   The Purkinje-Muscle Junction

The junctions between the terminal Purkinje fiber and ventricular muscle are electrophysiologically defined as sites where unipolar electrograms show a completely negative muscle deflection that is preceded by 2–5 ms by a Purkinje spike [142]. At non junctional sites where both Purkinje and muscle deflections are found, the muscle deflection is characterized by initial positivity ("R wave"). Unidirectional block has been shown to occur at Purkinje-muscle junctions, where conduction is maintained in a muscle-Purkinje direction but fails in the opposite direction [143, 144]. Mendez et al. proposed the "funnel" hypothesis in which "the narrow portion would correspond to a terminal Purkinje fiber whose conical part would be composed of a progressively increasing number of interconnected muscle fibers" [144]. In this view, the Purkinje network is seen as a branching cable, and at the Purkinje-muscle junction the "terminal" Purkinje fiber has to provide excitatory current to a three-dimensional mass of ventricular muscle. Joyner and co-workers suggested that the Purkinje network is better represented by a two-dimensional sheet that is coupled at discrete sites to the deeper muscle mass [142, 145, 146]. If coupling resistance at these sites is too low, the load that the large muscle mass imposes on the Purkinje network would prevent activation of the Purkinje sheet. If coupling resistance is too high, the Purkinje network could not deliver sufficient excitatory current to activate the muscle layers. A certain resistive barrier between the two tissues allows rapid propagation of the Purkinje layer over the endocardial surface to synchronize ventricular activation, facilitates ventricular activation, and maintains a longer action potential duration in the Purkinje layer as compared to ventricular muscle [145, 147]. Microelectrode recordings by Alanis and co-workers suggested that the delay between the Purkinje fiber and ventricular muscle was not due to slow conduction but to a "stop of the impulse in this region" [148]. Action potentials from junctional sites can be typical for Purkinje cells or ventricular muscle cells, or they can show upstrokes with multiple components. These latter action potentials were thought to arise from "transitional

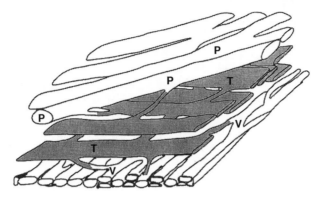

◻ Fig. 4.7

Schematic representation of the structure of a rabbit Purkinje-muscle junction. *P* Purkinje fibers, *T* transitional cells, *V* ventricular muscle (© Reproduced with permission from Tranum Jensen et al. [149])

cells" [148–150]. They show a slow foot and a dissociation of the upstroke into two or more components. This feature is consistent with the view that conduction at the junction is discontinuous and is compatible with the existence of one or several resistive barriers between Purkinje and muscle. Transitional cells in the rabbit heart are thin, broad, band-like cells (30–35 μm by 3–5 μm) arranged in one or two sheets in the subendocardium between Purkinje and muscle. Transitional cells are coupled via short, thin strands to both Purkinje and muscle fibers. Distances between Purkinje-transitional cell coupling sites and transitional cell-ventricular muscle coupling sites varied between 100 and 1,000 μm. This arrangement is schematically depicted in ❷ Fig. 4.7 [149]. In this structure there are two high resistance barriers: the thin connections between Purkinje fibers and transitional cells and those between the sheet of transitional cells and ventricular muscle. In the pig, another type of Purkinje-muscle junction was frequently observed, but only rarely in the rabbit. Here, a short linear segment of small transitional cells connected large-diameter Purkinje cells to ventricular muscle. This arrangement would be compatible with the "funnel" hypothesis.

4.12   The M Cell

Besides the cells of the specialized conduction system there appear to be other specialized cells in the ventricle. There is one report on the existence of a bundle of slowly conducting cells on the left septal surface of the normal human heart [151]. This report awaits confirmation by other studies, and the functional significance is unclear.

Another specialized cell is the midmural M cell [152–155]. Its most conspicuous feature is that its action potential duration is significantly longer than that of epicardial or endocardial cells, especially at (very) long cycle lengths. In addition, their maximal upstroke velocity is considerably greater than that of epicardial and endocardial cells. The slowly activating component of the delayed rectifier, IKs, is smaller in M cells than in epicardial and endocardial cells, and this may account for the longer action potential duration of M cells [156]. Most attention has been given to the role of M cells in ventricular repolarization, but the latter feature suggests that M cells may conduct the impulse faster than other ventricular myocardial cells. As already mentioned, on a macroscopic scale (i.e., electrodes 1 mm apart) no discontinuities in propagation from endocardium to epicardium have been found [63].

The existence of M cells in isolated cells and isolated in vitro preparations is well documented, although they could not be found in myocytes form the pig heart [157]. However, their role in the intact heart is uncertain. Electrotonic interaction between cells with intrinsically different action potential durations will shorten the long action potentials and prolong the short ones. As summarized by Tan and Joyner "the isolated rabbit ventricular cell is extremely sensitive to even a very small electrical load, with shortening of the action potential by 50% with electrical coupling to a model cell (of similar input resistance and capacitance to the ventricular cell) as high as 1,000 MΩ, even though the action potential amplitude and current threshold are very insensitive to the electrical load" [158]. In a review by Anyukhovsky et al. [159], literature data are summarized in their Fig. 4.9. The difference between longest and shortest action potential, or Activation-Recovery-Interval, are in the order of 20 ms for intact hearts, 40 ms for ventricular wedge preparations, 80 ms for thick myocardial slices, 120 ms for thin slices, and 90 ms for isolated cells. Most studies in intact hearts have failed to provide evidence for a midmyocardial layer with longer repolarization times. This was the case for studies in which refractory periods were measured at various depths in the left ventricular wall [160–164], and for studies in which Activation-Recovery-Intervals or repolarization times were measured at intramural sites in intact canine or human hearts [159, 165–168]. It therefore appears that in the intact heart, M cells have no functional significance.

References

1. Janse, M.J. and M.J. Davies, Generation and conduction of the heart beat and their disturbances, in *Diseases of the Heart*, 2nd ed., D.G. Julian, A.J. Camm, K.M. Fox, R.J.C. Hall, and P.A. Poole-Wilson, Editors. London, WB Saunders Company Ltd, 1996, pp. 88–114.

2. Kucera, J.P., A.G. Kléber, and S. Rohr, Slow conduction in cardiac tissue: II. Effects of branching tissue geometry. *Circ. Res.*, 1998;**83**: 795–805.

3. Shaw, R.M. and Y. Rudy, Ionic mechanisms of propagation in cardiac tissue. Roles of sodium and L-type calcium currents during reduced excitability and decreased gap junction coupling. *Circ. Res.*, 1997;**81**: 727–741.

4. Kléber, A.G., M.J. Janse, and V.G. Fast, Normal and abnormal conduction in the heart, in *Handbook of Physiology, section 2 The Cardiovascular System. Volume 1: The Heart*. New York, Oxford University Press, 2001, pp. 455–530.

5. Keith, A. and M. Flack, The form and nature of the muscular connections between the primary divisions of the vertebrate heart. *J. Anat. Physiol.*, 1907;**41**: 172–189.

6. Tranum-Jensen, J., The fine structure of the sinus node: a survey, in *The Sinus Node*, F.I.M. Bonke, Editor. The Hague, Nijhoff, 1978, pp. 149–165.

7. Opthof, T., The mammalian sinoatrial node. *Cardiovasc. Drugs Ther.*, 1988;**1**: 573–597.

8. Masson-Pévet, M., W.K. Bleeker, A.J.C. Mackaay, L.N. Bouman, and J.M. Houtkooper, Sinus node and atrial cells from the rabbit heart: a quantitative electron microscopic description after electrophysiological localization. *J. Mol. Cell. Cardiol.*, 1979;**11**: 555–568.

9. Bleeker, W.K., A.J.C. Mackaay, M. Masson-Pévet, L.N. Bouman, and A.E. Becker, Functional and morphological organization of the rabbit sinus node. *Circ. Res.*, 1980;**46**: 11–22.

10. Oosthoek, P.W., S. Viragh, A.E.M. Mayen, M.J.A. van Kempen, W.H. Lamers, and A.F.M. Moorman, Immunohistochemical delineation of the conduction system: I. The sinoatrial node. *Circ. Res.*, 1993;**73**: 473–481.

11. Verheijck, E.E., A. Wessels, A.C.G. van Ginneken, J. Bourier, M.W.M. Markman, J.L.M. Vermeulen, J.M.T. de Bakker, W.H. Lamers, T. Opthof, and L.N. Bouman, Distribution of atrial and nodal cells within the rabbit sinoatrial node. Models of sinoatrial transition. *Circulation*, 1998;**97**: 1623–1631.

12. Opthof, T., B. de Jonge, H.J. Jongsma, and L.N. Bouman, Functional morphology of the mammalian sinuatrial node. *Eur. Heart J.*, 1987;**8**: 1249–1259.

13. James, T.N., The sinus node. *Am. J. Cardiol.*, 1977;**40**: 965–986.

14. Opthof, T., B. de Jonge, A.J. Mackaay, W.K. Bleeker, M. Masson-Pévet, H.J. Jongsma, and L.N. Bouman, Functional and morphological organization of the guinea-pig sinoatrial node compared with the rabbit sinoatrial node. *J. Mol. Cell. Cardiol.*, 1985;**17**: 549–564.

15. Opthof, T., B. de Jonge, M. Masson-Pévet, H.J. Jongsma, and L.N. Bouman, Functional and morphological organization of the cat sinoatrial node. *J. Mol. Cell. Cardiol.*, 1986;**18**: 1015–1031.

16. Opthof, T., B. de Jonge, H.J. Jongsma, and L.N. Bouman, Functional morphology of the pig sinoatrial node. *J. Mol. Cell. Cardiol.*, 1987;**19**: 1221–1236.

17. Davies, M.J., Pathology of atrial arrhythmias, in *The Conduction System of the Heart*, M.J. Davies, R.H. Anderson, and A.E. Becker, Editors. London: Butterworths, 1983, pp. 203–215.

18. Alings, A.M.W., The aging sino-atrial node, Ph.D. thesis. University of Amsterdam, 1993.

19. Shiraishi, I., T. Takamatsu, T. Minamikawa, Z. Onouchi, and S. Fujita, Quantitative histological analysis of the human sinoatrial node during growth and aging. *Circulation*, 1992;**85**: 2176–2183.

20. Wybauw, R., Sur le point d'origine de la systole cardiaque dans l'oreillette droite. *Arch. Int. Physiol.*, 1910;**10**: 78–89.

21. Lewis, T., B.S. Oppenheimer, and A. Oppenheimer, The site of origin of the mammalian heart beat: the pacemaker in the dog heart. *Heart*, 1910;**2**: 147–169.

22. Trautwein, W. and K. Zink, Über Membran- und Aktionspotentiale einzelner Muskulfasern des Kalt-und Warmblüterherzens. *Pflug. Arch.*, 1952;**256**: 68–84.

23. West, T.C., Ultramicroelectrode recording from the cardiac pacemakers. *J. Pharmacol. Exp. Ther.*, 1955;**115**: 282–290.

24. Yanagihara, D. and H. Irisawa, Inward current activated during hyperpolarization in the rabbit sinoatrial node. *Pflüg. Arch.*, 1980;**385**: 11–19.

25. DiFrancesco, D. and C. Ojeda, Properties of the current if in the sino-atrial node of the rabbit compared with those of the current iK, in Purkinje fibers. *J. Physiol. (London)*, 1980;**308**: 353–367.

26. Reuter, H., Ion channels in cardiac cell membranes. *Annu. Rev. Physiol.*, 1984;**46**: 473–484.

27. DiFrancesco, D., A. Ferroni, M. Mazzanti, and C. Tromba, Properties of the hyperpolarizing-activated current (if) in cells isolated from the rabbit sino-atrial node. *J. Physiol. (London)*, 1986;**377**: 61–88.

28. Irisawa, H., H.F. Brown, and W. Giles, Cardiac pacemaking in the sinoatrial node. *Physiol. Rev.*, 1993;**73**: 197–227.

29. Trautwein, W. and K. Uchizono, Electrophysiologic study of the pacemaker in the sino-atrial node of the rabbit heart. *Z. Zell-forsch.*, 1963;**61**: 96–109.

30. Janse, M.J., J. Tranum-Jensen, A.G. Kléber, and F.J.L. van Capelle, Techniques and problems in correlating cellular electrophysiology and morphology in cardiac nodal tissue, in *The Sinus Node*, F.I.M. Bonke, Editor. The Hague: Nijhoff, 1978, pp. 183–194.

31. Sano, T. and S. Yamagishi, Spread of excitation from the sinus node. *Circ. Res.*, 1965;**16**: 423–431.

32. Steinbeck, G., M.A. Allessie, F.I.M. Bonke, and W.E.J.P. Lammers, The response of the sinus node to premature stimulation of the atrium studied with microelectrodes in isolated preparations of the rabbit heart, in *The Sinus Node*, F.I.M. Bonke, Editor. The Hague: Nijhoff, 1978, pp. 245–257.

33. Bouman, L.N., A.J.C. Mackaay, W.K. Bleeker, and A.E. Becker, Pacemaker shifts in the sinus node. Effects of vagal stimulation, temperature, and reduction of extracellular calcium, in *The Sinus Node*, F.I.M. Bonke, Editor. The Hague: Nijhoff, 1978, pp. 245–257.

34. Bouman, L.N. and H.J. Jongsma, Structure and function of the SA node: a review. *Eur. Heart J.*, 1986;**7**: 94–104.

35. de Haan, R.L., Discussion on models of entrainment of cardiac cells, in *Cardiac Rate and Rhythm*, L.N. Boumans and H.J. Jongsma, Editors. The Hague: Nijhoff, 1982, pp. 359–361.

36. Rook, M.B., B. de Jonge, and H.J. Jongsma, Gap junction formation and functional interaction between neonatal rat cardiocytes in culture. *J. Membr. Biol.*, 1990;**118**: 179–192.

37. Trabka, J.E., W. Coombs, M. Lemanski, M. Delmar, and J. Jalife, Immunohistochemical localization of gap junctional channels in adult mammalian sinus nodal cells- immunolocalization and electrophysiology. *J. Cardiovasc. Electrophysiol.*, 1994;**5**: 125–137.

38. Kodama, I. and M.R. Boyett, Regional differences in the electrical activity of the rabbit sinus node. *Pflug. Arch.*, 1985;**404**: 214–226.

39. Kirchhof, C.J., F.I.M. Bonke, M.A. Allessie, and W.E.J.P. Lammers, The influence of the atrial myocardium on impulse formation in the rabbit sinus node. *Pflug. Arch.*, 1987;**410**: 198–203.

40. Joyner, R.W. and F.J.L. van Capelle, Propagation through electrically coupled cells. How a small SA node drives a large atrium. *Biophys. J.*, 1986;**50**: 1157–1164.

41. Opthof, T., W.K. Bleeker, M. Masson-Pévet, H.J. Jongsma, and L.N. Bouman, Little-excitable transitional cells in the rabbit sinoatrial node: a statistical, morphological and electrophysiological study. *Experientia*, 1983;**39**: 1099–1101.

42. Meek, W.J. and J.A.E. Eyster, Experiments on the origin and propagation of the impulse in the heart. IV. The effect of vagal stimulation and cooling on the location of the pacemaker within the sino-atrial node. *Am. J. Physiol.*, 1914;**34**: 368–383.

43. Bouman, L.N., E.D. Gerlings, P.A. Biersteker, and F.I.M. Bonke, Pacemaker shift in the sino-atrial node during vagal stimulation. *Pflug. Arch.*, 1968;**302**: 255–267.

44. Mackaay, A.J.C., T. Opthof, W.K. Bleeker, H.J. Jongsma, and L.N. Bouman, Interaction of adrenaline and acetylcholine on sinus node function, in *Cardiac Rate and Rhythm*, L.N. Bouman and H.J. Jongsma, Editors. The Hague: Nijhoff, 1982, pp. 507–523.

45. Hariman, R.J., B.F. Hoffman, and R.E. Naylor, Electrical activity from the sinus node region in conscious dogs. *Circ. Res.*, 1980;**47**: 775–791.

46. Hariman, R.J., E. Krongrad, R.A. Boxer, F.O. Bowman, J.R. Malm, and B.F. Hoffman, Methods for recording electrograms from the sino-atrial node during cardiac surgery in man. *Circulation*, 1980;**61**: 1024–1029.

47. Boineau, J.P., R.B. Schuessler, C.R. Mooney, A.C. Wylds, C.B. Miller, R.D. Hudson, J.M. Borremans, and C.W. Brockus, Multicentric origin of the atrial depolarization wave: the pacemaker complex. Relation to dynamics of atrial conduction, P-wave changes and heart rate control. *Circulation*, 1978;**58**: 1036–1048.

48. Boineau, J.P., C.B. Miller, R.B. Schuessler, W.R. Roeske, L.J. Autry, A.C. Wylds, and D.A. Hill, Activation sequence and potential distribution maps demonstrating multicentric atrial impulse origin in dogs. *Circ. Res.*, 1984;**54**: 332–347.

49. Schuessler, R.B., J.P. Boineau, and B.I. Bromberg, Origin of the sinus impulse. *J. Cardiovasc. Electrophysiol.*, 1996;**7**: 263–274.

50. Cosio, F., A. Martín-Peňato, A. Pastor, A. Nuňez, M.A. Montero, C.P. Cantale, and S. Schames, Atrial activation mapping in sinus rhythm in the clinical electrophysiology laboratory: observations during Bachmann's bundle block. *J. Cardiovasc. Electrophysiol.*, 2004;**15**: 524–531.

51. Hoffman, B.F. and P.F. Cranefield, *Electrophysiology of the Heart*. New York: McGraw-Hill, 1960.

52. Rozanski, G.J. and S.L. Lipsius, Electrophysiology of functional subsidiary pacemakers in the canine right atrium. *Am. J. Physiol.*, 1985;**249**: H594–H601.

53. Kokobun, S., N. Nishimura, A. Noma, and H. Irisawa, The spontaneous action potential of rabbit atrioventricular node. *Jpn. J. Physiol.*, 1980;**30**: 529–539.

54. Vassalle, M., Electrogenic suppression of automaticity in sheep and dog Purkinje fibers. *Circ. Res.*, 1970;**27**: 361–377.

55. Glitsch, H.G., Electrophysiology of the sodium-potassium-ATPase in cardiac cells. *Physiol. Rev.*, 2001;**81**: 1791–1826.

56. Lewis, T., *Lectures on the Heart*. New York, Shaw and sons, 1915.

57. Tranum-Jensen, J., The fine structure of the atrial and atrioventricular (AV) junctional specialized tissues of the rabbit heart, in *The Conduction System of the Heart*, H.J.J. Wellens, K.I. Lie, and M.J. Janse, Editors. Leiden: Stenfert-Kroese, 1976, pp. 55–99.

58. Janse, M.J. and R.H. Anderson, Specialized internodal pathways: fact or fiction? *Eur. J. Cardiol.*, 1974;**2**: 117–136.

59. Puech, P., M. Esclavissat, D. Sodi-Pallares, and F. Cineros, Normal auricular activation in the dog's heart. *Am. Heart J.*, 1954;**47**: 174–191.

60. Yamada, K., M. Horiba, Y. Sakaida, M. Okajima, H. Horibe, H. Muraki, T. Kobayashi, A. Miyauchi, A. Oishi, A. Nonogawa, K. Ishikawa, and J. Toyama, Origination and transmission of impulse in right atrium. *Jpn. Heart J.*, 1965;**6**: 71–97.

61. Spach, M.S., T.D. King, R.C. Barr, D.E. Boaz, M.N. Morrow, and S. Herman-Giddens, Electrical potential distribution surrounding the atria during depolarization and repolarization in the dog. *Circ. Res.*, 1969;**24**: 857–873.

62. Hamlin, R.L., D.L. Smetzer, T. Senta, and C.R. Smith, Atrial activation paths and P waves in horses. *Am. J. Physiol.*, 1970;**219**: 306–313.

63. Durrer, D., R.Th. van Dam, G.E. Freud, M.J. Janse, F.L. Meijler, and R.C. Arzbaecher, Total excitation of the isolated human heart. *Circulation*, 1970;**41**: 895–912.

64. Goodman, D., A.B.M. van der Steen, and R.T.H. van Dam, Endocardial and epicardial activation pathways of the canine right atrium. *Am. J. Physiol.*, 1971;**220**: 1–11.

65. Spach, M.S., M. Lieberman, J.G. Scott, R.C. Barr, E.A. Johnson, and J.M. Kootsey, Excitation sequences of the atrial septum and the AV node in isolated hearts of dog and rabbit. *Circ. Res.*, 1971;**29**: 156–172.

66. Wittig, J.H., M.R. de Leval, and G. Stark, Intraoperative mapping of atrial activation before, during and after the mustard operation. *J. Thorac. Cardiovasc. Surg.*, 1977;**73**: 1–13.

67. De Ponti, R., S.Y. Ho, J.A. Salerno-Uriarte, M. Tritto, and G. Spadacini, Electroanatomic analysis of sinus impulse propagation in normal human atria. *J. Cardiovasc. Electrophysiol.*, 2002;**13**: 1–10.

68. Markides, V., R.J. Schilling, S.Y. Ho, A.W.C. Chow, D.W. Davies, and N.S. Peters, Characterization of left atrial activation in the intact human heart. *Circulation*, 2003;**107**: 733–739.

69. Betts, T.R., P.R. Roberts, and J.M. Morgan, High-density mapping of left atrial endocardial activation during sinus rhythm and coronary sinus pacing in patients with paroxysmal atrial fibrillation. *J. Cardiovasc. Electrophysiol.*, 2004;**15**: 1111–1117.

70. James, T.N., The connecting pathways between the sinus node and the A–V node and between the right and left atrium of the human heart. *Am. Heart J.*, 1963;**66**: 498–508.

71. Rossi, L., Interatrial, internodal, and dual reentrant atrioventricular nodal pathways: an anatomical update of arrhythmogenic substrates. *Cardiologia*, 1996;**41**: 129–134.

72. Sanchez-Quintana, D., D.W. Davies, S. Yen Ho, P. Oslizlok, and R.H. Anderson , Architecture of the atrial musculature in and around the triangle of Koch: its potential relevance to atrioventricular nodal reentry. *J. Cardiovasc. Electrophysiol.*, 1997;**8**: 1396–1407.

73. Inoue, S. and A.E. Becker, Posterior extensions of the human compact atrioventricular node: a neglected anatomical feature of potential clinical significance. *Circulation*, 1998;**97**: 188–193.

74. Chauvin, M., D.C. Shah, M. Haïssaguerre, L. Marcellin, and C. Brechenmacher, The anatomic basis of connections between the coronary sinus musculature and the left atrium in humans. *Circulation*, 2001;**101**: 647–652.

75. Moore, E.N., S.L. Jomain, J.H. Stuckey, J.W. Buchanan, and B.F. Hoffman, Studies on ectopic atrial rhythms in dogs. *Am. J. Cardiol.*, 1967;**19**: 676–685.

76. Moore, E.N., J. Melbin, J.F. Spear, and J.D. Hill, Sequence of atrial excitation in the dog during antegrade and retrograde activation. *J. Electrocardiol.*, 1971;**4**: 283–290.

77. Waldo, A.L., K.J. Vittikainen, and B.F. Hoffman, The sequence of retrograde atrial activation in the canine heart: correlation with positive and negative retrograde P waves. *Circ. Res.*, 1975;**37**: 156–163.

78. Thorel, C., Vorläufige Mitteilung über eine besondere Muskelverbindung zwischen dem Cava superior und die Hissischen Bundel. *Münch med Wschr* 1908;**56**: 2159–2164.

79. Bericht über die Verhandlungen der XIV Tagung der Deutschen pathologischen Gesellschaft in Erlangen vom 4-6 April 1910. *Z allg Path path Anat* 1910;**21**: 433–496.

80. Netter, F.H., *The Heart. The Ciba Collection of Medical Illustrations*, vol. 5, 1969, p. 13.

81. Pastelin, G., R. Mendez, and G.K. Moe, Participation of atrial specialized conduction pathways in atrial flutter. *Circ. Res.*, 1978;**42**: 386–393.

82. Janse, M.J. and R.H. Anderson, Specialized internodal atrial pathways. Fact or fiction? *Eur. J. Cardiol.*, 1974;**2**: 117–136.

83. Spach, M.S., W.T. Miller, R.C. Barr, and D.B. Geselowitz, Electrophysiology of the internodal pathways: determining the difference between anisotropic cardiac muscle and a specialized tract system, in *Physiology of Atrial Pacemakers and Conductive Tissues*, R.C. Little, Editor. Mount Kisco, New York: Futura Publishing Company, 1980, pp. 367–380.

84. Janse, M.J., R.H. Anderson, M.A. McGuire, and S.Y. Ho, "AV nodal" reentry: Part I: "AV nodal" reentry revisited. *J. Cardiovasc. Electrophysiol.*, 1993;**4**: 561–572.

85. Tawara, S., *Das Reizleitungssystem des Säugetierherzens. Eine anatomisch-histologische Studie über das Atrioventrikularbündel und die Purkinjeschen Fäden.* Jena: Fischer, 1906.

86. Anderson, R.H., Histologic and histochemical evidence concerning the presence of morphologically distinct cellular zones within the rabbit atrioventricular node. *Anat. Rec.*, 1972;**173**: 7–23.

87. Paes de Carvalho, A. and D.F. de Almeida, Spread of activity through the atrioventricular node. *Circ. Res.*, 1960;**8**: 801–809.

88. Becker, A.E. and R.H. Anderson, Morphology of the human atrioventricular junctional area, in *The Conduction System of the Heart: Structure, Function and Clinical Implication*, H.J.J. Wellens, K.I. Lie, and M.J. Janse, Editors. Philadelphia, PA: Lea and Febiger, 1976, pp. 263–286.

89. Anderson, R.H., M.J. Janse, F.J.L. van Capelle, J. Billete, A.E. Becker, and D. Durrer, A combined morphological and electrophysiological study of the atrioventricular node of the rabbit heart. *Circ. Res.*, 1974;**35**: 909–922.

90. McGuire, M.A., J.M.T. de Bakker, J.T. Vermeulen, A.F. Moorman, P. Loh, B. Thibault, J.L.M. Vermeulen, A.E. Becker, and M.J. Janse, Atrioventricular junctional tissue. Discrepancy between histological and electrophysiological characteristics. *Circulation*, 1996;**94**: 571–577.

91. Petrecca, K., F. Amellal, D.W. Laird, S.A. Cohen, and A. Shrier, Sodium channel distribution within the rabbit atrioventricular node and surrounding myocardium as analyzed with confocal microscopy. *J. Physiol.*, 1997;**501**: 263–274.

92. Spach, M.S., M. Lieberman, J.G. Scott, R.C. Barr, E.A. Johnson, and J.M. Kootsey, Excitation sequences of the atrial septum and the AV node in isolated hearts of the dog and rabbit. *Circ. Res.*, 1971;**29**: 156–172.

93. McGuire, M.A., J.M.T. de Bakker, J.T. Vermeulen, T. Opthof, A.E. Becker, and M.J. Janse, Origin and significance of double potentials near the atrioventricular node. Correlation of extracellular potentials, intracellular potentials, and histology. *Circulation*, 1994;**89**: 2351–2360.

94. Janse, M.J., F.J.L. van Capelle, R.H. Anderson, P. Touboul, and J. Billette, Electrophysiology and structure of the atrioventricular node of the rabbit heart, in *The Conduction System of the Heart*, H.J.J. Wellens, K.I. Lie, and M.J. Janse, Editors. Leiden: Stenfert Kroese, 1976, pp. 296–315.

95. Van Capelle, F.J.L., M.J. Janse, P.J. Varghese, G.E. Freud, C. Mater, and D. Durrer, Spread of excitation in the atrioventricular node of isolated rabbit hearts studied by multiple microelectrode recording. *Circ. Res.*, 1972;**31**: 602–616.

96. Janse, M.J., Influence of the direction of the atrial wave front on A–V nodal transmission in isolated hearts of rabbits. *Circ. Res.*, 1969;**25**: 439–449.

97. Mines, G.R., On dynamic equilibrium in the heart. *J. Physiol.*, 1913;**46**: 349–382.

98. White, P.D., A study of atrioventricular rhythm following auricular flutter. *Arch. Intern. Med.*, 1915;**16**: 517–535.

99. Scherf, D. and C. Shookhoff, Experimentelle Untersuchungen über die "Umkehr-Extrasystole" (reciprocating beats). *Wien Arch Inn Med* 1926;**12**: 501–529.

100. Moe, G.K., J.B. Preston, and H.J. Burlington, Physiologic evidence for a dual A–V transmission system. *Circ. Res.*, 1956;**4**: 357–375.

101. Rosenblueth, A., Ventricular "echoes." *Am. J. Physiol.*, 1958; **195**: 53–60.

102. Kistin, A.D., Atrial reciprocating rhythm. *Circulation*, 1965;**32**: 697–707.

103. Puech, P., La conduction réciproque par le noeud de Tawara. Bases expérimentales et aspects cliniques. *Ann. Cardiol. Angeiol.*, 1970;**19**: 21–40.

104. Schuilenburg, R.M. and D. Durrer, Atrial echo beats in the human heart elicited by induced atrial premature beats. *Circulation*, 1968;**37**: 680–693.

105. Schuilenburg, R.M. and D. Durrer, Ventricular echo beats in the human heart elicited by induced ventricular premature beats. *Circulation*, 1968;**40**: 337–347.

106. Bigger, J.T., Jr. and B.N. Goldreyer, The mechanism of supraventricular tachycardia. *Circulation*, 1970;**42**: 673–688.

107. Mendez, C., J. Han, P.D. Garcia de Jalon, and G.K. Moe, Demonstration of a dual AV conduction system in the isolated rabbit heart. *Circ. Res.*, 1965;**19**: 562–581.

108. Mignone, R.J. and A.G. Wallace, Ventricular echoes. Evidence for dissociation and reentry within the A–V node. *Circ. Res.*, 1966;**19**: 638–649.

109. Mendez, C. and G.K. Moe, Demonstration of a dual AV nodal conduction system in the isolated rabbit heart. *Circ. Res.*, 1966;**19**: 378–393.

110. Moe, G.K., W. Cohen, and R.L. Vick, Experimentally induced paroxysmal A–V nodal tachycardia in the dog. *Am. Heart J.*, 1963;**65**: 87–92.

111. Janse, M.J., F.J.L. van Capelle, G.E. Freud, and D. Durrer, Circus movement within the AV node as a basis for supraventricular tachycardia as shown by multiple microelectrode recordings in the isolated rabbit heart. *Circ. Res.*, 1971;**28**: 403–414.

112. Wit, A.L., B.N. Goldreyer, and A.N. Damato, An in vitro model of paroxysmal supraventricular tachycardia. *Circulation*, 1971;**43**: 862–875.

113. Coumel, P., C. Cabrol, A. Fabiato, R. Gourgon, and R. Slama, Tachycardie permanente par rythme réciproque. *Arch. Mal. Coeur Vaiss.*, 1967;**60**: 1830–1864.

114. McGuire, M.A., J.P. Bourke, M.C. Robotin, I.C. Johnson, W. Meldrum-Hanna, G.R. Nunn, J.B. Uther, and D.L. Ross, High resolution mapping in Koch's triangle using sixty electrodes in humans with atrioventricular nodal (AV nodal) reentrant tachycardia. *Circulation*, 1993;**88**: 2315–2328.

115. Sung, R.J., H.L. Waxman, S. Saksena, and Z. Juma, Sequence of retrograde atrial activation in patients with dual atrioventricular nodal pathways. *Circulation*, 1981;**64**: 1059–1067.

116. Ross, D.L., D.C. Johnson, A.R. Denniss, M.J. Cooper, D.A. Richards, and J.B. Uther, Curative surgery for atrioventricular junctional ("AV nodal") reentrant tachycardia. *J. Am. Coll. Cardiol.*, 1985;**6**: 1383–1392.

117. Haissaguerre, M., F. Gaita, B. Fischer, D. Commenges, P. Montserrat, P. d'Ivernois, P. Lemetayer, and J. Warin, Elimination of atrioventricular nodal reentrant tachycardia using discrete slow potentials to guide application of radiofrequency energy. *Circulation*, 1992;**85**: 2162–2175.

118. Ho, S.Y., J.M. McComb, C.D. Scott, and R.H. Anderson, Morphology of the cardiac conduction system in patients with electrophysiologically proven dual atrioventricular pathways. *J. Cardiovasc. Electrophysiol.*, 1993;**4**: 504–512.

119. Nikolski, V.P., S.A. Jones, M.K. Lancaster, M.R. Boyett, and I.R. Efimov, Cx43 and dual-pathway electrophysiology of the atrioventricular node and atrioventricular nodal reentry. *Circ. Res.*, 2003;**92**: 469–475.

120. Josephson, M.E. and J.M. Miller, Atrioventricular nodal reentry: evidence supporting an intranodal location. *Pacing Clin. Electrophysiol.*, 1993;**16**: 599–614.

121. Mendez, C., J. Han, P.D. Garcia de Jalon, and G.K. Moe, Some characteristics of ventricular echoes. *Circ. Res.*, 1965;**16**: 562–581.

122. Iinuma, H., L.S. Dreifus, T. Mazgalev, R. Price, and E.L. Michelson, Role of the perinodal region in atrioventricular nodal reentry: evidence in an isolated rabbit heart preparation. *J. Am. Coll. Cardiol.*, 1983;**2**: 465–473.

123. Mazgalev, T., L.S. Dreifus, J. Bianchi, and E.L. Michelson, The mechanism of AV junctional reentry: role of the atrionodal junction. *Anat. Rec.*, 1981;**202**: 179–188.

124. Loh, P., J.M.T. de Bakker, M. Hocini, B. Thibault, R.N.W. Hauer, and M.J. Janse, Reentrant pathway during ventricular echoes is confined to the atrioventricular node. *Circulation*, 1999;**100**: 1346–1353.

125. Loh, P., S.Y. Ho, T. Kawara, R.N.W. Hauer, M.J. Janse, G. Breithardt, and J.M.T. de Bakker, Reentrant circuits in the canine AV node during atrial and ventricular echoes: electrophysiologic and histologic correlation. *Circulation*, 2003;**108**: 231–238.

126. Bukauskas, F.F. and R.P. Veteikis, Passive electrical properties of the atrioventricular region of the rabbit heart. *Biofizika*, 1977;**22**: 499–504.

127. De Mello, W.C., Passive electrical properties of the atrioventricular node. *Pflug. Arch.*, 1977;**371**: 135–139.

128. Ikeda, N., J. Toyama, T. Shimizu, I. Kodama, and K. Yamada, The role of electrical uncoupling in the genesis of atrioventricular conduction disturbance. *J. Mol. Cell. Cardiol.*, 1980;**12**: 809–826.

129. Kokobun, S., M. Nishimura, A. Noma, and H. Irisawa, Membrane currents in the atrioventricular node. *Pflug. Arch.*, 1982;**393**: 15–22.

130. Kléber, A.G. and C.B. Riegger, Electrical constants of arterially perfused rabbit papillary muscle. *J. Physiol.*, 1987;**385**: 307–324.

131. Cranefield, P.F., B.F. Hoffman, and A. Paes de Carvalho, Effects of acetylcholine on single fibers of the atrio-ventricular node. *Circ. Res.*, 1959;**7**: 19–23.

132. Mazgalev, T., L.S. Dreifus, H. Iinuma, and E.L. Michelson, Effects of the site and timing of atrio-ventricular input on atrioventricular conduction in the isolated perfused rabbit heart. *Circulation*, 1984;**70**: 748–759.

133. Zipes, D.P., C. Mendez, and G.K. Moe, Evidence for summation and voltage dependency in rabbit atrioventricular nodal fibers. *Circ. Res.*, 1973;**32**: 170–177.

134. Gettes, L.S. and H. Reuter, Slow recovery from inactivation of inward currents in mammalian myocardial fibres. *J. Physiol.*, 1974;**240**: 703–724.

135. Billette, J., M.J. Janse, F.J.L. van Capelle, R.H. Anderson, P. Touboul, and D. Durrer, Cycle-length-dependent properties of AV nodal activation in rabbit hearts. *Am. J. Physiol.*, 1976;**231**: 1129–1139.

136. Truex, R.C., Comparative anatomy and functional considerations of the cardiac conduction system, in *The Specialized Tissues of the Heart*, A. Paes de Carvalho, W.C. De Mello, and B.F. Hoffman, Editors. Amsterdam: Elsevier, 1961, pp. 22–43.

137. Demoulin, G.C. and H.E. Kulbertus, Histopathological examination of concept of left hemiblock. *Brit. Heart J.*, 1972;**34**: 807–814.

138. Rosenbaum, M.B., M.V. Elizari, and J.G. Lazzari, *The Hemiblocks:New Concepts of Intraventricular Conduction Based on Human Anatomical, Physiological and Clinical Studies*. Oldsmar: Tampa Tracings, 1970.

139. Scher, A. and A.C. Young, Ventricular depolarization and the genesis of the QRS. *Ann. NY Acad. Sci.*, 1957;**65**: 766–778.

140. Le Grice, I.J., B.H. Smaill, L.Z. Chai, S.G. Edgar, J.B. Gavin, and P.J. Hunter, Laminar structure of the heart: ventricular myocyte arrangement and connective tissue architecture in the dog. *Am. J. Physiol.*, 1995;**269**: H571–H582.

141. Nagao, K., J. Toyama, I. Kodama, and K. Yamada, Role of the conducting system in the endocardial excitation spread in the right ventricle. *Am. J. Cardiol.*, 1981;**48**: 864–870.

142. Veenstra, R.D., R.W. Joyner, and D.A. Rawling, Purkinje and ventricular activation sequences of canine papillary muscle. Effects of quinidine and calcium on the Purkinje-muscle delay. *Circ. Res.*, 1984;**54**: 500–515.

143. Overholt, E.D., R.W. Joyner, R.D. Veenstra, D.A. Rawling, and R. Wiedmann, Unidirectional block between Purkinje and ventricular muscle layers of papillary muscle. *Am. J. Physiol.*, 1984;**247**: H584–H595.

144. Mendez, C., W.J. Mueller, and X. Urguiaga, Propagation of impulses across the Purkinje fiber-muscle junctions in the dog. *Circ. Res.*, 1970;**36**: 135–150.

145. Joyner, R.W., R.D.E. Veenstra, D.A. Rawling, and A. Chorro, Propagation through electrically coupled cells. Effects of a resistive barrier. *Biophys. J.*, 1984;**45**: 1017–1025.

146. Rawling, D.A., R.W. Joyner, and E.D. Overholt, Variations in the functional electrical coupling between the subendocardial Purkinje and ventricular layers of the canine left ventricle. *Circ. Res.*, 1985;**57**: 252–261.

147. Joyner, R.W., Effects of the discrete pattern of electrical coupling on propagation through an electrical syncytium. *Circ. Res.*, 1982;**50**: 192–200.

148. Alanis, J., D. Benitez, and G. Pilar, A functional discontinuity between the Purkinje and ventricular muscle cells. *Acta Physiol. Lat. Am.*, 1961;**11**: 171–183.

149. Tranum Jensen, J., A.A.M. Wilde, J.T. Vermeulen, and M.J. Janse, Morphology of electrophysiologically identified junctions between Purkinje fibers and ventricular muscle in rabbit and pig hearts. *Circ. Res.*, 1991;**69**: 429–437.

150. Martinez-Palomo, A., J. Alanis, and D. Benitez, Transitional cardiac cells of the conductive system of the dog heart. Distinguishing morphological and electrophysiological features. *J. Cell Biol.*, 1970;**47**: 1–17.

151. Kaneko, Y., Y. Taniguchi, T. Nakajima, M. Manita, T. Ito, M. Akiyama, and M. Kurabayahi, Myocardial bundles with slow conduction properties are present on the left interventricular septal surface of normal human hearts. *J. Cardiovasc. Electrophysiol.*, 2004;**15**: 1010–1018.

152. Sicouri, S. and C. Antzelevitch, A subpopulation of cells with unique electrophysiological properties in the deep subepicardium of the canine ventricle. The M cell. *Circ. Res.*, 1991;**68**: 1729–1741.

153. Sicouri, S., J. Fish, and C. Antzelevitch, Distribution of M cells in the canine ventricle. *J. Cardiovasc. Electrophysiol.*, 1994;**5**: 824–837.

154. Sicouri, S. and C. Antzelevitch, Electrophysiologic characteristics of M cells in the canine left ventricular free wall. *J. Cardiovasc. Electrophysiol.*, 1995;**6**: 591–603.

155. Anyukhovsky, E.P., E.A. Sosunov, and M.R. Rosen, Regional differences in electrophysiological properties of epicardium, midmyocardium, and endocardium: in vitro and in vivo correlations. *Circulation*, 1996;**94**: 1981–1988.

156. Liu, D.-W. and C. Antzelevitch, Characteristics of the delayed rectifier current (IKr and IKs) in canine ventricular epicardial, midmyocardial, and endocardial myocytes. *Circ. Res.*, 1995;**76**: 351–365.

157. Rodriguez-Sinovas, A., J. Cinca, A. Tapias, L. Armadans, M. Tresanchez, and J. Soler-Soler, Lack of evidence of m cells in porcine lefty ventricular myocardium. *Cardiovasc. Res.*, 1997;**33**: 307–313.

158. Tan, R.C. and R.W. Joyner, Electrotonic influences on action potentials from isolated cells. *Circ. Res.*, 1990;**67**: 1071–1081.

159. Anyukhovsky, E.P., E.A. Sosunov, R.Z. Gainullin, and M.R. Rosen, The controversial M cell. *J. Cardiovasc. Electrophysiol.*, 1999;**10**: 244–260.

160. Van Dam, R.Th. and D. Durrer, Experimental study on the intramural distribution of the excitability cycle and on the form of the epicardial T wave in the dog heart in situ. *Am. Heart J.*, 1961;**61**: 537–542.

161. Burgess, M.J., L.S. Green, K. Millar, R. Wyatt, and J.A. Abildskov, The sequence of normal ventricular recovery. *Am. Heart J.*, 1972;**84**: 660–669.

162. Janse, M.J., The effect of changes in heart rate on the refractory period of the heart, Ph.D. thesis. University of Amsterdam, Amsterdam, The Netherlands: Mondeel Offset Drukkerij, 1971.

163. Janse, M.J., A. Capucci, R. Coronel, and M.A. Fabius, Variability of recovery of excitability in the normal canine and ischemic porcine heart. *Eur. Heart J.*, 1985;**6**(Suppl. D): 41–52.

164. Bauer, A., R. Becker, K.D. Freigang, J.C. Senges, F. Voss, A. Hansen, M. Müller, H.J. Lang, U. Gerlach, A. Busch, J. Kraft, and W. Schöls, Rate-and site-dependent effects of propafenone, dofetilide, and the new IKs blocking agent chromanolol 293b on individual muscle layers of the intact heart. *Circulation*, 1999;**100**: 2184–2190.

165. Chinushi, M., M. Tagawa, H. Karai, T. Washizuka, A. Abe, H. Furushima, and Y. Aizawa, Correlation between the effective refractory period and activation-recovery-interval calculated from the intracardiac unipolar electrograms of humans with an without dl-sotalol treatment. *Jpn. Circ. J.*, 2001;**65**: 702–706.

166. Taggart, P., P.M. Sutton, T. Opthof, R. Coronel, R. Trimlett, W. Pugsley, and P. Kallis, Transmural repolarisation in the left

ventricle in humans during normoxia an ischaemia. *Cardiovasc. Res.*, 2001;**50**: 454–462.

167. Conrath, C., R. Wilders, R. Coronel, J.M.T. de Bakker, P. Taggart, J. de Groot, and T. Opthof, Intercellular coupling through gap junctions masks M cells in the human heart. *Cardiovasc. Res.*, 2004;**62**: 407–414.

168. Janse, M.J., E.A. Sosunov, R. Coronel, T. Opthof, E.P. Anyukhovsky, J.M.T. de Bakker, A.N. Plotnikov, I.N. Shlapakova, P. Danilo, J.G.P. Tijssen, and M.R. Rosen, Repolarization gradients in the canine left ventricle before and after induction of short-term cardiac memory. *Circulation*, 2005;**112**: 1711–1718.

5 Genesis of the Electrocardiogram

R.C. Barr · A. van Oosterom

P. W. Macfarlane et al. (eds.), *Basic Electrocardiology*, DOI 10.1007/978-0-85729-871-3_5,
© Springer-Verlag London Limited 2012

5.1 Introduction

In the beginning, Waller [1] measured voltage differences between two electrodes placed on the body surface and found that they changed in rhythm with the heartbeat. That was more than 100 years ago [2].

It is now known that electrocardiograms (ECGs) are possible because active tissues within the heart generate electrical currents that flow intensively within the heart muscle itself, and with lesser intensity throughout the entire body. The flow of current creates voltage differences between sites on the body surface where electrodes may be placed. These voltage differences, measured as a function of time, are called ECGs.

Since access to the body surface is much easier than access to the heart, it is not surprising that ECGs were measured extensively before an explanation of their origin, in terms of electrical events within the heart, could be obtained. What is more surprising is how productively ECGs were used before most of what are now considered the fundamental underlying principles were known. In fact, quantitative explanations for some significant electrocardiographic phenomena remain unavailable even today.

A consequence is that an understanding of the genesis of the ECG requires two frames of reference. The first derives from the colorful history of electrocardiography, which is the frame of reference from which most of the conventions of notation and practice, as well as a tremendous base of empirical knowledge, originated. Accordingly, a few salient points are presented in the section that follows. A more extensive history has been given in ❯ Chap. 1.

The second frame of reference is the base of knowledge available from studies of cardiac electrophysiology. Especially significant is the knowledge about the way currents flow in and around the cells of the heart as a whole. As with electrocardiography, important progress in cardiac electrophysiology has been accumulating for more than a century. However, only within the last 50 years have many central experimental methods been invented and used for the study of transmembrane potentials and currents within and throughout larger cardiac structures. A theoretical framework has been developed to assimilate and organize the experimental findings describing transmembrane and intracellular potentials, and how their associated currents flow and change with time. Many electrophysiological developments have come about largely independently of electrocardiographic viewpoints and conventions. The same applies to the insights stemming from the more recent biophysical studies in the field of electrocardiography. Much of the current electrocardiographic practice seems to be anchored more on the first 50 years than on the period thereafter.

This chapter aims at providing a link between the treatment of the fundamental aspects of electrocardiography found in clinical text books and the more advanced treatment of the same material discussed in detail in the other chapters of this volume.

5.2 Historical Summary

5.2.1 Electrocardiography

The curious history of electrocardiography was said by Burch and DePasquale [3] to be a history of errors and misconceptions, and by Johnson and Flowers [4] to be a "chronicle of wonder and discovery."

An immediate problem for the first electrocardiographers was that the capillary electrometer used by Waller gave tracings of poor quality. Electrocardiography advanced greatly when Einthoven invented the string galvanometer [5, 6] around 1900. Although heavy and bulky, the string galvanometer produced ECG waveforms (measurements of voltage versus time) that had a quality comparable to modern recordings. An electrocardiographic waveform as a whole was seen to consist of a series of deflections. For purposes of identification, Einthoven marked the peaks of the successive major deflections with the labels P, Q, R, S and T (❯ Fig. 5.1).

While the string galvanometer provided a means for recording ECGs, it did not provide an explanation of their genesis. There were substantial differences of opinion about the origin of the deflections, or even whether they had clinical significance. Einthoven demonstrated their clinical significance by showing differences between waveforms recorded from normal subjects and patients suffering from arrhythmias. For this work Einthoven received the Nobel prize in 1924.

There remained many questions and controversies about how electrocardiographic deflections originated within the heart. Thomas Lewis [7, 8] recognized that the temporal sequence of the deflections of the ECG occurred because there

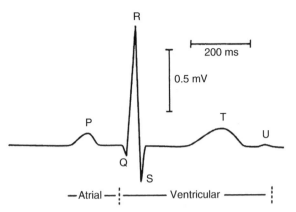

⬛ Fig. 5.1
P-Q-R-S-T-U peaks on a lead II waveform. While Einthoven's nomenclature implicitly emphasized the waveform's peaks, the durations of the intervals such as P-R and Q-T often are also carefully examined. The point where S rises to the baseline and abruptly changes slope is often identified as the J ("junctional") point

was a temporal sequence in which different cardiac structures became electrically active. To prove this thesis, Lewis measured the sequence of electrical excitation directly from the atria and ventricles of dogs, while simultaneously measuring ECGs from the body surface.

Because of the limited sensitivity of the original recording devices, early ECGs sometimes were measured from subjects whose hands or feet were placed in buckets of saline solution. The buckets of saline were "electrodes," which had a large contact area with the skin. As time went by, a system of "standard leads" evolved. The standard leads used measurements between specific limbs (❷ Fig. 5.2). For example, lead II uses the left leg as the positive input and the right arm as the negative input and so the signal observed by lead II represents the time course of the potential at the left leg minus that at the right arm.

Frank Wilson and others recognized the limitations in a system where all the electrodes were distant from the heart. They demonstrated the value of the precordial leads, which use electrodes placed on the chest. Voltages from the precordial leads are measured with respect to "Wilson's central terminal" (WCT), which is the average potential of the three limbs, right arm (RA), left arm (LA), and left leg (LL) [9]. This average was originally found by connecting the electrodes to the three limbs with 5,000 Ohm resistors. Under most circumstances, potentials ahead of an advancing excitation wave are more positive than the potential at Wilson's central terminal, and potentials behind the excitation wave are more negative. Combinations of standard leads and precordial leads measured with respect to Wilson's central terminal form the basis for the measurements of most ECGs even today. Lead theory and lead systems are discussed more extensively in ❷ Chaps. 10 and ❷ 11 respectively.

5.2.2 Electrophysiology

In 1949 Ling and Gerard introduced the glass microelectrode [10], a tool suitable for measuring potential differences across the membranes of individual cells, thereby greatly advancing the study of transmembrane potentials. This tool was rapidly adapted to cardiac studies. For example, in 1951 Woodbury, Hecht and Christopherson [11] reported on measurements from cardiac cells. In time, such methods allowed an extensive description of cardiac action potentials. Examples of their variation from structure to structure (nodes, atria, conduction system, ventricles) became available through sources such as Hoffman and Cranefield [12]. ❷ Figure 5.3 is a drawing of action potential wave forms of different cardiac structures [13].

The value of the transmembrane potential recordings was magnified by the mathematical descriptions put forward by Hodgkin and Huxley [14] to describe membrane currents in nerves. The Hodgkin-Huxley formulation provided a framework for the development of related mathematical descriptions for the cardiac muscle. An early example of this is the Beeler and Reuter model [15] and its later modifications, such as the one proposed in [16]; it assumes that only

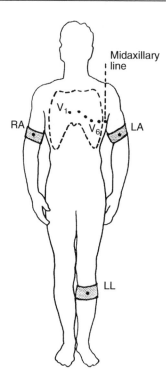

◘ Fig. 5.2
Electrode placement. Electrodes attached to the limbs are used for the "standard leads" I, II and III. For example, lead II measures the potential at electrode LL (connected to the positive input of the recorder) with reference to the potential on the electrode RA. "Unipolar" lead V_1 is measured with electrode V_1 located as shown on the chest, with reference to the average potential at electrodes RA, LA and LL. This configuration is called "Wilson's central terminal," WCT. The locations of the electrodes V_1-V_6 are indicated by dots on the chest. Potentials measured at these *electrodes* with reference to WCT are referred to as *leads* V_1-V_6

capacitative displacement current and sodium-channel current contribute during the time period of the action-potential upstroke. The model provides a quantitative description of the upstroke of the cardiac action potential using voltage-clamp data obtained from small spherical clusters of tissue-cultured heart cells. In a marked contrast are the much more comprehensive models of DiFrancesco-Noble [17] or Luo and Rudy [18] for ventricular myocardium, or those like that of Courtemanche et al. for the atria [19]. These include other channel currents and provide a much more comprehensive picture of the contribution of different ionic currents to the total membrane current.

A picture of the flow of currents within and around cells during the course of an action potential has emerged from these measurements and models. On the one hand, this picture can be used to examine in detail potentials and currents in the vicinity of active fibers and relate them to ionic movements through the membrane, as done, for example, by Spach and Kootsey [20]. The same picture can be used as a building block for models of larger segments of cardiac muscle, whether quantitatively, as with the bidomain model [21] (see also ❷ Chap. 7), or only qualitatively. Such models form the basis for much of the modern understanding of the genesis of the ECG. Cardiac electrophysiology is discussed more fully in ❷ Chap. 3.

5.2.3   Synthesis

Recent years have seen a renewed emphasis on unifying the electrocardiographic and electrophysiological frames of reference, a goal held from the beginnings of electrocardiography. The objective is to provide an explanation of the genesis of

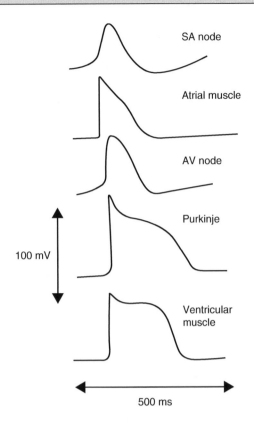

SA node

Atrial muscle

AV node

Purkinje

100 mV

Ventricular muscle

500 ms

⬛ Fig. 5.3
Characteristic action potentials drawn for different cardiac structures. Among the evident differences are the sloping base-lines for the SA and AV nodal traces, and the flat baselines elsewhere; the differences in duration; and the differences in rate of rise during depolarization, a characteristic associated with the velocity of propagating wave fronts, showing some of their characteristic differences. Striking color drawings of cardiac structures and their action potentials have been presented by Netter [13]

ECGs that is consistent with the underlying electrophysiology, quantitatively as well as qualitatively. For quantitative consistency, it is necessary to have mechanisms that are presented mathematically and then verified through measurements of sufficient precision; this ambitious goal remains to be accomplished in many important respects. More qualitatively, it is from the perspective of attempting to explain the genesis of the ECG in terms of the underlying cardiac events that the remainder of this chapter is presented.

5.3 Electric Current Sources and Their Potential Fields

How can the potentials and currents from individual fibers be related to those potentials observed some distance away? Such questions have been analyzed extensively elsewhere (as in [22]) and are examined in detail in ❷ Chaps. 6 and ❷ 7. Some central elements that relate to the genesis of the ECG are summarized here.

5.3.1 Source Character of a Single Fiber

The most basic building block for describing the cardiac electric generator is the single cardiac cell. Its properties are described in ❷ Sect. 6.3.1. Here we take it to be a single cardiac fiber along which, after being activated at one end, a process of local depolarization followed by repolarization propagates. Its properties as an equivalent electric source (❷ Sect. 2.5) are discussed from a different perspective in ❷ Sect. 6.3.1. The transmembrane potential V_m, is the difference between the potentials Φ_i and Φ_e at two points just inside and outside the membrane of cardiac cells or fibers, defined by convention as $V_m = \Phi_i - \Phi_e$. ❷ Figure 5.4 illustrates the potentials and currents generated during the propagation of an excitation along the fiber. This figure is drawn to illustrate the main concepts involved.

If the fiber is immersed in an extensive conducting medium the transmembrane current per unit length, i_m, (unit: A m^{-1}) acting as an equivalent line current source density for the extracellular compartment, may be approximated as

$$i_m(x,t) = \pi\, a^2 \sigma_i \frac{\partial^2 V_m(x,t)}{\partial x^2},$$

(5.1)

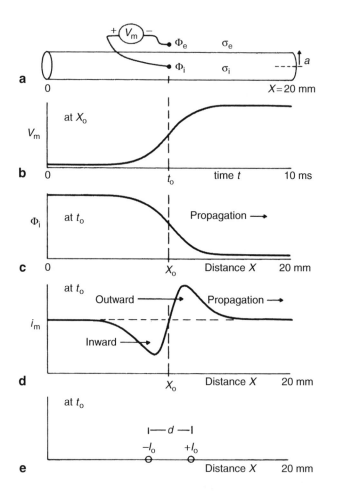

☐ **Fig. 5.4**

Potentials and currents of an action potential propagating to the right along a fiber. Part (a) identifies a site for measuring intracellular potential Φ_i and extracellular potential Φ_e with respect to a reference electrode located at an arbitrary point in the surrounding medium. V_m is the local transmembrane potential. The cylinder has radius a and intracellular and extracellular conductivities σ_i and σ_e. Part (b) shows a hypothetical tracing of V_m as a function of *time* at position x_o on the cylinder. Such a waveform might result from a previous excitation on the left. Because of the time scale used, only the depolarization phase is shown. Time t_o is taken to be near the middle of the upstroke of this waveform. Part (c) shows the value of Φ_i as a function of *distance* along the fiber at time t_o for the same fiber. Note that the potential declines to the resting value to the right. Part (d) shows the spatial distribution of the corresponding transmembrane current i_m along the fiber, defined as positive for outward flowing current and negative for inward flowing current with σ_i the intracellular conductivity and a the fiber radius. This expression is derived from the linear core-conductor model of the membrane processes along a single linear fiber [22]. It holds true quite generally, i.e., for the segments that locally depolarize, as well as for those that are repolarizing. Applying the potential profile along the fiber at time instant t requires taking the second spatial derivative of the function shown in ❷ Fig. 5.4c. This results in the distribution of the source strength i_m along the fiber at that same time instant t shown in ❷ Fig. 5.4d.

5.3.2   Extracellular Current Flow

In a segment of local depolarization, from the viewpoint of the extracellular space, the presence of an action potential in the fiber produces two major effects. First, there is a large current entering the extracellular space just ahead of the advancing excitation wave. Second, there is a large current sink just behind it. This is illustrated in ❷ Fig. 5.5. The potential field set up in the external medium is positive ahead of the wave front and negative behind it, both with reference to the potential at some remote reference point.

Inside the fiber, there is an axial gradient of the potential set up by the *active* processes at the cell membrane (❷ Fig. 5.4c). The intracellular current I_i flows "down" this gradient and is directed from the location of the (extracellular) sink to the (extracellular) source. Outside the strand, the *passive* return current flows from source to sink near the strand (along path A). It also flows, but less intensively, along pathways further away, such as path B. As a result, a potential field Φ_e is generated throughout the external volume by the current flow.

This current flow pattern can be understood intuitively in the following way. An approaching excitation wave drives large currents of magnitude I_0 out of the membrane, in effect, by discharging the membrane capacitance. (The ionic charge accumulation across the membrane is high because the membrane is thin and the polarizing voltages, at rest, are substantial.) Once the approaching excitation wave has depolarized the membrane past a threshold level, the membrane has a large sodium conductance, so large inward currents I_0 flow through the membrane. The inward currents are driven in part by the concentration gradient of sodium ions between the inside and the outside. The inward currents are also driven by the potential difference driving positive ions inward. Large intracellular potential differences exist along the fiber between the partially depolarized region where the current is entering, and the fully polarized regions ahead of the advancing excitation wave. These axial intracellular potential differences cause large intracellular axial currents, I_i. The intracellular currents then begin the process of discharge at the next portion of the membrane capacitance.

These processes occur within the membrane because of its ability to change conductivities in an ion-selective manner. They create relatively positive voltages on the outer surface of the membrane at the (extracellular) current source and a relatively negative voltage on the outer membrane near the sink. In contrast, the current flow through the intracellular and extracellular volumes (all the way out to the body surface) is essentially a passive current flow in the surrounding conducting medium.

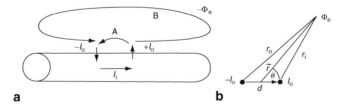

a   b

❑ Fig. 5.5

Current flow patterns in and around the fiber during depolarization. Intracellular longitudinal current I_i, transmembrane currents I_0, and extracellular current flowpaths A and B are shown. The flow of current throughout the extracellular volume creates the potential field Φ_e

5.3.3   Potential Field arising from Lumped Sources; Current Dipoles

For observation points in the external medium with electric conductivity σ_e, at some distance from the fiber the (infinite medium) potential field is indistinguishable from the one that results by lumping the inward currents together into a single current monopole $-I_0$ (sink) and all outward currents into a single current monopole I_0 (source) (❷ Sect. 2.5.1.1.), separated by a distance d.

At distances from the monopole pair that are much greater than d, the potential field in the external medium approaches the one generated by a current dipole $\vec{D} = I_0 \vec{d}$, ❷ Sect. 2.5.1.2. Vector $\vec{D}$ is called the dipole moment; its strength is proportional to the gradient of the transmembrane potential along the fiber. The potential field (generated in an infinite medium) at a field point $\vec{r}'$ with reference to the position of the dipole is,

$$\Phi_e(\vec{r}') = \frac{1}{4\pi\sigma_e} \frac{\vec{D} \bullet \vec{R}}{R^3}, \tag{5.2}$$

or, equivalently, as

$$\Phi_e(\vec{r}') = \frac{1}{4\pi\sigma_e} \frac{D \, \cos\varphi}{R^2} \tag{5.3}$$

This expression shows that the potential produced by the dipole depends on several factors. One is the dipole's magnitude D (unit: A m). Another is the cosine of the angle φ between the dipole direction (from sink to source) and a line from dipole location to the field point. A third is the reciprocal of the square of the distance R from the dipole location to the field point. See also ❷ Sect. 2.5.1.3.

5.3.4   Potential Field Around a Single Fiber

A more general expression for the external potential generated by the membrane processes of a fiber follows from the addition (superposition) of the contributions to the potential at field point (x', ρ') arising from elementary current monopoles $i_m(x, t) \, \Delta x$, with $i_m(x, t)$ as specified in (5.1) and Δx a small segment along the fiber. Based on (2.96) we have

$$\Phi_e(x', \rho'; t) = \frac{\pi a^2 \sigma_i}{4\pi\sigma_e} \int_{-\infty}^{\infty} \frac{1}{\sqrt{(x'-x)^2 + \rho'^2}} \frac{\partial^2 V_m(x; t)}{\partial x^2} dx, \tag{5.4}$$

in which ρ' denotes the distance from the external observation point to the fiber axis.

An alternative, equivalent expression, found by means of partial integration, is as follows

$$\Phi_e(x', \rho'; t) = \frac{-a^2 \sigma_i}{4\sigma_e} \int_{-\infty}^{\infty} \frac{x'-x}{\left((x'-x)^2 + \rho'^2\right)^3} \frac{\partial V_m(x; t)}{\partial x} dx \tag{5.5}$$

By introducing $\vec{S}(x) = \pi a^2 \vec{e}_x$ in (5.5), and since $\partial V_m(x, t)/\partial x$ has components along the fiber only, we may write

$$\Phi_e(x', \rho'; t) = \frac{-\sigma_i}{4\pi \, \sigma_e} \int_{-\infty}^{\infty} \frac{\partial V_m(x; t)}{\partial x} \frac{\vec{R}}{R^3} \bullet \vec{S}(x) dx, \tag{5.6}$$

with $\vec{R}$ the vector from source point $(x, 0)$ to field point (x', ρ'). By using (2.110) we find

$$\Phi_e(x', \rho'; t) = \frac{-\sigma_i}{4\pi \, \sigma_e} \int_{-\infty}^{\infty} \frac{\partial V_m(x, t)}{\partial x} \Omega(x, \vec{r}') dx, \tag{5.7}$$

with $\Omega(x, \vec{r}')$ the solid angle of the cross-section of the fiber at location x along the fiber subtended at field point (x', ρ') (❷ Sect. 2.2.12). This expresses the external potential field as the sum of the contributions from elementary double layers with strength $\Delta M_S = -\sigma_i(\partial V_m/\partial x)\,dx$, stacked up along the fiber and pointing in the direction of propagation at locations that are depolarizing.

Equation (5.7) has great significance for the description of the potential field generated by bioelectric sources. A more complete treatment of this topic is presented in ❯ Chaps. 6 and ❯ 7. In this chapter it is used mainly for source descriptions during the depolarization phase, for which the source strength (dipole density) is assumed to be uniform over the depolarization wave front.

Equations (5.4) and (5.7) involve the so-called convolution integrals. The first one is the convolution of a monopole source function derived from the second spatial derivative of the transmembrane potential along the fiber and the function $1/R$, and as can be seen from (5.7), the second that of a double layer with its strength proportional to the first spatial derivative and the function expressing the solid angle subtended by the wave front.

5.3.5   Source Description at Depolarization Wave Fronts; Uniform Double Layer Theory

What if there are many fibers rather than just one, as in some extensive part of the myocardium?

A first approximation is to compute the potential when many fibers are active, as the sum of the potentials generated by each one (superposition). At the depolarization wave front this can be viewed as a collection of elementary dipoles distributed over the surface $S(t)$ of the wave front at time t, as illustrated in ❯ Fig. 5.6.

The expression for the potential then reads

$$\Phi_e(\vec{r}';t) = \frac{1}{4\pi\,\sigma_e}\int_{S(t)}\frac{\vec{M}_S(\vec{r};t)\bullet\vec{R}}{R^3}\,dS(\vec{r}), \tag{5.8}$$

with $\vec{R} = \vec{r}' - \vec{r}$ the vector from source location $\vec{r}$ on S to field point $\vec{r}'$, with length R

(❯ Sect. 2.5.2.2). Note that, as a consequence of the propagation, the integration at different time instants t is taken over different surfaces $S(t)$.

Next, we assume the direction of the dipole density $M_S(\vec{r}';t)$ to be lined up with the direction of local propagation of the wave front. Then (5.8) becomes

$$\Phi_e(\vec{r}';t) = \frac{1}{4\pi\,\sigma_e}\int_{S(t)}M_S(\vec{r};t)\,d\omega(\vec{r}), \tag{5.9}$$

compare (5.7). If, moreover, M_S is a constant over the wave front $S(t)$, then (5.9) takes on a particularly simple form:

$$\Phi_e(\vec{r}';t) = \frac{M_S}{4\pi\sigma_e}\Omega(\vec{r}';t), \tag{5.10}$$

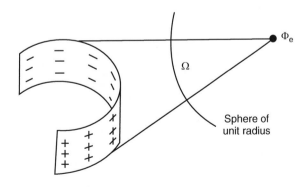

◻ Fig. 5.6

Depolarization wave front propagating towards an observer. The potential Φ_e generated by the distributed sources and sinks is proportional to the solid angle of the excitation wave as seen from the field point

where $\Omega(\vec{r}';t)$ is the solid angle subtended by the entire wave front $S(t)$ as seen from the field point, as illustrated in
❯ Fig. 5.6.

The source model based on the two assumptions of elementary dipoles lined up with the direction of the wave front propagation and having uniform strength is known as the uniform double layer (UDL). Based on (5.10), the theory of its application is referred to as the solid angle theory. It is a classic source model, originating from the work of Wilson et al. [23]. It is used in most basic texts on the relationship between electric cardiac sources and resulting potentials, as in the sequel. A particularly thorough demonstration of its usefulness has been published by Holland and Arnsdorf [24]. Note that this model is restricted to describing the major sources during depolarization only; its validity is discussed in
❯ Chap. 6.

5.3.6 The Effects of the Geometry of Torso Boundary and Inhomogeneous Tissue Conductivity

The expressions for the potentials Φ_e above assume implicitly that a uniform medium of infinite extent surrounds the active fibers. In reality, cardiac sources are immersed in a volume conductor containing regions of different conductivity. These include the blood within the heart, the lungs and skeletal muscle. Rather than having infinite extent, the volume conductor is sharply delimited at the body surface by the torso-air boundary. A cross-sectional drawing of the human torso identifying the locations of the heart and lungs within the torso is given in ❯ Fig. 5.7. The level corresponds to the fourth intercostal space, the level of electrodes V_1 and V_2. The position of the remaining four electrode placements, as projected into the plane of the figure are those proposed by Goldman [25]. The drawing shows the asymmetric placement of the ventricular muscle within the thorax. Note how closely the right ventricular (RV) free wall approaches the chest near V_1, and how much further V_6 is from the left ventricular (LV) free wall. In the preceding section, it was established that the distances between the cardiac sources and the sites of electrodes on the body surface was highly significant, in that potentials from the dipole sources declined as $1/R^2$. Gross inspection of ❯ Fig. 5.7 shows that moving around the thorax circumference, starting from the position of V_1, the length of R may vary by as much as a factor of 10, depending on the particular membrane that is active. That implies that the potentials may vary in magnitude by a factor of 100 because of distance effects alone. As a consequence, large deviations from normality may remain unnoticed in clinical recordings.

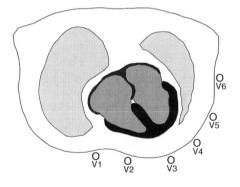

▧ Fig. 5.7

Superior view of a cross-sectional drawing of a human torso; derived from magnetic resonance images, showing, in increasingly darker shades, the lungs, the blood filled cavities, the atrial and ventricular myocardium. Circumferential locations of the six precordial electrodes as described by Goldman [25]. The transverse level is that of the fourth intercostal space, the level of electrodes V_1 and V_2; the remaining four are placed more inferiorly (❯ Fig. 5.2)

One way of mathematically taking into account the presence of boundaries and inhomogeneities is by the use of Green's theorem, as discussed in ❯ Sect. 2.6.4. An example of its use is the following equation for the potential on the body surface:

$$\Phi_B(\vec{r}') = \frac{\sigma_s}{\sigma_B}\Phi_{B,\infty}(\vec{r}') - \frac{1}{4\pi}\frac{\sigma_L - \sigma_B}{\sigma_B}\int_{S_L}\Phi_L d\omega_L - \frac{1}{4\pi}\int_{S_B}\Phi_B d\omega_B \qquad (5.11)$$

This expression is a specific form of (2.172), dedicated to its application to field points positioned at the body surface S_B. It describes the computation of the effect of the low conductivity of the lungs relative to that of other body tissues. It is assumed that bounding surfaces S_L can be drawn around "lungs" separating uniform regions of different conductivity inside and outside the boundaries (❯ Fig. 5.7). Potentials on the lung and body surfaces are designated by Φ_L and Φ_B respectively. Within the lung, and on the remaining parts of the body, the conductivities are given by σ_L and σ_B respectively.

The first term of (5.11) expresses the infinite medium potential of the source at field points on the torso surface, e.g., as in (5.9) placed in a medium with conductivity σ_s. In addition, (5.11) contains two integrals expressing the contributions of the secondary sources representing the effect of different conductivity values across the lung and torso interfaces. Note that if the conductivity values at both sides of the lung interface were taken as equal, then the contribution of the associated secondary sources would vanish.

The single, most dominating factor on the magnitude of the potentials on the body surface is the distance between source location and observation point (❯ Sects. 2.5.1.3 and ❯ 5.3.6). Next in rank is the effect of the torso boundary. To a first approximation, potential magnitudes are increased by a factor of 2 to 3 as a consequence (❯ Sect. 2.6.3.3).

As can be seen from an inspection of (5.11), the specific effects of the torso boundary or internal inhomogeneities are not described by a simple rule. Accordingly, extensive variations from these first approximations occur. Qualitative relationships between cardiac and body-surface events can often be accomplished satisfactorily even when volume-conductor effects are ignored, but the quantitative effects are quite substantial. Note that (5.11) as shown ignores other significant aspects of the volume conductor. These aspects include the inhomogeneity consisting of the highly conductive blood within the chambers, and the anisotropic nature of the conductivity of skeletal muscle. A more detailed treatment of this topic is presented in ❯ Chap. 8.

5.3.7 Depolarization Summary

Depolarization consists of a complex of excitation waves moving through the active tissue. Excitation waves correspond to the upstroke of the transmembrane action potential, moving by means of active propagation. From an extracellular viewpoint, excitation waves frequently consist of a source-sink pair, having a spacing of about one millimeter, traveling at a speed of the order of $0.4\,\mathrm{m\,s^{-1}}$ across the fiber measured in situ in the canine ventricle [26] and up to $1\,\mathrm{m\,s^{-1}}$ measured in vitro along the fibers of the strips of the cardiac muscle [27]. Using the mathematical equations above, it can be seen that during depolarization the magnitude of the extracellular potential Φ_e depends on the following:

(a) The intensity of the line density expressing the membrane current $i_{m(x,t)}$, discussed in ❯ Sect. 5.3.1 (unit: $\mathrm{A\,m^{-1}}$). This affects I_0 of ❯ Sect. 5.3.3 (unit: A) as well as M_S, the dipole layer strength (unit: $\mathrm{A\,m^{-1}}$). This intensity depends on the second spatial derivate of the intracellular potentials and, correspondingly on the magnitude of the action potentials (5.1).

(b) The distance R from the source of membrane current to the field point, i.e., the point where the extracellular potential, Φ_e, is being determined (5.3).

(c) The orientation of the source-sink pair with respect to the point where the extracellular potential, Φ_e, is being determined. The potential Φ_e is positive when the field point is on the source side of the pair.

(d) The number of fibers involved, i.e., the extent of the source region (5.9). Both the extent of the source region and the distance to it are taken into account in the solid angle Ω.

(e) The torso boundaries and inhomogeneities in conductivity within the volume conductor.

A more extensive treatment of linking the electrophysiology of the depolarization wave front with its expression in terms of an equivalent source description is contained in ❯ Chap. 6.

5.3.8   Repolarization Summary

Repolarization occurs when the action potential returns to its resting level. Current flow during repolarization can be analyzed in a fashion similar to that provided above for depolarization. However, significant differences between depolarization and repolarization include the following.

(a) Repolarization currents across the membrane and associated changes in the voltage of the membrane occur after a time delay following depolarization. Hence repolarization is not propagated in the same sense that depolarization is, although membrane currents at one site continue to be affected by events at neighboring sites.

(b) The time required for the membrane to repolarize is fifty or more times the length of the time required for depolarization. Hence the source distribution of the membrane current is much more widely dispersed in space than during depolarization. As a consequence the distribution cannot simply by represented in terms of the propagation of dipoles.

(c) As the sources and sinks are so much more widely separated, describing, specifically, the transition from (5.6) to (5.7) is no longer possible with good accuracy. For single fibers, the analysis requires a return to Eqns. (5.1–5.4), as was done, e.g., by Spach et al. [28].

(d) The intensity of the current emerging from (or entering) the membrane at any one site is much less during repolarization than during depolarization. Conversely, the current emerges (or enters) over a much wider region. These effects offset each other differently at varying distances from a strand of myocardial tissue. Near the tissue, deflections in electrograms taken at close distance from the myocardium during repolarization are small relative to those during depolarization. On the body surface, the T waves have magnitudes much more comparable to those of the QRS complexes.

The modeling of the electric sources for representing body surface potentials during repolarization has long been restricted to a single dipole. This type of source cannot easily be given an electrophysiological basis. A recent development has yielded the source description of the equivalent double layer, which has a clear link with electrophysiology, both during depolarization and repolarization. This topic is discussed in ❯ Chap. 7.

5.4   Attributes of the Deflections

The principles enumerated in the previous section provide a basis for understanding the attributes of each of the phases of the ECG, which are considered in turn. In each section, brief comments are included about the excitation of the underlying cardiac structures and about the resulting electrocardiographic deflections. Most topics presented here are analyzed in greater detail in other chapters of this volume. In this chapter, the main objective is to discuss linkages between what is happening within the heart and how this is expressed in the signals observed on the body surface.

5.4.1   Cautions

The mathematical relationships established above have served as a basis for many reports relating to body-surface potentials to currents and to potentials within the heart. In sequel, they are used as a guide to the qualitative relationships. Even so, it is important to realize that they ignore many aspects of the real tissue, including the anisotropy of the tissue, the different access of deep and superficial fibers to the extracellular volume, the blood within the cardiac chambers, and the anisotropy of the skeletal muscle.

Another concern is the fact that the electric potential as such does not relate in any way to the electric current sources expressing the electric activity of the heart (❯ Sect. 2.5). It is only the potential *differences* observed by at least two electrodes placed at some distance on the thorax that are related to such activity. In any recorded signal, if one of the electrodes involved is taken to be the reference, the potential at the reference is often tacitly assumed to be zero. Within a bounded volume conductor, this assumption is unjustified [29, 30], and is in fact incorrect. This also applies to the Wilson Central Terminal, the potential reference most frequently used in ECG recordings. In the documentation of any ECG signal the involved reference should be specified.

The qualitative explanations of QRS amplitudes and wave forms based on the solid angle theory, usually address the potential generated at the sensing electrode only. This implicitly assumes the solid angle of the wave fronts as seen by the reference electrode to be zero. For the correct application of the solid angle theory to the interpretation of the potential difference between two electrodes, the different solid angles subtended by the wave front as seen from the locations of the two electrodes should be subtracted [31].

The potential difference between any two different electrode locations reflects the integral of the component of the electric field along the path traveled from one electrode to the other. As a potential difference is a scalar, the route taken does not affect the outcome (❷ Sect. 2.5). The discussion on what is "seen" by either of the two electrodes, or which of the two electrodes acts at the reference [32] is meaningless and does not reflect basic physical principles [33]. The term reference electrode should be reserved for situations in which multiple signals are studied, all referred to a single location. Such signals are commonly referred to as unipolar leads, a complete misnomer that should preferably be replaced by "common reference signals."

5.5 P Wave

In a normal sinus rhythm, excitation begins at the "sinoatrial (SA) node and spreads in a pattern similar to that produced by dropping a stone into still water" (Scher [34]). James [35] has emphasized the different histological appearances of different atrial cells and suggested that different specialized pathways may exist in the atrium, in some fashion analogous to the conduction system of the ventricles (see ❷ Chap. 4 for further discussion of this point). However, measurements of the spread of the excitation, from the time of Peuch [36] to the measurements of Spach [37], differ. The measurements show that different velocities of excitation arise primarily from differences in the propagation velocity along and across atrial fibers. A review of this question was given by Sano [38].

From an electrocardiographic viewpoint (❷ Fig. 5.8), during the generation of the P wave, the active membrane is relatively distant from the electrodes on the torso surface. The extent of the sources will be small, since the atrial wall is

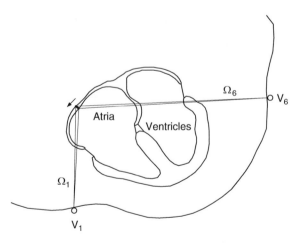

◻ Fig. 5.8

Solid angles during atrial excitation. A small region of atrial muscle is hypothesized to be active and identified by a bold line. Propagation is in the direction of the arrow. Solid angles from V_1 and V_6 are indicated by the straight lines drawn. Note that the solid angle concept in fact relates to 3D space. The drawing indicates that the area of the active surface is small and the distances from either body surface site relatively long. Both these effects will lead to a small solid angle and thereby small potentials during the P wave

thin, and the muscle is excited by propagation proceeding tangentially to the wall. The dominant active electric sources are few during depolarization. The consequence is that the corresponding manifestation of atrial activity on the body surface, the P wave, normally has a low magnitude (in the range of 60–120 μV).

As excitation proceeds from the SA node, the leading (positive) side of the excitation wave front will be leftward and downward. The contribution of the small front shown in ❷ Fig. 5.8 produces a negative deflection in lead V_6 and positive deflection in lead V_1. The total excitation process usually produces positive apex P wave values in lead VF, and negative ones in lead VR. The duration of atrial excitation, and therefore the duration of the P wave, is about 100 ms.

In the past, the fact that the magnitude of the P wave was often frequently not much higher than the noise level of ECG recorders, has introduced considerable imprecision into P-wave standards as documented in the literature. These were restricted mainly to P wave amplitudes and durations. As a consequence the P wave has been mainly used to provide the relative timing between atrial and ventricular events. With the advances in recording technology (lower noise levels), and the current interest in atrial electric activity during atrial flutter or atrial fibrillation, efforts are directed towards extracting more information about atrial electric activity from the ECG.

5.6   PQ Segment

On an ECG recorded with standard methods, the P wave is followed by an interval of about 70 ms leading on to the onset of depolarization of the ventricles: the PQ segment. Because of the small magnitudes of potential differences on the thorax generated during this interval, this period is usually considered to be electrically silent. However, early applications of the body surface mapping technique have identified clear, non-zero patterns of potential differences on the thorax during this period, with magnitudes that are about one third of those during depolarization of the atria [39, 40]. The time course of these patterns is almost the reverse of those during depolarization, suggesting that these potentials relate to the repolarization of the atria, with a very small dispersion of the durations of the action potentials of atrial myocytes [41, 42]. At the moment of onset of ventricular depolarization, these potential differences may have magnitudes up to 30 μV. The locations showing maximal potential differences are not included in the electrodes of the standard 12-lead ECG [41].

In a normal heart, atrial excitation initiates excitation of the atrioventricular (AV) node, which in turn initiates excitation of the ventricular conduction system. As the diameter of the fibers of the AV node is small, the conduction velocity through them is low (about 0.05 m s^{-1}). Conversely, the fibers of the ventricular conduction system are large, so conduction is much faster (about 2 m s^{-1}).

Though excitation is progressing through the AV node and conduction system, excitation includes a small number of fibers, distant from the surface. The potentials observed during the PQ segment have also been attributed to this process. On the body surface these are in the range of 1–10 μV peak-to-peak. In 1973 and 1974, Berbari et al. [43], Flowers et al. [44] and others began publishing a series of papers that indicated that recordings could be obtained from the body surface, during the PR interval. In 1983, Flowers et al. [45] presented an analysis of PR intervals in normal subjects and patients with abnormalities of the conduction system. Their recordings showed a biphasic deflection during the PQ segment, having a magnitude of about 2.5 μV. Earlier studies in animals, as well as recordings from humans with normal and abnormal AV conduction, support the hypothesis that these signals arise from the His-Purkinje system, primarily through the temporal linkages between the His-Purkinje waveforms and those known to arise from the ventricles.

5.7   QRS Complex

The QRS deflections arise from the excitation of the ventricular muscle. In normal excitation, the conduction system causes excitation of the muscle to begin more or less simultaneously at a number of right and left ventricular endocardial sites. (Detailed maps are presented in ❷ Chap. 4.) One consequence is that excitation has a substantial radial as well as tangential direction throughout the excitation of much of the ventricular wall.

There are a number of general characteristics about the electrocardiographic effects of ventricular excitation that arise from the overall geometric relationships between ventricular and body-surface points as they interact with the gross features of ventricular excitation. Several of these are illustrated in ❷ Fig. 5.9, in which the two heavy lines represent excitation waves, one in the right ventricle (❷ Fig. 5.9a) and one in the left (❷ Fig. 5.9b). Both advance toward the epicardium. Electrode sites are identified on the body surface at V_1 and V_6. Suppose the potential at V_1 and V_6 are measured with respect to Wilson's central terminal the following should be noted.

(a) An electrode at point V_1 or V_6 on the body surface "sees" a solid angle Ω_1 associated with the excitation wave in the right ventricle (left panel) or from the excitation wave in the left ventricle (right panel). The solid angle reflects the entire excitation surface in three dimensions that results from the excitation wave extending above and below the plane of the figure, not simply the cross-sectional line drawn there. The solid angles at V_1 and V_6 are different, because the distance and orientation of V_1 from either excitation wave differs from that of V_6. Moreover, for the wave fronts shown, their signs differ.

(b) If both activation fronts are present, the potential at V_1 or V_6 is the algebraic sum of the potentials produced by each of the excitation waves separately. In ❷ Fig. 5.9, a positive voltage is produced at V_1 by the RV excitation wave, and a negative voltage by the LV excitation wave. The sum is probably slightly positive. The fact that the sum is algebraic means that the sum is lower in magnitude than would be the case if either excitation wave were present separately. This phenomenon is called *cancellation* [46] in the electrocardiographic literature. One consequence is that if only one excitation wave is present, the magnitude of the body surface deflection is higher than if two are present. A similar effect is seen at V_6.

(c) As the right ventricle is closer to an electrode on the anterior chest, such as V_1, than to the left ventricle, a right ventricular excitation wave will have a greater solid angle, and therefore produce a greater voltage at V_1, than an excitation wave of the same extent and orientation in the left ventricle.

(d) Excitation waves in either ventricle extend over greater distances when excitation is predominantly in the endocardial to epicardial direction than when excitation proceeds in a direction tangential to the surface of the walls.

(e) The right ventricular excitation wave generally starts somewhat later than the one initiated at the left ventricular aspect of the septum. Moreover, the right ventricle is relatively thin and, once activated, its excitation is for the greater part directed along the right ventricular wall and ends later than that of the left ventricle. The consequence is that the earliest part of the QRS deflection normally reflects septal activation, the middle part a combination of left and right ventricular activity, while the final part reflects predominantly the excitation of the basal part of the right ventricle.

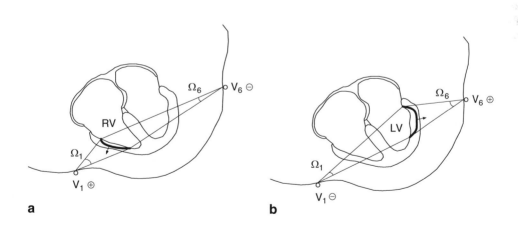

a   b

◻ Fig. 5.9

Solid angles during ventricular excitation. An excitation wave is drawn in (*left panel*) the right ventricle and (*right panel*) the left ventricle. Comparison with ❷ Fig. 5.8 shows the solid angles to be much larger during QRS than during P, so that larger potentials are to be expected. The *larger solid angles* occur mostly because of the greater extent of either excitation wave, since excitation proceeds radially as well as tangentially in a normal sequence. Conversely, note that the orientation of the RV and LV excitation waves shown produces potentials of opposite sign at either V_1 or V_6. If both excitation waves are present simultaneously their effects will tend to cancel

(f) The conduction system "programs" normal excitation of the ventricles in such a way that excitation is completed relatively rapidly. RV and LV excitation overlap extensively (with electrical cancellation). Many cardiac abnormalities (e.g., conduction system defects) tend to produce body-surface waveforms that are longer and of greater magnitude, because the normal "program" is lost. In later chapters the specific electrocardiographic changes arise from the presence of conduction defects, infarction, hypertrophy and other clinical conditions.

5.8   ST Segment

Following the QRS deflections, the ECG has a relatively quiescent period before the large deflection of the T wave occurs. A simple qualitative explanation of this phenomenon is as follows

(A model based interpretation of the ST-T signals is given in ❷ Chap. 7). Consider ❷ Fig. 5.10. Suppose there are two electrodes located on the endocardial and epicardial surfaces of the ventricular wall (electrodes 1 and 2, ❷ Fig. 5.10a). Suppose further that the wave forms of the transmembrane potentials (TMPs) at the endocardial and epicardial sites are identical (as illustrated by the stylized shape of ❷ Fig. 5.10b). A difference of excitation between the endocardial and epicardial sites results in the situation shown in ❷ Fig. 5.10c.

There are periods during which the overlapping tracings have the same potential value. One is the baseline phase (identified as b on ❷ Fig. 5.10c). Another is the plateau phase, denoted as p, of the action potentials. During period p there is no intracellular potential difference between sites 1 and 2. Therefore, no intracellular current flows between these sites during interval p. Consequently, no extracellular (or electrocardiographic) potential differences are generated in the case of the stylized TMPs.

Similarly, if the TMPs throughout the entire ventricle have the same baseline and plateau voltages, and if there is a period of time following excitation (QRS) during which the plateau voltages throughout the ventricles overlap, then during this period of time (the ST segment) the observed electrocardiographic voltages return to the baseline, i.e., are zero.

Available evidence indicates that neither condition is precisely satisfied in normal human hearts, though both exist, more or less. Measurement of body-surface potential distributions [47] during the ST segment in chimpanzees and in normal human subjects show that there is no period of time following excitation when either epicardial or body-surface potentials return uniformly to the baseline. Instead, there is a period of overlap between the potentials that arise from the last portions of muscle to be excited and repolarization potentials from other regions. This period may last for 10 ms or more. However, in a normal sequence, both the potentials at the end of depolarization and the beginning of repolarization are small, so the ECG does return to a voltage near the baseline.

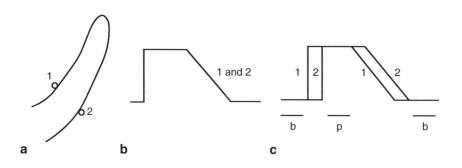

❏ Fig. 5.10

ST segment with identical transmembrane potential waveforms. Part (a) identifies two electrodes across a portion of the ventricular wall. Part (b) shows a single TMP shape hypothesized to be present at all ventricular sites. Part (c) shows the TMPS if excitation at site 2 occurs later than at site 1. Nonetheless, there are periods of time, identified b (baseline) as p (plateau phase), when both action potentials at endocardium and epicardium are the same. During this time there are no intracellular potential differences among sites and therefore no intracellular or extracellular currents

The J point of the ECG is identified as the time when a tracing changes slope abruptly at the end of the S wave. The J point is sometimes used as a marker for the end of excitation. Comparison of the electrocardiographic waveform with the complete body-surface potential distribution or, when available, epicardial electrograms, shows that the J point marks the end of excitation only approximately. Again the approximation occurs because of the overlap of potentials at the ending of depolarization and the beginning of repolarization [47].

Changes in the cardiac excitation sequence or changes in the action-potential wave shape can be expected to change the amplitude and wave form of the electrocardiogram during the ST time period.

If the amplitude or the wave form of the TMP changes in a region of muscle, then the situation portrayed in ❯ Fig. 5.11 arises. Electrodes 1 and 2 are again sites on the endocardium and epicardium respectively. Suppose the TMP from site 1 differs in its time course, as well as at its time of onset, as compared to that at site 2. In ❯ Fig. 5.11a, it is assumed that the TMP at site 1 has half the magnitude of that at site 2, but otherwise is the same.

As the TMPs differ, there is no longer a period of time during the plateau when no potential difference exists between sites 1 and 2. Consequently, a current will flow intracellularly from site 2 to site 1 at time t_p, as shown diagrammatically in ❯ Fig. 5.11b. (Whether the current will flow all the way from the epicardium to the endocardium, or only across a much narrower region, will depend on the potential distribution between sites 1 and 2.) As there now exists an intracellular current, currents will flow extracellularly as well, as indicated by the flow I_e in ❯ Fig. 5.11b.

In the example shown, the current flow pattern will cause the extracellular potential to be relatively positive on the endocardium near site 1, and relatively negative on the epicardium near site 2 (❯ Fig. 5.11c). Consequently, ECGs recorded from a region overlying site 2 will be seen to have "ST-segment depression." Interpretations based on this kind of analysis are often used to explain ECGs recorded in patients with ischemic muscle regions and in those with recent infarctions. A widely examined analysis of ST potentials in relation to infarct size was developed by Maroko et al. [48].

It is worth noting that in ❯ Fig. 5.11a the action potentials also differ in potential during the baseline segments. Elevations or depressions of the "baseline" during the T-P interval with opposite polarity to those during the ST segment therefore occur [49]. However, most electrocardiographic recording systems use ac-coupled amplifiers. (Such amplifiers filter out dc voltages of tens of millivolts that are created at the electrochemical interface between the skin and body-surface electrodes.) Consequently, electrocardiographic records do not indicate whether voltages between surface electrodes are present during the "baseline" period. Analysis of ECGs is often based on conventions that assume that no currents or potentials exist prior to the P wave. Assuming that such potentials are not present when they are has the effect of increasing the magnitude of the change said to be present during the ST segment. An exaggerated change during ST comes about because individual tracings show correctly the difference between the baseline voltage and that during the ST segment (❯ Sect. 12.4.4.4.)

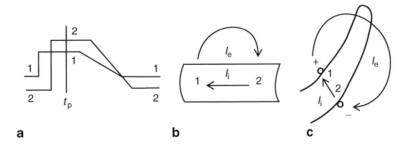

❑ Fig. 5.11
ST segment with non-uniform action potentials. (a) shows that site 2 has the same action-potential waveform as used in ❯ Fig. 5.10. In contrast, site 1 has an action potential that is reduced in magnitude, but otherwise the same. Now there is no time during the plateau when all intracellular sites have the same voltage. Consequently (b) shows an intracellular longitudinal current I_i; and extracellular current I_e flow at time t_p. If action potentials with reduced amplitude are present throughout an endocardial region near electrode 1, then (c) negative potentials will occur over the epicardial region and positive potentials over the endocardial one

5.9   T Wave

5.9.1   T Wave in the Case of Uniform Action Potential Duration

Repolarization of ventricular muscle fibers from active to resting transmembrane voltages produces the T wave. Since the voltage changes of repolarization traverse the same range as those of depolarization, except in the reverse direction, it is tempting to think of the T wave as depolarization in reverse. However, if this were true, all ECG wave forms observed during repolarization should have a reversed polarity compared to those during depolarization, with a lower amplitude and slower time course due to the much slower rate of repolarization (❯ Chap. 7). As this is not in agreement with experimental observations, this simple hypothesis must be rejected.

5.9.2   Normal T Waves

Because the signs of the T waves in the ECG do not all have the reversed polarity of the corresponding QRS complexes, the hypothesis of a uniform duration for all TMP wave forms must be wrong. What would be an alternative? Clearly this must be related to non-uniformity and/or local differences in TMP wave forms throughout the myocardium. The weight of available measurements from intact animals indicates that the duration of the action potential varies from endocardium to epicardium. More specifically, it appears that action potentials nearer the endocardium are longer. Moreover, Burgess et al. [50], using refractory period measurements in dogs, found that repolarization normally occurs later at the apex than toward the base. Somehow, based on such data, the notion has emerged that the timing of repolarization at the epicardium precedes that on the endocardium. However, the correct statement is that, generally, epicardial action-potential durations (APD) are shorter than those of the endocardium. The differences involved are not uniform for different parts of the ventricular myocardium, as it depends on the timing of depolarization and are different between LV and RV. More recently, different experimental studies have shown regression lines of APD as a function of local activation time having a slope of about −0.4 [51, 52]. The full consequence of this complexity in a full 3D model of the ventricular myocardium can only be worked out by using an advanced model of the sources during repolarization. An example of such a model-based analysis of T wave properties [53] is described in ❯ Chap. 7.

5.9.3   Intrinsic, Primary and Secondary T Waves

As described above, the excitation sequence interacts with the variation in action-potential duration from place to place.

What if there were no such interaction? In concept, the "intrinsic" T wave is the T wave that results if all cells in the ventricle depolarize simultaneously. An intrinsic T wave can be created experimentally by applying a large stimulus to the entire muscle simultaneously. The intrinsic T wave thereby occurs because of differences in action-potential duration from site to site.

Conversely, the "secondary" T wave was defined by Abildskov et al. [54] as the one necessary to make the ventricular gradient (see below) equal to zero, a condition that will be fulfilled if all myocytes have the same APD. Thereby, the secondary T wave occurs because of differences in action-potential onset. The secondary T wave, not a naturally occurring waveform, can be constructed numerically.

The "primary" T wave was defined by Abildskov et al. [54] as the difference between the actual T wave and the secondary T wave. Like the secondary T wave, it can be constructed numerically. If the actual T waves occur because of a mixture of the effects of the depolarization sequence and the effects of variations in action-potential duration, and if subtracting the secondary T wave is equivalent to subtracting the effects from the depolarization sequence, then it seems intuitively reasonable that the "primary T wave" is the same as the "intrinsic T wave." Horan et al. [55] examined the question of whether they were identical and found that the primary T wave approached identity with the intrinsic T wave. Failure of absolute congruence was attributed to the lack of a precise marker to provide precise time alignment between all waveforms.

At the present time, the intrinsic, primary, and secondary T waves are used mostly as concepts and constructions made in the course of better understanding the source of the actual T waves, rather than as waveforms routinely constructed for physiological or clinical interpretation.

5.9.4 Ventricular Gradient

Closely related to the different T waves discussed in the preceding section is the concept of the ventricular gradient. In 1934, Wilson et al. [56] introduced the idea that the area under the ventricular deflections of the ECG had a significance beyond that provided from a moment-by-moment evaluation. They determined the area under electrocardiographic curves during QRST, the ventricular deflections. In determining the area, "due care" was used to construct a baseline, as doing so was "a matter of greatest importance." Then the net area between the waveform and the baseline was found. Those portions of the area that lay below the baseline were considered negative and subtracted, while those that lay above the baseline were considered positive and added.

Wilson et al. concluded that if all action potentials had the same shape, magnitude and duration, the net area under each electrocardiographic deflection was zero. However, many waveforms showed net areas that were nonzero. In analyzing these waveforms, Wilson et al. looked principally at excitation sequences where action potentials from region to region varied at the onset and duration, but not otherwise. They concluded that any net area was a "measure of the effects produced by local variations in the excitatory process, and particularly by local variations in the duration of the excited state."

To analyze the differences in areas, Wilson et al. made use of Einthoven's triangle. In concept, ECGs were obtained from electrodes at the apices of an equilateral triangle, centered on the heart. (Actual electrodes were on the limbs.) Wilson et al. considered the vector formed by replacing the waveform at each apex with the waveform's net area. The vector was the one whose projection onto each side of the triangle gave the observed difference between apices. They considered, for example, the vector produced by a uniform gradient in the duration of the excited state. They concluded that the vector that "represents the effects produced by this gradient will point from the end of the fiber where the systole is longer to the end where it is shorter, and will have a length proportional to the difference in the length of systole at the two ends." Further, the vector remained unchanged for any excitation sequence if the duration of the excited systole at each site remained unchanged.

The idea that the differences in action-potential duration can be determined from body-surface waveforms has proved an intriguing object of theoretical study, as in the work of Burger [57] and Geselowitz [58]. Experimentally, QRST areas have been determined from many body-surface leads [59], aimed at relating these areas to arrhythmias. Over the years these investigations have refined the ventricular gradient concept, often presenting the refinements more unambiguously than the text descriptions of Wilson et al.

A mathematically precise presentation of the concepts of the ventricular gradient is as follows [60]. It is based on the well-founded notions on the genesis of bioelectric potentials listed below. These are referred to here as "properties."

- The generation of the potential differences outside a cell stems from biochemical processes at the cell membranes.
- The nature of these sources is that of a current generator [61].
- The volume conduction properties of tissues, however complex, are linear: the superposition principle applies.
- At any moment in time, any field generated in the extra-cellular domain stems from the spatial gradients of the TMPs, denoted as $V_m(\vec{r}, t)$, at source locations $\vec{r}$ [23].
- If all cells are completely polarized (at a constant value) the electric field set up by the sources in the surrounding medium is zero [23].

Taking the gradient of any scalar function involves computing spatial differences of the TMPs of individual cells, which is a linear operation. The application of the superposition principle is, again, a linear operation. Hence, the potential differences in the extra-cellular domain stem from a linear operator (superposition) acting on a linear operator (taking the gradient) acting on the TMPs. The cascade of two linear operations is also linear, hence: all external fields arise from a linear (spatial) operator acting on the TMPs of all myocytes. Expressing the strengths of all myocytes by matrix $\mathbf{V}_m$, with its rows representing the time courses of all individual TMPs, and its columns their instantaneous strengths, the linear operation involved, conveniently denoted by a matrix multiplication (❷ Sect. 2.A.1.3), is

$$\Phi = \mathbf{A} \mathbf{V}_m \tag{5.12}$$

This equation expresses the potentials in the extra-cellular domain, Φ, as the (matrix) multiplication of the TMPs $\mathbf{V}_m$ by the transfer matrix $\mathbf{A}$. Matrix $\mathbf{A}$ expresses all volume conduction effects, be it inhomogeneous or homogenous, isotropic or anisotropic. In words: the potential in any observation point ℓ (c.q. lead position), $\phi_l(t)$, is found to be a linear combination of the TMPs at that same instant of time. The weighting factors are the element of row ℓ of matrix $\mathbf{A}$.

From Prop.5 it follows that the sum of all elements of any row ℓ of this matrix is zero. Hence, when "feeding" the transfer matrix $\mathbf{A}$ with any constant column vector $\mathbf{c}$, a vector having identical elements c, the resulting potential is zero for all observation points, expressed in matrix terms:

$$\mathbf{A} \mathbf{c} = 0 \tag{5.13}$$

We now consider the integration over time (QRST interval) applied to the TMPs of all myocytes. The integral over time, the area under the curve, of the TMP of myocyte n is denoted as v_n, and the entire set of these integrals of all myocytes as the column vector $\mathbf{v}$. The effect of the corresponding integration over time of the potentials observed in lead ℓ, row ℓ of matrix Φ, (5.12), is denoted as $IQRST_\ell$. The set of all integrals constitutes a column vector $\mathbf{i}_{QRST}$. The result of the integration over time applied to both sides of (5.12) can thus be expressed as

$$\mathbf{i}_{QRST} = \mathbf{A} \mathbf{v} \tag{5.14}$$

Each myocytes n is assumed to be activated at depolarization time δ_n and, by taking the time of its maximal downward slope as a marker, to repolarize at time instant ρ_n. The corresponding activation recovery interval, ARI [62], is denoted as $\alpha_n = \rho_n - \delta_n$. For each myocyte, integral v_n depends on the value of its resting potential r_n, the magnitude of the upstroke of its action potential, u_n and its ARI value $\alpha_n = \rho_n - \delta_n$.

By considering action potentials having approximately the same shape (Assumption.1) it follows that for the integral of the TMP curve we may write $v_n = \alpha_n (r_n + u_n)$. In situations where both the upstroke (Assumption 2) and the resting potentials (Assumption 3) may be taken to have uniform values, each with integral c, it follows that for the complete set of QRST integrals at the field points we have

$$\mathbf{i}_{QRST} = c \mathbf{A} \boldsymbol{\alpha}, \tag{5.15}$$

which shows that, within the validity of the assumptions of uniform general shape, uniform upstroke and uniform resting potential, integrals over time of lead potentials are a linear combination of the individual ARI values of all myocytes.

The previous formulation can be refined. To this end we write the ARIs' column vector, $\boldsymbol{\alpha} = \bar{\boldsymbol{\alpha}} + \Delta\boldsymbol{\alpha}$ in which $\bar{\boldsymbol{\alpha}}$ denotes a column vector having all elements equal to the mean, $\bar{\alpha}$, of the individual values α_n, and $\Delta\boldsymbol{\alpha}$ denotes the column vector of all individual deviations α_n from their mean. Substitution of $\boldsymbol{\alpha} = \bar{\boldsymbol{\alpha}} + \Delta\boldsymbol{\alpha}$ into (5.15) then yields

$$\mathbf{i}_{QRST} = c \mathbf{A} (\bar{\boldsymbol{\alpha}} + \Delta\boldsymbol{\alpha}) = c \mathbf{A} \Delta\boldsymbol{\alpha} \tag{5.16}$$

Note that $\mathbf{A} \bar{\boldsymbol{\alpha}} = 0$ because of (5.13).

This analysis, (5.16), identifies the QRST integral of each lead signal as a linear combination of the elements of $\Delta\boldsymbol{\alpha}$. The weights are lead specific. The vector $\Delta\boldsymbol{\alpha}$ is the full representation of the total dispersion of APDs of all myocytes, and so the refinement of the statement following (5.15) is that the QRST integral of a lead signal is a linear combination of the elements of the dispersion of the action potential durations of all myocytes. The weights are lead specific.

In the case of the ventricular gradient introduced by Wilson, the "areas under the curve," $\mathbf{i}_{QRST}$ were derived from three signals only. The result was expressed as the ventricular gradient, a vector in 3D space. Equation (5.16) is a generalization of this concept, constituting a vector in L dimensional space. The concept of the ventricular gradient is seen to be meaningful only within the assumptions used in this analysis. The analysis may be extended to the interpretation of the QRS and STT integrals separately [60].

The magnitudes of the vectors representing the (QRS)(T)-integrals, are influenced by the transfer of the volume conductor: (differences in) heart position and orientation, as well as by thorax geometry. Since both vectors have passed through one and the same filter (matrix A), the angles involved are less sensitive to inter-individual differences in geometry. The angle β between any two L-dimensional vectors a and b in the plane they share follows from

$$\cos(\beta) = (a \cdot b)/(a \cdot b), \tag{5.17}$$

in which the dot indicates the sum of the product of all corresponding elements of vectors a and b, and a and b their lengths. If vectors a and b are referred to zero mean, the right hand side of (5.17) is the linear correlation coefficient between the elements of a and b. Both the angle β [63] and its cosine [64] have been tested as markers of repolarization abnormality.

5.10   U Wave

The U wave is a low amplitude, usually mono-phasic, ECG deflection directly following, and partly merged with, the T wave. Until recently, it has not received much attention in electrocardiographic literature. Many considered it a rarity, but in fact, by applying proper baseline correction procedures, it can be observed in almost all healthy subjects. Reasons for it having escaped notice are its low magnitude and a baseline correction performed at a premature timing.

Surawicz [65]described the U wave as a separate deflection of relatively low amplitude, usually detectable at slow or moderate heart rates, with an apex occurring about 100 ms following the end of the T wave. The U wave coincides with isovolumic relaxation. The presence, genesis and significance of the U wave have been a source of controversy. In part, the controversy has arisen because it is often hard to see U waves in experimental recordings in the presence of noise, as there is no clear demarcation between the end of T and the beginning of U or the onset of the P wave in the waveform of a given lead. The experimental difficulties are great, once causing Lepeschkin [66], who studied the U wave extensively, to remark jovially that the main question about the U wave is whether it exists or not.

In addition, differences of opinion have existed about the genesis of the U wave because various diastolic deflections recorded in local electrograms do not necessarily have the same timing as the U wave in human surface ECGs [66]. Such discrepancies are significant because the genesis of most other electrocardiographic deflections has been determined by comparing the timing of deflections on electrograms with those on the surface ECG.

There are two classic theories of U-wave genesis. Kishida et al. [67] describe these as follows. One theory attributes U-wave genesis to the repolarization of Purkinje fibers. The other theory attributes the U wave to potentials generated during relaxation of the ventricular myocardium.

Hoffman and Cranefield [12] argued in favor of the former-theory, saying "the action-potential of Purkinje fibers is considerably longer than that of ventricular muscle, and the phase of rapid repolarization of Purkinje fibers is coincident in time with the U wave."

Lepeschkin [66] discussed both theories extensively, but favored the latter, as did Surawicz [65]. Surawicz said that mechano-electrical coupling was the most likely cause of the U wave, because "it has been shown that stretch prolongs terminal repolarization in single fibers" [68], and "therefore may be expected to produce an ECG deflection after the T wave." Changes from a more stressed apex to a less stressed base, the "stretch gradient theory," are thought to result in different potentials between those regions, and thereby the U wave.

More recently, explanations based on the expression of mid-cardial myocytes [69], after-potentials [70] and late repolarization [71] have appeared in the literature.

Whatever its origin, Kishida et al. [67] described a negative U wave as highly specific for the presence of heart disease, most commonly systemic hypertension, aortic and mitral regurgitation, and ischemic heart disease.

5.11   Vectorial and Other Interpretations of the ECG

Analysis of the generation of ECGs has been accomplished within a number of frameworks having substantial conceptual differences. Most have focused on QRS. Many investigators from the time of the early electrocardiographers until the present day have analyzed ventricular excitation from the viewpoint of thinking of the electrical activity of the heart as coming from a single "equivalent" dipole. This is a hypothetical current source that, when placed inside a homogeneous volume conductor, would generate the potential field on the surface of the thorax that most closely resembles the measured field. To this end its position, strength and orientation are tuned.

That the field generated by a complex current generator such as the heart can be approximated by that of a single dipole stems from the theory of multipoles [72]. That theory shows that an "equivalent dipole" will closely approximate the infinite medium potentials at distances like that of the body surface as the heart itself. However, because some of the cardiac surface comes close to the chest, the theory can be applied only as a first approximation. It appears that many early investigators considered the errors involved in approximating real cardiac potentials with those from a single equivalent dipole to be small [73]. For the full time course of the potential field during the QRS complex, the relative difference RD, defined as the RMS difference between the potentials generated by the equivalent dipole and the measured ones relative to the RMS value of the measured ones, is of the order of $RD = 0.2$. For more obese subjects the error tends to be lower, for lean subjects it is higher.

In more recent years, experimental evidence, particularly from body-surface maps [74], has demonstrated unequivocally that no single dipole can be "equivalent" in the sense of accurately reproducing the body-surface observations. As a result, multiple-dipole models of cardiac excitation were proposed, particularly by Barber and Fischman [75] and Selvester et al. [76]. Multiple-dipole models conceptually divide the ventricular muscle into several regions. Such models envisage each imaginary dipole as functioning "equivalently," in an electrical sense, to one region. Such models have been used very effectively, as by Ritsema van Eck [77] and, later, Miller and Geselowitz [78]. In this way it was shown how electrocardiographic changes observed on the body surface result from plausible alterations in cardiac action potentials and their timing. An interactive simulation package for studying such effects, including a demonstration of vector properties, has been made available from the internet [79].

A major weakness of both single- and multiple-dipole models springs from their being imaginary "equivalent" entities. The equivalence is, even in concept, an equivalence at a distance from the source only. This follows directly from (5.3), which shows that close to the dipole the potential may be infinite. Consequently, the currents and potentials near the active muscle may behave quite differently from those of an equivalent dipole, even if there may be a fair "equivalence" on the body surface. For a full discussion on this point, see ❷ Chaps. 8 and ❷ 9.

5.12 Evaluation

The fact that electrocardiography has been in use for more than a century leads one to think that most aspects of the relationships between the electrocardiographic waveforms and the underlying cardiac events would have been fully established by now. However, that is not the case. One of the main reasons is that acquiring accurate measurements of what is taking place electrically within the heart remains very difficult. This is particularly so when the volume conductor is intact. Recent years have seen marked changes in the recognition of the importance of anisotropies within the cardiac muscle, the quality of the quantitative descriptions of volume conductor behavior and the ability to link together such knowledge by means of numerical models. As the full weight of an improved understanding of the genesis of ECGs comes to bear fruit, further significant improvements in the quality and value of electrocardiographic interpretation are to be expected.

References

1. Waller, A., A demonstration on man of the electromotive changes accompanying the heart's beat. *J. Physiol.*, 1887;**8**: 229–234.
2. Einthoven; 100 Years of Electrocardiography, in M.J. Schalij, M.J. Janse, A. van Oosterom, V.D.W.E.E. and H.J.J. Wellens, Editors. Leiden: The Einthoven Foundation, 2002, pp. 616.
3. Burch, G.E. and N.P. DePasquale, *A History of Electrocardiography*, Chicago: Illinois, 1964.
4. Johnson, J.C. and N.C. Flowers, History of electrocardiography and vectorcardiography, in *The Theoretical Basis of Electrocardiology*, C.V. Nelson, and D.B. Geselowitz, Editors. Oxford, Clarendon Press, 1976.
5. Einthoven, W., Un nouveau galvanometer. *Arch. Neerl. Sci. Exactes Nat.*, 1901;**6**: 625–633.
6. Einthoven, W. and K. de Lint, Ueber das normale menschliche Elektrokardiogram und Uber die capillar-elektrometrische

Untersuchung einiger Herzkranken. *Pflugers Arch. Ges. Physiol.*, 1900;**80**: 139–160.

7. Lewis, T., J. Meakins, and P.D. White, The excitatory process in the dog's heart. Part I-The auricles. *Phil. Trans. R. Soc. London Ser. B.*, 1914;**205**: 375–420.

8. Lewis, T. and M.A. Rothschild, The excitatory process in the dog's heart. Part II. *Phil. Trans. R. Soc. London Ser. B.*, 1915;**206**: 181–226.

9. Wilson, F.N., F.D. Johnston, A.G. MacLeod, and P.S. Barker. Electrocardiograms that represent the potential variations of a single electrode. *Am. Heart. J.*, 1934;**9**: 447–458.

10. Ling, G. and R.W. Gerard, The normal membrane potential of frog sartorius fibers. *J. Cellular Comp. Physiol.*, 1949;**34**: 383–396.

11. Woodbury, L.A., H.H. Hecht, and A.R. Christopherson, Membrane resting and action potentials of single cardiac muscle fibers of the frog ventricle. *Am. J. Physiol.*, 1951;**164**: 307–318.

12. Hoffman, B.F. and P.F. Cranefield, *Electrophysiology of the Heart*. New York: McGraw-Hil, 1960.

13. Netter, F.H., *Heart*, vol **5**. New York: CIBA, 1969.

14. Hodgkin, A.L. and A.F. Huxley, A quantitative description of the membrane current and its application to conduction and excitation in nerve. *J. Physiol.*, 1952;**117**: 500–544.

15. Beeler, G.W. and H. Reuter, Reconstruction of the action potential of ventricular myocardial fibers. *J. Physiol. (London)*, 1977;**268**: 177–210.

16. Ebihara, L. and E.A. Johnson, Fast sodium current in cardiac muscle. A quantitative description, *Biophysical Journal*, 1980;**32**: 779–790.

17. DiFrancesco, D. and D. Noble, A model of cardiac electrical activity incorporating ionic pumps and concentration changes. *Phil. Trans. R. Soc. London Ser. B.*, 1985;**307**: 353–398.

18. Luo, C. and Y. Rudy, A dynamic model of the cardiac ventricular action potential. I. Simulation of ionic currents and concentration changes. *Circ. Res.*, 1994;**74**: 1071–1096.

19. Courtemanche, M., R.J. Ramirez, and S. Nattel, Ionic mechanisms underlying human atrial action potential properties: Insights from a mathematical model. *Am. J. Physiol.*, 1998;**275**: 301–321.

20. Spach, M.S. and M.J. Kootsey, Relating the sodium current and conductance to the shape of transmembrane and extracellular potentials by simulation: Effects of propagation boundaries. *IEEE Trans. Biomed. Eng.*, 1985;**BME-32**: 743–755.

21. Plonsey, R. and R.C. Barr, Mathematical modeling of electrical activity of the heart. *J. Electrocardiol.*, 1987;**20**: 219–226.

22. Plonsey, R. and R.C. Barr, *Bioelectricity: A Quantitative Approach*. New York: Springer, 2007.

23. Wilson, F.N., A.G. Macleod, and P.S. Barker, The distribution of action currents produced by the heart muscle and other excitable tissues immersed in conducting media. *J. Gen. Physiol.*, 1933;**16**: 423–456.

24. Holland, R.P. and M.F. Arnsdorf, Solid angle theory and the electrocardiogram: physiologic and quantitative interpretations. *Prog. Cardiovasc. Dis.*, 1977;**19**: 431–457.

25. Goldman, M.J., *Principles of Clinical Electrocardiography*, 10 ed. Los Altos: Lange, 1979.

26. Scher, A.M., A.C. Young, A.L. Malmgren, and R.R. Paton, Spread of electrical activity through the wall of the ventricle. *Cardiovasc. Res.*, 1953;**1**: 539–547.

27. Sano, T., N. Takayama, and T. Shimamoto, Directional differences of conduction velocity in the cardiac ventricular syncytium studied by microelectrodes. *Circ. Res.*, 1959; **VII**: 262–267.

28. Spach, M.S. and R.C. Barr, Origin of epicardial ST-T wave potentials in the intact dog. *Circ. Res.*, 1976;**39**(4): 475–487, (1978).

29. Burger, H.C., The zero of potential: A persistent error. *Am. Heart J.*, 1955;**49**: 581–586.

30. Geselowitz, D.B., The zero of potential. *IEEE Engineering in Medicine and Biology Magazine*, 1998;**17**: 128–132.

31. van Oosterom, A., Solidifying the solid angle. *J. Electrocardiol.*, 2002;**35S**: 181–192.

32. Kondo, M., V. Nesterenko, and C. Antzelevitch, Cellular basis for the monophasic action potential. Which electrode is the recording electrode? *Cardiovasc. Res.*, 2004;**62**: 635–644.

33. Vigmond, E.J., The electrophysiological basis of MAP recordings. *Cardiovasc. Res.*, 2005;**68**: 502–503.

34. Scher, A.M., and Excitation of the heart, in *The theoretical basis of electrocardiology*, C.V. Nelson, and D.B. Geselowitz, Editors. Oxford: Clarendon Press, 1976: 44–69

35. James, T.N., The connecting pathways between the sinus node and A-V node and between the right and the left atrium in the human heart. *Am. Heart J.*, 1963;**66**: 498–508.

36. Puech, P., *L'activite electrique auriculaire normale et pathologique*, Paris: Masson et Cie, 1956.

37. Spach, M.S., M. Lieberman, J.G. Scott, R.C. Barr, E.A. Johnson, and J.M. Kootsey, Excitation sequences of the atrial septum and the AV node in isolated hearts of the dog and rabbit. *Circ. Res*, 1971;**29**: 156–172.

38. Sano, T., Conduction in the heart, in *The theoretical basis of electrocardiology*, C.V. Nelson and D.B. Geselowitz, Editors. Oxford: Clarendon Press, 1976.

39. Spach, M.S., R.C. Barr, R.B. Warren, D.W. Benson, A. Walston, and S.B. Edwards, Isopotential body surface mapping in subjects of all ages: emphasis on low-level potentials with analysis of the method. *Circulation*, 1979;**59**: 805–821.

40. Mirvis, D.M., Body surface distribution of electrical potential during atrial depolarization and repolarization. *Circulation*, 1980;**62**: 167–173.

41. Ihara, Z., A. van Oosterom, and R. Hoekema, Atrial repolarization as observable during the PQ interval. *J. Electrocardiol.*, 2006;**39**(3): 290–297.

42. van Oosterom, A. and V. Jacquemet, Genesis of the P wave: Atrial signals as generated by the equivalent double layer source model. *Europace*, 2005;**7**: S21–S29.

43. Berbari, E.J., R. Lazzara, P. Samet, and B.J. Scherlag, Noninvasive technique for detection of electrical activity during the PR segment. *Circulation*, 1973;**48**: 1005–1013.

44. Flowers, N.C., R.C. Hand, P.C. Orander, C.B. Miller, M. Walden, and L.G. Horan, Surface recording of electrical activity from the region of the bundle of His. *Am. J. Cardiol.*, 1974;**33**: 384–389.

45. Flowers, N.C., V. Shvartsman, H.L.G.P. Palakurthy, G. S. Som, and M. R. Sridharan, Analysis of PR subintervals in normal subjects and early studies in patients with abnormalities of the conduction system using surface His bundle recordings. *J. Am. Coll. Cardiol.*, 1983;**2**: 939–946.

46. Helm, R.A., Electrocardiographic cancellation. Mathematical basis. *Am. Heart J.*, 1960;**60**: 251–265.

47. Spach, M.S., R.C. Barr, D.W. Benson, Walston, and S.B. Edwards, Body surface low-level potentials during repolarization with analysis of the ST segment. *Circulation*, 1979; **59/4**: 822–836.

48. Maroko, P.R., P. Libby, J.W. Covell, B.E. Sobel, J.J. Ross, and E. Braunwald, Precordial S-T segment elevation mapping: An atraumatic method for assessing alterations in the extent of myocardial ischemic injury. *Am. J. Cardiol.*, 1972;**29**: 223–230.

49. Janse, M.J., F.J.L.V. Capelle, H. Morsink, A.G. Kléber, F. Wilms-Schopman, C.N. d'Alnoncourt, and D.D. Durrer, Flow of injury current and patterns of excitation during ventricular arrhythmias in acute regional myocardial ischemia in isolated porcine and canine hearts. *Circ. Res.*, 1980;**47**: 151–165.

50. Burgess, M.J., L.S. Green, K. Millar, R. Wyatt, and J.A. Abildskov, The sequence of normal ventricular recovery. *Am. Heart J.*, 1972;**84**(5): 660–669.

51. Franz, M.R., K. Bargheer, W. Rafflenbeul, A. Haverich, and P.R. Lichtlen, Monophasic action potential mapping in a human subject with normal electrograms: Direct evidence for the genesis of the T wave, *Circulation*, 1987;**75**/2: 379–386.

52. Cowan, J.C., C.J. Hilton, C.J. Griffiths, S. Tansuphaswadikul, J.P. Bourke, A. Murray, and R.W.F. Campbell, Sequence of epicardial repolarization and configuration of the T wave. *Br. Heart J.*, 1988;**60**: 424–433.

53. van Oosterom, A., Genesis of the T-wave as based on an equivalent surface source model. *J. Electrocardiol.*, 2001;**34S**: 217–227.

54. Abildskov, J.A., M.J. Burgess, M.J. Millar, R. Wyatt, and R. Baule, The primary T wave- a new electrocardiographic waveform. *Am. Heart J.*, 1971;**81/2**: 242–249.

55. Horan, L.G., R.C. Hand, J.C. Johnson, M.R. Sridharan, T.B. Rankin, and N.C. Flowers, A theoretical examination of ventricular repolarization and the secondary T wave. *Circ. Res.*, 1978;**42/6**: 750–757.

56. Wilson, F.N., A.G. Macleod, P.S. Barker, and F.D. Johnston, The determination and significance of the areas of the ventricular deflections of the electrocardiogram. *Am. Heart J.*, 1934;**10**: 46–61.

57. Burger, H.C., A theoretical elucidation of the notion: Ventricular gradient. *Am. Heart J.*, 1957;**53/2**: 240–246.

58. Geselowitz, D.B., The ventricular gradient revisited: Relation to the area under the action potentials. *IEEE Trans. Biomed. Eng.*, 1983;BME-**30/1**: 76–77.

59. Abildskov, J.A., P. Urie, R. Lux, M.J. Burgess, and R. Wyatt, Body surface distribution of QRST area. *Adv. Cardiol.*, 1978;**21**: 59–64.

60. van Oosterom, A., Reflections on T waves, in *Advances in Electrocardiology*, M. Hiraoka, S. Ogawa, I. Kodama, I. Hiroshi, H. Kasnuki, and T. Katoh, Editors. New Jersey, World Scientific, 2005, pp. 807–815.

61. Plonsey, R., An extension of the solid angle formulation for an active cell. *Biophysical J.*, 1965;**5**: 663–666.

62. Haws, C.W., and R.L. Lux, Correlation between in vivo transmembrane action potential durations and activation-recovery intervals from electrograms. *Circulation*, 1990;**81/1**: 281–288.

63. Kardys, I., J.A. Kors, I.M. van der Meer, A. Hofman, D.A.M. van der Kuip, and J.C.M. Witteman, Spatial QRS-T angle predicts cardiac death in a general population. *Eur. Heart J.*, 2003;**24**: 1357–1364.

64. Zabel, M., B. Acar, T. Klingenheber, M.A. Franz, S.H. Holenlozer, and M. Malik, Analysis of 12-lead T-wave morphology for risk stratification after myocardial infarction. *Circulation*, 2000;**102**: 1252–1257.

65. Surawicz, B., U wave - the controversial genesis and the clinical significance. *Jpn. Heart J.*, 1982;**23**(suppl.I): 17–22.

66. Lepeschkin, E., Physiologic basis of the U wave, in *Advances in Electrocardiography*, R.C. Schlant and J.W. Hurst, Editors. New York, Grune and Stratton, 1972.

67. Kishida, H., J.S. Cole, and B. Surawicz, Negative U wave: A highly specific but poorly understood sign of heart d disease. *Am. J. Cardiol.*, 1982;**49**: 2030–2036.

68. Lab, M.J., Mechanically dependent changes in action potentials recorded from the intact frog ventricle. *Circ. Res.*, 1978;**42**: 519–528.

69. Antzelevitch, C., and S. Sicouri, Clinical relevance of cardiac arrhythmias generated by after-depolarsations: Role of M-cells in the generation of U-waves, triggered activity and torsade de pointes. *J. Am. Coll. Cardiol.*, 1994;**23**: 259–277.

70. di Bernardo, D., and A. Murray, Origin on the electrocardiogram of U-waves and abnormal U-wave inversion. *Cardiovasc. Res.*, 2002;**53**: 202–208.

71. Ritsema van Eck, H., J.A. Kors, and G. van Herpen, The U wave in the electrocardiogram: A solution for a 100-year-old riddle. *Cardiovasc. Res.*, 2005;**67**: 256–262.

72. Geselowitz, D.B., Multipole representation for an equivalent cardiac generator. *Proc. IRE*, 1960, pp. 75–79.

73. Frank, E., Absolute quantitative comparison of instantaneous QRS equipotentials on a normal subject with dipole potentials on a homogeneous torso model. *Circ. Res.*, 1955;**3**: 243–251.

74. Taccardi, B., Distribution of heart potentials on the thoracic surface of normal human subjects. *Circ. Res.*, 1963;**12**: 341–352.

75. Barber, M.R., and E.J. Fischmann, Heart dipole regions and the measurement of dipole moment. *Nature*, 1961;**192**: 141–142.

76. Selvester, R.H., J.C. Solomon, and T.L. Gillespie, Digital computer model of a total body electrocardiographic surface map. An adult male-torso stimulation with lungs. *Circulation*, 1968;**38**: 684–690.

77. Ritsema van Eck, H.J., *Digital Simulation of Cardiac Excitation and Depolarization*, PhD. thesis. Halifax, NS, Canada, Dalhousie University, 1972.

78. Miller, W.T., and D.B. Geselowitz, Simulation studies of the electrocardiogram. I. The normal heart. *Circ. Res.*, 1978;**43**: 301–315.

79. van Oosterom, A., and T.F. Oostendorp, ECGSIM: An interactive tool for studying the genesis of QRST waveforms. *Heart*, 2004;**90**: 165–168.

Part III

Mathematical Modeling

6 Macroscopic Source Descriptions

A. van Oosterom

P. W. Macfarlane et al. (eds.), *Basic Electrocardiology*, DOI 10.1007/978-0-85729-871-3_6,
© Springer-Verlag London Limited 2012

6.1   Introduction

Throughout the cardiac cycle, the cells of the heart deliver varying amounts of electric current to the surrounding tissues. The effect of these currents at the body's surface is the production of potentials which change continuously during the course of a heartbeat. In attempting to understand the nature of these body-surface potentials, various models have been postulated. These models describe the electrical sources and the volume conductor in which these sources are embedded, i.e., the human torso.

The computation of the potential distribution at the body surface based on such modeling assumptions is called the "forward problem of electrocardiography" (❯ Chap. 8). Its solution is a prerequisite for the solution of a problem of more direct clinical interest, the so-called "inverse problem of electrocardiography." By this is meant the study of the electrical state of the heart through analysis of the potentials at the body surface (❯ Chap. 9). Since this problem has no unique solution, it is imperative that constraints be imposed on the description of the source, i.e., the electrical generators of the heart.

Two different classes of source descriptions can be distinguished. The first class is that of the equivalent generators of physics (❯ Chaps. 2 and ❯ 8) in which sources like the single dipole (vectorcardiography), the single moving dipole, multiple dipoles or multipoles are used. Theoretically, these generator models allow a unique determination of their strength from observed body-surface potentials but the link with cellular electrophysiology is not straightforward (❯ Sect. 5.11).

The second class is that of macroscopic source descriptions. These form an *intermediate* step between the cellular activity and the electric field within the heart muscle at a scale of, say, 1 cm, which is small in comparison with heart size but large in comparison with cell size. The justification for this approach is that the total number of cells involved in the genesis of the ECG is so large (10^{10}) that it prohibits the consideration of the contribution by each individual cell. Formulations of macroscopic equivalent generators aim at representing as much as is feasible (and known) of cellular morphology in a source description of the potential field at a distance that is, say, ten times that of the length of a single myocyte.

This class of macroscopic source descriptions is the subject of this chapter. A major part of the chapter is devoted to the discussion of the classic model for the description of the electric sources during ventricular depolarization: the uniform double layer (UDL). The expression of the potential field is worked out by using the solid angle theory. The objective of the detailed analysis of this classic source model is to illustrate the potential fields and associated signals that are generated by this source. This forms the essential background for a discussion on its validity and usefulness.

A generalization of the UDL source model that permits the modeling of the sources during repolarization, is discussed in ❯ Chap. 7.

The formulations are mainly cast in terms of homogeneous, isotropic configurations. The effect of anisotropy is discussed only briefly. More complete models, in which the anisotropy of the ventricular wall is incorporated, are treated in ❯ Chap. 8.

6.2   Estimation of Macroscopic Cardiac Sources

The true cellular electrical generators are the biochemical processes that are active at the level of the cell membrane (❯ Chap. 3). A macroscopic equivalent source model is a description of the cellular electrical generator which results in a potential field in the exterior of the cell which, on a macroscopic scale, is indistinguishable from the observed potential field. From a known description of the electric sources, the potentials at some distance from the sources can be determined by applying the laws of electric current flow. The implied so-called forward problem of finding the potentials has a unique solution that can be computed for all types of source complexity.

The current sources actually generating the observed potentials are in general not amenable to direct observation, they need to be *derived* from observed potential differences.

The slow progress that has been made in the application of source models can be linked to the fact that the corresponding inverse computation, the determination of sources from the observed potentials, generally does *not* have a unique solution. This doom that lies over the inverse problem is fundamental and cannot be solved, as was pointed out as early as 1853 by von Helmholtz [1], even long before electrocardiology was "invented." The only way out of this problem is to postulate *in advance* a source description, a source *model*, and to merely be content with establishing the parameters (specifications) of this source on the basis of the observed potentials. The inverse problem subsequently constitutes a parameter estimation problem.

The transfer between the sources and the potentials is dominated by the geometry of the source-observation point configuration and by the entire spatial distribution of the electric conductivities of the body tissues. The doom on the inverse problem [1] now crops up again: the spreading out of electric currents diminishes the potentials in the medium and diffuses the image of the sources the further one moves away from the sources. This doom not only lies on the interpretation of potentials observed on the body surface but also on those observed inside the heart (myocardium; cavities).

For a diagnostic application, the source description should preferably have a direct physiological significance and, hence, one would like to include as much as is possible of the complexity of the relevant physiological details that have become available through invasive studies. However, the further one moves away from the source, the more sober the a priori source specification has to be, demanding a parsimonious use of source parameters. If a more abundant source specification is postulated, the correspondence – in forward computations – between observed data and computed potentials may improve, but in the related inverse problem the confidence intervals of the estimated parameters become unacceptably large. Although one may wish to include the reality of rotating, non-uniform, anisotropic myocardial conductivity in the analysis, in the ultimate, clinical application of the models the accuracy of the relevant parameters values is usually insufficient.

The analysis presented in this chapter relates to sober source descriptions, with parameters derived from sober models of the conducting medium surrounding the source while computing the potential field.

6.3 Equivalent Sources of the Membrane

6.3.1 The Single Cell

We first consider a model for the potential field generated by a single cell situated in an infinite medium of homogeneous, isotropic electrical conductivity σ_e (unit: S m^{-1}), ❯ Fig. 6.1, and we take the potential at infinity to be zero (❯ Sect. 2.5).

The interior of the cell (the axoplasma) is assumed to be a passive conductor having a homogeneous, isotropic electrical conductivity σ_i. The interior and exterior of the cell are separated by the membrane, which is bounded by two surfaces: S_i and S_e. All active (biochemical) electric sources are considered to be lying between these two surfaces. Using standard results from potential theory and realistic estimates of the membrane properties, it can be shown [2–4] that the potential $\Phi(\vec{r}')$ at a field point $\vec{r}'$ (observation point, with reference to the origin at $\vec{O}$) in the exterior medium is

$$\Phi(\vec{r}') = -\frac{1}{4\pi\sigma_e} \int_S (\sigma_i \Phi_i - \sigma_e \Phi_e) d\omega \tag{6.1}$$

The surface S lies just between the surfaces S_i and S_e. It specifies the entire configuration since, at a macroscopic scale, the membrane can be considered to be infinitesimally thin. The potentials Φ_i and Φ_e denote the potentials just inside

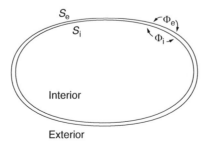

❑ Fig. 6.1
Configuration of a single cell, used for evaluating the external potential field

6

and outside this surface, respectively. The term $d\omega$ of (6.1) is the solid angle of element dS of the membrane surface S subtended at $\vec{r}'$, $\frac{\vec{R} \bullet d\vec{S}}{R^3}$, with $d\vec{S}$ pointing outward and $\vec{R} = \vec{r}' - \vec{r}$ directed from the source locations $\vec{r}$ on the membrane to field point $\vec{r}'$ (❯ Sect. 2.5.2.2).

The expression $\sigma_i\Phi_i - \sigma_e\Phi_e$ in (6.1) is a generalization of the concepts introduced by Wilson et al. [5], which formed the basis for the solid angle theory as used in theoretical electrocardiography. The expression can be identified as the strength of an (equivalent) double layer. It expresses a current dipole density per unit area M_S; with unit: A m^{-1}, as discussed in ❯ Sect. 2.5.2.2. This shows that the basic cardiac electric generator must be viewed as a *current* source [3], which justifies the use of the superposition principle when computing the potential field generated by multiple sources. When placed in an infinite medium, this virtual, equivalent double layer determines the potential field external to the cell. The double layer is directed normal to the membrane surface and has a strength that depends on transmembrane potential differences *as well as* on differences in the electric conductivities at either side of the membrane.

When an isolated cell is completely polarized, the transmembrane voltage $V_m = \Phi_i - \Phi_e$ is constant ($V_m \sim -80\,\text{mV}$) over the entire closed surface of the membrane and the double-layer strength is uniform over this surface. Hence, in the exterior region the potential field is zero. This follows from

$$\Phi(\vec{r}') = \frac{-1}{4\pi\sigma_e}(\sigma_i\Phi_i - \sigma_e\Phi_e)\int_S d\omega = 0 \tag{6.2}$$

since $\int_S d\omega = 0$ for any observation point $\vec{r}'$ exterior to any closed surface S, as is discussed in ❯ Sect. 2.5.1.2.

Similarly, when the cell is completely depolarized, V_m is uniform over the closed surface of the membrane ($V_m \sim 5\,\text{mV}$), and the potential in the exterior region is, again, zero.

When the cell is partly depolarized, the potential in the exterior region can only be determined through integration as in (6.1). An instructive approximation of this case is to consider the field due to an elongated membrane, with an idealized transmembrane potential that is constant over both the depolarized section and over the section which is still at rest, i.e., polarized, with potential values of $V_d \sim +5\,\text{mV}$ and $V_p \sim -80\,\text{mV}$, respectively (❯ Figs. 5.5 and ❯ 6.2).

In this case, the potential in the region exterior to the cell is approximately equal to that generated (in the homogeneous medium) by a double-layer source of strength $(V_d - V_p)\sigma_i$ placed at cross-section A. The exterior potential at $\vec{r}'$ generated by this equivalent source is

$$\Phi(\vec{r}') = \frac{1}{4\pi\sigma_e}\sigma_i(V_d - V_p)\,\Omega\,(\vec{r}'), \tag{6.3}$$

with $\Omega(\vec{r}')$ the solid angle subtended by cross-section A, with area A, at observation point $\vec{r}'$ (❯ Fig. 6.3). The membrane is shown by dashed lines, as a reminder that the equivalent source at cross-section A is active in the infinite medium. Since V_p is negative, $V_d - V_p$ is positive and the equivalent dipole has the same direction as the propagation.

The approximation involved assumes $\sigma_i\Phi_i \gg \sigma_e\Phi_e$. For this situation (6.3) can be explained as follows. We first place virtual double layers of equal strength V_d, but having opposite orientations, at cross-section A. One of these two has the same strength as that of the membrane to the left of A. Together these form a closed surface, which produces a zero external potential field. Next we repeat the same process for the region to the right of A, now with virtual double-layer

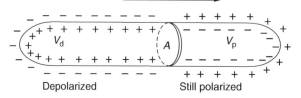

■ Fig. 6.2

Simplified diagram of an elongated cell which is activated from left to right. The cross-section A closes the depolarized zone (*left*) and the region still at rest (*right*)

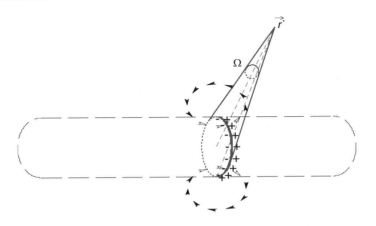

◼ Fig. 6.3
Equivalent source for the partly depolarized cell shown in ❷ Fig. 6.2. The arrowheads indicate the direction of local current flow

strengths of V_p. Here again, one of these virtual layers forms a closed surface, now to the right of A, having a uniform strength and, hence, producing a zero external field. The remaining two virtual double layers form the double layer as shown in ❷ Fig. 6.3, having the effective source strength implied in (6.3).

For distal observation points this expression (6.3), may be simplified further by using the approximation

$$\Omega\left(\vec{r}'\right) \sim \frac{\vec{A} \bullet \vec{R}}{R^3},$$

with $\vec{R}$ a vector of magnitude R pointing from the center of the disk A to observation point $\vec{r}'$, and $\vec{A}$ a vector of magnitude A directed towards the region of the cell that is still polarized. In this case,

$$\Phi(\vec{r}') = \frac{1}{4\pi\sigma_e} \frac{\sigma_i\left(V_d - V_p\right)\vec{A} \bullet \vec{R}}{R^3} \qquad (6.4)$$

The term $\sigma_i\left(V_d - V_p\right)\vec{A}$ can be identified as a current dipole $\vec{D}$ (❷ Sect. 2.5.1.2), pointing towards the zone that is still at rest; thus

$$\Phi(\vec{r}') = \frac{1}{4\pi\sigma_e} \frac{\vec{D} \bullet \vec{R}}{R^3} \qquad (6.5)$$

The plus and minus signs in ❷ Figs. 6.2 and ❷ 6.3 serve to indicate the sign of local potential differences across the membrane and the virtual double layer, respectively. In some text books on this subject the associated membrane charge is erroneously used to explain the external field in terms of electrostatics, rather than in the required terms of equivalent current generators demanded by electrical volume conduction theory (❷ Chap. 2).

6.3.2   The Single Fiber

The conditions for the application of (6.3) are not usually met in practice. For long fibers, the situation is never such as depicted in ❷ Fig. 6.2, but much more like that indicated in ❷ Fig. 6.4 for propagated activation along a fiber, where the transmembrane potential is different along the length of the fiber. At the time instant shown the segment on the left is in different stages of recovery of polarization, in the middle part various, successive stages of depolarization are present; the segment on the right is still at rest, i.e., polarized.

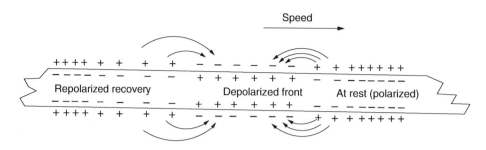

□ Fig. 6.4
Schematized, propagating depolarization and repolarization along an elongated fiber

To find the potential at $\vec{r}'$ in this situation we return to the general expression (6.1), while assuming the transmembrane potential difference to be a function of the distance ℓ along the fiber only (axial symmetric distribution). Moreover, we define $M_S(\ell)$ as

$$M_S(\ell) = -(\sigma_i \Phi_i(\ell) - \sigma_e \Phi_e(\ell)) \tag{6.6}$$

The term $d\omega$ of (6.1) relates to the membrane element $\vec{R} \bullet d\vec{S}/R^3$, with $d\vec{S}$ an element of the membrane defined as pointing outward, and $\vec{R}$ directed from the source locations on the membrane to field point $\vec{r}'$, so we need to evaluate

$$\Phi(\vec{r}') = \frac{1}{4\pi\sigma_e} \int_S M_S(\ell) \frac{\vec{R}}{R^3} \bullet d\vec{S} \tag{6.7}$$

To this end we apply Gauss' divergence theorem (2.26), to the integral in (6.7), which yields

$$\int_S M_S(\ell) \frac{\vec{R}}{R^3} \bullet d\vec{S} = \int_V \nabla \bullet \left(M_S(\ell) \frac{\vec{R}}{R^3} \right) dv = \int_V \nabla M_S(\ell) \bullet \frac{\vec{R}}{R^3} dv + \int_V M_S(\ell) \nabla \bullet \frac{\vec{R}}{R^3} dv \tag{6.8}$$

(using (2.29)). The second integral on the right is zero since

$$\nabla \bullet \frac{\vec{R}}{R^3} = \nabla \bullet \nabla \frac{1}{R} = \nabla^2 \frac{1}{R},$$

and any integral including the latter is zero for non-zero values of R, which is the case for external observation points (❯ Sect. 2.6.4.1), and so we find

$$\Phi(\vec{r}') = \frac{1}{4\pi\sigma_e} \int_V \frac{\partial M_S(\ell)}{\partial \ell} \frac{\ell' - \ell}{R^3} dv = \frac{1}{4\pi\sigma_e} \int_L \int_{S_\ell} \frac{\partial M_S(\ell)}{\partial \ell} \frac{\ell' - \ell}{R^3} dS \, d\ell \tag{6.9}$$

where ℓ' is the coordinate of the external field point $\vec{r}'$ along an axis parallel to the fiber. The first integral is taken over length L of the fiber, the second one over the cross-section of the fiber at location ℓ.

We now take the gradient of the function $M_S(\ell)$ to be uniform over the cross-section S_ℓ and, hence, the integration over this surface yields $\Omega(\ell; \vec{r}')$, the solid angle subtended at an external field point $\vec{r}'$ by S_ℓ, a disk with an area of πa^2, with a the radius of the fiber (❯ Sect. 5.3.4), and so (6.9) reduces to

$$\Phi(\vec{r}') = \frac{1}{4\pi\sigma_e} \int_L \frac{\partial M_S(\ell)}{\partial \ell} \Omega(\ell; \vec{r}') \, d\ell \tag{6.10}$$

Equation (6.10) generally holds true, and may also be used if the fiber is curved. In these circumstances the variable ℓ must be taken to be the length traveled along the fiber.

For remote field points and a straight fiber, the solid angle $\Omega(\ell; \vec{r}')$ may be approximated by

$$\Omega(\ell; \vec{r}') \approx \pi a^2 \frac{\ell' - \ell}{R^3}, \tag{6.11}$$

in which $R = \sqrt{(\ell' - \ell)^2 + y'^2 + z'^2}$, with the fiber coordinate ℓ taken to be lined up along the x-axis.

The result expressed by (6.10), which was derived from general membrane properties (6.1), is identical to the result expressed by (5.7), derived from the linear core-conductor model expressed by (5.1).

6.3.3 Electrograms Generated by a Single Fiber

Equation (6.1) may be used to describe the electrograms recorded by electrodes placed near a fiber along which electric activity is propagating. However, the computation of the integral involved demands the full spatio-temporal specification of the intra and extracellular potentials at the membrane of the full length of fiber. Such data is generally not available. One of the more interesting applications of simplified fiber models is as follows. We assume:

1. Fiber length to be much greater than the electrode to fiber distance;
2. The approximation $\sigma_i \Phi_i \gg \sigma_e \Phi_e$ to be justified, and hence $M_S(\ell) = -(\sigma_i \Phi_i(\ell) - \sigma_e \Phi_e(\ell)) \approx -\sigma_i V_m(\ell)$;
3. A transmembrane potential that propagates along the fiber at constant velocity v.

The assumption of constant velocity implies that the time course of the transmembrane potential is identical for all points along the fiber, although exhibiting its upstroke at increasingly later time instances for locations more to the right. At location ℓ along the fiber, this function is denoted as $V_m(\ell, t)$. At time instant t during propagation, the corresponding expression for the transmembrane potential as a function of space (along the fiber) then reads

$$V_m(\ell; t) = \widetilde{V}_m(t - \ell/v), \tag{6.12}$$

substitution of $M_S(\ell, t) = -\sigma_i \widetilde{V}_m(t - \ell/v)$ in (6.10) yields

$$\Phi(\ell'; t) = \frac{-\sigma_i}{4\pi\sigma_e} \int_{-\infty}^{\infty} \frac{\partial \widetilde{V}_m(t - \ell/v)}{\partial \ell} \Omega(\ell' - \ell) \, d\ell \tag{6.13}$$

Finally, by introducing τ as $\tau = \frac{\ell}{v}$, which invokes a change of variables, we find

$$\Phi(\ell'; t) = \frac{\sigma_i}{4\pi\sigma_e} \int_{-\infty}^{\infty} \frac{\partial \widetilde{V}_m(t - \tau)}{\partial \tau} \Omega(\ell' - v\tau) \, d\tau \tag{6.14}$$

For fixed observation points, ℓ', the integral in (6.14) can be recognized as the convolution, in the temporal domain, of the *first* derivative of $\widetilde{V}_m(t - \tau)$ representing the source and a weighting function $\Omega(\ell' - v\tau)$ representing the volume conduction effects in the temporal domain. As is discussed in ❯ Sect. 5.3.4, an equivalent expression can be formulated in terms of the convolution of the *second* derivative of $\widetilde{V}_m(t - \tau)$ and the function $1/R(\ell' - v\tau)$. An early paper on this topic claimed just the second type of source description to be the correct one [6]. However, both can be justified.

A graphical illustration of the result expressed by (6.14) is shown in ❯ Fig. 6.5. Panel A depicts the time course of a stylized transmembrane potential (TMP), the function $\widetilde{V}_m(t)$. The activation propagates along a fiber with radius $a = 0.5$ mm at velocity $v = 0.1$ m/s. For the duration of the action potential shown (APD), about 150 ms, the instantaneous, spatial extent of the TMP is 15 mm. The TMP function shown is the product of two logistic functions, one representing the fast depolarization phase and the other the repolarization phase [7]. The maximum slopes of the logistic functions were set at 100 and -2 mV/ms, respectively. The corresponding duration of the upstroke of the TMP is about 3 ms. The solid line depicts the derivative of $\widetilde{V}_m(t)$. The right panel shows the function $\Omega(\tau)$ for observation point $(\ell' = 0, \rho' = a)$ on the

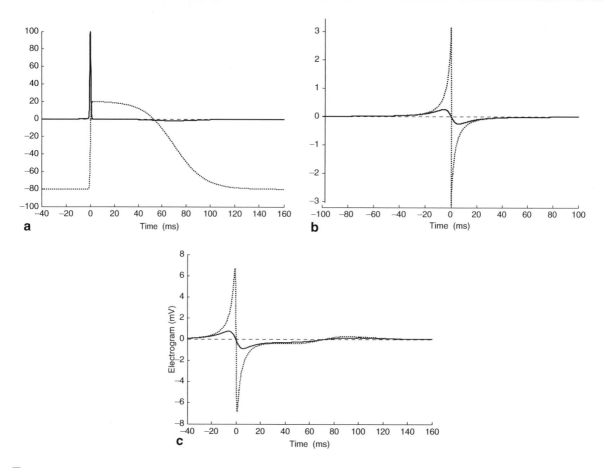

■ **Fig. 6.5**
Simulated electrograms based on (6.14). **Panel A**: *dotted line*: stylized transmembrane potential $\widetilde{V}_m(t)$, vertical scale in mV; *solid line*: its derivative; **panel B**: *dotted line*: solid angle function $\Omega(\tau - \tau')$ for field point on the fiber, $\rho' = a = 0.5$ mm (*dotted line*) and at distance $\rho' = 2\,a = 1$ mm (*solid line*); note its extreme values of $\pm\pi$; **panel C**: corresponding electrograms; *dotted line*: at field point $\rho' = a$, *solid line*: at $\rho' = 2\,a$; vertical scale in mV

outside of the membrane, as well as for $(\ell' = 0, \rho' = 2\,a)$. The lower panel shows the electrograms at $\ell = 0$ resulting from the convolution of $\frac{\partial \widetilde{V}_m(t-\tau)}{\partial \tau}$ with the two functions shown in Panel B. The ratio σ_i/σ_e, the parameter scaling the magnitude of the electrograms, was set at 0.4. All parameter settings were aimed at endowing the illustration in ❷ Fig. 6.5 of some general aspects of the genesis of electrograms. Note that for an APD of 400 ms of a TMP traveling at a transmural velocity of 0.5 m/s (ventricular myocardium) the spatial extent of the TMP would be 20 cm.

Inspection of (6.14) and the resulting wave forms (❷ Fig. 6.5) leads to the following conclusions, all valid within the limitations of the assumptions listed in the first part of this section.

1. The equivalent source strength of a propagating TMP is proportional to the derivative of the TMP. As a consequence, the mean level of the TMP does not influence the electrograms.
2. For field points with $\rho' = a$ (on the outside of the membrane) the solid angle function (SA) exhibits a jump of $2\,\pi$, independent of the fiber radius. As a consequence, the magnitude of the electrogram at that location is independent of the radius of the fiber.
3. The duration (e.g., its half-width w) of the SA curve for $\rho' = a$ (dotted line in ❷ Fig. 6.5, Panel B), is proportional to a/v.

4. If the upstroke of the TMP takes far less time than the half-width w of the SA curve, as is the case in ❷ Fig. 6.5, the shape of the solid angle curve dominates the wave form of the fast deflection in the electrogram.

5. For distal field points the amplitude of the SA curve is proportional to a^2 / ρ'^2.

6. For field points (ℓ', ρ') on the line parallel to the fiber for which $\ell' \gg \rho'$, the solid angle subtended by a cross-section of the fiber at $\ell = 0$ is approximately equal to $\frac{1}{4} a^2 / (\ell'^2 + \rho'^2) \approx \pi a^2 / \ell'^2$. Since this value is independent of ρ' the two curves shown in Panel B merge beyond, say, $|t| = 25$ ms. As a consequence, the magnitudes as well as wave forms of the two signals shown in Panel C are very similar during repolarization. See also point (d) of ❷ Sect. 5.3.8.

6.3.4 Estimating Sources from Electrograms

The model of the genesis of an electrogram discussed in ❷ Sect. 6.3.2 assumes a uniform potential profile that propagates at a uniform velocity along an infinite fiber placed in an infinite medium. The fiber is taken to have a uniform diameter.

The validation of this model requires a documentation of all relevant parameters such as: (1) fiber diameter, (2) propagation velocity along the fiber, (3) the transmembrane potential at all points along the fiber, (4) values for the intra and extracellular conductivity of the fiber, assumed to be uniform along the fiber. Moreover, the fact that the fiber (necessarily) is of finite length and that the medium in which it is situated is finite needs to be accounted for. The latter necessitates the use of a well-defined potential reference (❷ Sect. 5.4.1).

If all modeling assumptions do not strictly hold true, the more general expression of (6.1) should be used as the source term, supported by the handling of the volume conduction effects by methods like the ones discussed in ❷ Chap. 2.

6.4 Macroscopic Source Descriptions During Depolarization

Equation (6.14) may be applied to the description of potentials arising from the fibers of the conduction system. The application of (6.12) and its consequence (6.14), for describing the potential distribution arising from the electrical activity of the muscle cells of the myocardium is not possible: the cells are too short to justify the assumptions used in deriving these equations. Moreover, the external medium in the direct vicinity of the cell is not homogeneous, but is formed by all neighboring cells, some of which are in direct contact with the cell considered (❷ Chap. 3). Any attempt to account for all details of the possible interactions between these cells in terms of their intrinsic generator characteristics and of the volume conduction configuration is not feasible.

To circumvent this problem, a source description can be used which is derived from the observed macroscopic potential distribution within the ventricular myocardium, the sole object of which is to serve as a source description for the genesis of the potentials at the body surface (the ECG). Over the years, several such source descriptions have been put forward. The best known of these is that of the uniform double layer (UDL), first implied in the work of Wilson et al. [5].

Following a local stimulus in the myocardium, the cells in the direct vicinity of the stimulus are activated. The interiors of these cells are coupled through several low-resistive connections to neighboring cells. As a result, these cells are activated as well and in turn activate their (previously passive) direct neighbors. At a macroscopic level, this can be described in terms of an activation boundary which propagates like a wavefront through the myocardium.

As discussed in ❷ Sect. 5.3.5, the UDL theory postulates a double-layer current of uniform strength at the surface separating myocytes that are depolarized and those that still at rest, i.e., polarized: the activation wavefront. Following an initiation of the activation at one or more sites, one or more wavefronts propagate throughout the myocardium and, barring early repolarization, the UDL sources form the major generator of the currents during this period, which ends when all myocytes have been activated.

For many years, the UDL model has served to explain in a qualitative way the shapes of the various ECG waveforms during the depolarization phase of the ventricles [8, 9]. In later years its validity has been questioned, as is discussed in ❷ Sect. 6.4.4.1. This has triggered off the search for alternative source descriptions in which the anisotropy of the generator characteristics and of the conductivity of the medium in which these generators are situated is incorporated at different levels of complexity. As a result of the difficulty in the analysis of these problems, some of the attempts have been restricted to the analysis of monolayers of cardiac cells [10]. There have been some attempts at deriving a description for the full three-dimensional source configuration which might serve to replace, or improve on, the uniform double layer. Three such alternative source descriptions are described in ❯ Sect. 6.6. But first, to appreciate to what extent these predictions differ from those based on the UDL, the properties of the UDL are discussed in detail. As it is the most simple source description, this also makes it suitable for introducing the concepts involved.

The analysis of the potentials generated by the UDL source is based on a series of models of source extent and volume conductors with step-wise increasing complexity.

6.4.1   Potentials Generated by Basic Wavefront Geometries Carrying a UDL Source

In this classic UDL source description, the sources are assumed to be of a (current) dipolar nature: each surface element ΔS of the activation wave front is assumed to carry an elementary dipole of strength $\Delta \vec{D} = M_S \Delta \vec{S}$, which is directed towards the myocytes still at rest. The strength M_S of this dipole layer is assumed to be uniform over the entire activation boundary. We start by considering the situation with the source placed inside an infinite medium, and taking the reference potential at infinity to be zero. As shown in ❯ Sect. 5.3.5 the source yields a potential field

$$\Phi(\vec{r}') = \frac{M_S}{\sigma} \frac{\Omega}{4\pi},$$

for which we now write

$$\Phi(\vec{r}') = \frac{M_S}{\sigma} \frac{\Omega}{4\pi} = V_D \frac{\Omega}{4\pi} \tag{6.15}$$

The variable V_D is the potential difference across the double layer (compare (6.3)) and Ω is the solid angle subtended by the wave front at the observation point (compare (6.3)). Throughout this section the value $V_D = 40\,\text{mV}$ is used, a value that was based on intramural recordings of the canine ventricle, as is discussed in ❯ Sect. 6.4.3.2.

The simplicity of (6.15) is partly the reason for its popularity as a source description. The potentials predicted by this source description will now be shown in some illustrative cases, which differ only with respect to the shape and extent of the double layer.

6.4.1.1   A Circular Disk

We first consider the potential field of a double layer that has the shape of a flat circular disk of radius R (❯ Fig. 6.6(a)). This configuration was introduced for studying basic membrane properties as early as 1933 by Wilson et al. [5], who also described the solution.

The solid angle subtended by the disk at a field point on the x-axis is given by (2.112). Inserting this expression into (6.15) yields as the potential distribution (potential profile) along the x-axis

$$\Phi(x) = \frac{1}{2} V_D \left(\frac{x}{|x|} - \frac{x}{\sqrt{x^2 + R^2}} \right) = 20\,(\pm 1 - \cos\alpha) \quad (\text{mV}) \tag{6.16}$$

with α the top angle of the cone specified by the observation point $(x, 0, 0)$ as its top and the passing through the rim of the disk. A plot of this potential profile, expressed in units V_D, for $R = 1$ is shown in ❯ Fig. 6.6 (right panel). Note the potential jump of magnitude V_D when crossing the disk at $x = 0$.

6.4.1.2   A Hemisphere

Next we consider a double layer having the shape of a hemispherical shell of radius R (❯ Fig. 6.7 (left panel)). This is the simplest possible equivalent model for the source strength of a wavefront inside a myocardial layer (bounded by the

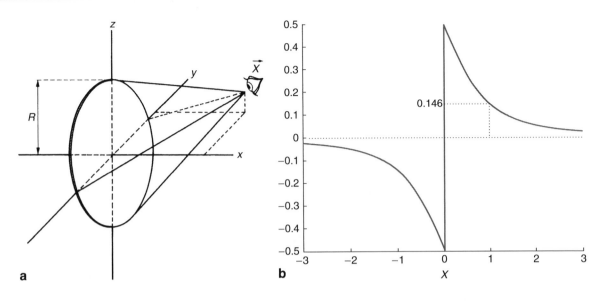

◘ Fig. 6.6
Left: Double layer having the shape of a disk of radius R viewed by the eye drawn at field point $\ddot{x}$; *right*: resulting potential profile along the x-axis according to (6.16), expressed in units $V_D = 40\,\text{mV}$; $R = 1$, x and R in the same arbitrary unit

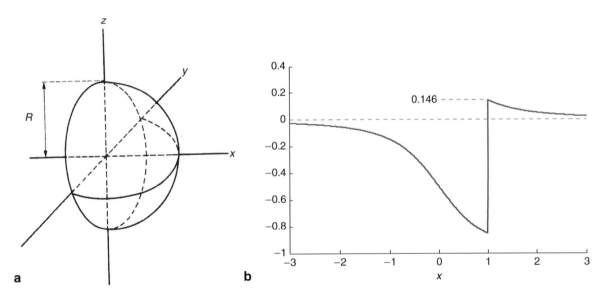

◘ Fig. 6.7
Left: Double layer having the shape of a hemispherical shell of radius $R = 1$; *right*: resulting potential profile along the x-axis according to (6.17), expressed in units $V_D = 40\,\text{mV}$; x and R are expressed in the same, arbitrary unit

plane $x = 0$) that has progressed in radial fashion following a stimulus at $x = 0$. The potential field follows, again, from the solid angle subtended by the hemisphere. To this end, we consider two disks with radius R that close the hemisphere, carrying the same strengths as that of the hemisphere, but with opposite polarity. One of these disks combined with the sources on the hemisphere form a closed double layer, which has a zero external field (❷ Sect. 2.2.12). The potential exterior to the closed source configuration is, hence, identical to the field of the remaining disk. For interior field points this also holds true, but here the solid angle of the closed hemispherical shell is -4π (❷ Sect. 2.2.12). As a consequence, we now have

$$\Phi(x) = \frac{1}{2} V_D \left(\frac{x-R}{|x-R|} - \frac{x}{\sqrt{x^2+R^2}} \right),$$
(6.17)

this potential profile is depicted in ❷ Fig. 6.7 (right panel).

A comparison of (6.16) and (6.17) leads to an interesting interpretation. The first terms, $\frac{1}{2} V_D \frac{x}{|x|}$ in (6.16) and $\frac{1}{2} V_D \frac{x-R}{|x-R|}$ in (6.17), describe the potential jump while crossing the double layer, reflecting its *local* strength. The second term, $-\frac{1}{2} V_D \frac{x}{\sqrt{x^2+R^2}}$, describes the *global* properties of the double layer, i.e., its spatial extent, which is completely specified by the surface closing the hemisphere. For the hemisphere the jump in the potentials by V_D now occurs at $x = R$, starting from the level of $-\frac{1}{2} V_D \left(1 + 1/\sqrt{2}\right)$. An initial oversight in the need for inclusion of the first term in (6.17), as can be observed in [11], initiated a discussion on the validity of this type of equivalent source description.

No simple expression is available for evaluating the potential field off-axis. However, numerical methods are available. A particularly effective method is the one in which the surface involved is tessellated by triangular elements. The solid angle is found by adding up the solid angles of these elements, each computed by means of an analytical expression [12]. This method can be used for double layers having an arbitrary shape. It was used to draw ❷ Fig. 6.8, which depicts the potential field for the source configuration shown in the left panel of ❷ Fig. 6.7 in the plane $y = 0$.

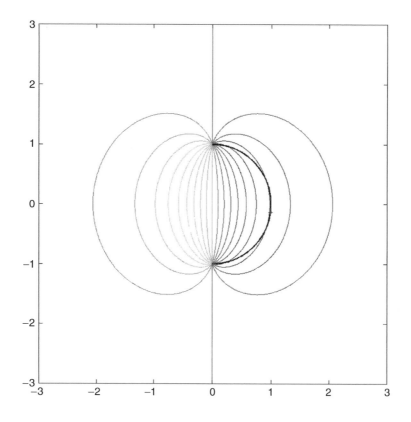

■ **Fig. 6.8**
Potential field in the plane $y = 0$ generated by the hemispherical double layer shown in ❷ Fig. 6.7. Isopotential lines drawn at $V_D/10 = 4$ mV intervals; the heavy solid line is the cross-section of the plane with the double layer. Potentials to the right of the double layer are positive, elsewhere they are negative. The potential profile along x-axis is shown in the *right* panel of ❷ Fig. 6.7. Position of absolute minimum of -34.12 mV indicated by an asterisk; maxima of 9.08 mV near the edge of the hemisphere

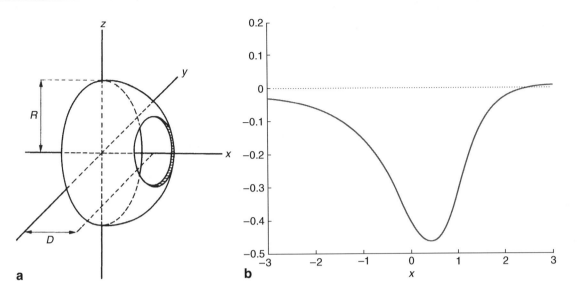

■ Fig. 6.9

Left: Double layer having the shape of a de-capped hemisphere of radius *R*; *right*: the resulting potential profile along the *x*-axis according to (6.18), expressed in units $V_D = 40\,\text{mV}$; $R = 1.25$; $D = 1$; *x, R* and *D* expressed in the same arbitrary unit

6.4.1.3   A De-Capped Hemisphere

Here the sources are again on a hemisphere of radius R but now the top has been lifted, leaving a layer of width D (6.9 (left panel)). This models a similar situation to the one described in the previous subsection, but now at the – later – stage where the wavefront has broken up at a boundary of the myocardium. The potential distribution in this case is easily found (using the superposition principle) by subtracting the potentials arising from the cap from those described for Case 2. The potentials from the cap are identical to those of hypothetical double layer sources on a disk with a radius $R_c = \sqrt{R^2 + D^2}$ closing the cap. For points on the x-axis the potential thus reads

$$\Phi(x) = \frac{1}{2}\,V_D\left(\frac{x - D}{\sqrt{(x - D)^2 + R_c^2}} - \frac{x}{\sqrt{x^2 + R^2}}\right) \tag{6.18}$$

This potential profile is shown in the right panel of ❷ Fig. 6.9. Note that the x-axis here does *not* cross the actual double layer, and so no potential jump of magnitude V_D comes into view along this axis.

6.4.1.4   A Dispersed Double Layer

The equivalent source double associated with ventricular depolarization is not a double layer in the mathematical sense described in ❷ Sect. 6.3.1. When crossing the wavefront the successive myocytes passed are at different stages of depolarization. As a consequence, the equivalent sources and sinks of electric current are spread out along the normal of the activation boundary and extend over a distance of the order of 1 mm, the length of about ten myocytes. The potential profile across the activation boundary shows a smooth, S-shaped curve rather than the jump that is seen in ❷ Fig. 6.7. For the purpose of modeling this local property of the potential profile different functions may be used. Here we will use the simple expression

$$S(x) = \frac{x}{\sqrt{x^2 + w^2}},$$

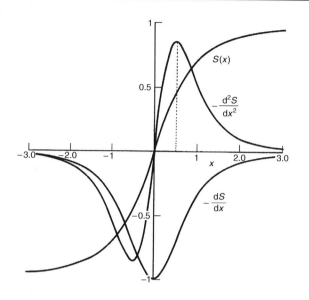

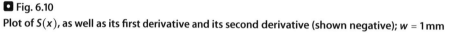

◻ Fig. 6.10

Plot of $S(x)$, as well as its first derivative and its second derivative (shown negative); $w = 1\,\text{mm}$

with w (of the order of 1 mm) specifying the distance of the current source distribution along the normal of the activation boundary. This function is merely an empirical function, chosen to represent the dispersed nature of the sources; it will now be taken to represent the local properties of the double layer and so it can replace the term $\frac{x}{|x|}$ in (6.16). This function is depicted in ❷ Fig. 6.10, $S(x)$, as well as the plots of its first and second derivative with respect to x.

In those cases where the local curvature of the activation surface is small, or zero in the case of a planar wavefront, the second derivative can be interpreted as representing the current-source volume density along the normal to the wavefront. In that case, but in that case only, Poisson's equation (❷ Sect. 2.6.1.1),

$$\nabla^2 \Phi = \frac{-i_v}{\sigma},$$

with i_v the current source volume density (units: A m^3) impressed by the biochemical processes at the membranes and

$$\nabla^2 \Phi = \frac{\partial^2 \Phi}{\partial x^2} + \frac{\partial^2 \Phi}{\partial y^2} + \frac{\partial^2 \Phi}{\partial z^2},$$

can be approximated as

$$\nabla^2 \Phi \approx \frac{d^2 \Phi}{dx^2} = \frac{-i_v}{\sigma},$$

the distance between the maximum (current source) and the minimum (current sink) of d^2S/dx^2 for this $S(x)$ is w. The expression for the potential profile of the hemispherical dispersed UDL along the x-axis, replacing (6.17), now reads

$$\Phi(x) = 20 \left(\frac{x - R}{\sqrt{(x - R)^2 + w^2}} - \frac{x}{\sqrt{x^2 + R^2}} \right) \text{(mV)}, \tag{6.19}$$

the shape of this profile is plotted in ❷ Fig. 6.11 (solid line) in which the corresponding potential profile of the mathematical double layer (❷ Fig. 6.7 (right panel)) is also drawn (dashed line). Note that the distal profile is not affected by the

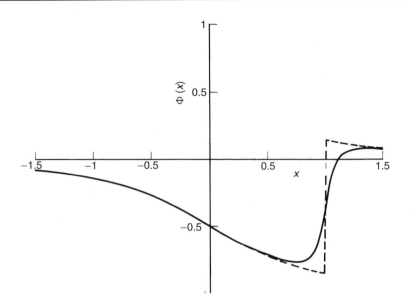

Fig. 6.11
Potential (in units: V_D = 40 mV) along the *x*-axis (units: cm) of a hemisphere, like in ❷ Fig. 6.7, but now carrying a dispersed double layer (*solid line*); w = 1 mm, R = 1 cm. The *dashed line* replicates the potential generated by the mathematical double layer (❷ Fig. 6.7 (*right* panel))

distributed nature of the sources. The difference between the maximum and minimum of the potential profile is reduced. This means that if this difference were taken as an estimate of V_D (as has been done), it would be an underestimation; the wider the sources are spread out, that is the larger w, the greater the underestimation will be.

6.4.2   Potentials Generated by the UDL at a Propagating Wavefront

The setting of the UDL source used in the previous section implies planar boundaries of the myocardium at the endocardium and the epicardium. We now consider the more realistic configuration of uniform myocardial tissue contained in a thick-walled spherical shell. Based on this model, electrograms and potential profiles generated by the UDL source are illustrated, resulting from the propagation of wavefronts initiated at either an endocardial or an epicardial site. The velocity of the propagation is put at a uniform value of 1 m/s. The wavefronts shown correspond to the traveling time from stimulus point while propagating through the myocardium (Huygens principle). The sequences of the resulting wavefronts are shown in ❷ Fig. 6.12. Note that in the right panel the direction of the total wavefront reverses after about 22 ms; the terminal wave fronts resulting from the endocardial and the epicardial stimulus site are highly similar.

We now consider a selection of potentials generated by the sequence of activation wavefronts shown in ❷ Fig. 6.12. The double-layer strength V_D is put at 40 mV. The stimulus is at time t = 5 ms. The field points involved are documented in ❷ Fig. 6.13. Owing to the axial symmetry of the problem, the field points situated in the plane of ❷ Fig. 6.13 suffice. The field points chosen are A(1)–A(13) on the endocardium; B(1)–B(13) on the epicardium and a series of 12 points along straight lines from the center of the sphere passing through the wall. Such field points are similar to those at intramural electrode arrays used in electrophysiological studies, also known as "plunge" electrodes [13].

6.4.2.1   Infinite Medium Potentials

We start by examining the infinite medium potentials generated by the sequence of activation wavefronts shown in ❷ Fig. 6.12, i.e., the potentials are generated assuming the electric conductivity of the entire, infinite medium to be uniform.

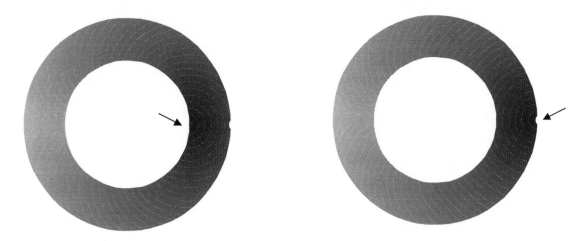

Activation wavefronts inside a thick-walled spherical shell *model* of myocardial tissue, drawn in the plane symmetry, resulting from a single, local stimulus. *Left* panel: endocardial stimulus; *right* panel: epicardial stimulus. *Arrows* indicate stimulus sites. Isochrones drawn at 2.5 ms intervals. Assumed uniform propagation velocity of 1 m/s. Radius of outer sphere (epicardium) 4 cm; radius of inner sphere (endocardium) 2.4 cm. Total duration of the propagation 83.5 and 93.5 ms for endocardial and epicardial stimulus sites, respectively

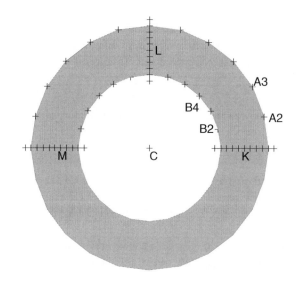

◘ Fig. 6.13
Locations of epicardial field points (**a**), endocardial field points (**b**), field points at needle electrodes (K,L,M) and one at the center of the spherical shell (**c**). Note that the needle electrodes include field points external to the wall, one just inside the cavity and another one just outside the wall. 13 epicardial and 13 endocardial field points are labeled anti-clockwise; 11 points along the needle electrodes are labeled inside outward. Stimulus sites as used in ❷ Fig. 6.12 are along needle K

In ❷ Fig. 6.14 a sequence of the potential profiles along the line from center C to the line K (❷ Fig. 6.13). Time instants shown, at 4 ms intervals, correspond to the initial stages of the propagating UDL front. The dotted lines represent the infinite medium potentials. The left panel relates to an endocardial stimulus, in the right panel to a stimulus at the epicardium. Note that, in both situations, the potential jump at the wavefront remains constant right up to the moment

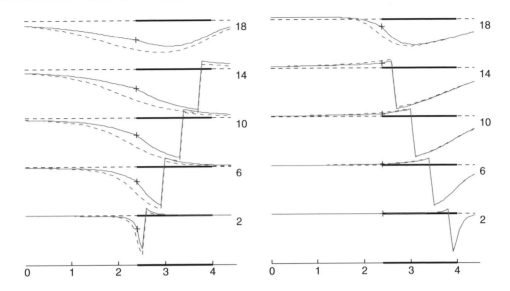

Fig. 6.14

Sequence of potential profiles along a line from center C passing through line K shown in ❯ Fig. 6.13. Time instants shown, at 4 ms intervals, are selected during the initial stages of the propagating UDL front. *Dotted lines*: infinite homogeneous medium; *solid lines*: potentials in the presence of higher conductivity inside the cavity. *Left*: stimulus at endocardial electrode of needle K; *right*: stimulus at epicardial electrode of needle K. Distance along horizontal axis in cm. The *heavy lines* along the horizontal axes mark the location of electrode K, as well as the zero level of individual potential profiles. Potential reference is at infinity. Vertical spacing of the profiles corresponds to 40 mV, thus calibrating the potential. Figures next to the profiles denote the time from stimulus in ms

of breakthrough of the wavefront. Following that moment, the sharp jump in the potential is no longer present, and the profiles (not shown) become increasingly flat with time. Note that these potential profiles imply a common reference for the potential specified at all field points considered. Here, in the infinite medium model used, the zero reference was set at infinity.

Traditionally, intramural electrograms have been recorded and studied rather than the transmural potential profiles shown in ❯ Fig. 6.14. To facilitate a direct comparison between predicted and recorded potentials, the results of the same computations are now shown as electrograms at the field points specified in ❯ Fig. 6.13. The electrograms simulated at the 11 terminals of the intramural electrode K shown in ❯ Fig. 6.13, are presented by the dotted lines in ❯ Fig. 6.15. The electrograms at the 13 endocardial field points B and 13 epicardial field points A are shown in ❯ Figs. 6.16 and ❯ 6.17, respectively. Note, by comparing ❯ Fig. 6.15 with ❯ Figs. 6.16 and ❯ 6.17, that the magnitude of potential jump at field points at the boundary of the myocardium is 20 mV, i.e., one half that of the value $V_D (= 40 \text{ mV})$ at intramural field points. Interestingly, the progression of electrogram wave forms along the epicardium in the right panel of ❯ Fig. 6.16 is from the rS to the Rs configuration of standard electrocardiographic terminology.

6.4.2.2 The Effect of Inhomogeneous Conductivity; the Brody Effect

The electric conductivity of blood is higher than that of the isotropic representation of myocardial tissue. The effect of this on the potential field is generally known as the Brody effect [14]. To evaluate its significance for the UDL source model, all potentials arising from the propagating wavefronts shown in ❯ Fig. 6.12 were also computed for the situation that the conductivity of the inner sphere, representing a blood-filled cavity, is threefold that of the (infinite) medium around it. The results are presented by the solid lines in ❯ Figs. 6.14–6.17, alongside those pertaining to the homogeneous situation, the dotted lines. The computations involved were carried out by means of the boundary element method (BEM), ❯ Sect. 2.6.4.

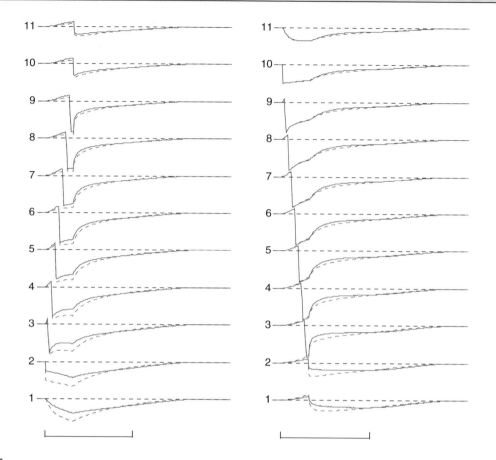

◻ Fig. 6.15

Electrograms at electrodes 1–11 of intra-mural electrode K indicated in ❷ Fig. 6.13. Potential reference at infinity. *Dotted lines*: infinite homogeneous medium; *solid lines*: potentials in the presence of higher conductivity inside the cavity. *Left*: stimulus at endocardial electrode of needle K; *right*: stimulus at epicardial electrode of needle K. Time bar 50 ms. Vertical spacing of the profiles corresponds to 40 mV, and calibrates the potential

In ❷ Fig. 6.14 the effect can be seen most clearly at the endocardial field point. In the potential profile a discontinuity in its slope can be observed at this location. The value of this slope multiplied by the local conductivity is equal to the current density $J_n(\mathrm{A\,m^{-2}})$ normal to the boundary. This density is continuous across any boundary (2.128), so where the conductivity is large the slope should be small, as is indeed observed. On the profiles, the discontinuity is marked by the + sign. On the endocardium the higher conductivity reduces the potential jump of 20 mV over the wavefront as found for the homogeneous situation by a factor of 2, as expected on the basis of the conductivity ratio at the interface (❷ Sect. 2.6). This leaves 10 mV as the theoretical maximum jump that can be expected for $V_D = 40$ mV. Inside the myocardium, the potential jump at the wavefront is unaffected by the inhomogeneity, as can be expected from the UDL model. The inhomogeneity does affect the level at which the jump takes place. On the epicardium the reduction factor for the passing (but not crossing) wavefront is less than 2, which can be explained by a larger distance from the inhomogeneous region. For the more realistic situation of dispersed sources at the wavefront, as discussed in ❷ Sect. 6.4.1.4, the potential gradients at the wavefront set up by the global distribution of the sources interact with the local gradients.

In ❷ Sect. 2.6 it is shown that the effect of local discontinuities in the conductivity may be described by virtual sources at the interfaces where the conductivity occurs. For field points that are relatively far away from such interfaces, the effect of the local gradient of the potential field is mainly limited to the setting of the overall level of the local potential. This explains the relatively minor effect of the inhomogeneous cavity on the early profiles shown in the right panel of

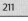

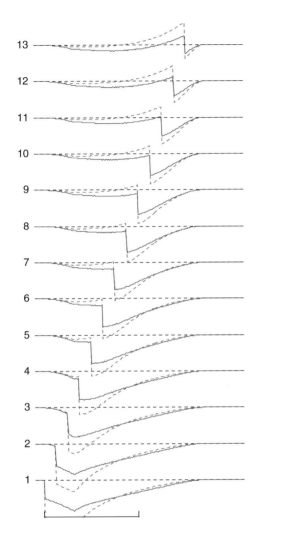

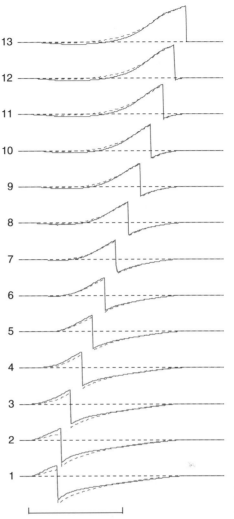

Fig. 6.16
Electrograms along endocardium; field points B1–B13 indicated in ❯ Fig. 6.13. Potential reference at infinity. *Dotted lines*: infinite homogeneous medium; *solid lines*: potentials in the presence of higher conductivity inside the cavity. *Left*: stimulus at endocardial electrode of needle K; *right*: stimulus at epicardial electrode of needle K. Time bar 50 ms. Vertical spacing of the profiles corresponds to 20 mV, and calibrates the potential. *Note that scaling differs* by a factor 2 from what is used in ❯ Fig. 6.15

❯ Fig. 6.14, as well as on the electrograms shown in ❯ Figs. 6.16 and ❯ 6.17. An overall evaluation of the Brody effect on the potential field confirms its significance, but also that it can not be represented by a single scaling factor [15].

6.4.2.3 Bounding the Medium; the Influence of the Reference

The expression of the cardiac electric activity is invariably observed in a bounded medium, be it the thorax or some fluid-filled container used during in vitro experiments.

In both circumstances the effect of these bounds may be limited, mainly restricted to setting the overall level of the potential field, similar to what is described in the previous section with regard to the Brody effect.

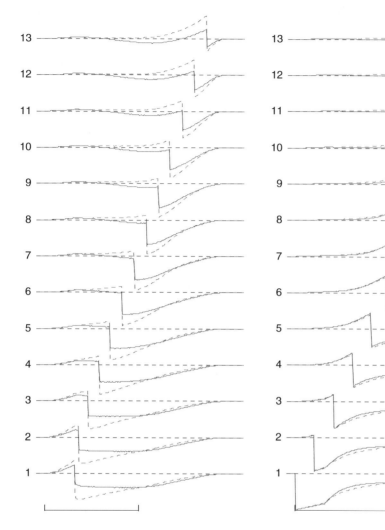

◘ Fig. 6.17
Electrograms along epicardium; field points A1–A13 indicated in ❷ Fig. 6.13. Potential reference at infinity. *Dotted lines*: infinite homogeneous medium; *solid lines*: potentials in the presence of higher conductivity inside the cavity. *Left*: stimulus at endocardial electrode of needle K; *right*: stimulus at epicardial electrode of needle K. Time bar 50 ms. Vertical spacing of the profiles corresponds to 20 mV, and calibrates the potential. *Note that scaling differs* by a factor 2 from plots in ❷ Fig. 6.15. The epicardium in the *right* panel of ❷ Fig. 6.16 is from the rS to the Rs configuration of standard electrocardiographic terminology

Of greater significance is the fact that one of the two the electrodes essential for measuring potential differences, commonly called the reference electrode, can no longer be set at infinity (❷ Sect. 5.4.1). If the dimension of the myocardial tissue is small compared to that of the volume conductor (thorax, container) holding it, the potential gradients set up at the boundary by the electric sources will be small relative to those close to the tissue, the ones as picked up by the sensing electrode. This will cause the observed potential differences between sensing electrode and reference electrode to be largely independent of the location of the reference on the boundary. However, the dimensions of the heart relative to its distance from the torso boundary cannot taken to be small, and so the selection of any reference will influence the observed ECG wave forms. The same applies to potential differences observed between a micro electrode placed inside a cell and a reference electrode placed nearby. The location of the latter may greatly influence the magnitudes and wave forms of the observed potential differences.

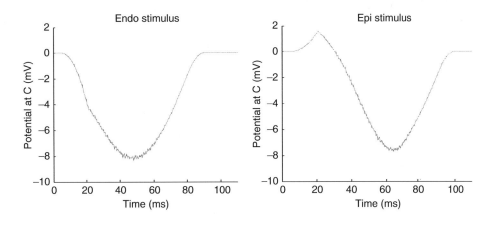

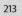

▣ Fig. 6.18
Electrograms at field point C, the center of the spheres indicated in ❷ Fig. 6.13. Superposition of infinite medium potentials and potential including Brody effect. *Left*: stimulus at endocardial electrode of needle K; *right*: stimulus at epicardial electrode of needle K

To illustrate this point, first, in ❷ Fig. 6.18, electrograms at field point C of ❷ Fig. 6.13 are shown. This location is similar to the cavity reference used in some of the early mapping of cardiac electric activity. The electrograms shown are those inside the infinite homogeneous medium, and superimposed those including the Brody effect at this field point. The timing of the wavefronts is shown in ❷ Fig. 6.12. Note that for the source configuration considered, the magnitude of the electrograms is about one fifth of the assumed double-layer strength $V_D (= 40\,\mathrm{mV})$, and that the effect of the higher conductivity of blood at the center of the sphere is very small. The initial positivity following the epicardial stimulus reflects the initial orientation of the total wavefront in 3D space toward C (right panel ❷ Fig. 6.12) having, correspondingly, the total solid angle of the wavefront is positive. After about 25 ms point C views the rear of the wavefront only (negative total solid angle). Following the endocardial stimulus, field point C views the rear exclusively. This indicates that the predominant negativity as observed experimentally may be explained by the solid angle theory, in combination with the predominantly convex geometry of the myocardium.

Next, in ❷ Fig. 6.19, the effect for the inhomogeneous situation (Brody effect) is illustrated that result if the potential at field point C is used as the reference. The comparison is documented for the endocardial stimulus, for which the electrograms based on the infinite medium reference are shown by the solid lines in the left panels of ❷ Figs. 6.16 and ❷ 6.17. In ❷ Fig. 6.19 these results are reproduced, with superimposed (dashed lines) the corresponding electrograms based on taking the potential at field point C as the reference. Since the infinite medium potentials at the endocardium have magnitudes that are similar, the effect of using the reference at C can be seen more clearly in the endocardial signals.

6.4.2.4 Discussion

The model study presented in the previous sub-sections permits the analysis of the fields generated by the UDL model in isolation of a multitude of unknown, or poorly specifiable factors affecting the data observed during electrophysiological measurements.

All potential profiles and electrograms shown in the previous sub-sections are based on the simple model of UDL source, isotropic electric conductivity, and a Huygens type of propagation assuming uniform velocity. In spite of this, a wide variety of wave forms can be observed. The qualitative nature of the signals corresponds well to experimental observations. Being based on the UDL source at propagating wavefronts, all effects of ongoing repolarization effects were excluded, which resulted in a return to baseline at the termination of propagation for all signals. Any decay towards the baseline, hence, relate to depolarization currents only, with details of the decay being related to the time course of the total solid angle of the wavefront subtended at the field point; sharp deflections signify a passing wavefront.

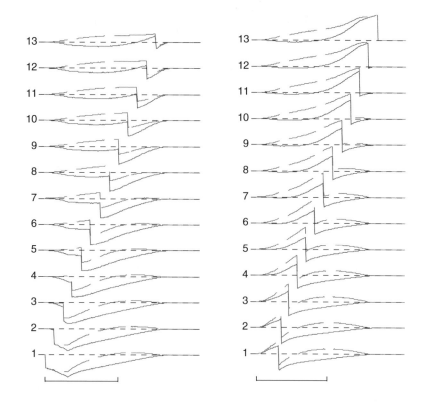

◘ Fig. 6.19

Electrograms in the presence of the Brody effect, following an endocardial stimulus. *Solid lines*: potential reference at infinity; *dashed lines*: reference at the center of the spheres (field point C). *Left*: endocardial field points B1–B13; *right*: epicardial field points A1–B13. Time bar 50 ms; vertical spacing of the profiles corresponds to 20 mV, and calibrates the potential

The simulated signals at the needles L and M demonstrated a regular, gradual progression of the wave forms along the needles between those documented for the endocardial side and the epicardial side. For needle L, all fast down slopes occurred almost simultaneously, in agreement with the isochrones shown in ❷ Fig. 6.12. Without the full knowledge of the position of these wavefronts, any interpretation of the observed data may easily lead to incorrect interpretations of such data.

The relevance of the potential at the reference electrode can be seen to be quite significant. A different location of the reference than that of C shown in ❷ Fig. 6.13 yields different effects than those visible in, e.g., ❷ Fig. 6.19.

Initially, electrophysiological studies relied on data presented in the form of electrograms. The study discussed in ❷ Sect. 6.4.3.1 introduced the method of studying potential profiles along the intra mural electrodes. More recently, mapping the potentials transmural potential field or potential fields on the heart surface have been used, as shown, e.g., in [11, 16]. These methods are complementary, and form essential tools in the understanding of the complex spatio-temporal nature of the electric activity of the heart.

6.4.3　Electrophysiology Based UDL Parameters

The validation of any source model entails a comparison of the potentials (potential differences) generated by the model and those observed experimentally. As is discussed in ❷ Sect. 6.3.4 for the single fiber, this demands the matching of the complexity of the experimental setup and those used in the computations. In the case of the source modeling of the entire heart, this requirement cannot easily be fulfilled. Below, experimentally observed potentials are interpreted in terms of the UDL model.

6.4.3.1 Potentials Recorded Inside the Canine Myocardium

The potentials along a linear multi-terminal intramural electrode array (IME; plunge electrode), following an endocardial stimulus, have been recorded in the free part of the canine left ventricular wall [17]. The electric properties of the canine myocardium have been shown to be comparable to that of the human myocardium. The animals were anesthesized using 20 mg Nembutal per kg body mass. Respiration was maintained artificially through tracheal intubation. The thorax was opened by median sternotomy. Following the insertion of the IMEs, different series of recordings were made. In some of these, the part of the ventricular myocardium studied was exposed to air, in other ones the thorax was closed as tightly as possible, while filling up any remaining gaps with a fluid having approximately the same electric conductivity as the mean conductivity of body tissues [18]. The results shown in this section pertain to the latter configuration. The diameter of the IME was 1 mm, as was the inter-electrode distance. The IME was surrounded by four other IMEs, inserted into the wall at distances of about 1 cm from the central one. The simultaneously recorded potentials at these flanking IMEs served as a check on the nature of the propagation along the central IME. In particular, the possible involvement of activity initiated by the Purkinje fibres needed to be ruled out. The potentials along the central IME are shown in ❯ Fig. 6.20. In the left column electrograms are shown that were recorded with respect to a common reference at the aortic root. Such signals with a common reference are commonly, but incorrectly, referred to as unipolar leads, one of the many unfortunate misnomers in the field of electrocardiography.

Evaluation

The electrograms can be compared with the simulations as depicted in the left panel of ❯ Fig. 6.15. However, note that, inevitably, the simulated potentials have a different common reference. The middle column depicts the corresponding bipolar signals: the potential differences observed between pairs of successive electrodes along the IME: the potential at any electrode minus that of its neighbor situated closer to the cavity. The right column depicts the corresponding sequence of recorded transmural potential profiles at successive time instants; time increases from top to bottom. These can be compared to the simulated profiles shown in the left panel of ❯ Fig. 6.14. The discontinuity of the slope at the endocardial electrode, resulting from the Brody effect, can be clearly seen, in particular for time instances between 22 and 44 ms.

The electrograms measured inside the ventricular wall following the stimulus artifact, shown in the left column of ❯ Fig. 6.20, display the progression of a negative deflection, which passes along at uniform velocity, consistent with conditions used in generating model signals (❯ Fig. 6.15). The magnitude of the down slope of the experimental data is uniform along the IME. The same conclusion can be drawn from the bipolar signals and potential profiles shown in ❯ Fig. 6.20.

In the full report on this study [18] it was reported that the same qualitative correspondence between potentials observed experimentally and those based on the UDL source was observed for potentials during spontaneous activity sinus beat in the free wall of the left ventricle. In that situation, the potentials observed at the flanking IMEs revealed a more planar nature of the wavefront, traveling transmurally from endocardium to epicardium. No significantly different details were observed in the profile for mid-myocardial locations of the wavefront compared to locations close to either endocardium or epicardium. Other observed signals and profiles, such as following an epicardial stimulus, transmural data in the septum and in the right ventricular free wall, could be described well on the basis of the UDL source. This was taken as a justification of the use of this source model.

The exampled shown in ❯ Figs. 6.6–6.19 all relate to an axial symmetric distribution of the sources, the axis being, e.g., the line through needles K and M in ❯ Fig. 6.13. If anisotropic propagation is involved any of the circular configuration, like the one shown in ❯ Fig. 6.6 the on an elliptical shape. The potential profiles along the axis, like the one shown in ❯ Fig. 6.7, are different, but only in a minor way, even if the ratio of the longest and the shortest axes of the ellipse is a high as 8.

6.4.3.2 Parameters of the UDL Source Estimated from Measured Potentials

Based on the experimentally observed transmural potential profiles described in ❯ Sect. 6.4.3.1, the parameters V_D and w of the UDL have been estimated. These were found to be of the order $V_D = 40$ mV and $w = 0.7$ mm.

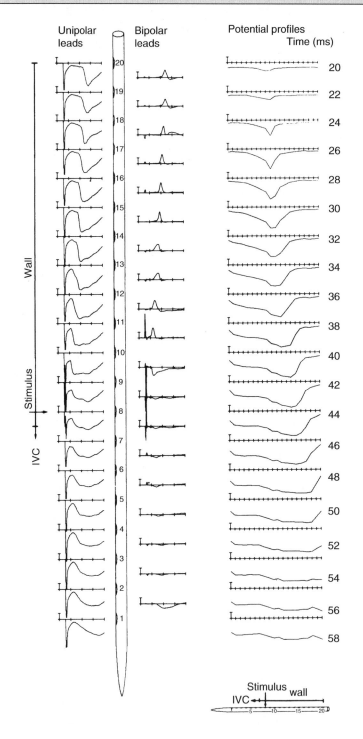

Fig. 6.20

Potentials measured inside canine ventricular myocardium following endocardial stimulation. The *left* column shows common reference electrograms and bipolar electrograms, respectively. The *right* column depicts the corresponding potential profiles along 1 mm spaced electrodes along an IME at the time instants indicated on the *right*. The stimulus site on the electrode is indicated; the stimulus is delivered at *t* = 10 ms. The *abscissae* of the *left* and middle columns are marked at 20 ms/div; those in the *right* column are marked at 1 mm/div. IVC denotes intra ventricular cavity

The observed value of w indicates (using the observed transmural propagation velocity of $0.4\,\mathrm{m\,s^{-1}}$) that the duration of the passage of the depolarization phase of the dispersed sources across the wavefront is of the order of

$$t \cong \frac{2w}{v} = \frac{1.4 \times 10^{-3}}{0.4} = 3.5\ \mathrm{ms},$$

the associated dipole surface density (6.15) was computed by taking some realistic value for the overall macroscopic conductivity of the cardiac tissue. Taking $\sigma = 0.16\,\mathrm{Sm^{-1}}$, it follows that $M_S = \sigma V_D = 6.4 \times 10^{-3}\,\mathrm{Am^{-1}}$.

The electric field strength, $E = -\mathrm{d}\Phi/\mathrm{d}x$, along the profile can be derived from (6.19) as

$$E(x) = -\frac{1}{2}\,V_D\left(\frac{w^2}{\left((x-R)^2 + w^2\right)^{3/2}} - \frac{R^2}{\left(x^2 + R^2\right)^{3/2}}\right),$$

at the activation boundary $x = R$ the field strength has a maximum value of

$$E_{\max} = -\frac{1}{2}\,V_D\left(\frac{1}{w} - \frac{1}{R}\right),$$

if $R \gg w$ this results in $E_{\max} = 28\,\mathrm{V\,m^{-1}}$. The condition stated, $R \gg w$, illustrates the interaction of the local and the global properties of the source. Only for a planar front were $(R = \infty)$ does the second derivative along the axis of the potential profile exclusively represent the local macroscopic source properties. For wave fronts set up just following a stimulus, its apparent strength is smaller than its actual strength.

For the associated impressed current density, $J = \sigma E$, its maximum value can now be estimated as

$$J_{\max} \cong -4.5\ \mathrm{Am^{-2}},$$

the impressed macroscopic current source volume density i_v can be estimated in the approximation $(R \gg w)$

$$\nabla^2\Phi \cong \frac{\mathrm{d}^2\Phi}{\mathrm{d}x^2} = \frac{-i_v}{\sigma},$$

the maximum value of i_v occurs at $x = \frac{1}{2}w$ (❯ Fig. 6.10), for which

$$i_{v;\max} = \frac{0.43\,\sigma\,V_D}{w^2} \cong 5.8 \times 10^3\,\mathrm{Am^{-3}},$$

the above are gross overall estimates of the various ways in which the macroscopic cardiac sources can be specified by physical parameters. They are interrelated by the assumed potential distribution of the dispersed uniform double layers (6.19). They characterize the in situ situation of intact, healthy cardiac tissue during an activation sequence which is predominantly transmural. During spontaneous ventricular activation, the main activation sequence at the free wall of the left ventricle is from endocardium to epicardium (❯ Chap. 4). The UDL source during such an activation sequence can be quantified by the parameter values described in this sub-section.

6.4.4 Validity of the UDL Source Model

The validation (i.e., non-falsification) of any source model entails a comparison of the potentials (potential differences) generated by the model and those observed experimentally. This demands the matching of the complexity of the experimental setup and that used in the computations. Even for the single fiber, as is discussed in ❯ Sect. 6.3.4, this requirement cannot easily be fulfilled, and even less for the source modeling of the entire heart, this.

For many years the uniform double-layer model has served to explain in a qualitative fashion the potentials recorded at the body surface. The most thorough presentation of its potential for this qualitative description was given by Holland and Arnsdorf [9].

In several quantitative studies, involving approaches to the "forward problem of electrocardiography" (❷ Chap. 8), the implied cellular model for healthy cardiac tissue is that of the uniform double layer [19, 20]. The results described in ❷ Sects. 6.3.3 and ❷ 6.3.4 also suggest that the uniform double layer describes the macroscopic potentials inside the ventricular wall during a transmural activation sequence in healthy myocardium quite well. However, several other studies have led to severe criticisms about the validity of the uniform double layer [21], in particular in view of the well-established anisotropic nature of the electric properties of myocardial tissue. These studies gave rise to the formulation of several alternative models, which are necessarily more complex in nature. A discussion on the use of the UDL model was described in [22]. The main arguments exposed in that paper are as described in ❷ Sect. 6.4.4.1. Throughout, the essentially anisotropic nature of myocardial tissue [23, 24] needs to be kept in mind.

6.4.4.1   The UDL Model Criticized

The critique on the UDL was initiated by a group that had previously been advocating its use [8]. In a report published in 1976 [25] it was shown forward computations based on the UDL and on the observed activation data failed to produce potentials comparable to those observed on the surface of a cylinder containing a conducting fluid into which a canine heart was submerged. The possibility that this might be due to an insufficient accuracy of a) the recorded geometry, b) the depolarization sequence as estimated from the spatial sampling implied in the use of the intramural electrodes, or c) the calculations performed, was not discussed. Hence, their doubt about the validity of the UDL source model remained. As an alternative, the axial model, described in ❷ Sect. 6.5, was postulated.

However, more recent studies have demonstrated a close correspondence between UDL-based forward simulations and observations made under similar conditions [26]. A significant, all be it indirect, support of the UDL source model came from a study, in which the UDL was used to estimate (inverse problem) the individual depolarization sequences of three human subjects. These inverse computations used, separately for each subject, MRI data that specified the relevant interfaces of regions with different conductivity. Next, the estimated depolarization sequence was used (forward problem, ❷ Chap. 8) in a straight forward procedure, to compute the magnetocardiograms (MCG). This was done prior to the recording of the magnetic data. Without applying any tuning or fitting procedure, the subsequently recorded MCGs showed a great similarity with the simulated data, regarding both gross wave form morphology and their magnitude.

In 1976, in an attempt to explain the poor simulation results, potentials inside the canine myocardium recorded by means of a (limited) number of intramural "plunge" electrodes were processed to represent instantaneous potential distributions throughout the ventricular wall [11]. The UDL "predictions" were computed in the infinite medium approximation (Fig. 7a of [11]) and were found to be essentially different from the observed data. The observed field showed a gradient across the wavefront, which the simulation did not. In a more recent publication on this point (Fig. 6a of [21]), the correct field produced by the hemispherical UDL is shown, similar to the one originally like the one shown in [18], and drawn here as ❷ Fig. 6.8.

An analysis (❷ Sect. 6.5.1) of the alternative axial model that was proposed by the group demonstrates that this source model also fails to produce the potential wavefronts across the wavefronts.

Additional experimental data fuelling the dispute came from the Scher group. Based on potential readings on a restricted area of the epicardium as well as within the myocardium directly below, their data initially [27, 28] stressed anisotropy. However, from a later paper [29] support for the UDL can be distilled.

A major impetus for the concern regarding validity of the UDL came from an increasing insight into the anisotropic nature of the myocardium. In a much quoted study by Clerc [30] the work of Weidmann on propagation and conductivities along fibers was extended to the transverse fiber situation. For the interpretation of his data Clerc used the one-dimensional (cable) model applied to a configuration of closely packed cylinders.

His results on various conductivity values reported in the along fiber direction are in agreement with those of Weidmann [31]. For the transverse fiber direction Clerc's interpretation of the experimental data led him to state conductivity values, which gave rise to high values for the anisotropy ratios, the ratios of intra and extracellular conductivity.

In [32], Clerc's interpretations of his transverse fiber experimental data were criticized, as were the resulting estimates of the various anisotropy ratios. Up until now, no complete, and completely validated set of values for the (anisotropic) conductivities has become available [33]. Compare the data listed in Tables 1 and 2 of [32].

After studying the potentials recorded by Taccardi and his group at small distances from the epicardium of a dog heart submerged in a cylindrical bath, the importance of anisotropy was stressed by Colli-Franzone et al. [34]. Here in the observed epicardial potential distribution, in the region exterior to the approximately ellipsoidal depolarized region following an epicardial stimulus, a small region of positive values were found ahead of the wavefront. The observation was accentuated by drawing about as many isopotential lines around the small positive peak as were used for the large negativity overlying the depolarized area. Here the effect of the conductivity of the bath, which was much lower than that of the myocardium, creating secondary sources, may have played a part in exaggerating the apparent anisotropy.

The same phenomenon was stressed in later publications by the group [16]. Following an epicardial stimulus, local maxima of about 5 mV were observed ahead of the wavefront, whereas the depolarized region exhibited values of up to 33 mV. The observations were made on the epicardium in a region exposed to air. In the presence of this type of boundary the UDL source in an otherwise homogeneous medium does not create local maxima on the boundary ahead of the wavefront.

The results shown in ❯ Fig. 6.19 stress the significance of the position of the reference electrode [35].

6.4.4.2 The Strength of the UDL Source Model

The above examples demonstrate the difficulty in evaluating simplified source models from observed potentials. For a correct evaluation the full spatial extent of the source distribution and a full account of the passive conduction properties is required. Anisotropy is an inherent property of fiber structure. It dominates the propagation of activity as well as electric conductivity and, hence, current spread. In spite of this, the UDL source model has been shown to be a useful concept [36]. A simplified argument as to why this may work is as follows. In the macroscopic approach, the local double-layer source, with strength V_D, is taken to feed currents generated at the membranes of the myocytes into the tissue. As shown in ❯ Sect. 6.3.2, $M_S = -(\sigma_i \Phi_i - \sigma_e \Phi_e) \approx -\sigma_i V_m$. The isotropic, homogeneous medium with conductivity σ_e, and combined with $V_D = M_S/\sigma_e$, this yields an extra-cellular potential field,

$$\Phi(\vec{r}\,') = V_D \frac{\Omega}{4\pi} \sim \frac{\sigma_i V_m}{\sigma_e} \frac{\Omega}{4\pi} \tag{6.20}$$

Anisotropy will affect all of the 3 factors of the first fraction shown in this expression. The scalar conductivities become tensors and the membrane potential V_m has to be replaced by a variable having directional properties. When the bi-domain approach [37] is applied (❯ Chap. 8) to the problem of finding the potential field reduces to a mono-domain formulation if an equal anisotropy ratios for intracellular and extracellular domain is assumed. Considerations with regards to cell coupling and cell geometry support this assumption; insufficient experimental evidence has been put forward to reject it [32]. The experimental values of $V_D = 40$ mV for the transverse fiber source strength [17] and $V_D = 51$ mV for along fiber source strength [38] are the ones most closely corroborating the equal anisotropy ratio assumption and, indirectly, the UDL source model.

A further explanation as to why the UDL works is the following. For the entire heart, anisotropy is not uniform, because of the complex lining up of overlaying muscle layers of the myocardium. This tends to fudge the overall effect of anisotropy, in particular when the potentials observed are those on the body surface.

Based on the experimental data discussed in ❯ Sect. 6.4.3.1, the value for the strength of the UDL was taken to be 40 mV [17, 18]. It is in agreement with the order of magnitude found for the fast deflection of the down slope of intramural electrograms found in early electrophysiological studies [13, 39]. The analysis presented ❯ Sect. 6.4.2 shows that this would result in a maximum value of 20 mV, the down slope of an electrogram generated by a wavefront passing along the epicardium in contact with a conductive medium with conductive properties similar to that of the myocardium. This is similar to values observed experimentally (Fig. 2 of [16]). In the latter study the shape of the wavefront was elliptical rather than circular as is implied in ❯ Sect. 6.4.2. On the epicardium exposed to air the potential difference across the wavefront following from an epicardial stimulus can be expected to be of the order of 40 mV, provided the wavefront has not yet broken through the endocardium. On the other hand, if the myocardium is in direct contact with a medium that has a conductivity that is higher than that of the myocardium, the potential differences are smaller. Assuming the conductivity of blood to be threefold that of myocardial tissue, a twofold reduction can be expected, leaving about 10 mV as the expected maximum amplitude of an electrogram recorded on the endocardium. This value is in agreement with experimental observations in the ventricles as well as in the atria.

6.5 Anisotropic/Non-Uniform Models

In the uniform double-layer model, both the strength of the double layer and the conductivity of the medium in which this equivalent source is located are assumed to be independent of the direction in which the cardiac fibers are aligned within the myocardium. In reality, the elementary sources may be expected to depend, with regard to strength and in direction, on fiber orientation. The conductivity of the medium is known to be dependent on fiber orientation; the electrical current in passive myocardium is conducted more easily in the fiber direction than in a direction across the fibers. As a consequence, at a macroscopic local level the conductivity is a tensor rather than a scalar. This means that the conductivity should be specified by the components:

1. longitudinal conductivity σ_ℓ, the conductivity along fibers;
2. transverse conductivity σ_{t1}, the conductivity across fibers, in a direction perpendicular to fiber orientation, tangent to the ventricular wall; and
3. transverse conductivity σ_{t2}, the conductivity in a direction perpendicular to fiber orientation as well as to the ventricular wall.

The latter two transverse conductivities are usually assumed to be equal: $\sigma_{t1} = \sigma_{t2} = \sigma_t$.

As a consequence of fiber orientation, the elementary dipole strengths of a depolarization wavefront, the conductivity of the medium, or both may be assumed to be anisotropic and the inclusion of this aspect necessarily leads to an anisotropic, possibly non-uniform, source model.

6.5.1 The Axial Model

The first attempt to replace the uniform double layer was described by Corbin and Scher in 1977 [28]. The assumptions of their model are as follows.

A large section of myocardium is considered in which all fibers are aligned in parallel (❯ Fig. 6.21). Let $\vec{\ell}$ be a (dimensionless) unit vector in the fiber direction. All surface elements $d\vec{S}$ of a depolarization wavefront within this tissue are assumed:

a. To carry a current dipole having a strength proportional to $\vec{\ell} \bullet d\vec{S}$
b. To point in the local fiber direction, toward the tissue still at rest
c. To be situated within a homogeneous tissue of isotropic conductivity

The elementary dipoles $\vec{D}$ involved can be expressed as $\vec{D} = p(\vec{\ell} \bullet d\vec{S})\,\vec{\ell}$, with p the dipole surface density, which is assumed to be uniform. Since the conductivity of the medium was taken to be homogeneous and isotropic, the potential $\Phi(\vec{r}')$ generated by an elementary dipole $p\,d\vec{S}$ at some observation point $\vec{r}'$ is

$$\Phi(\vec{r}') = \frac{1}{4\pi\sigma}\frac{p\,\vec{\ell}\bullet d\vec{S}\ \vec{\ell}\bullet\vec{R}}{R^3} \tag{6.21}$$

with $\vec{R}$ the vector pointing from the dipole location to the observation point, and R its length. The potential at $\vec{r}'$ generated by all sources on the depolarization boundary S can be found by using the superposition principle, as the sum (integral) of the contributions of all elementary dipoles:

$$\Phi(\vec{r}') = \frac{p}{4\pi\sigma}\int_S \frac{\vec{\ell}\bullet\vec{R}\ \ \vec{\ell}\bullet d\vec{S}}{R^3} \tag{6.22}$$

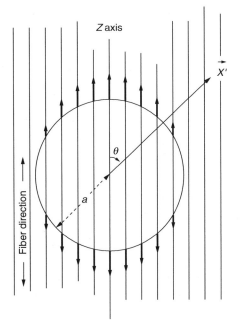

◘ Fig. 6.21
Spherical depolarized region inside the myocardium. Axial source strength is lined up exclusively with the fiber direction (*z*-axis). Elementary source strength at the spherical surface proportional to the cosine of the angle between fiber direction and the vector pointing from the center of the sphere and the observation point

The corresponding expression for the UDL source model is (5.8) (see also ❷ Sect. 2.5.2.2).

The axial model prescribes all elementary dipoles to point in the fiber direction. Their strength is maximal for a wavefront propagating in the fiber direction, is zero for propagation across fibers and, in general, is proportional to the cosine of the angle between the direction of propagation of the wavefront and local fiber direction. Note, once more, that the conductivity of the tissue itself was taken to be the scalar, which implies an isotropic conductivity.

6.5.1.1 Potentials Generated by the Axial Model

The potentials generated by an arbitrarily-shaped depolarization wavefront based on the axial model can be found from (6.22), taking into account the particular shape of the wavefront *S*. In general this integral can only be solved numerically but there is one interesting exception. When the wavefront is assumed to be a closed sphere, the integral can be solved analytically. The resulting potential distribution can be used to assess the character of the axial model.

In [40] it is shown that the potential at an observation point $\vec{r}'$ that lies at a distance R from the center of a sphere of radius a carrying a source distribution corresponding to the axial model is

$$\Phi(R,\theta) = -\frac{p}{3\sigma}, \quad 0 \leq R < a, \tag{6.23}$$

$$\Phi(R,\theta) = \frac{p}{3\sigma}\left(\frac{a}{R}\right)^3 \left(2\cos^2\theta - 1\right), \quad R > a, \tag{6.24}$$

with θ the angle between R and the fiber direction. When crossing the activation boundary at an angle θ with respect to the fiber direction, the potential jumps by $\Delta V = (p\cos^2\theta)/\sigma$, which is zero for across-fiber propagation.

These analytical results can be compared with the corresponding results for a uniform double layer with the same geometry, which are

$$\Phi(R) = -V_D, \quad 0 \leq R < a, \tag{6.25}$$

$$\Phi(R) = 0, \quad R > a, \tag{6.26}$$

independent of θ.

The assumed source configuration can be studied experimentally by delivering an epicardial stimulus under the conditions of an epicardium exposed to air. The volume conduction effects of this exposure on the potentials set up inside the myocardium can, in the planar wall approximation, be treated by introducing a virtual source distribution that is the mirror image of the actual, hemispherical or hemi-ellipsoidal wavefront. This mirror image, combined with the actual source, forms a closed surface to which the preceding result ((6.23) and (6.24)) may be applied. Note that this is a valid description only as long as the wavefront has not yet broken through at the endocardium.

As shown by (6.24) the axial model predicts that ahead of the wavefront in a direction close to that of the fibers (small values of θ), small positive potentials are expected. These have been observed experimentally. The (mathematical) uniform double-layer model is incapable of explaining these. When looking at the transmural, transverse (across fiber) part of the activation wavefront, matters are entirely different. Here, the axial model predicts the absence of a potential jump across the wavefront, which is incorrect since major, nonzero potential jumps are clearly present for transmural, transverse propagation (❷ Fig. 6.20).

6.5.2 The Oblique Dipole Model

The discussions about which model is preferable have led to the formulation of a new model, the "oblique dipole model" [34], which can be considered as a synthesis of the classical uniform double-layer model and the axial model. As in the previously discussed models, the medium in which this source description is situated is assumed to be a homogeneous, isotropic, infinite medium. The anisotropy of the fibers is exclusively assigned to the source description. In the oblique dipole model, in addition to the axially oriented sources of the axial model, dipole sources are postulated, which are oriented exclusively in the transverse direction. It is therefore necessary to distinguish between the surface tissue dipole densities p_ℓ for the longitudinal or fiber directions and p_t for the transverse direction. The contributions to the potential generated by the transverse sources alone now can be expressed as

$$\Phi(\vec{X}) = \frac{p_t}{4\pi\sigma} \int_S \frac{\vec{t} \bullet \vec{R} \; \vec{t} \bullet d\vec{S}}{R^3} \tag{6.27}$$

where $\vec{t}$ is a (dimensionless) unit vector in the plane defined by $\vec{R}$ and fiber direction $\vec{\ell}$, pointing across fibers, towards the tissue still at rest (compare (6.21)).

In general, the combination of the axial and the transverse components is not perpendicular, i.e., oblique, to the surface elements dS of the depolarization wavefront S, from which property the name of this model was derived.

The combined axial and transverse dipolar sources yield the potential distribution

$$\Phi(\vec{X}) = \frac{1}{4\pi\sigma} \int_S \frac{[p_t(\vec{t} \bullet \vec{R}) \, \vec{t} + p_l(\vec{l} \bullet \vec{R}) \, \vec{\ell}] \bullet d\vec{S}}{R^3} \tag{6.28}$$

When $p_\ell = p_t = p$ this equation reduces to

$$\Phi(\vec{X}) = \frac{p}{4\pi\sigma} \int_S \frac{\vec{R} \bullet d\vec{S}}{R^3}, \tag{6.29}$$

The expression for the UDL, since in that case, p can be moved in front of the integral and $(\vec{t} \bullet \vec{R})\vec{t} + (\vec{\ell} \bullet \vec{R})\vec{\ell}$ represents $\vec{R}$ as the vector sum of its projections on $\vec{t}$ and $\vec{\ell}$. For this situation, the oblique model reduces to the classic uniform double-layer model. When $p_t = 0$ the oblique model reduces to the axial model.

An alternative way of expressing the potential due to the oblique dipole model results by substituting $p_t = p_u$ and $p_\ell = p_a + p_u$ in (6.28). By using

$$p_t(\vec{t} \bullet \vec{R})\vec{t} + p_\ell(\vec{\ell} \bullet \vec{R})\vec{\ell} = p_u(\vec{t} \bullet \vec{R})\vec{t} + (p_a + p_u)(\vec{\ell} \bullet \vec{R})\vec{\ell} = p_u \vec{R} + p_a(\vec{\ell} \bullet \vec{R})\vec{\ell}$$

this shows that the potential generated by the oblique dipole model can be viewed as the sum of

$$\Phi_u(\vec{X}) = \frac{p_u}{4\pi\sigma} \int_S \frac{R \bullet d\vec{S}}{R^3},$$

contributed by a purely uniform source, and

$$\Phi_a(\vec{X}) = \frac{p_a}{4\pi\sigma} \int_S \frac{(\vec{\ell} \bullet R)\vec{\ell} \bullet d\vec{S}}{R^3},$$

the contribution of a purely axial source [34].

The application of the oblique dipole model to the interpretation of recorded potentials generated by myocardial tissue now demands a potential jump at the activation boundary of $\Delta V_\ell = (p_u + p_a)/\sigma$ for propagation in the longitudinal direction, and of $\Delta V_t = p_t/\sigma$ in the transverse direction.

In some experimental studies, values of $\Delta V_\ell = 74$ mV and $\Delta V_t = 43$ mV were reported. In terms of the oblique dipole model, this indicates that the contribution of purely axial sources, required to supplement those of the uniform double layer, are quite substantial, i.e., roughly of the same magnitude. However, in experiments carried out by the authors of the oblique dipole model [34] in which the potential distribution generated by a perfused heart contained in a large container was accurately measured, the ratio p_ℓ/p_t required for an optimal fit of the computed to the observed potentials was found to be even much larger (> 15). This discrepancy is probably caused by the experimental conditions of the latter experiments. In particular, the fact that the conductivity of the fluid in the bath containing the heart was much larger than that of the myocardial tissue may have influenced these results.

6.5.3 Fully Anisotropic Models

All source models described in the previous paragraphs, modeling the potential distribution in the myocardium and the surrounding medium, are macroscopic source models, which have in common that they are taken to feed the current that they generate into a medium of isotropic conductivity. All of these fail, in one way or another, to account completely for the potentials observed experimentally. The anisotropy of the sources as expressed in the axial model and in the oblique dipole model solved by no means all problems: anisotropy is reflected in source strength only. To derive any further improvement, the obvious next step is not only to consider the source anisotropy but also the anisotropy in the conductivity of the myocardial tissue, caused by the same fiber structure. There have been several studies aimed at achieving this goal [11, 28, 29, 34, 36, 41]. In particular, the study by Roberts and Scher [29] should be consulted to see how far this approach can lead. One of their conclusions is that the full treatment of anisotropy is definitely needed to account for the potential distribution inside the ventricular wall. It is, however, complicated by the complex architecture of cardiac fibers which are not all neatly lined up in parallel [23, 24]. The more complete handling of this problem is based on the so-called bi-domain theory [4, 37, 41, 42]. This topic is treated in ❷ Chap. 8 (❷ Sect. 8.3.2) and in ❷ Chap. 7, "Appendix: The EDL and Bidomain Theory".

6.6 Evaluation

When describing the potential in the region outside the heart, for some applications of the uniform double layer, being the simplest of all models, may still be used. This applies certainly to qualitative description of QRS waveforms [9] and also to some quantitative approaches to the genesis of the electrocardiogram [19, 20, 43, 44]. It has been mainly applied to the modeling of ventricular activity. It has been found to serve well as an entry to the inverse computation of the timing of ventricular activation sequence [43, 45–49]. The latter problem is currently referred to as activation time imaging. At present the accuracy of parameters specifying anisotropy is insufficient for the inclusion of the complexity of the fiber structure in inverse procedures.

This chapter is restricted to the modeling of the sources during depolarization, and in particular to the properties and usefulness of the UDL model. In the next chapter a generalization of this source model is described that provides a means for modeling the sources during repolarization. It may also be used for the modeling of the electric sources of the atria.

References

1. von Helmholtz, H., Ueber einige Gezetze der Verteilung elektrischer Ströme in körperliche Leitern mit Anwendung auf die thierisch-elektrischen Versuche. Pogg. *Ann. Physik und Chemie*, 1853;**89**: 211–233; 353–377.

2. Plonsey, R., *Bioelectric Phenomena*. New York: McGraw-Hill, 1969.

3. Plonsey, R., An extension of the solid angle formulation for an active cell. *Biophys. J.*, 1965;**5**: 663–666.

4. Plonsey, R., and R.C. Barr, *Bioelectricity: A Quantitative Approach*. New York: Kluwer Academic/Plenum Press, 2000.

5. Wilson, F.N., A.G. Macleod, and P.S. Barker, The distribution of action currents produced by the heart muscle and other excitable tissues immersed in conducting media. *J. Gen. Physiol.*, 1933;**16**: 423–456.

6. Spach, M.S., et al., Extracellular potentials related to intracellular action potentials in the dog Purkinje system. *Am. Heart J.*, 1972;**30**: 505–519.

7. van Oosterom, A. and V. Jacquemet, A parameterized description of transmembrane potentials used in forward and inverse procedures, in *International Conference on Electrocardiology*. Gdansk, Poland: Folia Cardiologica, 2005.

8. Scher, A.M. and A.C. Young, Ventricular depolarization and the genesis of the QRS. *Ann. NY Acad. Sci.*, 1957;**65**: 768–778.

9. Holland, R.P. and M.F. Arnsdorf, Solid angle theory and the electrocardiogram: physiologic and quantitative interpretations. *Prog. Cardiovasc. Dis.*, 1977;**19**: 431–457.

10. Spach, M.S., et al., Extracellular potentials related to intracellular action potentials during impulse conduction in anisotropic canine cardiac muscle. *Circulation. Res.*, 1979;**45**: 188–204.

11. Scher, A.M., L.V. Corbin, and A.C. Young, *Cardiac cell-to-cell conduction in electrocardiographic modelling*, in *Measuring and Modelling of the Cardiac Electric Field*. Slowak Acc. Science; Bratislava: VEDA, 1980.

12. van Oosterom, A. and J. Strackee, The Solid Angle of a Plane Triangle. *IEEE Trans. Biomed. Eng.*, 1983;**BME-30**(2): 125–126.

13. Durrer, D. and L.H. van der Tweel, Spread of activation in the left ventricular wall of the dog. *Am. Heart J.*, 1953;**46**: 683–691.

14. Brody, D.A., A theoretical analysis of intracavitary blood mass influence on the heart-lead relationship. *Circ. Res.*, 1956;**IV**: 731–738.

15. van Oosterom, A. and R. Plonsey, The Brody effect revisited. *J. Electrocardiol.*, 1991;**24**: 339–348.

16. Taccardi, B., et al., Effect of myocardial fiber direction on epicardial potentials. *Circulation*, 1994;**90–96**: 3076–3090.

17. van Oosterom, A. and R.T. van Dam, Potential distribution in the left ventricular wall during depolarization. *Adv. Cardiol.*, 1976;**16**: 27–31.

18. van Oosterom, A., Cardiac Potential Distributions. Department of Medical Physics,University of Amsterdam: Amsterdam, The Netherlands, 1978.

19. Ritsema van Eck, H.J., Digital Simulation of Cardiac Excitation and Depolarization. Dalhousie University: Halifax, NS, 1972.

20. Miller, W.T. and D.B. Geselowitz, Simulation studies of the electrocardiogram. I. The normal heart. *Circ. Research.*, 1978;**43**: 301–315.

21. Scher, A.M., Validity of the uniform double layer in the solution of the ECG forward problem. *J. Electrocardiol.*, 1995;**27**(Suppl.): 163–169.

22. van Oosterom, A., Solidifying the solid angle. *J. Electrocardiol.*, 2002;**35S**: 181–192.

23. Greenbaum, R.A., et al., Left ventricular fibre architecture in man. *Br. Heart J.*, 1981;**45**: 248–263.

24. Streeter, D.D.J., et al., Fiber orientation in the canine left ventricle during diastole and systole. *Circ. Res.*, 1969;**24**: 339–347.

25. Scher, A.M., Excitation of the heart, in *The Theoretical Basis of Electrocardiology*, C.V. Nelson and D.B. Geselowitz, Editors. Oxford: Clarendon Press, 1976, pp. 44–69.

26. Oostendorp, T.F., R. MacLeod, and A. van Oosterom, Non-invasive determination of the activation sequence of the heart validation with invasive data. Proc. 19-th IEEE/EMBS Conf, 1997, IEEE-Engineering in Medicine Society. CDROM: pp 335–338.

27. Ramirez, I.F., et al., Effects of cardiac configuration, paddle placement and paddle size on defibrillation current distribution: a finite element model. *Med. Biol. Eng. Comput.*, 1989;**27**: 587–594.

28. Corbin, L.V. and A.M. Scher, The canine heart as an electrocardiographic generator. *Circ. Res.*, 1977;**41/1**: 58–67.

29. Roberts, D.E. and A.M. Scher, Effect of tissue anisotropy on extracellular potential fields in canine myocardium in situ. *Circ. Res.*, 1982;**50**: 342–351.

30. Clerc, L., Directional differences of impulse spread in trabecular muscle from mammalian heart. *J. Physiol.*, 1976;**255**: 335–346.

31. Weidmann, S., Electrical constants of trabecular muscle from mammalian heart. *J. Physiol.*, 1970;**210**: 1041–1054.

32. Plonsey, R. and A. van Oosterom, Implications of macroscopic source strength on cardiac cellular activation models. *J. Electrocardiol.*, 1991;**24/2**: 99–112.

33. Roth, B.J., Electrical conductivity values used with the bidomain model of cardiac tissue. *IEEE Trans. Biomed. Eng.*, 1997;**BME-44**: 326–328.

34. Colli-Franzone, P., et al., Potential fields generated by oblique dipole layers modeling excitation wavefronts in the anisotropic myocardium: comparison with potential fields elicited by

paced dog hearts in a volume conductor. *Circ. Res.*, 1982;**51**: 330–346.

35. Taccardi, B., et al., ECG waveforms and cardiac electric sources. *J. Electrocardiol.*, 1996;**29S**: 98–100.

36. van Oosterom, A., Anisotropy and the double layer concept, in *Progress in Electrocardiology*, P.W. Macfarlane, Editor. Tunbridge Wells: Pitman Medical, 1979, pp. 91–97.

37. Henriquez, C.S., Simulating the electrical behavior of cardiac tissue using the bidomain model. *Crit. Rev. Biomed. Eng.*, 1993;**21**(1): 1–77.

38. Kléber, A.G. and C.B. Riegger, Electrical constants of arterially perfused rabbit papillary muscle. *J. Physiol.*, 1987;**385**: 307–324.

39. Scher, A.M., et al., Spread *of electrical activity through the wall of the ventricle. Cardiovasc. Res.*, 1953;**1**: 539–547.

40. van Oosterom, A., Cell models – macroscopic source descriptions, in *Comprehensive Electrocardiology*, P.W. Macfarlane and T.T.V. Lawrie, Editors. Oxford: Pergamon Press, 1989, pp. 155–179.

41. Muler, A.L. and V.S. Markin, Electrical properties of anisotropic nerve-muscle syncytia-II, spread of flat front of excitation. *Biophysics*, 1977;**22**: 536–541.

42. Gulrajani, R.M., *Bioelectricity and Biomagnetism*. New York: Wiley, 1998.

43. Cuppen, J.J.M. and A. van Oosterom, Model studies with the inversely calculated isochrones of ventricular depolarization. *IEEE Trans. Biomed. Eng.*, 1984;**BME-31**: 652–659.

44. van Oosterom, A. and T.F. Oostendorp, ECGSIM: an interactive tool for studying the genesis of QRST waveforms. *Heart*, 2004;**90**(2): 165–168.

45. Greensite, F., Y.J. Qian, and G.J.M. Huiskamp, Myocardial activation imaging: a new theorem and its implications, in Basic and Applied Biomedical Engineering, Building blocks for health care. *Proceedings of the 17th Annual International Conference of the IEEE Engineering in Medicine and Biology Society*, 1995.

46. Huiskamp, G.J.M. and A.V. Oosterom, Forward electrocardiography based on measured data, in Images of the Twenty-First Century. *Proceedings of the Annual International Conference of the IEEE Engineering in Medicine and Biology Society*, Y.K.A.F.A. Spelman, Editor. New York: IEEE Publishing Services, 1989, pp. 189–190.

47. Huiskamp, G.J.M., et al., Invasive confirmation of the human ventricular activation sequence as computed from body surface potentials. in *Computers in Cardiology '92*. Los Alamitos, CA: IEEE Computer Society Press, 1993.

48. Huiskamp, G.J.M., et al., The depolarization sequence of the human heart surface computed from measured body surface potentials: confrontation with invasive measurements. in *Electrocardiology'88*. Wiesbaden: Elsevier, 1989.

49. Modre, R., et al., Atrial noninvasive activation mapping of paced rhythm data. *J. Cardiovasc. Electrophysiol.*, 2003;**13**: 712–719.

7 The Equivalent Double Layer: Source Models for Repolarization

A. van Oosterom

P. W. Macfarlane et al. (eds.), *Basic Electrocardiology*, DOI 10.1007/978-0-85729-871-3_7,

7.1   Introduction

The modeling of the electric current sources during depolarization by means of the uniform double layer (UDL) is described in general terms in ❷ Chap. 5, and in greater detail in ❷ Chap. 6. It is linked to the electrophysiology of wave fronts propagating through the myocardium. Some decades ago [1, 2], studies appeared that exploited the equivalence between the actual double layer at the wave fronts and a source description on the heart surface, the surface bounding the myocardium. This source description has been found to be very effective in the inverse determination of the timing of depolarization on the basis of observed body surface potentials (❷ Chap. 9), a method now commonly referred to as activation time imaging.

Around the same period [3], the development of a source model started in which the equivalent cardiac electric generator is expressed in terms of the electric potentials on a surface encompassing the myocardium, similar to the pericardium. In most related studies the surface involved is referred to as the epicardium. Such voltage sources are based on the theoretical unique one-to-one relationship between the voltage on the surface bounding a volume conductor and those on some interior surface, on condition that the surface is *closed* and that no primary sources are present in between. All active sources are assumed to lie within the inner surface. Inverse methods based on this relationship aim at obtaining a "closer look" at the sources without assuming any a priori knowledge about the nature of these sources (❷ Chap. 9).

Both source models can be classed as being equivalent surface source models (ESS). In the case of the extended UDL variant the current sources are of the double layer type, in the second approach the electric current sources stem from a specification of the potential distribution on the epicardium.

This chapter describes the properties of the first source model: the equivalent current double layer surface source, which will be referred to here as the EDL model. This model has the potential of describing the cardiac electric generator during the depolarization phase (QRS segment) as well as during the repolarization phase of the cardiac cycle (STT segment), both in a manner that is related to the underlying electrophysiology. As such, it has been claimed to be promising in serving to explain STT wave morphology [4].

There is a direct link between the UDL and the EDL source model, which is based on the solid angle formulation, as is explained in ❷ Sect. 7.2. Next, in ❷ Sect. 7.3 a recent development of the theory is described, which justifies the handling of the sources during repolarization by means of the EDL. The development is based on a theoretical formulation derived by Geselowitz [5, 6]. The section describes only the most essential parts of this development. A more complete recapitulation of the theory is presented in Appendix. In ❷ Sect. 7.4 some types of STT wave morphology are shown based on the EDL source. ❷ Sect. 7.5 lists and discusses some of the major inferences on the STT wave forms as generated on the basis of the model. Finally, ❷ Sect. 7.6 discusses some potentials and limitations of the EDL source model.

7.2   Linking the UDL to the EDL

The direct link between the UDL source for modeling the sources at the wave fronts to the equivalent representation on the surface S_h stems directly from the properties of the solid angle Ω appearing in the fundamental expression that links wave front shape and extent to the resulting potential field $\Phi(\vec{r}')$ in the infinite medium,

$$\Phi(t;\vec{r}') = V_D \frac{\Omega(t)}{4\pi} \tag{7.1}$$

This is the expression discussed in ❷ Sect. 6.3.1 (6.15), here with the temporal behavior of the solid angle wave front shown explicitly. In the EDL formulation, the surface S_h considered is the closed surface encompassing the entire myocardium; for the ventricles: the epicardium and endocardium, as well as their connection at the base. The essence is explained by using the diagrams shown in ❷ Fig. 7.1.

We first consider panel A. It depicts the situation where, following a stimulus at the endocardium, the shaded region has been depolarized. The wave front carrying the UDL source is indicated by the heavy solid line. In 3D space its shape is as depicted in ❷ Fig. 6.7. The front is denoted by S_{UDL}. The field points are taken to lie outside the myocardium. For such field points the potential field generated by UDL sources on S_{UDL} is exactly the same as that generated by an equivalent UDL source, having the same strength as the one at the wave front, placed on the segment of the endocardial surface,

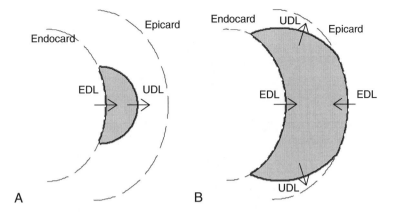

Fig. 7.1
Schematic diagram illustrating the link between UDL and EDL. *Shaded region* represents depolarized myocardium; *arrows* denote polarity of UDL and EDL double strength. *Heavy solid lines and dotted lines* represent UDL and EDL locations, respectively. *Panel A*: Early stage of depolarization following an endocardial stimulus. *Panel B*: later stage of depolarization; wave front previously broken through at the epicardium

S_{endo}, bounding the depolarized region (heavy, dashed line). This follows from the fact that for an exterior observation point both surfaces subtend the same solid angle. The same holds true for all other wave fronts lying entirely within the myocardium that have a different shape, while having an identical intersection with the endocardium: the border of the wavefront at S_{endo}. Hence, for the external field points, the UDL source at the wave front may be replaced by an equivalent (UDL type) source at S_{endo}. In ❷ Fig. 7.1A, this source is marked by the arrow EDL. Note that it points into the depolarized region, whereas the UDL source at the wave front points away from that region.

Next, the situation depicted in Panel B is treated. A break-through of the wave front has occurred and its shape may be similar to that depicted in ❷ Fig. 6.9: the de-capped hemisphere. In ❷ Fig. 7.1B the direction of the UDL sources at the wave front is identified by the two arrows labeled UDL, as always, pointing away from the depolarized region. Let the closed surface bounding the depolarized region be S_D. The latter is the union of the surface S_{UDL} of the wave front, its intersection with the endocardium S_{endo}, and its intersection with the epicardium, S_{epi}:

$$S_D = S_{UDL} \cup S_{endo} \cup S_{epi}$$

As an entry to the introduction of the EDL, we consider the effect of the placing on S_D of an extra, virtual double layer with strength V_{Dvir}. Being a closed surface, this does not generate an external field, and for external field points we find, based on (2.47) of ❷ Sect. 2.2.12 and on (7.1),

$$4\pi \, \Phi(\vec{r}') = V_D \Omega(S_{UDL}) + V_{Dvirt} \left(\Omega(S_{UDL}) + \Omega(S_{endo}) + \Omega(S_{endo}) \right),$$

an expression that holds true for any value of V_{Dvir} In particular, by choosing $V_{Dvirt} = -V_D$, the two terms involving $\Omega(S_{UDL})$ cancel, and so is found that

$$\Phi(\vec{r}') = \frac{1}{4\pi} V_D \Omega(S_{UDL}) = \frac{-1}{4\pi} V_D \left(\Omega(S_{endo}) + \Omega(S_{epi}) \right) \tag{7.2}$$

By once more using (2.47) and defining $S_{dep}(t)$ as $S_{endo}(t) \cup S_{epi}(t)$, representing the segment of the total heart surface S_h overlaying tissue that has been depolarized prior to the time t considered in ❷ Fig. 7.1b, it can be seen that a straightforward generalization of (7.2) reads

$$\Phi(t, \vec{r}') = \frac{-1}{4\pi} V_D \Omega(S_{dep}(t)) \tag{7.3}$$

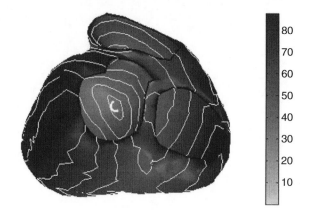

☐ **Fig. 7.2**
Activation sequence spreading over the S_h of a human ventricle is shown by means of the isochrones of the local activation time τ. The heart is depicted in a superior-right-posterial view. The activation is initiated in the middle of the left ventricular aspect of the septum (*small circle*). The sequence shown propagates at a constant velocity of 1.1 m/s through the myocardial tissue. The isochrones are drawn at 10 ms intervals

The minus sign relates to the convention of using the outward normal of S_h in the definition of the solid angle (❷ Sect. 2.2.12), as well as to the change in the direction of the virtual double, as expressed by the arrows labeled EDL shown in ❷ Fig. 7.1b. Equation (7.3) can be seen to cover likewise the situation depicted in ❷ Fig. 7.1a.

An expression that is mathematically equivalent to (7.3) reads

$$\Phi(t,\vec{r}\,') = \frac{-1}{4\pi} V_D \int_{S_h} H\left(t - \tau(\vec{r})\right) \, d\omega(\vec{r}), \tag{7.4}$$

in which the function H denotes the Heaviside step function expressed on S_h, which is zero if $t < \tau(\vec{r})$, the time of local depolarization, and equal to one otherwise. It describes the successive switching on of the contribution of elementary double layer source elements on S_h at location $\vec{r}$ at time instants $\tau(\vec{r})$. During normal propagation, all parts of S_h are successively depolarized: depolarization spreads over S_h like an oil-slick over water. Correspondingly, at the end of depolarization we have $H = 1$ over the entire closed surface S_h. At this time the integral represents the solid angle of a closed surface for an exterior field point, which is zero (2.50), as is the external field. An example of the propagation over the ventricles following a single stimulus in the middle part of the septum facing the left ventricular cavity is presented in ❷ Fig. 7.2. The isochrones shown are drawn at equal distances from the stimulus site while traveling through the myocardium [7]. At any moment in time $t = \tau(\vec{r})$ the source strength H in the region ahead of any isochrone τ is zero; at that same moment it is equal to one in the area previously depolarized, i.e., having lower values τ.

7.2.1   Discussion

If the transmural spread of the depolarizarion wave is known, the UDL source present at the wave front and its representation by the UDL source on the heart surface S_h generate exactly the same exterior potential fields, as is shown in the preceding section. For the evaluation of the forward problem there can, hence, be no advantage in using either expression (7.1) or its equivalent, variant (7.4). However, for the inverse problem of estimating the timing of depolarization from observed field potentials the situation is different. As discussed in ❷ Sect. 7.1, within the context of the UDL source, the potential fields generated by different wave fronts that have the same intersection with the surface S_h are identical. As a consequence, the actual location of the wave front inside the myocardium can not be estimated on the basis of observed potential fields.

In contrast, by using the boundary S_h as the location of the UDL sources as in (7.4), a unique inverse exists [8]. The uniqueness holds true provided that the surface S_h is known. It forms the most essential prior information required for solving the associated inverse problem (❯ Chap. 11). From the introduction of (7.4) onward, magnetic resonance imaging has been used as the technique for documenting S_h [1].

Equation (7.4) expresses the most basic variant of the equivalent double layer source EDL: a double layer distribution over the surface S_h that has zero strength until the local region depolarizes, after which the local strength is one. An alternative formulation reads

$$\Phi(t, \vec{r}') = \int_{S_h} A(\vec{r}', \vec{r})\, S(t, \vec{r})\, \mathrm{d}S(\vec{r}),\qquad(7.5)$$

where $S(t; \vec{r}) = H(t - \tau(\vec{r}))$, and the double layer strength V_D as well as the remaining variables of (7.4) are represented by the transfer from sources at location $\vec{r}$ to the potential at the field point $\vec{r}'$: $A(\vec{r}', \vec{r})\, \mathrm{d}S(\vec{r})$. The function $S(t, \vec{r})$ is dimensionless, expressing the spatio-temporal character of the EDL source. An overall scaling factor, specifying its nature (elementary current dipole density) and overall strength, is incorporated in the transfer function $A(\vec{r}', \vec{r})$.

7.3 Generalization of the EDL

The EDL source as described in the previous section is an equivalent expression for the UDL sources at the propagation wave fronts during depolarization. The effect of repolarization, which starts right from the moment of the first local depolarization, is disregarded. As a consequence, as is described above, after depolarization is complete, no external potential field remains. In the ECG this is taken to be the moment at the end of the QRS complex, the J point. However, although in the normal ECG the potential differences observed on the thorax around the J point are small, they are invariably non-zero. A more complete model of the sources of the ECG would therefore require the inclusion of the repolarization phenomena. This holds all the more true since the time interval following the J point, the STT segment, has been long recognized as yielding highly relevant diagnostic information. The generalization of the EDL source described in the next section provides a valuable model for describing (modeling) the current sources of the ECG throughout the entire cardiac cycle.

7.3.1 Linking EDL Source Strength to Transmembrane Potentials

In this section the generalization of the EDL is described in its most basic form, using the general character of impressed current density of individual cells and the various notations introduced in ❯ Chap. 2. The derivation shown here is an alternative to the one presented by Geselowitz [5, 6]. A more complete treatment is included in the appendix to this chapter.

We start from the field of an individual cell as discussed in ❯ Sect. 6.3.1, in particular from (6.1), which is recapitulated here as

$$\Phi(\vec{r}') = \frac{1}{4\pi\sigma_e} \int_S -(\sigma_i \Phi_i - \sigma_e \Phi_e)\, \mathrm{d}\omega \qquad(7.6)$$

The surface S is the cell membrane (❯ Fig. 6.1). By reintroducing the notation $M_S = -(\sigma_i \Phi_i - \sigma_e \Phi_e)$ for the strength of the equivalent dipole surface density directed along the outward normal of S (6.6), and using

$$\mathrm{d}\omega = \frac{\vec{R}}{R^3} \bullet \mathrm{d}\vec{S} = \nabla \frac{1}{R} \bullet \mathrm{d}\vec{S}$$

(2.48 and 2.33), we see that

$$\Phi(\vec{r}') = \frac{1}{4\pi\sigma_e} \int_S M_S \nabla \frac{1}{R} \bullet \mathrm{d}\vec{S} \qquad(7.7)$$

Next, we apply Gauss' law (2.26) to the integral on the right. For the (virtual) vector field

$$M_S(\vec{r}) \nabla \frac{1}{R(\vec{r})}$$

this yields

$$\int_S M_S \nabla \frac{1}{R} \bullet d\vec{S} = \int_V \nabla \bullet \left(M_S(\vec{r}) \, \nabla \frac{1}{R(\vec{r})} \right) dV = \int_V \nabla \bullet M_S(\vec{r}) \, \nabla \frac{1}{R(\vec{r})} \, dV$$
$$+ \int_V M_S(\vec{r}) \, \nabla^2 \frac{1}{R(\vec{r})} \, dV \qquad (7.8)$$

The second integral on the right is zero, because R is non-zero for exterior field points $\vec{r}'$.

Equation (2.161); the integration is over the internal source locations within the cell volume V. With the remaining first integral applied to (7.7) we see that

$$\Phi(\vec{r}') = \frac{1}{4\pi\sigma_e} \int_S M_S \, \nabla \frac{1}{R} \bullet d\vec{S} = \frac{1}{4\pi\sigma_e} \int_V \nabla \bullet M_S(\vec{r}) \, \nabla \frac{1}{R(\vec{r})} \, dV, \qquad (7.9)$$

which identifies $\nabla \bullet M_S(\vec{r})$ as a (virtual) volume source density throughout cell volume V (❯ Sect. 2.5.3).

With the potential field generated by a single cell now being expressed by (7.9), we may compute the potential for field points outside the myocardium by taking the volume V to represent the entire myocardial tissue. However, this volume also includes the interstitial space. This may be accounted for by introducing a local volume fraction $0 \le f_v(\vec{r}) \le 1$, the fraction of space occupied locally by the cell volume. For densely packed myocardial cells this fraction is of the order of 0.8.

Inserting this (scalar) factor in (7.9) and reversing the derivation along (7.7)–(7.9) leads to the interpretation of surface S in (7.7) as representing the surface bounding the myocardium. The expression for the external potential field then reads

$$\Phi(\vec{r}') = \frac{1}{4\pi\sigma_e} \int_{S_h} f_v(\vec{r}) M_S(\vec{r}) \, d\omega(\vec{r}', \vec{r}) \qquad (7.10)$$

Note that both the volume fraction and the virtual double layer source density in this expression relate to their values at S_h (only). In the applications of this expression shown in the next section, the approximation $M_S = -(\sigma_i \Phi_i - \sigma_e \Phi_e) \approx -\sigma_i V_m$ is used, leading to

$$\Phi(\vec{r}') = \frac{-1}{4\pi\sigma_e} \int_{S_h} f_v \sigma_i V_m d\omega \qquad (7.11)$$

Finally, if σ_i and f_v are assumed to be uniform over S_h, and by reintroduction of the temporal nature of the transmembrane potential, we have

$$\Phi(t, \vec{r}') = \frac{-f_v \sigma_i}{4\pi\sigma_e} \int_{S_h} V_m(t, \vec{r}) \, d\omega(\vec{r}', \vec{r}), \qquad (7.12)$$

which may be cast in the same form as in (7.5) by writing

$$\Phi(t, \vec{r}') = \int_{S_h} A(\vec{r}', \vec{r}) V_m(t, \vec{r}) \, dS(\vec{r}), \qquad (7.13)$$

with all scaling factors, including the negative sign, now absorbed in the (solid angle) transfer function A. The overall scaling factor used in the sequel is taken such that, by assigning a shape to V_m that is identical to that of the function S used in ❯ Sect. 2.1 in (7.5) during depolarization, the potential field resulting from using (7.13) is the same as the one based on (7.5). The value of the scaling factor used in the sequel corresponds to taking the effective double layer strength inside a medium of unit conductivity to be 40 mV, an overall value previously deduced from experimental studies [9–11].

7.3.2   Discussion

Equation (7.13) defines the spatio-temporal potentials in the infinite medium. For a bounded medium, the same basic formulation can be used. In this situation the potential field can be found by applying the spatial linear filter expressing all volume conductor effects, as is explained in ❷ Sect. 2.6.4.3. This yields as the final, most direct expression for the potential field of the EDL

$$\Phi(t, \vec{r}') = \int_{S_h} B(\vec{r}', \vec{r}) V_m(t, \vec{r}) \, dS(\vec{r}), \tag{7.14}$$

with $B(\vec{r}', \vec{r})$ the linear function expressing the full transfer between EDL source elements around $\vec{r}$ on S_h to the potential at field points $\vec{r}'$ inside the bounded medium external to S_h. Note that this also handles the situation where the conductivity outside S_h has a conductivity $\sigma_o \neq \sigma_e$.

If either f_v or σ_i are non-uniform over S_h, (7.11) needs to be used instead of (7.12), which requires a full specification of these variables.

Interestingly, within the various assumptions implied in deriving (7.14), the EDL source model indicated that any sources *within* S_h do not directly influence the external potential field. However, the activity of such internal sources does affect the propagation of all depolarization waves that may be simultaneously propagating within the myocardium and thus the wave form and timing of the sources at S_h. The same applies to the subsequent repolarization process.

The effectiveness of the EDL source model in describing ECGs as well as electrograms, both during depolarization and repolarization, is illustrated in the next section.

7.4 ECG Signals Generated by the EDL

The properties of the EDL source model are illustrated here in an application to simulating ECG wave forms on the thorax and electrograms on the heart surface S_h. As discussed in ❷ Sect. 7.3.2 (7.14), this requires the computation of the transfer function $B(\vec{r}', \vec{r})$ describing the volume conduction properties, the surface S_h carrying the EDL and the spatio-temporal transmembrane potential over S_h. Simulations of this type have been described in the literature both for the ventricles [12, 13] and for the atria [14]. Here, an application to ventricular activity is shown. The evaluation of (7.14) was carried out numerically, in which the field potentials transfer $\Phi(t, \vec{r}')$, the transfer matrix $B(\vec{r}', \vec{r})$ and the $V_m(t, \vec{r})$ were represented by matrices $\mathbf{\Phi}$, $\mathbf{B}$ and $\mathbf{V}_m$, respectively. The numerical variant of (7.14) then reads

$$\mathbf{\Phi} = \mathbf{B}\mathbf{V}_m, \tag{7.15}$$

an expression similar to (5.12) in ❷ Sect. 5.9.4. As discussed in that same section, the sum of all elements of any row of matrix $\mathbf{B}$ equals zero.

7.4.1 Source Specification

The shape of S_h is shown in ❷ Fig. 7.2. It was obtained from magnetic resonance images (MRI) taken from a healthy male subject. The image shown is that of a triangulated version of S_h, specified by $N = 1,500$ evenly distributed nodes. Realistic transmembrane potentials were assigned to each node n. Their wave forms are based on an analytical function involving logistic curves [15]. The parameters of this function were fixed, apart from a parameter δ_n specifying, for each individual node n, the local timing of the maximum upslope during depolarization, and a parameter ρ_n specifying the timing of the maximal downslope during repolarization. The difference $\alpha_n = \rho_n - \delta_n$ represents the local duration of the transmembrane potential, a measure similar to the activation recovery interval (ARI) introduced in the work of Haws and Lux [16]. The variety of wave forms of the assigned TMPs is illustrated in ❷ Fig. 7.3, by showing the TMPs of the nodes having maximum δ_n, ρ_n and α_n values, as well as of those having minimum δ_n, ρ_n and α_n values. Maps of local depolarization times δ_n and repolarization times ρ_n on the heart surface S_h used for the demonstration of the properties of the EDL source model are shown in ❷ Fig. 7.4. The numerical expression of the entire source configuration is that of a matrix $\mathbf{V}_m$. Its $N = 1,500$ rows represent the individual TMPs at all nodes on S_h. Each row expresses a TMP sampled at 1 ms intervals, comprising $T = 500$ samples. The descriptive statistics of the basic parameters of all 1,500 nodes are as shown in ❷ Table 7.1.

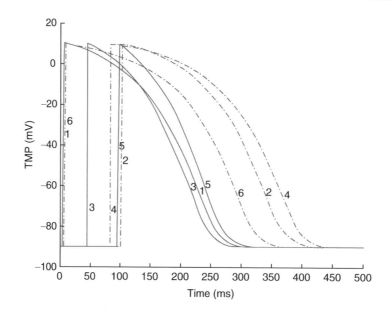

Fig. 7.3

Stylized transmembrane potentials of six nodes on S_h. Labels shown to the right of the traces near maximum upslope (timing δ_n), maximal downslope (timing ρ_n) of the TMPs. Labels refer to the TMPs with (1) earliest δ_n, (2) latest δ_n, (3) earliest ρ_n, (4) latest ρ_n, (5) shortest α_n, and (6) longest α_n

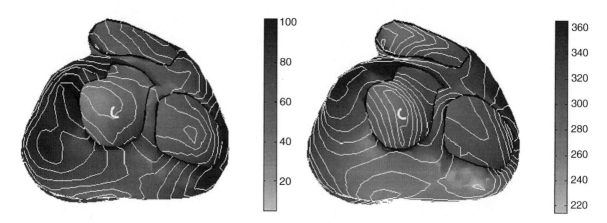

Fig. 7.4

Left: Timing of depolarization times δ_n of 1,500 nodes on S_h of a human ventricle, used in EDL based simulation of QRST wave forms. *Right*: corresponding values for the local repolarization times ρ_n. The isochrones are drawn at 10 ms intervals. The heart is depicted in a superior-right-posterior view. The small semicircle marks the site on the septum where depolarization was earliest

7.4.2 The Transfer Function B

The numerical expression of $B(\vec{r}', \vec{r})$ (7.14), the linear function expressing the full transfer related to the volume conduction effects inside the thorax, can be represented by a matrix **B**. Each of its elements expresses the transfer between an individual EDL source element at node n of S_h to the potential at any of L locations (field points) of interest. These

Table 7.1

TMP parameters of all 500 nodes on S_h

	Mean	SD	Min	Max	Range (max–min)
dep δ (ms)	52.2	19.7	4.95	102	97
rep ρ (ms)	276	21.7	214	367	152
ARI α (ms)	225	24.4	142	285	143

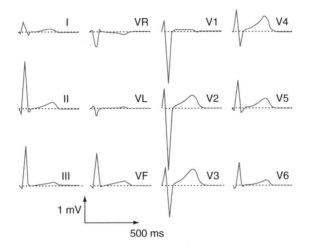

Fig. 7.5

Superposition of measured standard 12-lead ECG (*dash-dot line*) and the EDL based simulations (*solid lines*). The high quality of the simulated signals causes the traces in the two line styles to be almost indistinguishable. Note that the signals at the extremity electrodes, VL, VR and VF, are shown in an unaugmented scaling, which emphasizes their equal footing with the precordial signals V1–V6, all nine being referred to the same reference (WCT)

matrix elements were computed by using the boundary element method (❯ Sect. 2.6.4.3) applied to an MRI documentation of the geometry of thorax, lungs and the blood filled cavities of the subject for whom the EDL properties are discussed in this chapter. These compartments constitute the inhomogeneous representation of the most relevant, significant inhomogeneities inside the thorax.

For any desired set of L locations (field points) the EDL based wave forms of potentials on the thorax or any other set of field points outside the myocardium, such as electrograms on endocardium or epicardium, can be computed from (7.15).

The matrix Φ representing the simulated potentials has L rows (L wave forms), specified at T subsequent time instances. Dedicated versions of the transfer matrix $\mathbf{B}$ may be computed for the field points of interest, lying, e.g., on the thorax surface or on the surface S_h. In the following two sections examples are shown for ECGs and electrograms.

7.4.3 Standard 12-Lead ECG

The matrix Φ of the EDL based simulated potentials at the electrode positions of the standard 12-lead ECG is shown in ❯ Fig. 7.5. The simulated signals are superimposed on the signals measured on the subject studied.

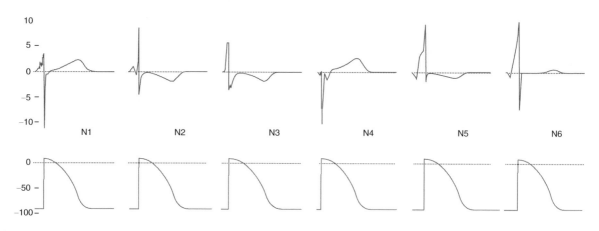

Fig. 7.6

Upper traces: EDL based electrograms at six nodes of S_h. *Lower traces*: TMPs (local EDL source strength) at these nodes. Note the fast downward deflection in the electrograms, with their timing coinciding with the fast upstroke of the TMPs. Time interval: 500 ms; vertical scale in mV

Table 7.2

TMP parameters and electrogram features of 6 of the 1,500 nodes on S_h shown in Fig. 7.6

	Node					
	N1	N2	N3	N4	N5	N6
Location	epi RV	endo RV	septal RV	septal LV	endo LV	epi RV
δ_n (ms)	59	60	34	25	86	82
ρ_n (ms)	268	287	273	240	294	284
α_n (ms)	208	227	239	215	208	202
Amplitude fast negative deflection electrograms (mV)	14.7	13.2	9.22	10.7	11.2	18.4
Apex T wave electrogram (mV)	2.24	−1.89	−1.83	2.71	−1.16	0.576

7.4.4   Endocardial and Epicardial Electrograms

EDL based electrograms simulated at six of the 1,500 nodes on S_h are illustrated in Fig. 7.6. The nodes were selected along the intersection of a straight line, crossing the myocardium, from N1 (epicardial node at the free wall of the right ventricle) to N6 (epicardial node on the free wall of the left ventricle). The remaining four nodes are: node N2: the RV endocardial node closest to node N1, node N3: the node at the intersection of the line and RV aspect of the septum, node N4: the node at the intersection of the line and the LV aspect of the septum, node N5: the node on the endocardium of the LV closest to N6. The potential reference was the mean of the potentials at all nodes. The TMP parameters of the six nodes and some of the features of the electrograms are listed in Table 7.2.

7.4.5   Discussion

The realism of the signal wave forms shown in Figs. 7.5 and 7.6 demonstrates the power of the EDL source model for modeling electrocardiographic signals. Being based on apparently minor differences in the TMP wave forms, the morphology of the signals arises from the geometry of the myocardium (S_h), the timing of depolarization and repolarization at S_h and the transfer expressing volume conduction effects.

The high correlation between the simulated and the measured potentials is no guarantee that the source model as such is valid. A proper validation would also require the various model components to be realistic. The major emphasis here lies on the realism of the timing of depolarization δ_n and repolarization ρ_n. The timing used in the simulations, shown in ❷ Fig. 7.4, are based on an inverse procedure, similar to the one described in [17]. The realism of the resulting depolarization times has been established by comparing them with those found in invasive studies, notably the study by Durrer et al. published in 1970 [18]. The timing of repolarization has, similarly, been derived from a dedicated adaptation of the inverse procedure [13]. Here no complete set of reference data derived from invasive measurements is available, but the sparse data that is available seems to agree with the global nature of the isochrones shown in the right panel of ❷ Fig. 7.4 [19, 20]. For a more complete discussion of this topic, see [4].

The wave forms of electrograms on the epicardium, with the heart placed inside an infinite homogeneous medium, were simulated by Simms and Geselowitz. The surface source model implied is the EDL. The global morphology and magnitudes of their results, documented during depolarization only, are in full agreement with those described for the spherical shell discussed in ❷ Chap. 6. In the study by di Bernardo and Murray of the genesis of the T wave [21], the implied source model was also the EDL. The examples shown here relate to ventricular activity only. However, the application of this source model to the electric activity of the atria has also proved to be effective [14].

7.4.6 T Waves as Explained in Standard Text Books

Most ECG textbooks include some notions related to the genesis of the T wave. Correct as these may be in a general sense, they do not do justice to the complexity of the problem. In this chapter the full spatio-temporal character of the sources is represented by an equivalent surface source situated at the boundary of ventricular tissue. The local source strength is assigned the characteristic wave form of the transmembrane potentials of ventricular muscle cells. The simulated potentials shown in ❷ Figs. 7.5 and ❷ 7.6 were derived from a linear combination of a large number of assigned transmembrane potentials.

In contrast, in ECG textbooks the morphology of the T wave is explained by subtracting just two typical transmembrane wave forms. Differences in timing in agreement with the general concepts of electrophysiology are assigned to it [22]. An example of this approach is shown in ❷ Fig. 7.7. In the upper traces, paired TMP potential wave forms of the type shown in ❷ Fig. 7.6 are depicted. The solid lines were assigned all upstrokes at $\delta = 30$ ms; the timing of the maximal downslope is at $\rho = 290$ ms. The dash-dot lines all have their upstroke at $\delta = 40$ ms, and ρ values, from left to right: 250, 270, 290, 310 and 330 ms.

The lower traces depict the differences between the paired electrograms shown above them (solid traces minus dash-dot traces). These may be likened to the wave forms of either electrograms or basic ECGs. Here we will refer to these wave forms as electrograms.

1. As a consequence of the applied subtraction, the amplitude of their "QRS" complexes would be 100 mV, a value that is clearly unrealistic. In practice the involved scaling depends on the volume conductor configuration, in particular the distance between source and field points.
2. For the TMPs shown, the baseline of the electrograms is zero: a common resting potential of the TMPs does not become expressed.
3. The sign of the T wave reflects the sign of the difference between the repolarization times of the two TMPs: $\Delta\rho = \rho_{solid} - \rho_{dash-dot}$. Similarly, $\Delta\delta = \delta_{solid} - \delta_{dash-dot}$ corresponds to the sign of the "QRS." This results in QRS and T waves having the same polarity (concordant signs) if the signs of $\Delta\rho$ and $\Delta\delta$ as defined above, are the same. Non-concordant signs result if the order of the sequence of depolarization is the same as that of repolarization.
4. The timing of the apex of the T wave shown is [268 280 X 299 307], which is approximately equal to the mean of the repolarization times ρ_{solid} and $\rho_{dash-dot}$. The X corresponds to the situation of the third pair: since both TMP repolarize simultaneously, no T wave is generated.
5. The absolute value of apex T is proportional to $\Delta\rho$. In particular, if $\Delta\rho = 0$ the amplitude of the T wave is zero.

In basic textbooks on electrocardiography the justification for the approach of subtracting two slightly different TMPs and taking the difference to represent ECG morphology is usually not discussed. The EDL theory can be used for this purpose, while also pinpointing the limitations of the simple approach, as is shown below.

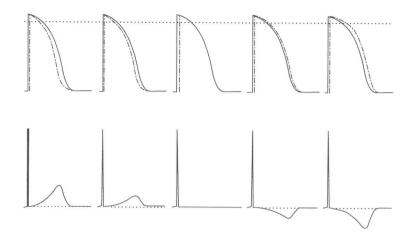

Fig. 7.7

Upper traces: TMP wave forms similar to the ones shown in ❯ Fig. 7.6; *solid lines*: timing upstroke: 30 ms for all five traces from left to right; timing maximal downslope 290 ms for all traces. *Dash-dot lines* timing upstroke: 40 ms for all five traces; timing maximal downslope (from left to right) 250, 270, 290, 310 and 330 ms. *Lower traces*: subtraction of the respective two TMPs (*solid traces – dash-dot traces*) shown above. Time interval: 500 ms; Upstroke TMP's from −90 to +10 mV; Vertical scale of lower traces in arbitrary units. *Dotted lines* drawn at zero level

The subtraction method, resulting in an electrogram $\phi_\ell(t)$ can be formulated as

$$\phi_\ell(t) = 1 \times V_{m,1}(t) + (-1) \times V_{m,2}(t), \tag{7.16}$$

which expresses the electrogram as a linear combination of two transmembrane potentials. The weights of the linear combination are 1 and −1, respectively. This, in turn, can be written as

$$\mathbf{\Phi} = \mathbf{B}\mathbf{V}_m, \tag{=(7.15)}$$

with the matrix $\mathbf{B}$ here being the row vector $[1\ {-}1]$. The motivation for highlighting this parallel is that, as is evident, the sum of the elements of the row is zero, similar to that which holds true for volume conduction effects acting on transmembrane potentials derived sources (❯ Sect. 5.9.4), as is the EDL.

In some studies, electrograms were considered in their relationship to two subtracted transmembrane potentials [23, 24]. The signals were observed on a small part of myocardial tissue (referred to as a wedge) placed in a small perfusion chamber (bath). The potential difference was recorded between two electrodes in the bath, each placed at some distance from two opposing sides of the tissue, the endocardial side and the epicardial side. This signal was referred to as the ECG. In addition, two intracellular traces were shown, one recorded at the endocardial and one at the epicardial aspect of the tissue. The question here is: what type of source model can be proposed to justify this procedure? How could a local transmembrane potential act as the source for an external electrogram?

This question can be answered on the basis of by the EDL. In the study, the sources were assumed to lie on the endocardial aspect, S_1, and on the epicardial aspect, S_2, of the surface S bounding the tissue. Any sources on the remaining part of S were ignored. Moreover, all "sources" on the endocardium were implicitly assumed to have the same strength (TMP): $V_{m,1}(t)$, those on the epicardium $V_{m;2}(t)$. Under these conditions, let $\phi_1(t)$ denote the potential at the electrode in the bath facing S_1 and $\phi_2(t)$ the potential at the electrode facing S_2 based on (7.12). By writing

$$c = \frac{f_v \sigma_i}{4\pi\,\sigma_e}$$

we see that

$$\phi_1(t) = -c\left(V_{m,1}(t)\,\Omega_{1,1} + V_{m,2}(t)\,\Omega_{1,2}\right) \tag{7.17}$$

Similarly, the potential at field point 2 reads

$$\phi_2(t) = -c\left(V_{m,1}(t)\,\Omega_{2,1} + V_{m,2}(t)\,\Omega_{2,2}\right) \tag{7.18}$$

Note that $\Omega_{i,j}$ is the solid angle subtended by the entire surface S_j at field point i, $(i,j = 1, 2)$. If the thickness of the preparation is discarded we have, in fair approximation, $\Omega_{1,1} = -\Omega_{1,2} \triangleq \Omega_1$ and $\Omega_{2,1} = -\Omega_{2,2} \triangleq \Omega_2$ and, hence the potential difference between the field points, taken to be the electrogram $E(t)$ follows, by subtracting (7.18) from (7.17), as

$$E(t) = \phi_1(t) - \phi_2(t) = -c\left(\Omega_1 + \Omega_2\right)\left(V_{m,1}(t) - V_{m,2}(t)\right) \tag{7.19}$$

Within the assumed validity of the ELD source, this indeed justifies taking the electrogram to be the (scaled) difference between two transmembrane potentials, but only if the rim of the wedge may be assumed to be very thin, which allows the contribution to the potential of any "activity" on the rim to be ignored. Moreover, both faces (epicardial and endocardial) need to be activated uniformly. In all other circumstances, like that of the intact heart, (7.12) needs to be evaluated in full detail, involving multiple sub-segments of the surface, each having their individual transmembrane potential.

The scaling factor depends on the conductivities and solid angles involved: $-c\left(\Omega_1 + \Omega_2\right)$. The individual solid angles are larger for observation points closer to the surface of the tissue, with 2π being their maximum magnitude for a planar surface (2.52).

This analysis also emphasizes that, when applying the solid angle theory to electrocardiography, at least two solid angles need to be considered. The first one is the solid angle subtended by the EDL source at the observation point. The second one is its solid angle subtended at the reference point. Any observed electrogram or body surface potential relates to the *difference* between these two solid angles. The analysis remains valid when the effect of the finiteness and/or inhomogeneity of the volume conductor is included, since this effect can be viewed a linear operator acting on the infinite medium potentials (❯ Sect. 2.6.4.3).

7.5 EDL Based Inferences for Basic STT Parameters

A discussion of T wave features derived from completely general physical and physiological principles is presented in ❯ Sect. 5.9.4. The resulting fundamental, basic expressions, (5.12) and (5.13) are the same as shown in this chapter for the EDL. In ❯ Sect. 5.9.4, the matrix $\mathbf{V}_m$ represents the transmembrane potentials of all myocytes, acting as the source. In this chapter the matrix $\mathbf{V}_m$ represents the transmembrane potentials at the surface bounding the myocardium. Within the limitations of this approximation, the inferences drawn from (5.12) and (5.13) may be carried over to the T waves as generated by the EDL. Some additional inferences of T wave morphology as derived from the EDL based signals, as previously published [13, 25], are as follows.

The first three points apply in general:

1. Rather than being a weighted sum (the difference) of two TMPs, the ECG is a weighted sum of numerous transmembrane potentials. The weighting coefficients relate to the positions of the field points relative to the heart as well as to volume conduction effects. For any field point, the sum of the weighting coefficients is zero, as is the case for the two weights ($+1$, -1) expressing a subtraction.
2. Both depolarization (QRS) and repolarization (STT) morphology will generally not be monophasic if resulting from the subtraction of two TMPs as shown ❯ Fig. 7.7, but rather biphasic or triphasic as shown in ❯ Fig. 7.5, involving numerous, slightly different TMPs.
3. The notion that the timing of local epicardial repolarization precedes that of local endocardial repolarization may be true in the statistical sense (❯ Table 7.2) but is not necessarily valid at all transmural locations (❯ Table 7.1 and ❯ Fig. 7.4).

The remaining remarks apply to the situation discussed in ❯ Sect. 5.9.4: the TMPs acting as the source for the EDL are assumed to have a similar shape, differing mainly in the timing of local depolarization δ_n and repolarization ρ_n only. Moreover, the individual deviations from the mean repolarization time, $\Delta\rho_n = \rho_n - \bar{\rho}$, being the full expression of dispersion of the timing of repolarization, are assumed to be small relative to the duration of the downslope of the

TMPs [13, 25, 26]. These assumptions apply to the healthy myocardium of subjects at rest. Deviations from it show up as differences in the features listed below. All weights mentioned below are lead specific and depend on the volume conductor properties of the thorax.

1. The individual T wave morphologies of any lead is a weighted sum of the derivative of a mean transmembrane potential, $\bar{V}_m(t)$. The function $-\bar{V}_m(t)$ has been named the Dominant T wave [25]. The negative sign was included to bring its polarity in line with that of the T wave polarity observed in most of the precordial standard leads.
2. The timing of the Dominant T wave is equal to the mean repolarization time $\bar{\rho}$ [16, 25]. Note that this is a generalization of what is found when subtracting just two TMPs (❷ Sect. 7.4.6).
3. The integral over time of any lead potential reflects a weighted sum of the individual $\Delta\rho_n$ values.
4. The magnitude of the apex value of an individual T wave is a weighted sum of the $\Delta\rho_n$ values. Note that this is a generalization of what is found when subtracting just two TMPs (❷ Sect. 7.4.6).
5. The width of individual T waves reflects the duration of the downslope of the mean TMP.

7.6   Discussion

The most general expression of the use of the EDL source model discussed in this chapter is (7.13) or, in its discretized form, (7.15). The way in which the EDL is introduced in ❷ Sects. 7.2 and ❷ 7.3 is through its link with the classic UDL source model. However, a far more general variant, expressed in its numerical form, is

$$\Phi = BS, \qquad (7.20)$$

in which matrix $\mathbf{S}$ specifies the strength of an equivalent double layer (current dipole layer) on any surface S bounding all active, primary sources (❷ Chap. 2). Based on the general laws of volume conduction theory (❷ Chap. 2) it can be shown that such a source description provides a unique specification of the potential field in the region exterior to S [8].

The EDL variant discussed in this chapter takes S to coincide with S_h, the surface bounding all myocytes. Moreover, its strength is taken to be proportional to the local transmembrane potential $\mathbf{V}_m(t)$ at S_h. In view of the realism of the wave forms based on this source model, ❷ Fig. 7.5 for ECG wave forms and ❷ Fig. 7.6 for electrograms, it can be concluded that the source model appears to be appropriate for describing the genesis of ECG during the repolarization phase of the cardiac myocytes. The wave forms shown relate to healthy myocardium of a subject at rest. The dispersion of the timing of repolarization was small, ischemia was absent and individual TMP wave forms were assumed to have a similar shape.

Other simulations based on the EDL have been reported in the literature, e.g., [12, 27–29]. The interactive simulation package ECGSIM [30] in fact uses the EDL as the source model. Such simulations reveal that by reducing local transmembrane potentials on S_h the effect of acute ischemia on STT wave forms can be studied in individual leads.

It may seem to be puzzling that only the myocytes close to S_h are involved as elements of the EDL, thus discarding any contributions of mid-myocardial myocytes. The main explanation for this is that the effective source strength derived from local mid-myocardial myocytes is proportional to local differences (the divergence, ❷ Sect. 2.2.7) of the gradients of their TMPs. These tend to cancel for mid-myocardial myocites, but not for myocytes at S_h. Even so, the EDL source model must be considered as an effective first order approximation. This topic is treated in greater detail in the Appendix. The treatment is relevant only for circumstances in which the EDL source $\mathbf{S}$, as in (7.20), can be taken to be the local transmembrane potential $\mathbf{V}_m(t)$ at S, as in (7.15), with S coinciding with the heart surface S_h. In all other situations the general expression for the EDL source strength $\mathbf{S}$, as in (7.20), may still be used in a forward simulation. This requires $\mathbf{S}$ to be known.

Appendix: The EDL and Bidomain Theory

The equivalent double layer source on the closed surface S_h bounding the myocardium can be used to represent the potential field outside S_h as generated by all myocytes within S_h. The derivation of the EDL presented in ❷ Sect. 3.1 uses the approximation $-(\sigma_i\Phi_i - \sigma_e\Phi_e) \approx -\sigma_i V_m$, which expresses the double layer strength generating the field of a single cell placed inside a large container [31, 32]. The approximate nature of this step is clear when computing the contribution to the potential field of an individual myocyte surrounded by closely packed neighbors: the presence of such neighbors will affect the external potential field.

General Formulation

An alternative derivation may be based on the bidomain theory [33–38] (❯ Sect. 8.3.2), which is a macroscopic description of the potential field based on the concept of two interpenetrating domains: one representing the intercellular space, the other the extracellular space [38]. Both are treated as being homogenized, having effective conductivities $\mathbf{G_i}$ and $\mathbf{G_e}$, respectively. The latter differs from the "normal" conductivity in that the geometry of the cellular compartment and the interstitial space is taken into account. The notation using bold capitals stresses the fact that most biological tissues exhibit anisotropic conductivity as a consequence of their fiber structure. This needs to be expressed by a tensor rather than by a scalar. The tensor involved can be expressed by a symmetric 3×3 matrix.

Although the membranes as such are not represented explicitly, the electric sources at the membranes are accounted for by impressed currents. The derivation of the EDL source as based on the bidomain theory, and explained by using lead field concepts (❯ Chap. 10) was formulated by Geselowitz [5, 6]. Below, the essential steps are presented in a condensed form, exclusively derived from the bidomain theory.

The full bidomain based expression (compare (8.10)) for computing the extracellular potential from $\nabla V_m(\vec{r})$ reads

$$\nabla \bullet ((\mathbf{G_i}(\vec{r}) + \mathbf{G_e}(\vec{r}))\nabla \phi_e(\vec{r})) = -\nabla \bullet (\mathbf{G_i}(\vec{r})\nabla V_m(\vec{r})) \tag{7.21}$$

Recall that the nabla operator, ∇, acting on a scalar function produces a gradient field, the vector consisting of the three spatial partial derivatives. The divergence operator, $\nabla \bullet$ acting on a vector, sums the spatial derivatives of its (vector) argument, thus producing a scalar field (❯ Sects. 2.2.6 and ❯ 2.2.7).

The solving of (7.21) needs to be carried out numerically. Its complexity hampers the drawing of inferences from the formulation as such. In order to proceed, some simplifying assumptions are made, the realism and validity of which are discussed at the end of this appendix.

Equal Anisotropy Ratio Assumption

We first assume the ratio of the extracellular and intracellular conductivity tensors to be a constant κ, independent of position:

$$\mathbf{G_e}(\vec{r}) = \kappa \, \mathbf{G_i}(\vec{r}) \tag{7.22}$$

For elements of the conductivity tensors along (L) fiber direction or transverse to it (T) this corresponds to assuming $g_{eL} = \kappa \, g_{iL}$, $g_{eT} = \kappa g_{iT}$ and, hence, $g_{eL}/g_{eT} = g_{iL}/g_{iT}$. Based on this, the assumption is referred to as the "equal anisotropy ratio assumption."

Inserting (7.22) in (7.21), leads to

$$\nabla \bullet (\mathbf{G_e}(\vec{r})\nabla \phi_e(\vec{r})) = -\nabla \bullet \left(\frac{\kappa}{1+\kappa}\mathbf{G_i}(\vec{r})\nabla V_m(\vec{r})\right) = -\nabla \bullet (\mathbf{G_\kappa}(\vec{r})\nabla V_m(\vec{r})), \tag{7.23}$$

with

$$\mathbf{G_\kappa} \triangleq \frac{\kappa}{1+\kappa}\mathbf{G_i}$$

Equation (7.23) applies to the medium inside S_h, the myocardium. Outside S_h we want to find the potential field ϕ_0, while assuming a local conductivity $\mathbf{G_0}$. Since no primary sources are present outside S_h we have

$$\nabla \bullet (\mathbf{G_0}\nabla \phi_0) = 0 \tag{7.24}$$

With no primary sources present on S_h, the standard continuity conditions of current flow (2.127) and (2.128) apply at S_h, and so we have for field points on S_h:

$$\phi_0 = \phi_e \quad \text{and} \quad \vec{e}_n \bullet (\mathbf{G}_0 \nabla \phi_0) = \vec{e}_n \bullet (\mathbf{G}_e \nabla \phi_e) \tag{7.25}$$

We now introduce potential field ϕ, and define it to be equal to ϕ_0 outside S_h and equal to ϕ_e inside S_h. The potential field is taken to be present in a medium with conductivity $\mathbf{G}(\vec{r}) = \mathbf{G}_0(\vec{r})$ in the region outside S_h, and $\mathbf{G}(\vec{r}) = \mathbf{G}_e(\vec{r})$ inside S_h. Correspondingly, we have $\mathbf{G}_\kappa(\vec{r}) = \mathbf{G}(\vec{r})/(1 + \kappa)$. It can be seen that a function ϕ that is a solution to

$$\nabla \bullet (\mathbf{G}(\vec{r}) \nabla \phi(\vec{r})) = \nabla \bullet \vec{J}^i \tag{7.26}$$

in which

$$\vec{J}^i = -\mathbf{G}_\kappa(\vec{r}) \nabla V_m(\vec{r}) \tag{7.27}$$

satisfies the continuity equations (7.25) as well as (7.23) and (7.24).

The solution to (7.26) links the impressed volume conduction density $i_v = -\nabla \bullet \vec{J}^i$, a scalar function (unit: A m^{-3}), to the desired potential field $\phi(\vec{r}')$, which is also a scalar function (unit: V) (❯ Sect. 2.5.3). Based on the linearity of the conductive medium, the superposition principle may be applied, with the integral adding up the contributions of the elementary sources. This may be expressed as

$$\phi(\vec{r}') = \int\limits_{vol} Z(\vec{r}', \vec{r}) \, i_v(\vec{r}) \, \mathrm{d}V = - \int\limits_{vol} Z(\vec{r}', \vec{r}) \, \nabla \bullet \vec{J}^i(\vec{r}) \, \mathrm{d}V \tag{7.28}$$

The scalar function $Z(\vec{r}', \vec{r})$ represents the transfer between individual point sources $i_v(\vec{r}) \, \mathrm{d}V$ (unit: A) and the potential. Through Ohm's law, it has as its unit: Ohm. It is the solution to the variant of the basic problem to be solved, (7.26),

$$\nabla \bullet (\mathbf{G}(\vec{r}) \nabla Z(\vec{r}', \vec{r})) = -\delta(\vec{r}', \vec{r}), \tag{7.29}$$

with $\delta(\vec{r}', \vec{r})$ the 3D Dirac delta function (❯ Sect. 2.6.4.1) expressing the source density of a point source at $\vec{r}$.

Equation (7.28) applies completely generally, irrespective of any inhomogeneity or anisotropy. In complex volume conductor configurations the function $Z(\vec{r}', \vec{r})$ may not easily be computed. The derivation of the EDL shown utilizes the general nature of (7.28).

The application of the divergence theorem (2.26) to the vector field $Z(\vec{r}', \vec{r}) \vec{J}^i(\vec{r})$ shows that

$$\int\limits_{vol} \nabla \bullet (Z(\vec{r}', \vec{r}) \, \vec{J}^i(\vec{r})) \, \mathrm{d}V = \int\limits_{S_h} Z(\vec{r}', \vec{r}) \, \vec{J}^i(\vec{r}) \bullet \mathrm{d}\vec{S} = 0$$

The integral on the right is zero since the boundary condition used for the internal domain is $\vec{J}^i(\vec{r}) \bullet \mathrm{d}\vec{S} = 0$ at S_h. From the above, we have

$$\int\limits_{vol} \nabla \bullet (Z(\vec{r}', \vec{r}) \, \vec{J}^i(\vec{r})) \, \mathrm{d}V = \int\limits_{vol} \nabla Z(\vec{r}', \vec{r}) \bullet \vec{J}^i(\vec{r}) \, \mathrm{d}V$$

$$+ \int\limits_{vol} Z(\vec{r}', \vec{r}) \, \nabla \bullet \vec{J}^i(\vec{r}) \, \mathrm{d}V = 0$$

and (7.28) is seen to be equivalent to

$$\phi(\vec{r}') = - \int\limits_{vol} \vec{J}^i(\vec{r}) \bullet \nabla Z(\vec{r}', \vec{r}) \, \mathrm{d}V = - \int\limits_{vol} \mathbf{G}_\kappa(\vec{r}) \nabla V_m(\vec{r}) \bullet \nabla Z(\vec{r}', \vec{r}) \, \mathrm{d}V \tag{7.30}$$

Since, like all conductivity tensors, $\mathbf{G}_\kappa$ is symmetric equation (7.30) may be written as

$$\phi(\vec{r}') = -\int_{vol} \nabla V_m(\vec{r}) \bullet (\mathbf{G}_\kappa(\vec{r})\nabla Z(\vec{r}',\vec{r}))\, dV, \tag{7.31}$$

Next, we consider the following identity

$$\nabla \bullet (V_m(\vec{r})\, \mathbf{G}_\kappa(\vec{r})\nabla Z(\vec{r}',\vec{r})) = \nabla V_m(\vec{r}) \bullet (\mathbf{G}_\kappa(\vec{r})\nabla Z(\vec{r}',\vec{r}))$$
$$+ V_m(\vec{r})\nabla \bullet (\mathbf{G}_\kappa(\vec{r})\, \nabla Z(\vec{r}',\vec{r}))$$

which is used to replace the integrand in (7.31). This results in

$$\phi(\vec{r}') = -\int_{vol} \nabla \bullet (V_m(\vec{r})\, \mathbf{G}_\kappa(\vec{r})\nabla Z(\vec{r}',\vec{r}))\, dV + \int_{vol} V_m(\vec{r})\nabla \bullet (\mathbf{G}_\kappa(\vec{r})\nabla Z(\vec{r}',\vec{r}))\, dV$$

The first volume integral can be converted to an integral over the bounding surface S_h by applying the divergence theorem. In the second integral we substitute $\mathbf{G}_\kappa(\vec{r}) = \mathbf{G}(\vec{r})/(1+\kappa)$, and use the delta function properties of $\nabla \bullet (\mathbf{G}(\vec{r})\nabla Z(\vec{r}',\vec{r}))$ resulting from the equation defining $\nabla Z(\vec{r}',\vec{r})$, (7.29). The resulting final expression for the potential reads

$$\phi(\vec{r}') = -\frac{1}{1+\kappa}\int_{S_h} V_m(\vec{r})(\mathbf{G}(\vec{r})\nabla Z(\vec{r}',\vec{r})) \bullet d\vec{S} - \frac{1}{1+\kappa}V_m(\vec{r}')\chi(\vec{r}'), \tag{7.32}$$

with $\chi(\vec{r}') = 1$ for field points within S_h and $\chi(\vec{r}') = 0$ otherwise.

Equation (7.32) mainly replicates (11) shown in [6]. Its notation is more general in that it stresses the anisotropy as well as the dependency on the source location of all variables involved. For field points outside S_h the second term on the right of (7.32) is zero. The remaining part of this appendix relates to external field points only.

By using the symmetric nature of $\mathbf{G}$ we now have

$$\phi(\vec{r}') = -\frac{1}{1+\kappa}\int_{S_h} V_m(\vec{r})\, \nabla Z(\vec{r}',\vec{r}) \bullet \mathbf{G}(\vec{r})\, d\vec{S} \tag{7.33}$$

The conductivity tensor expresses the effect of the fibrous structure of the myocardium. Within this context two different constituents may be identified: the one along the local fiber direction, g_ℓ, and one in the direction normal to the fibers, the transverse conductivity, g_t. Note that the distinction between intra- and extra-cellular values is not required as a consequence of the assumed equal anisotropy ratio. By introducing the local fiber direction in 3D space by the unit vector $\vec{a} = \vec{a}(\vec{r})$ it can be shown [39] that

$$\mathbf{G} = g_t\mathbf{I} + (g_\ell - g_t)\mathbf{A}, \tag{7.34}$$

with $\mathbf{A}$ denoting the tensor derived from the fiber direction $\vec{a}$ (the rank one matrix $\vec{a}\vec{a}^{\mathrm{T}}$, with $\vec{a}$ interpreted as a column vector and $\vec{a}^{\mathrm{T}}$ as a row vector), and $\mathbf{I}$ the 3×3 identity matrix. Since fiber direction $\vec{a}$ and surface normal $d\vec{S}$ are orthogonal at S_h the substitution of (7.34) in (7.33) yields

$$\phi(\vec{r}') = -\frac{1}{1+\kappa}\int_{S_h} g_t(\vec{r})\, V_m(\vec{r})\, \nabla Z(\vec{r}',\vec{r}) \bullet d\vec{S} \tag{7.35}$$

Equation (7.35) indicates that, in the case of a uniform, equal anisotropy ratio, all variables determining the external potential field are expressed by their values at S_h only and are permitted to be inhomogeneous throughout the myocardium. This pertains both to the "active" variable $V_m(\vec{r})$ and to the remaining ones that describe the passive electric volume conduction properties of the medium.

The Final Step

The application of (7.35) requires the function $\nabla Z(\vec{r}',\vec{r})$ to be known. As indicated while introducing the function $Z(\vec{r}',\vec{r})$ (7.28), this function is the solution to (7.29) and expresses the infinite medium potential at field point $\vec{r}'$ generated by a point source at $\vec{r}$, now restricted to a position *on* S_h, but still inside a medium in which an inhomogeneous, anisotropic medium (the region within S_h) is present. In this final step of the discussion we use the approximation

$$Z(\vec{r}',\vec{r}) = \frac{c}{4\pi\sigma_0}\frac{1}{R},\tag{7.36}$$

with R the length of the vector $\vec{R} = \vec{r}' - \vec{r}$. As shown in ❷ Sect. 2.5.1, the spatial behavior of this function is that of the potential field generated by a current monopole with unit strength placed inside an infinite medium with homogeneous isotropic conductivity σ_0. The constant c is included to express the presence of the passive electrical properties of the medium inside S_h. Inserting this approximation in (7.35) gives

$$\phi(\vec{r}') = -\frac{c}{4\pi\sigma_0(1+\kappa)}\int_{S_h} g_t(\vec{r})\,V_m(\vec{r})\,\nabla\frac{1}{R}\bullet d\vec{S}$$

$$= -\frac{c}{4\pi\sigma_0(1+\kappa)}\int_{S_h} g_t(\vec{r})\,V_m(\vec{r})\,d\omega\tag{7.37}$$

Finally, if $g_t(\vec{r})$ is taken to be uniform at S_h we see that the external field potential is

$$\phi(\vec{r}) = -\frac{c\,g_t}{4\pi\sigma_0(1+\kappa)}\int_{S_h} V_m(\vec{r})\,d\omega,\tag{7.38}$$

which is a weighted sum of the local transmembrane potential at S_h, with weights that are proportional to the elementary solid angles $d\omega = d\omega(\vec{r};\vec{r}')$. As discussed in ❷ Sect. 7.4.2, the effect of the bounded nature of the volume conduction inside the thorax, as well as that of any inhomogeneities present may be accounted for by a dedicated transfer function acting on the infinite medium potentials (7.14).

Evaluation

The ECG signals as generated by the EDL source as described in ❷ Sect. 7.4 are based on (7.12), which has the same structure as that of (7.38). The derivation of (7.12) uses the approximation $-(\sigma_i\Phi_i - \sigma_e\Phi_e) \approx -\sigma_i V_m$ for the impressed current dipole surface density (A m^{-1}) assumes the medium inside S_h to be homogeneous and isotropic. In contrast, the derivation of (7.38) is based on the bidomain theory, with $\vec{J}^i = -\mathbf{G}_\kappa(\vec{r})\nabla V_m(\vec{r})$ expressing an impressed current density (A m^{-2}). If the full anisotropic nature of both domains representing the passive medium inside S_h is taken into account the computation of the potential field must be found by solving (7.21).

By assuming a constant anisotropy ratio for both domains the potential field in the external medium can be found from (7.35). This, interestingly, allows the active sources to be inhomogenous throughout the myocardium (interior of S_h), and demands its value to be known at S_h only. The same holds true for the term $g_t(\vec{r})\,\nabla Z(\vec{r}',\vec{r})$ that describes the passive conductive tissue properties. The final expression (7.38) assumes a uniform value of the transverse conductivity at S_h and approximates the conductivity of the medium inside takes the tissue inside S_h to be homogeneous and isotropic, but only for computing $Z(\vec{r}',\vec{r})$. Note that in the case of a completely isotropic passive medium we have

$$\phi(\vec{r}) \doteq \int_{S_h} g_t(\vec{r})\,V_m(\vec{r})\,d\omega\tag{7.39}$$

and if, moreover, the transverse conductivity is taken to be uniform at S_h

$$\phi(\vec{r},t) \doteq \int_{S_h} V_m(\vec{r},t)\,d\omega,\tag{7.40}$$

which expresses the basic aspects of the classic UDL source model (solid angle theory) as well as its generalization in the form of the EDL (the inclusion of a source description during repolarization).

The equal anisotropy assumption used in this appendix serves as an essential step in the derivations shown. Direct validation of the assumption is difficult because of the wide range of the values of g_{eL}, g_{iL}, g_{eT} and g_{iT} reported in the literature [10]. More recent publications on this point have not led to a clarification on this point [40, 41]. Indirect support for using the equal anisotropy assumptions came from the experimentally observed values of the potential difference across wave fronts propagating either purely transverse or along fibers. For the correct interpretation of such data the local shape of the wave front needs to be planar. Experimental studies in which this condition was satisfied yielded values of about 40 mV for both the propagation in the transverse direction and along fibers [9, 10, 42]. Recent large scale simulation experiments revealed only minor differences between the results obtained using the bi-domain formulation and those of the monodomain formulation based on the equal anisotropy assumption [35].

If the full complexity of the distribution of the inhomogenous anisotropy of the conductivity tensor is desired to be taken into account, this demand should be confronted with the limited accuracy with which such data would be available, as well as with the reality of the complete complex morphology of the myocardial tissue. The inclusion of such data in the interpretation of the ECG of individual subjects does not seem to be feasible.

References

1. Cuppen, J.J.M. and A. van Oosterom, Model studies with the inversely calculated isochrones of ventricular depolarization. *IEEE Trans. Biomed. Eng.*, 1984;**BME-31**: 652–659.

2. Salu, Y., Relating the multipole moments of the heart to activated parts of the epicardium and endocardium. *Ann. Biomed. Eng.*, 1978;**6**: 492–505.

3. Martin, R.O., *Inverse Electrocardiography*. Duke, NC: Duke University, 1970.

4. van Oosterom, A., The equivalent surface source model in its application to the T wave, in *Electrocardiology'01*. University Press São Paolo, 2002.

5. Geselowitz, D.B., On the theory of the electrocardiogram. *Proc. IEEE*, 1989;**77/6**: 857–876.

6. Geselowitz, D.B., Description of cardiac sources in anisotropic cardiac muscle. Application of bidomain model. *J. Electrocardiol.*, 1992;**25**(Suppl.): 65–67.

7. van Oosterom, A. and P. van Dam, The intra-myocardial distance function as used in the inverse computation of the timing of depolarization and repolarization, in *Computers in Cardiology*. France: Lyon, 2005.

8. Cuppen, J.J.M., Calculating the isochrones of ventricular depolarization. *SIAM J. Sci. Stat. Comput.*, 1984;**5**: 105–120.

9. van Oosterom, A. and R.T. van Dam, Potential distribution in the left ventricular wall during depolarization, in *Adv. Cardiol.*, 1976;27–31.

10. Plonsey, R. and A. van Oosterom, Implications of macroscopic source strength on cardiac cellular activation models. *J. Electrocardiol.*, 1991;**24/2**: 99–112.

11. Roberts, D.E. and A.M. Scher, Effect of tissue anisotropy on extracellular potential fields in canine myocardium in situ. *Circ. Res.*, 1982;**50**: 342–351.

12. Simms, H.D. and D.B. Geselowitz, Computation of heart surface potentials using the surface source model. *J. Cardiovasc. Electrophysiol.*, 1995;**6**: 522–531.

13. van Oosterom, A., Genesis of the T-wave as based on an equivalent surface source model. *J. Electrocardiol.*, 2001;**34S**: 217–227.

14. van Oosterom, A. and V. Jacquemet, Genesis of the P wave: atrial signals as generated by the equivalent double layer source model. *Eurospace*, 2005;**7**(Suppl. 2): S21–S29.

15. van Oosterom, A. and V. Jacquemet, A parameterized description of transmembrane potentials used in forward and inverse procedures, in *International Conference on Electrocardiology*. Gdansk; Poland: Folia Cardiologica, 2005.

16. Haws, C.W. and R.L. Lux, Correlation between in vivo transmembrane action potential durations and activation-recovery intervals from electrograms. *Circulation*, 1990;**81/1**: 281–288.

17. Huiskamp, G. and A. Van Oosterom, The depolarization sequence of the human heart surface computed from measured body surface potentials. *IEEE Trans. Biomed. Eng.*, 1989;**35**(12): 1047–1058.

18. Durrer, D., et al., Total excitation of the isolated human heart. *Circulation*, 1970;**41**: 899–912.

19. Franz, M.R., et al., Monophasic action potential mapping in a human subject with normal electrograms: direct evidence for the genesis of the T wave. *Circulation*, 1987;**75/2**: 379–386.

20. Cowan, J.C., et al., Sequence of epicardial repolarization and configuration of the T wave. *Br. Heart J.*, 1988;**60**: 424–433.

21. di Bernardo, D. and A. Murray, Explaining the T-wave shape in the ECG. *Nature*, 2000;**403**: 40.

22. Harumi, K., M.J. Burgess, and J.A. Abildskov, A theoretic model of the T wave. *Circulation*, 1966;**XXIV**: 657–668.

23. Yan, G.X., W. Shimizu, and C. Antzelevitch, Characteristics and distribution of M cells in arterially perfused canine left ventricular wedge preparation. *Circulation*, 1998;**98**: 1921–7.

24. Antzelevitch, C., et al., The M-cell: its contribution to the ECG and to normal and abnormal electrical function of the heart. *J. Cardiovasc. Electrophysiol.*, 1999;**10**: 1124–52.

25. van Oosterom, A., The dominant T wave and its significance. *J. Cardiovasc. Electrophysiol.*, 2003;**14**(Suppl. 10): S180–S187.

26. van Oosterom, J., The singular value decomposition of the T wave: its link with a biophysical model of repolarization. *Int. J. Bioelectromagnetism*, 2002;**4**: 59–60.

27. Hooft van Huysduynen, B., et al., Dispersion of repolarization in cardiac resynchronization therapy. *Heart Rhythm*, 2005;**2**: 1286–1293.

28. Huiskamp, G.J.M., Simulation of depolarization and repolarization in a membrane equations based model of the anisotropic ventricle. *IEEE Trans. Biomed. Eng.*, 1998;**BME-45/7**: 847–855.

29. Hooft van Huysduynen, B., et al., Validation of ECG indices of ventricular repolarization heterogeneity. *J. Cardiovasc. Electrophysiol.*, 2005;**16**: 1097–1103.

30. van Oosterom, A. and T.F. Oostendorp, ECGSIM: an interactive tool for studying the genesis of QRST waveforms. *Heart*, 2004;**90**(2): 165–168.

31. Wilson, F.N., A.G. Macleod, and P.S. Barker, The distribution of action currents produced by the heart muscle and other excitable tissues immersed in conducting media. *J. Gen. Physiol.*, 1933;**16**: 423–456.

32. Plonsey, R., An extension of the solid angle formulation for an active cell. *Biophys. J.*, 1965;**5**: 663–666.

33. Muler, A.L. and V.S. Markin, Electrical properties of anisotropic nerve-muscle syncytia-II, Spread of flat front of excitation. *Biophysics*, 1977;**22**: 536–541.

34. Geselowitz, D.B. and W.T.I. Miller, A bi-domain model for anisotropic cardiac muscle. *Ann. Biomed. Eng.*, 1983;**11**: 191–206.

35. Potse, M., et al., A comparison of monodomain and bidomain reaction-diffusion models for action potential propagation in the human heart. *IEEE Trans. Biomed. Eng.*, 2006;**53**(12): 2425–2435.

36. Gulrajani, R.M., *Bioelectricity and Biomagnetism*. New York: Wiley, 1998.

37. Henriquez, C.S., Simulating the electrical behavior of cardiac tissue using the bidomain model. *Crit. Rev. Biomed. Eng.*, 1993;**21**: 1–77.

38. Schmitt, O., Biological information processing using the concept of interpenetrating domains, in *Information Processing in the Nervous System*, K.N. Leibovic, Editor. New York: Springer, 1969.

39. Panfilov, A.V., Modelling of re-entrant patterns in an anatomical model of the heart, in *Computational Biology of the Heart*, A.V. Panfilov and A.V. Holden, Editors. Chistester, UK: Wiley, 1997.

40. Gabriel, R.W. and L. Gabriel, The dielectric properties of biological tissues. (II) Measurements in the range of 10 Hz to 20 GHz, Phys. Med. Biol., 1996;**41**: 2251–2269.

41. Roth, B.J., Electrical conductivity values used with the bidomain model of cardiac tissue. *IEEE Trans. Biomed. Eng.*, 1997;**BME-44**: 326–328.

42. Kléber, A.G. and C.B. Riegger, Electrical constants of arterially perfused rabbit papillary muscle. *J. Physiol.*, 1987;**385**: 307–324.

8 The Forward Problem of Electrocardiography

Rob MacLeod · Martin Buist

P. W. Macfarlane et al. (eds.), *Basic Electrocardiology*, DOI 10.1007/978-0-85729-871-3_8,
© Springer-Verlag London Limited 2012

8.1 Introduction

In this chapter we describe a class of problems known collectively as the "forward problem of electrocardiography," which all share the goal of describing cardiac and torso electrical potentials starting from some description of electrical sources within the heart. To solve this forward problem, these electrical sources must be known beforehand, which may suggest a certain degree of artificiality, or at least impracticality, when viewed from the clinical context. The goal of clinical electrocardiography is to use the body-surface potentials from a patient to extract relevant parameters of the cardiac sources, which is the essence of the inverse problem of electrocardiography discussed in the following chapter. The forward problem, in contrast, has a more fundamental role in that it must capture the entire relationships between some description of the sources and the remote manifestations of cardiac bioelectricity.

In its full scope, the forward problem begins with the membranes of the cardiac myocytes and goes to the body-surface potentials; more limited formulations can start, for example, with potentials or activation times on the epicardial and endocardial surfaces, while others can start with descriptions of extracellular tissue potentials and predict epicardial electrograms. In all cases, a practical forward solution must first describe the sources, ideally in some way that strikes a compromise between spatial/temporal fidelity and tractability, i.e., it should be possible to measure or compute the values of interest. The forward solution must also capture in adequate detail the effect of the volume in which the sources are located, the "volume conductor," as its shape and electrical conductivity will determine the currents and potentials that form the solution of the forward problem.

In this chapter, we present a rather broad view of the forward problem, one that includes all four components of a "versatile, present-day heart model" that Gulrajani outlined [1] and are reflected in the goals of the Physiome and Cardiome projects [2]. These components include the anatomical and physical substrate of the heart, the transmembrane action potential as the elemental bioelectric source of activation, the spread or propagation of this activation from cell to cell or element to element within the heart, and, finally, a volume conductor (typically the thorax) through which bioelectric currents pass from the heart to the outer surface, where they generate the electrocardiogram (ECG). One can examine each component of the complete problem with a range of approaches that include experiments with living tissues or mathematical and computational simulations, and complete coverage of all these options is well beyond the scope of this chapter. In this regard, our emphasis will be on mathematical and numerical approaches, although there will be some description of relevant findings from experiments.

A notable challenge of a forward problem is its multiscale nature, i.e., a complete forward solution encompasses information from the scale of the ion-channel protein to the complete human thorax and from the nanosecond to minutes or even hours of time. One can measure or simulate transmembrane potentials from a cardiac cell (myocyte) or even unitary currents through single channels of a cell membrane; however, both these approaches are intractable when the goal is to capture the behavior of the whole heart – there are thousands of ionic channels in a myocyte and billions of myocytes in a heart. Although mathematical models can include larger numbers of points to represent the heart than is possible with direct measurements, the density and complexity of representation are also limited by computer memory and computational capacity. Hence, one must accept simplifications and approximations that lead to workable formulations at the cost of detail and accuracy. Thus, for example, direct electrical measurements of the heart can come from extracellular potentials, sometimes only from the accessible surface(s), and at spacings in the range of millimeters to centimeters. At millimeter spatial resolution, the measurements can cover only small portions of the complete organ; to achieve more complete coverage results in a spatial resolution in the range of centimeters even with the most advanced measurement systems. Mathematical formulations of the forward problem are somewhat less restricted in the number of spatial locations that they can include but are also constrained in this case by computational resources.

It is a general observation common to most biological system that the extreme complexity of the physiology of the heart at each scale requires simplification. It is not feasible to use the same detailed model of membrane behavior suitable for a simulation of a single cell when the goal is to study cardiac arrhythmias in a heart that contains billions of such cells. As a result, the choice of specific source representation and volume conductor resolution derive from the type of behavior one wishes to simulate and the questions such simulations might answer. In this chapter, we describe, for example, formulations that predict potentials on the body surface from those on the epicardial surface and that solve the resulting equations using a boundary element approach. There is simplification in that the problem includes only potentials on these two surfaces, which, in turn, has the advantage that we can represent each of these surfaces with a large number of points (high spatial resolution) before exceeding the memory capacity of the computer. On the other hand, such a formulation forfeits direct information about cells or ionic channels or even the effects of the blood in the chambers of the heart.

Although one pictures the forward solution as a physically or anatomically outwardly directed process, this is not necessarily the case. It is possible to formulate an inwardly directed forward problem in which the sources are located in the heart tissues and the goal is to compute the electric potentials in the blood volume. This formulation is perhaps especially notable because it leads to a tractable inverse formulation that is the basis for a device that is the most widely used clinical application of the cardiac inverse problem [3].

The development of the forward problem has relied on both experimental and mathematical results and each approach has its respective strengths and limitations. The advantages of experimental approaches include the preservation, without simplification, of heart geometry and physiology, e.g., action potentials and spread of activation, and the ability to impose changes in this physiology through the use of drugs, artificial stimulation, temperature, mechanical load, or reduced coronary blood flow. Although experimental models contain the full complexity of the living tissues, measuring the parameters of interest is limited by physical access and the maximum number – and thus spatial resolution and coverage – of simultaneous measurement channels. For example, it is not possible to capture a truly complete image of the time-dependent potentials or currents within a whole heart. Even measurements limited to, for example, the epicardial potentials can only occur invasively, thus disrupting the integrity of the physiologic volume conductor and the resulting body-surface ECG.

Mathematical approaches remove the limitations of access and, to a certain extent, the number of parameters that one can monitor. The main challenge then becomes how to represent the true physiology in a realistic manner. Analytical approaches to mathematical solutions to the forward problem calculate the remote potentials from closed-form expressions for the cardiac sources. They offer great numerical precision, complete access at any desired resolution, and continuous variation of parameters. However, they are only possible under the most simplified geometric assumptions, e.g., that the heart and body are perfectly spherical or that lungs completely surround the heart in a concentrically spherical shape. They also implement an often highly simplified representation of the action potentials or spread of activation and sometimes compute body surface potentials not as time signals (ECG's) but rather as sparse snapshots in time under specific conditions during which simple sources adequately capture cardiac fields.

Numerical approximations of forward problems are certainly the most flexible and potentially powerful of all the options because they can, at least in principle, represent any sort of geometry in the form of discrete polygonal models and also any conceivable representation of bioelectric sources and spread of activation. Numerical forward problems in electrocardiography are generally unique in the sense that a specific set of source conditions leads to one and only one set of body-surface or epicardial potentials. As we describe in the following chapter, the same is not generally true of the inverse solution, e.g., multiple sets of cardiac source conditions can lead to the same set of body-surface potentials so that it may be impossible to determine which of the source conditions is correct. The presence of uniqueness should not, however, suggest that solving forward problems is trivial; there are considerable technical challenge and effort required to create the necessary geometric models, biophysical formulations, and numerical approximations. The geometry of the body is complex and contains regions of varying and even anisotropic electrical conductivity and there are many nonlinear relationships among relevant parameters. The complexity of simulations is also limited by computer capacity so that even relatively simplified simulations may take hours or even days to generate. Thus the main areas of research in numerical forward problems involve the creation of realistic geometric models, the choice of appropriate simplifications of complex electrophysiology, and the search for more efficient means of implementing them.

Although all three of these approaches – experimental, analytical, and numerical – have contributed to the knowledge of the forward problem, the dominant form in contemporary research is clearly the numerical simulation approaches with experimental results serving the essential role of validation. As we shall describe, this research has led to many recent findings and also encouraged the development of publicly available software and experimental data sets to allow non-experts to carry out forward solutions using modest computational resources and time.

The content of the rest of this chapter will address in more detail all the aspects of the problem outlined above and will seek to capture the current state of understanding and research in the area of forward problems in electrocardiography. We begin with a discussion of each of the three main approaches to solving the forward problem in electrocardiography, including at least brief overviews of the generation of action potentials and propagation simulations. We then continue with a section on the computational aspects of capturing the geometry and solving the forward problem using numerical approaches. The chapter ends with a list of the major research challenges that we have identified. We have chosen to emphasize contemporary themes at the expense of the rich history in the field and refer to the previous edition of this chapter for readers interested in more detailed coverage of this history [4]. In choosing the topics and literature to include in the chapter, we have tried to be comprehensive and balanced, however, we extend apologies for inevitable omissions.

To describe the choice of physical formulation, especially in mathematical terms, we will draw heavily on the concepts of ❯ Chaps. 2, ❯ 6, and ❯ 7, which cover the underlying physics of bioelectricity and cardiac sources, respectively. ❯ Chap. 5 provides a valuable overview of bioelectric sources and their links to the body-surface ECG and therefore contains information required to appreciate fully this chapter. This chapter, in turn, should serve as source of background information for the chapter that follows, which is dedicated to the electrocardiographic inverse problem.

8.2   Experimental Approaches

There is a close link in the field of electrocardiography – and electrophysiology in general – between breakthroughs in measurement technology and new insights into the structure and mechanisms of the underlying behavior. This link exists at all levels of scale and has influenced the development of diverse forward problems in electrocardiography. The first ECG recordings were from Waller in the late nineteenth century [5], but the real breakthroughs in ECG analysis and interpretation came, more than 20 years later, at least in part, because of Einthoven's improvements to the string galvanometer that allowed rapid recordings from patients located remotely from the equipment [6]. Near the other end of the size spectrum, the understanding of ion-channel function was first suggested by Hodgkin and Huxley based on their implementation of voltage clamp methods [7] and then later expanded greatly because of the information that came from patch-clamp methods developed by Neher and Sakmann [8]. The importance of such experimental techniques is further underscored by the fact that each of these breakthroughs resulted in a Nobel Prize for its innovators.

From the enormous richness of experimental approaches and findings that have advanced electrocardiography and forward problems, we highlight here just a tiny sample of findings and information that is most relevant. Because of the large scope of the modern view of forward problems, such coverage must include cellular, tissue, whole heart, and thorax components. As we shall see, each of these fields of experimentation has a naturally synergistic counterpart in the domain of simulation and modeling and one cannot imagine contemporary research without close coupling between these domains.

8.2.1   Cellular Electrophysiology

The broad goals of electrophysiological measurements at the cellular level are to determine the resting and dynamic electric potentials across the cell membrane and to measure the associated currents that flow through the membrane. This current flow occurs through hundreds to thousands of ion channels, each of which belongs to one of tens of channel types. Each channel is composed of an opening or pore, surrounded by complex amino-acid helices that form several separate proteins of largely known composition. It is the characteristics of these proteins and the changes in structure that they undergo that ultimately give rise to ionic currents, changes in membrane voltage, and the driving forces for bioelectricity in the heart and thorax. These channel types differ in terms of their selectivity for particular ions, their electrical conductivity, and their time and voltage-dependent activity. The characterization of these features in normal and diseased channels forms the central theme of a great deal of experimental studies.

Measurements of transmembrane potential generally occur by means of electrodes placed inside individual cells, much as one measures potential difference between two locations in a circuit. Because cells in the myocardium are relatively small (roughly brick shaped with 100 μm length and 10–20 μm sides), electrodes are created from small pieces of glass tubing pulled under heat to a diameter of under 1 mm [9]. Measurements of individual ion currents typically occur by means of slightly larger glass microelectrodes that attach to the membrane and isolate small numbers and even single channels. The measurements in this case are of the currents that flow through the small patch of membrane under the electrode tip [8].

For use in forward problems, the most important variation on this basic theme is the voltage-clamp configuration, which uses either two separate electrodes or one that switches between functions at a frequency high enough for it to

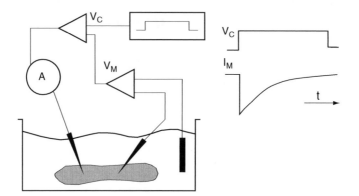

⬤ Fig. 8.1

Schematic diagram of the voltage clamp procedure. Two electrodes impaled in the cell provide membrane potentials measurement and current injection. Comparison of the membrane voltage V_m and the command potential V_c creates a difference signal that injects measured current into the cell in order to maintain $V_c = V_m$. Time signals indicate the response of time- and voltage-dependent current to a step pulse of the control potential

carry out the roles of both separate electrodes [10]. As shown in ⬤ Fig. 8.1, the purpose of the voltage clamp paradigm is to hold, or clamp, the transmembrane voltage at a chosen value and then measure the ionic current required to maintain this potential. Because the voltage is held constant across the membrane, i.e., the voltage-dependent behaviors are fixed, the resulting current measurements reveal the temporal behavior of the channels.

Another essential tool for studying cellular electrophysiology is a set of drugs that selectively block individual ion-selective currents. Hodgkin and Huxley made use of TTX, a toxin derived from the puffer fish that very selectively blocks Na^+ channels (and still causes many deaths each year among puffer-fish gourmands) and TEA, a blocker of some types of potassium channels [11]. With selective channel blockers, it is possible to isolate individual currents and use voltage clamp to determine their unique voltage and time dependence. Thus, it was that Hodgkin and Huxley were able to determine the time- and voltage-dependent characteristics of sodium and potassium channels in the squid giant axon and both formulate and test their Nobel-prize winning approaches to mathematically modeling the behavior of ion channels [12].

The widespread availability of techniques from molecular biology and knowledge of the protein sequence of ion channels continues to shape the contemporary approach to cellular electrophysiology. It is now possible to alter in very controlled ways the sequence of amino acids that make up ion channels and to them embed these modified channels into selected cell types and then study their behavior. In this way, it is possible to address questions in basic cellular electrophysiology and also to create experimental models of a wide range of disease states. Such changes in structure are possible through direct cloning of ion channels, but also by manipulating the genetic code of (usually) mice to create viable transgenic species lines that exhibit specific disease states. As just one example of this powerful approach, researchers altered the structure of the sarcolemmal ATP-sensitive potassium (KATP) channels and compared them with normal (wild type) channels in cells and intact transgenic mice [13]. These studies showed that the KATP channel is primarily responsible for the changes in action potential morphology during myocardial ischemia that lead to the shifts in body-surface ST-segment potentials that are the most common diagnostic feature for myocardial ischemia and infarction.

8.2.2   Tissue and Whole Organ Experiments

The science and technology of experimental approaches for myocardial tissue and the whole hearts is enormous and includes applications in both basic research and day-to-day clinical practice (see, for example, Lux et al. for one recent review [14]). Here we outline the general conceptual framework for such measurements as they relate to the description of bioelectric sources and to some specific approaches that are relevant to any discussion of the electrocardiographic forward problem.

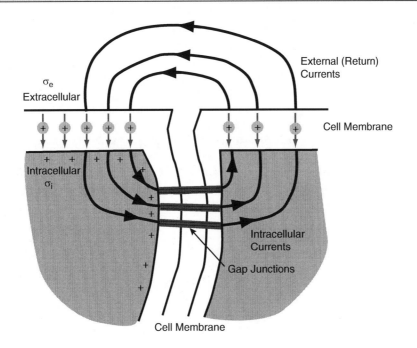

◘ Fig. 8.2
Schematic diagram of currents flowing between cells. The figure shows the interface between two cells with cell membrane and gap junctions linking the ends of cells. The left-hand cell is depolarized so that its intracellular space becomes positive with respect to the right-hand cell; hence, current flows directly from one intracellular space to the other through the gap junctions. Extracellular currents form the necessary return path for these currents. Conductivities σ_i and σ_e characterize the intracellular and extracellular space, respectively

The main goal of experimental approaches at the tissue and whole-organ level is to measure features of cell-to-cell coupling and observe behaviors that arise from the integration of many cells into the complex, three-dimensional structure of the heart. The measured quantity is almost invariably voltage coming from the extracellular current, i.e., the return current that flows between cells through the extracellular space. In fact, it is the qualitative appreciation of the difference between intracellular and extracellular measurements and currents that is perhaps most relevant to any discussion of the electrocardiographic forward problem. This conceptual framework provides the bridge between ionic currents and the macroscopic bioelectric fields that is central to any discussion of cardiac sources, which we describe in ❷ Sect. 8.3.

❷ Figure 8.2 shows schematically the relationship between ionic currents and the passive currents that flow between cells and into the extracellular space. In the figure, the left-hand cell is depolarized while the right-hand cell is at rest, thus producing the potential difference that is *always* necessary for current to flow from cell to cell, and by extension, from one part of the heart to another. Current is able to flow easily between neighboring cells because of the presence of gap junctions so that the downstream cell then also begins to accumulate charge. This initial charge accumulation, in turn, provides capacitive current that appears to flow (as all capacitive currents *appear* to flow – there is no ion flow across the membrane but rather a movement of ions on both sides that is the current) into the extracellular (interstitial) space. This extracellular, or return, current flows through the interstitium, which has a discrete conductivity, σ_e, and thus generates local voltage differences that one can measure.

8.2.2.1   Lead Systems and Electrode Arrays

There are two basic approaches to measuring cardiac activity: *unipolar* and *bipolar* leads. Both have physical implementations in the form of contact electrodes. A *lead* is the potential-difference time-signal recorded between two locations in or around the heart or body; signals from the body surface are *electrocardiograms* (ECG's) and signals from the heart are *electrograms* (EG's). Unipolar leads in measurements of cardiac bioelectricity represent the potential difference between one site on or near the heart and a reference, or *indifferent* electrode typically located remotely from the heart. The actual electrodes can be a small metal pellets, disks, or uninsulated lengths of wire, placed in direct contact with myocardium (see ❷ Fig. 8.4). The electrode is connected to the noninverting input of an electronic differential amplifier, while the inverting (negative) inputs of all the amplifiers are connected to the indifferent electrode. Thus, the potential measured by each amplifier represents the difference of voltage between an individual electrode recording site and the reference site. The main advantages of unipolar leads is that they share a common reference and thus provide the necessary information for comparing values over different leads and hence over space. The recording of voltage over space is known as *cardiac potential mapping*. A disadvantage of unipolar leads is that the signals contain both local information, attenuated fields from remote events, and measurement noise, and one often wishes to separate local from remote events. The signals in Panels A and B in ❷ Fig. 8.3 are examples of unipolar electrograms.

Bipolar leads consist of two, closely spaced electrodes, with one connected to the inverting and the other to the noninverting input of an amplifier and have the advantage of increased sensitivity to local activity while reducing the effects from distant activity and noise. The bipolar signal represents the algebraic difference between the unipolar signals that would have been recorded from the separate electrodes. This subtraction removes common information or similarities in the two unipolar signals, leaving only those aspects of the unipolar signals that are different. Such differences, in turn, are the result of local events so that bipolar leads emphasize the passage of the activation wavefront and may improve

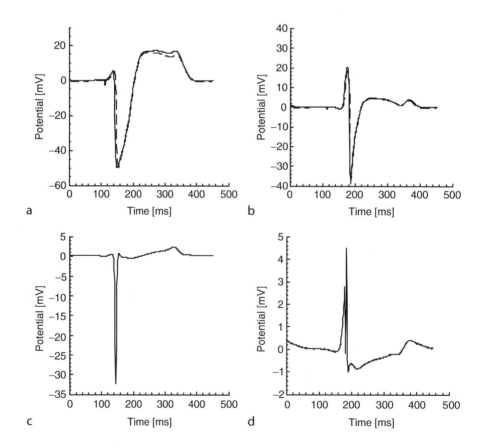

◻ Fig. 8.3

A sample of unipolar electrograms and the bipolar leads derived from their difference. (**a** and **b**) each contain two very similar unipolar electrogram from neighboring sites in a 1,200-lead epicardial array. (**c** and **d**) contain the bipolar leads derived from the two unipolar signals in (**a** and **b**) respectively. Note the different vertical scales in each plot (From [14] with permission)

detection of activation. One weakness of bipolar leads is that they do not share a common reference and thus cannot be compared with other leads in any sort of mapping based on amplitude or time course of the signals. ❷ Figure 8.3 shows two pairs of unipolar EGs recorded from closely spaced electrodes (Panels A and B) as well as their differences – the bipolar signals that would have been recorded from them (Panels C and D).

From the perspective of the electrocardiographic forward problem, another salient features of lead type is that unipolar and bipolar leads sense different information and each type provides data for a different formulation of the forward problem, as we shall see in ❷ Sect. 8.3.2. Unipolar leads recorded from the epicardial surface(s) of the heart provide direct information for the form of the forward problem based on surface potentials sources. Bipolar leads, on the other hand, provide direct source information for forward models based on activation times. It is imperative to note that one can fairly easily derive activation times from unipolar electrograms [15–19], but that it is impossible to derive potential maps from bipolar leads.

A fundamental question in any mapping and forward or inverse modeling application is the number and location of electrodes required. From a purely experimental perspective, the best number/location configuration of electrodes is based on a combination of features such as the desired biomedical goal, the accessibility of the heart to measurements, the types of electrodes available, and the capabilities of the acquisition system. The question of the minimum required spatial resolution has not been resolved completely, but current consensus indicates that a spacing of ≈ 2.5 mm is required to capture the details of cardiac activation [20]. This resolution assumes simple linear interpolation between measurement sites, either through explicit interpolation or implicitly in the visualization or signal processing required to identify features of interest. There are, however, more sophisticated forms of interpolation that allow, for example, lower density measurements (≈ 10–15 mm) on the epicardial surface and are still capable of reconstructing activation wavefronts [21, 22]. In an even more extreme case, if a set of high-resolution training data is available, it is possible using statistical estimation techniques to reconstruct activation maps on the entire ventricular surface from a very unevenly spaced set of only 10–40 electrodes restricted to the coronary veins [23, 24].

A selection of typical electrode configurations of unipolar and bipolar lead configurations used in contemporary electrophysiology, a subset of which is shown schematically in ❷ Fig. 8.4, includes the following:

1. Epicardial arrays sewn into nylon socks that cover some or all of the ventricles;
2. Rigid plaque arrays with regular electrode spacing that cover 1–10 cm^2 areas of the ventricles or atria;
3. Sets of transmural plunge needles with 3–12 electrodes in each needle;
4. Catheters with 1–16 electrodes that are placed in the ventricles, atria, or coronary veins;
5. Basket catheters consisting of 4–6 strands, each containing 4–8 electrodes for insertion into the right or left atrium; and
6. An inflatable, multielectrode balloon or large bore catheter with 10–80 electrodes that can be introduced into the ventricles through an incision or through the coronary vessels.

8.2.3 Physical Models and Phantoms of the Thorax

Physical models of cardiac sources and volume conductors have existed almost as long as the field of electrocardiography and much of the original understanding of the electrocardiographic field came from studies with such models. One can argue whether the ultimate goal of such models has been to solve the forward problem or the inverse problem of electrocardiography; investigators simply set out to understand the relationship between some form of cardiac source and the resulting potentials and currents on and in the torso volume conductor. ❷ Chapter 9 also includes coverage of this topic, and here, we introduce the topic with some results and interpretation. We also refer to other recent reviews of the topic [25, 26].

One of the earliest and certainly most thorough evaluations of a physical model based on a single bipolar source in a realistically shaped three-dimensional torso model was that of Burger and Van Milaan [27, 28]. The physical model of the torso was an electrolytic tank made out of a michaplast shell molded on a statue of a supine human. The tank split horizontally to provide access to the interior, which was filled with copper sulfate solution and equipped with copper foil electrodes fixed to the inner surface (see ❷ Fig. 8.5). The heart source model was a set of copper disks oriented along one of the body axes and adjustable from outside the tank by means of a rod. The first model used only the electrolyte as the

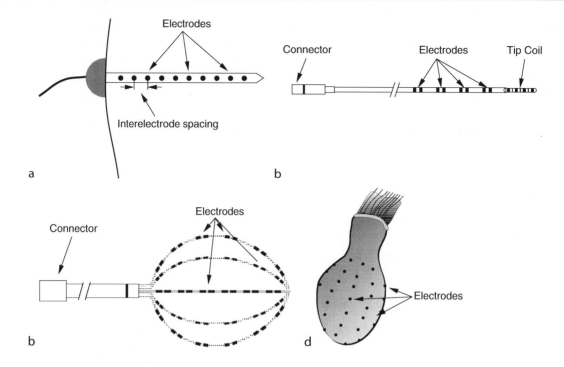

◘ Fig. 8.4

A sample of electrode arrays commonly used in cardiac mapping. (a) plunge needle with ten individual electrodes; (b) multi-electrode catheter arranged in four bipolar pairs; (c) basket catheter with six wands, each containing six bipolar pairs; and (d) inflatable sock array for surgical insertion into the left ventricle (From [14] with permission)

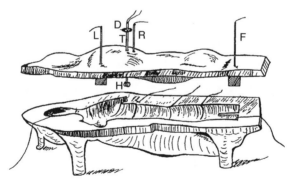
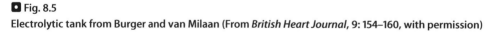

◘ Fig. 8.5

Electrolytic tank from Burger and van Milaan (From *British Heart Journal*, 9: 154–160, with permission)

homogeneous volume conductor [27], but subsequent versions incorporated inhomogeneous regions constructed from cork and sand bags for spine and lungs respectively [28].

It is relevant at this point to note that the source of the forward problem in these and many subsequent studies was the single dipole, described in ❷ Chap. 2. The dipole is also the basis for the lead field concept described in detail in ❷ Chap. 10. Burger and van Milaan were able to derive both algebraic and geometric forms of this relationship for each of the standard limb leads by fitting their measurements of limb lead potentials for known heart vector positions to a simple linear equation,

$$\phi_i = \vec{p} \cdot \vec{L}_i, \tag{8.1}$$

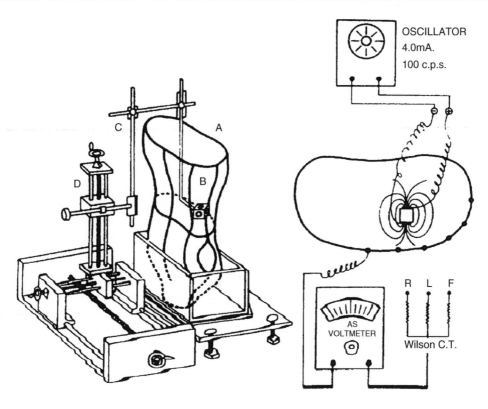

◘ Fig. 8.6
Electrolytic tank from Nagata (From *Japanese Heart Journal*, 11(2): 183–194, with permission)

where ϕ_i is the potential for a particular lead i, $\vec{p}$ represents the dipole moment vector, and $\vec{L}_i$ is the lead vector corresponding to the specific lead (❷ Sect. 10.3). To explore the effects of the volume conductor, they repeated the derivation after including various inhomogeneities in the tank and observing the effect on the weighting coefficients of the algebraic expressions. Theirs and subsequent studies by Grayzel and Lizzi, who used conductive paper (Teledeltos) to create two-dimensional inhomogeneous models of the human thorax [29, 30], were among the first to recognize the importance to the ECG not only of volume-conductor shape but also of the role of inhomogeneities in the volume conductor.

Another major breakthrough in the sophistication of physical models came from Nagata, who described several further refinements of artificial source and volume conductor models and subsequently introduced the use of biological sources rather than dipoles [31, 32]. In a preliminary study, Nagata placed a bipolar source in 27 different locations and measured the torso tank surface potentials at electrode sites equivalent to eight different lead systems in common usage at that time [31]. Like Burger and van Milaan, Nagata used a torso geometry based on a three-dimensional human thorax (see ❷ Fig. 8.6) and made measurements both in the homogeneously conducting tank as well as (in a subsequent study) with inflated dog lungs and agar gel models of human lungs inserted into the tank [32]. The goal of the studies was to derive the lead vector – expressed here as the "impedance transform vector" – from measurements over a wide variety of bipole source locations and lead systems. A second goal was to evaluate the effects of torso boundaries and inhomogeneities on the shape of the lead vector field. The limitations of this study lay in the lead field approach, which represents the heart as a single dipole rather than a distributed source of bioelectric current.

The later study by Nagata was notable also because he introduced a significant improvement over all previous studies by replacing the synthetic bipolar source with a perfused dog heart, thus achieving a much higher degree of realism than available with simple current bipoles [32]. Nagata did not measure cardiac potentials directly and therefore had no means of describing the real heart quantitatively. Instead, his study focused on the relationship between ECG signal parameters such as R-wave amplitude and signal morphology and the presence or absence of torso inhomogeneities.

There followed then several studies with the goal of evaluating the suitability of the single dipole as a representative source model. De Ambroggi and Taccardi carried out very careful studies of the electrocardiographic field from two bipoles in a two-dimensional electrolytic bath [33]. Their aim was to establish whether it was possible to characterize sources composed of two eccentrically placed bipoles based on potentials measured at sites distributed throughout the bath. Hence, it was not a validation of a quantitative forward solution but more a qualitative evaluation of the relationship between cardiac sources and body surface potentials. Subsequent studies by Mirvis et al. set out to address this same question with rabbit hearts placed inside spherical electrolytic tanks [34–36]. They found that a single moving dipole was not an adequate representation of the heart's electrical activity but that any of three different higher order discrete sources they tested did virtually equally well at reproducing the potentials on the surface of the tank in which the hearts were suspended. The important result of this study was to demonstrate from an experimental model that the single heart dipole model of electrocardiography was incomplete. A new source description was necessary.

It was Barr et al. who provided the new source description when they proposed representing the heart in terms of its epicardial potentials [37, 38]. This also led to a new series of validation studies based on this formulation, the first of which Barr et al. carried out not using an electrolytic tank, but instead an instrumented complete animal model [39]. This preparation included surgical implantation of 75 epicardial electrodes, re-closure of the chest wall in order to restore the integrity of the thoracic volume conductor, and, after a 2-week recovery period, measurement of both epicardial and 150 body-surface potentials with a 24-channel acquisition system. To record geometric information, the thorax of the animal was later sliced and photographed to create a model consisting of the electrode locations on the epicardial and torso surfaces. This landmark study provided data that have been used by several other investigators to validate their forward and inverse solutions [40, 41]. The major limitation of this validation model was that the spatial resolution of the geometric model was modest (the geometric model consisted of only the electrical measurement sites). Furthermore, because of the limited number of recording channels available (20), the potential measurements were performed in sequence and then time aligned, increasing the risk that changes occurring on a beat-to-beat basis or over the time of the measurements would be captured in only a subset of the recordings. ❷ Chap. 9 describes the most modern version of this form of physical studies by Nash et al. using an intact pig with instrumented epicardial surface and (re-)closed chest [25, 42].

Most of the experimental phantom studies performed since those of Barr et al. have been of the hybrid type pioneered by Nagata using an isolated heart either with an electrolytic tank [43–63] or with endocardial and catheter measurements for the endocardial inverse solution [64–66]. The main advantages of this type of preparation over instrumented whole animal experiments are the relative ease of carrying out the experiments and the increased level of control they provide. The isolated heart is more directly accessible when suspended in an electrolytic tank, which permits manipulations of its position, pacing site, coronary flow, temperature, etc. as well as the injection of drugs. The simplified geometry of the (usually homogeneous) tank also makes constructing customized geometric models simpler and faster than when a complete medical imaging scan is required for a whole animal.

A contemporary example of the isolated dog heart and human-shaped electrolytic tank preparation is shown in ❷ Fig. 8.7 (see also ❷ Chap. 9). This preparation uses a second dog to provide circulatory support for the isolated heart, which achieves very stable physiologic conditions over many hours. With the isolated heart, it is also possible to cannulate individual arteries and then regulate the coronary flow rate, blood temperature, and the infusion of cardioactive drugs in order to examine the effects of physiologic change on forward and inverse solutions [55, 59, 61–63, 67–69].

The advantages of physical models include the extreme level of control and intervention that is possible with such preparations. One has excellent access to the source and the volume conductor and can induce changes in either, in some cases within seconds, and can then measure the resulting changes in bioelectric potentials. The source especially can be very realistic with live, perfused, beating hearts available, albeit in most cases with compromised (through anesthesia and surgery) or even absent autonomic nervous systems. In the closed chest animal preparations, there is even a certain degree of realism to the volume conductor, although again with caveats of surgery and anesthesia. One of the challenges of these models is measuring and controlling for geometric details, at least for parts of the preparation. A rigid torso-shaped tank has a very precisely known geometry but the same is not true, for example, in the case of a re-closed chest cavity in a pig. Even with the rigid torso tank, the location and shape of the heart can be challenging to determine with high precision. As we shall see in the following section, obtaining precise geometry is one of the emerging themes of the forward problem and contemporary research in this area. One final challenge, common to all animal experiments and especially with artificial sources of cardiac bioelectricity, is that although the results may be useful to develop and evaluate problem formulations, one must use great care in extrapolating the physiological findings to humans.

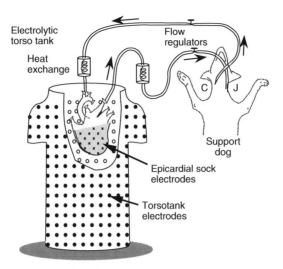

◘ Fig. 8.7
Physical model of forward problem originally devised by Taccardi et al. with an isolated, perfused dog heart suspended in the electrolytic tank. Recording electrodes consist of 192–384 tank surface electrodes and a 64–490 lead epicardial sock array

8.3   Modeling Cardiac Bioelectricity

Creating and using simulations of cardiac bioelectricity has a long and rich history and also covers an enormous range of scale and mathematical sophistication. In this chapter, we provide only a brief overview of this material and focus on the methods that are most relevant in the contemporary research and that drive the forward problem in electrocardiography. As we have defined it, the scope of the forward problem is also very large, and therefore, we include at least some coverage over the complete spectrum from ionic channels to whole hearts.

The unifying goal of simulating cardiac sources is to represent in some compact and mathematically defined way the currents and electric potentials that the heart produces. These representations may be based on explicit anatomical information and even require geometric models of cells, tissue, or the whole heart. Source models may, however, also bear little resemblance to realistic anatomy, but be abstractions of real biophysical sources that are useful only when the distances from the source are large compared with the extent of the source. One can view such a range of representations as similar to describing a source of light either in terms of the actual filament shape of the bulb or, simplified, as a point source radiating equally in all directions; both representations are useful at some scale but not usually across the full range of possible scales. Similarly, representations of cardiac bioelectricity even at the same scale may differ in degree of accuracy or sophistication and they may also vary in terms of the range of situations they can simulate. For example, a source model may create highly realistic potentials for a normal heart beat but be completely inadequate for pathological states. In all cases, source representations are approximations and hence reflect some degree of compromise, usually in order to be mathematically or computationally tractable.

8.3.1   Models of Cardiac Myocytes

The requirement of a model of cardiac cells is that they simulate with acceptable fidelity both the resting and dynamic behavior of the cell. Resting potentials depend on the concentrations of ions on both sides of the cell membrane and on the resting conductivity of ion channels, and a complete model of the cell will reflect these dependencies and even allow for variations in these parameters that reflect pathophysiology, e.g., a cell model should allow the resting potential to rise (depolarize) with elevation in extracellular potassium ($[K_e^+]$), as a real cell does during acute ischemia. Accurate representation of the action potential of the cell is a much more challenging requirement, especially given that, again, this behavior must reflect a wide range of variations in all the relevant ion channels and their time and voltage dependence. The action potential of a myocyte is the sum of tens of different types of channels arranged in densities that vary with the cell type, species, and even location in the same heart. Each ion channel, in turn, opens and closes in a stochastic manner and thus allows current to flow in a complex time, voltage, and ligand dependent manner, described ultimately by the set of proteins that make up the channel structure. An ideal model of the cell would allow predictions of ionic currents and action potential shape on the basis of variation in the underlying protein structure, i.e., the sequence of amino acids that make up the proteins, determined by the DNA of the cell nucleus.

Such a complete model does not yet exist but there do exist frameworks in which to approach the required (or desired) sophistication. Moreover, there are formalisms that are based on at least reasonable simplifications and ensemble averages of the individual ion channel characteristics that seek to predict the behavior of pieces of cell membrane and whole cells. Even more simplified models also exist that approximate the essential parameters of action potential behavior and are driven by empirical mathematical formulations. Here, we describe briefly these first category of cell models as they represent the far dominant form in forward solution formulations.

8.3.1.1   Biophysically Based Models

There are two levels of biophysically based modeling approaches in common use today: one that describes the opening and closing of individual ion channels and the other that computes currents and voltages for the entire cell. Both of them share the characteristic that they appeared before there was clear experimental proof of the behavior and especially the structure that they attempt to simulate. In this sense they illustrate one of the most powerful applications of simulations, that is to start with a concept of the underlying mechanism and then create a quantitative model that reflects this concept as a means of testing it against measured data.

The Hodgkin–Huxley formalism was the result of breakthroughs in both measurement and theory that occurred in the period of rapid progress that followed World War II. Hodgkin and Huxley made use of the electronic circuitry and devices developed during the war to implement and then apply the voltage-clamp technique described in ❷ Sect. 8.2.1 to the squid giant axons [7]. In order to describe first conceptually and then quantitatively the results of these experiments, they proposed the idea of ion channels, that is, openings in the axon membrane that were selective to specific ions and that had time and voltage dependencies that voltage clamp allowed them to investigate. Starting from first-order kinetic equations common in physical chemistry and ordinary differential equations frequently used to describe simple rate dependencies, they adjusted parameters in order to fit the measured data and presented calculations to support these concepts [11, 12, 70]. Subsequent experiments, requiring numerous technological breakthroughs and performed by their successors, proved that the concept of ion channels was sound and led to a Nobel Prize for Hodgkin and Huxley. This simulation formalism is still central to most modern membrane and cell models and there are excellent descriptions in many review articles and even text books [71–73].

❷ Figure 8.8 is a schematic circuit diagram that shows the essentials of the Hodgkin–Huxley formalism applied to the cardiac myocyte. Components include an expression for membrane potential expressed as the product of ionic currents and the capacitance of the lipid bilayer that makes up cellular membranes. The original models of Hodgkin and Huxley applied only to nerve axon and included single Na^+ and K^+ currents; to represent cardiac action potentials substantial modifications are necessary.

The basic equation from the circuit in ❷ Fig. 8.8 that drives all models based on the formalism of Hodgkin and Huxley is

$$\frac{\partial V_m}{\partial t} = -\frac{1}{C_m}\left(I_{ion} + I_{stim}\right), \tag{8.2}$$

where V_m is the membrane potential, C_m is the membrane capacitance, I_{ion} is the sum of the active ion currents, and I_{stim} is a stimulus current (usually) required to depolarize the cell to reach threshold.

The ionic current is the sum of individual currents that flow through ion-selective channels driven by an equilibrium potential and regulated by a time- and voltage-dependent conductance, expressed as

$$I_{ion} = I_{Na} + I_K + I_{Ca}\dots, \tag{8.3}$$

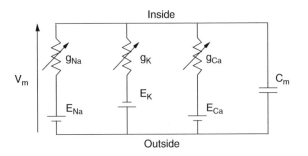

Inside

Outside

◻ Fig. 8.8
Circuit diagram for the Hodgkin–Huxley formalism applied to cardiac myocytes. The parallel circuit of membrane capacitive current and individual ion currents passing through variable resistors captures the essence of the electrical behavior of the cell

where ... indicates that the list of individual currents is variable and may include different subspecies of currents for the same ion, each having a different time and voltage dependence. Each individual current, in turn, can be expressed according to the circuit diagram as the product of a voltage difference and a conductivity

$$i_X(V,t) = (V_\mathrm{m} - E_X)g_X(V,t), \tag{8.4}$$

where I_X is the current for ion X, which flows whenever membrane voltage V_m diverges from the equilibrium potential for the particular ion, E_X, and the conductivity for that ion, g_X, is non-zero. The equilibrium potential, E_X, is a function of the relative concentrations of the particular ion on both sides of the semipermeable membrane and is predicted by the Nernst equation:

$$E_X = \frac{RT}{Z_X F} \ln\left(\frac{[X]_\mathrm{e}}{[X]_\mathrm{i}}\right), \tag{8.5}$$

where R is the gas constant constant, T is temperature, Z_X is the valance of ion species X, F is the Faraday constant, and $[X]_\mathrm{e}$ and $[X]_\mathrm{i}$ are the extracellular and intracellular concentrations respectively, of ion species X. Conceptually, the Nernst potential is the membrane potential difference at which there is no incentive for net movement of a particular ion, i.e., the voltage at which, at least for a particular ion, there is equilibrium between inward and outward currents. At any other membrane potential, each ion will experience a net *driving force* equal to $V_\mathrm{m} - E_X$ that will move ions across the membrane if the membrane has adequate permeability to that ion.

With this formulation, the descriptions of individual ion currents reside essentially in the time and voltage dependence of the conductivities. As part of their original formulation, Hodgkin and Huxley developed simple expressions for these conductivities based on first-order rate equations that in some way capture their idea of the underlying channel behavior. They fitted the parameters of these equations in order to agree with experimental voltage-clamp results. The resulting formalism remains the most commonly used in modern simulation of electrically active membranes.

The first model of cardiac membranes was by Noble et al. in 1962 and there are at least 30 different variations on this theme known in the literature today [73]. Each model varies in terms of the number and type of individual ion channels included and the animal species for which individual parameters are known from experimental studies. Perhaps, most commonly used are the models from Luo and Rudy [74, 75], which include not only ion channels but (in the 1994 edition) also support for intracellular buffering of calcium. Sachse has recently summarized very well the state of membrane simulation models, including both electrical and mechanical models [73].

From the perspective of the electrocardiographic forward problem, the choice of membrane simulation model is always sharply constrained by the limits of computation. We describe in ❷ Sect. 8.3.2 models of cardiac tissue, some of which include individual membrane models as the primary drivers. Because of the desire to simulate pieces of myocardium up to the size of whole heart, it is necessary to discretize the tissue into hundreds of thousands, even millions, of tiny elements, each of which contains its own membrane model. In order to then be able to compute electrical activity for even a reasonable part of a single heart beat, it is necessary to find efficient, simplified ion-channel models. This simplification in model comes at a cost of accuracy but is an acceptable compromise, in part, because the very existence of tissues reduces the impact of individual cells or small groups of cells on the overall behavior of the simulation.

8.3.2   Models of Cardiac Tissue

In this section, we step from the cellular level to the tissue and whole heart and describe models that capture aspects of their electrical behavior that are relevant to the forward problem. As with the cell, some models of myocardium represent a biophysical approach and are based on accurate anatomical features of the heart. Others are parametric in that they use abstractions of some sort to capture the essential features of the electric fields from myocardium, often requiring a certain distance between the source and the observation location. In general, such parametric representations are less accurate but much simpler to compute; their other major weakness is that it is rarely possible to measure them directly or even to uniquely associate their parameters to anatomical or physiological characteristics of the real heart.

8.3.2.1   Discrete Source Models

The simplest and best known means of representing the electrical activity from the heart is the heart dipole, first described and applied to the heart by Einthoven [6, 76] and still the description with the largest impact on clinical education and the interpretation of the ECG [77]. While simple to grasp physically and to compute numerically, the single dipole is only a barely adequate description of the electrical activity of the heart and even at the body surface cannot explain certain features of potential distributions and the ECG [78]. If anything, it is remarkable that a representation encapsulated by only six parameters can do as well as it does and this fact is perhaps the best evidence of the attenuation, smoothing, and smearing effects of the volume conductor that we explore in more depth in ❷ Sect. 8.5. However, for the purpose of quantitative simulation and the detailed study of almost any aspect of normal or abnormal cardiac electrophysiology, the dipole is an inadequate model and hence is rarely considered in contemporary research studies.

There are other forms of discrete sources, based on combinations of dipoles or other higher order forms of this basic current source. Some have proved useful in very special circumstances, such as representing the earliest phase of an ectopic beat, when it resembles a pair of waves moving in opposite directions and hence as a pair of dipoles or a quadrapole [79]. The occurrence of an accessory pathway connecting the atria and ventricles as it arises in the Wolff–Parkinson–White (WPW) syndrome has also been modeled as a discrete dipole that is active only for a few milliseconds [80–86]. This accessory pathway is a tissue band that links the atria with the ventricles and thus forms a connection secondary to that via the atrio-ventricular (AV) node. This connection can create a circular pathway of excitation that goes from atria to ventricles back to atria and thus a reentrant circuit that can be the substrate for ventricular arrhythmias and even death [86, 87]. During the instant in which the excitation travels through the accessory pathway, this bioelectric source is very focal and discrete, and the electric field from this source resembles that of a single current dipole. There have also been many reported studies in which a set of distributed dipoles, each with unique orientation and activation times has represented the potentials from the heart – as we will see, this is still a representation that allows models of propagation to generate extracardiac fields (❷ Sect. 8.4). One such model was even the source for a complex inverse solution expressed in terms of on time and off times for a multiple dipole source [88].

In the contemporary context, there are more accurate and sophisticated formulations that are both more accurate, and through modern computers, tractable sources of cardiac bioelectricity. The rest of this section focuses on these, but for more detail on discrete models, the review by Gulrajani is an excellent resource [1].

8.3.2.2   Bidomain Method

One of the most successful and perhaps initially confusing approaches to representing the electrical activity of the myocardium is the bidomain technique, first conceived by Schmitt [89], proposed by Miller and Geselowitz [90] and

Tung [91] for the heart, and later expanded and used by others to examine all facets of cardiac excitation and stimulation [92–97]. We present here only a brief overview of the method and refer to an excellent review by Henriquez for more details [98].

The main goal of the bidomain approach is to simplify through a process of "homogenization" the features of an aggregate of individual myocytes so as to enable feasible computations of pieces of heart tissue and ultimately the entire heart. Computation that did not employ such a simplification but instead included every cell of the heart would require approximately 10 billion sets of parameters for each time instant, where each set of parameters could include as many as 30 variables, clearly beyond the scope of any computer. The bidomain approach makes explicit use of the fact that the heart is essentially a syncytium, that is, every cell connects via its immediate neighbors to all other cells. This means that, in principle, stimulating a single cell will eventually lead to all cells firing an action potential (and contracting) in a sequence. The bidomain then describes the heart as composed of two domains, one for all intracellular space and the other for all extracellular space, both coexisting in the same physical space (the myocardium). Thus, what is actually a discrete syncytium of many individual cells, each with their its transmembrane voltage, becomes two continuous domains. Intracellular potential and extracellular potential then become continuous functions of space, as does their difference, the transmembrane voltage. Similarly, other parameters of the tissue, most notably electrical resistance, become continuous functions in the intracellular and extracellular spaces. Joining the two domains of the bidomain is the membrane, which in the classic bidomain has no volume but is likewise distributed everywhere throughout the tissue. Most importantly, the membrane contains the ionic channels represented by voltage- and time-dependent currents that generate action potentials within the cells. ❷ Figure 8.9 shows schematically the organization of intracellular and extracellular spaces with a membrane linking the two. Also visible in the figure is the current that leaves the extracellular space and travels into the extramyocardial volume conductor; it is this current that is ultimately responsible for the torso and body-surface potentials (ECG).

As with other aspects of the forward problem, *analytical* expressions in terms of continuous functions are rarely available so that *numerical* approaches or discrete approximations of myocardial geometry are necessary. Thus, somewhat paradoxically, what starts as a discrete arrangement of myocytes eventually becomes a discrete organization of small pieces of tissue, each small enough to be treated as uniform with regard to potentials and ionic currents. We describe this process of homogenization and subsequent discretization in the following section.

The derivation of the governing equations of bidomain techniques begins with the statement of Ohm's Law in terms of conductivities for the intracellular and extracellular spaces as

$$\vec{J}_i = -\sigma_i \nabla \phi_i$$
$$\vec{J}_e = -\sigma_e \nabla \phi_e,$$

(8.6)

where the subscripts i and e on each of $\vec{J}$, σ, and ϕ indicate intracellular or extracellular spaces respectively.

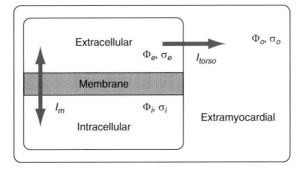

■ Fig. 8.9

Schematic view of the bidomain method of describing myocardium. The heart contains intracellular and extracellular spaces that are linked by a membrane. Currents from the extracellular space (I_{torso}) flow into the extramyocardial volume conductor to produce body-surface potentials

Conservation of current requires that whatever current leaving the intracellular domain must enter the extracellular: a condition that is possible because both domains are assumed to exist at the same point in space. This allows one to write

$$\nabla \cdot \vec{J}_i = -\nabla \cdot \vec{J}_e \tag{8.7}$$

Substituting (8.6) into (8.7) provides a conservation equation in terms of the intracellular and extracellular potential fields as

$$\nabla \cdot (\sigma_i \nabla \phi_i) = -\nabla \cdot (\sigma_e \nabla \phi_e) \tag{8.8}$$

We can now make use of the definition of the transmembrane potential

$$V_m = \phi_i - \phi_e \tag{8.9}$$

to express (8.8) in terms of V_m and ϕ_e by subtracting $\nabla \cdot (\sigma_i \nabla \phi_e)$ from both sides to obtain

$$\nabla \cdot ((\sigma_i + \sigma_e) \nabla \phi_e) = -\nabla \cdot (\sigma_i \nabla V_m) \tag{8.10}$$

This equation is the first of the two bidomain equations and calculates the extracellular potential field, given a transmembrane potential distribution. Note that this is essentially a form of Poisson's equation with a source term based on the current density associated with the transmembrane potential field. In fact, the extracellular domain of the bidomain is contiguous with the passive regions outside the heart so that one could consider the whole torso to be a bidomain in which the contributions from V_m are only non-zero in the heart region.

As shown in ❷ Fig. 8.9, any transfer of current between the intracellular and extracellular domains must pass through the intervening membrane so that

$$\nabla \cdot \vec{J}_i = -\nabla \cdot \vec{J}_e = A_m I_m \tag{8.11}$$

Here A_m is known as the surface-to-volume ratio of the bidomain membrane and essentially describes how much membrane surface area is present per volume of tissue. The function I_m describes the current flow across the membrane per unit of membrane area. It is the sum of a time-dependent capacitive current and a second current, I_{ion}, representing the flow of ions through selectively permeable channels in the membrane as described in ❷ Sect. 8.3.1:

$$I_m = C_m \frac{\partial V_m}{\partial t} + I_{ion}, \tag{8.12}$$

where C_m now denotes the membrane capacitance per unit area.

Combining (8.11) and (8.12) gives

$$\nabla \cdot (\sigma_i \nabla \phi_i) = A_m \left(C_m \frac{\partial V_m}{\partial t} + I_{ion} \right), \tag{8.13}$$

in which I_{ion} is a function of V_m, and therefore, it is common (but not universal) practice to re-state the left hand side of (8.13) in terms of V_m by adding and subtracting $\nabla \cdot (\sigma_i \nabla \phi_e)$ and again imposing the definition of V_m to write

$$\nabla \cdot (\sigma_i \nabla V_m) + \nabla \cdot (\sigma_i \nabla \phi_e) = A_m \left(C_m \frac{\partial V_m}{\partial t} + I_{ion} \right) \tag{8.14}$$

Equation (8.14) is the second bidomain equation and from it, one can calculate the transmembrane potential.

It is possible for an external stimulus current to be applied to either domain (I_{s1} and I_{s2}); this allows the two bidomain equations to be written as

$$\nabla \cdot ((\sigma_i + \sigma_e) \nabla \phi_e) = -\nabla \cdot (\sigma_i \nabla V_m) + I_{s1}, \tag{8.15}$$

$$\nabla \cdot (\sigma_i \nabla V_m) + \nabla \cdot (\sigma_i \nabla \phi_e) = A_m \left(C_m \frac{\partial V_m}{\partial t} + I_{ion} \right) - I_{s2}, \tag{8.16}$$

where I_{s1} and I_{s2} are the stimulus currents.

These two equations are highly coupled and indeed solutions can prove to be computationally prohibitive over large domains and/or on high resolution meshes. If either the extracellular domain is assumed to be highly conducting ($\sigma_e \sim \infty$) or the domains are assumed to be equally anisotropic ($\sigma_i = k\sigma_e$), it is possible to reduce the bidomain system to a single equation with a significant reduction in computational complexity. The result is known as the monodomain equation,

$$\nabla \cdot (\sigma \nabla V_m) = A_m \left(C_m \frac{\partial V_m}{\partial t} + I_{ion} \right) - I_s, \tag{8.17}$$

in which σ is defined by $\sigma^{-1} = \sigma_e^{-1} + \sigma_i^{-1}$. This expression is essentially a nonlinear cable equation when reduced to its one-dimensional form. Thus one can think of the bidomain approach as a multidimensional generalization of the nonlinear cable equation.

8.4 Simulating Propagation

To simulate a full heart beat, it is necessary to have bioelectric sources that vary with time, ideally over more than one beat if the goal is to study arrhythmias or other effects related to heart rate. The most realistic way to generate time-varying sources is to simulate the spread of excitation within tissue, and there are many approaches to describing such propagation in the heart. As with all simulation components, there exists a range of levels of sophistication and degrees of realism and flexibility that such a model can simulate.

There are two stages to this type of simulation and multiple approaches to both. The first step is to predict the sequence in which different regions of the tissue depolarize, the actual spread of excitation. The result is a set of activation and/or repolarization times, parameters which are immediately useful to address some highly relevant questions. The second step is to use the timing values of the excitation and repolarization to generation potentials either within the tissue, or more often, on the epicardium and endocardium. In the context of the forward problem, one usually wishes to generate such potentials at the body surface (although we leave this last step to the section on volume conductors). As described in ❯ Sect. 8.3.2, a common approach to calculating potentials is to represent different regions of the heart as dipole sources and use the activation wavefronts to provide their orientation and active/repolarization times and thus determine their timing. Another approach, described in detail in ❯ Chaps. 6 and ❯ 7, is to represent the sources as moving double layers, with timing and path determined from the propagation parameters. Rather than explicitly computing the spread of excitation, it is also possible to assume knowledge of this sequence, e.g., to acquire it from experiments, and then generate extracardiac potentials from this information.

We use this approximate taxonomy of stages to describe and categorize specific models and begin with simulation approaches that generate the *sequence of activation* or *spread of excitation*, which we take as equivalent expressions. Here, again, we emphasize the intuition of each approach over its mathematical description and solution and refer readers to other sources for more detail.

8.4.1 Physiology Background

We begin with a qualitative description of the process by which excitation travel through the heart. Like all organs, the heart comprises a large number of cells, each of which must be stimulated (partially depolarized) in order to generate an action potential. At the tissue level, the question arises as to how the impetus to depolarize passes from one cell to the next. The answer is via Ohm's Law and gap junctions. Ohm's Law ($I = V/R$) states that current will flow when a potential difference arises and the resistance between regions at different potentials is low enough. Thus, if one cell depolarizes, it will become more positive than its neighbors so that current will flow, providing there is a conductive pathway. The conductive pathway is provided by what are known as "gap junctions". Gap junctions are a form of protein channel embedded in the cell membrane that form direct connections between the interior of one cell and the interior of a neighboring cell through which charged ions may flow – each one represents a resistor with relatively low resistance compared with surrounding tissue. While return currents do flow in the extracellular space, the gap junction connections are the primary means of transferring electrical information between cardiac cells. ❯ Figure 8.2 in ❯ Sect. 8.2.2 shows schematically the relationship between two cells coupled by gap junctions, the primary current pathway through the gap junctions, and the return current through the extracellular space.

There are some characteristic features of propagation in myocardium that follow from these mechanisms and any attempt at simulating propagation must also take them into account. In fact, appreciation of these features can lead to simplified formulations of propagation, as we will show. The first notable feature is syncytial nature of the heart described in ❯ Sect. 8.3.2, by which each cell is connected to all other cells by means of a series of neighbors – a single depolarized cell will eventually cause all cells to depolarize as long as there is a path to each cell. Similarly, all paths from one cell to a nonneighboring cell must go through intermediary cells, i.e., there are generally no short cuts or direct connections between remote regions of the heart. The exception to this rule is a set of special cells, superimposed and only partially connected to the rest of the heart, that are typically noncontractile and preferentially carry extrication more rapidly than surrounding tissues. This *conduction system* is responsible for the coordination and timing of the spread of excitation, ensuring, for example, through a branching network of fibers that most of the subendocardial regions of the ventricular septum are stimulated almost simultaneously. Not all elements of the conduction system accelerate the spread of excitation. In fact, the atrio-ventricular (AV) node is the only electrical link between atria and ventricles – in a normal heart, at least – and it exhibits especially slow conduction speed because of weak intercellular coupling and smaller, rather slowly rising action potentials of the cells. A complete propagation model of the heart must incorporate all these behaviors, or at least must be able to mimic them in some form.

We will now describe some of the more common forms of simulating propagation in physical and mathematical terms and also direct the reader to ❯ Chap. 6 of this volume for a discussion of the specific example of double layer sources.

8.4.2 Cellular Automata

The concept of cellular automata dates back to the 1940s and two scientists, Stanislas Ulam and John von Neumann, but by far the most widely recognized use is John Conway's *Game of Life* [99]. Moe et al. adopted this approach in the early 1960s [100] and the methods still find great popularity today due to its computational efficiency [101–107]. A cellular automata approach divides the electrical wave propagation problem into two components. First, the domain of interest is divided up into a regular grid. Each point on the grid has a set of neighboring points, the number of which depends on the dimension of the problem and the topology of the grid. The second component is the automaton that is used to represent the behavior of a single cell and is so named because its actions are solely determined by a set of internal rules. Note that because of computational constraints, an element or cell of the grid in this context is usually substantially larger than a physical cardiac cell.

In its simplest form, a cell in a cellular automata model would have two states, resting and excited (essentially on and off) plus a set of rules to describe the transition from one state to the other and back again. This system mimics a piecewise approximation of an action potential. To then replicate the behavior necessary for propagation, there are rules that determine how the state of one cell affects those of its neighbors. Typically, a cell may transition to the excited state a fixed time after it senses that one or more of its neighbors have been excited. The same cell would then have a rule whereby it returns to the resting state after some further period of time has elapsed, thus encapsulating the ordered cell-by-cell coordination prescribed by the underlying physiology.

More complex – and realistic – cellular automata incorporate additional states in order to capture, for example, refractory properties. One example of such a model from Bailie et al. [108] includes three states: quiescent (Q), excited (E), or refractory (R). In addition there are a total of six rules that govern the transition into and out of each state, summarized in ❯ Table 8.1.

Starting from a quiescent state, a cell makes the transition to the excited state if it detects that one or more of its neighbors are in an excited state. Next, after a prescribed time period, the cell transitions to the refractory state, and then after another period of time, returns to the initial quiescent state. ❯ Figure 8.10 shows the initial stages of propagation using this simple automaton.

We present here a few examples of the many modern applications of cellular automata models, each of which has added notable features in order to better replicate real spread of excitation (and in some cases repolarization) in normal and diseased tissue. A summary of earlier examples can be found in the review of Saxberg [109].

□ Table 8.1

Rules governing a simple three state cellular automata model

State(t)	Count(t)	Neighbor(t)	State(t+1)	Count(t+1)
Q	(any)	0	Q	0
Q	(any)	≥ 1	E	1
E	< E_T	(any)	E	Count(t)+1
E	E_T	(any)	R	1
R	< R_T	(any)	R	Count(t)+1
R	R_T	(any)	Q	1

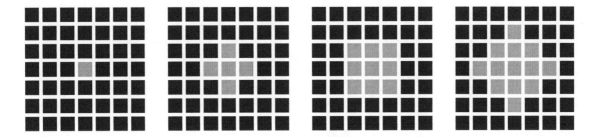

□ Fig. 8.10

Propagation from a point source using a cellular automata approach. Initially, one cell is set to be in an excited state (*light*) while the remainder are quiescent (*dark*). Subsequent images show neighboring cells making the transition to the excited state

Leon et al. described in a series of studies a cellular automata model that incorporated anisotropic propagation in a human ventricle model by altering the rules of interaction among cells [103, 110, 111]. In order to change from resting to activated state, each target cell received inputs from all neighboring cells, each with its contribution weighted by the direction between the target cell and each neighbor relative to the local fiber direction. In this way, neighboring cells that lie along the local fiber direction have more influence on a target cell than neighbors that lie in the cross-fiber direction. They then used this model to simulate reentrant propagation and to illustrate some of the effects of rotational anisotropy on conduction in a very realistic heart model with 1 mm resolution.

Wei et al. constructed an anatomically based heart mesh that included descriptions of the atria and ventricles, using approximately 50,000 connected elements [112]. The structure was such that each element was connected to 12 adjacent neighbors. The authors divided the heart into 16 cell types with different properties and simulated a normal cardiac excitation pattern. At each time step 54 dipolar sources were constructed from the transmembrane potential distribution and these were used to simulate the ECG and also the vectorcardiogram. WeiXue et al. used CT images to construct a 65,000 element heart model at a resolution of 1.5 mm [113]. The hexahedral elements were arranged in a cubic close-packed structure meaning that each was connected to 26 neighbors. Again a cellular automata approach was used to model propagation and in this case the primary interest was in the epicardial and body surface potential distributions associated with Wolff–Parkinson–White syndrome. Hren et al. developed even more finely resolved cellular automata models with 0.5 mm cell size and used it to simulate various forms of arrhythmia and determine a functional limit of the resolving power of body surface potentials, and to investigate their use in guiding radio-frequency ablation procedures [114, 115].

Following the success of the Visible Human Project [116], there has been much interest in using this high-resolution data source in biomedical computations. Sachse et al. segmented the cardiac geometry from the Visible Man [117], and like Weixue et al. [113], used the pixelated structure as a template for a cellular automata solution. In their study, the transmembrane potential distribution at each time point was used to construct ECG signals from both normal sinus rhythm and also a number of conduction pathologies. Freudenberg et al. also constructed a heart model but in this case using the Visible Female data set [118]. The resolution of the original images was scaled down by a factor of two in each direction to limit the number of variables that the computation had to encompass.

The main advantage of the cellular automata approach over more biophysically detailed models is the computational speed; whole heart simulations are possible without the need for expensive supercomputing facilities. There are, however, drawbacks to this approach. For most implementations, the shape of the resulting wavefront is dependent on the topology of the grid – a mesh tiled with squares produces a topologically square wavefront [109]). Although it is possible to generate curved wavefronts [118], these are restricted by the need for a characteristic dimension for the curvature. The cellular automata approach is also unsuitable for simulations in which dynamic cellular activity is important, such as the onset of ischemia, as they do not include realistic cellular electrophysiology and hence cannot respond to most external stimuli.

Huygens' Principle Models

From a macroscopic perspective, one can consider the spreading electrical excitation passing through the heart as a wave and therefore look toward other wave representations to model the phenomena. Huygens' principle, also known as Huygens' wavefront method, originated in the 1600s with the Dutch physicist Christian Huygens and his studies of the wave theory of light. The idea is conceptually simple and based on an assumption of constant wave speed. From a given time point and knowing the wave speed, one can construct the location of the wavefront at the next time point by simply drawing circles (or spheres in three dimensions) of an appropriate size along the existing wavefront as shown in ❷ Fig. 8.11. From a point source, the Huygens' principle is essentially like dropping a pebble into a pond and observing the path of the first wave.

Numerically for a Huygens' wave simulation, the heart tissue is usually divided into regular pieces, each on a scale much larger than a single myocyte. The activation sequence is best described with reference to ❷ Fig. 8.11, in which the dark grey cells behind the wavefront have been previously activated. As the wave moves from its initial position (solid line) to its final position (dashed line), it moves over the centers of the light grey squares and these are then added to the list of active cells. Ahead of the wavefront the white cells indicate that the tissue is yet to be activated.

Early examples of this idea in the cardiac field date back to the 1960s, for example, Okajima et al. [119], who constructed a model of the ventricles using 27,000 cubes and solved it under the assumption of isotropic conduction within this geometry. Resolutions quickly increased with Solomon and Selvester publishing a ventricular model with 750,000 points giving a spatial resolution of 1 mm [120].

Huygens' principle simulations can also incorporate anisotropy by assuming that the wave speed differs depending on local fiber orientation. Lorange et al. developed such a model but did not align wave speeds with realistic fiber orientation so that the resulting elliptical wavefronts did not match experiments [121]. Later models did include this alignment and incorporated fiber rotations in two and three dimensions, including an anatomically based ventricular geometry [122]. More details on this form of propagation model are available in an excellent review by Plonsey and Barr [123].

In general, the Huygens' approach describes only the location of the activation wavefront and cannot describe repolarization. This limitation can be circumvented by a cellular automata-like set of rules to return each cell to its original state after a predetermined period of time has elapsed since the initial activation. Besides the lack of a biophysical basis

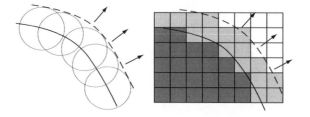

❑ Fig. 8.11

Huygens' wavefront method uses a constant wave speed approach. The new position of the wavefront can be found by placing *circles* of an appropriate diameter on the existing wavefront (*left*). With previously excited cells drawn *dark grey* and quiescent cells *white*, the cells which will become active as the wavefront moves forward are shown in *light grey* (*right*)

for this approach, the main limitation of this model is that propagation is restricted to occur in a finite number of directions (perpendicular to the wavefront) – in other words, the curvature of the wavefront has no effect on the speed of propagation.

8.4.3 Eikonal Curvature

An eikonal equation will generate the position of the wavefront in a manner that does allow the wavefront curvature to influence the speed of propagation. Essentially, a concave wavefront creates a current density that is higher than that of a plane wave, because the wave is propagating into a smaller area (see ❷ Fig. 8.12) and this causes the wave to accelerate. The opposite is true for a convex wavefront in which the wave moves into a larger area of resting tissue, which causes the wave to decelerate.

Mathematically a general eikonal equation has the form

$$|\nabla u (x)| = F (u (x)),\tag{8.18}$$

where $u(x)$ is the travel time, or eikonal, from the source to the point x. The equation governing the propagation of a Huygens' wavefront is actually a simplification of (8.18) where $F(u(x)) = 1$. To correct for the dependence of the wave speed on the wavefront curvature, (8.18) can be written as

$$|\nabla u (x)| = 1 + \nabla^2 u (x)\tag{8.19}$$

This is an elliptic equation, and therefore, the wavefront position at all times can be calculated in a single step. There are a small number of variations on this equation in the literature, including some based on parabolic representations; however, the essential feature is the inclusion of the Laplacian term, which allows wavefront curvature to influence the wave speed.

There are two classes of Eikonal equation based studies of cardiac propagation: those for which the position of the wavefront is the desired outcome and those for which it is an intermediate step. As an example of the former class, Keener developed a parabolic eikonal model that he solved using a finite difference approach and applied it to investigate microstructural effects [124]. More recently Hooks et al. used a finite element method to solve an eikonal equation over an orthotropic canine ventricular geometry [125]. The final model required only 180 tricubic Hermite elements to describe the wavefront position. For examples of the second class of models, Colli-Franzone and his colleagues have made many

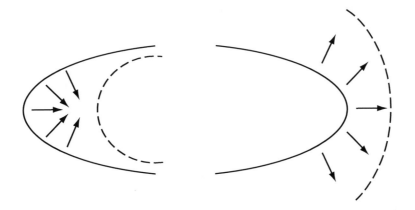

■ Fig. 8.12
A concave wavefront creates a high local current density that causes the wavefront to accelerate and flatten out as it propagates (*left*). A convex wavefront creates a low local current density that causes the wavefront to decelerate and flatten out (*right*)

outstanding contributions and have developed what is probably the current state of the art in eikonal models [126–131]. Their studies include models of the spread of activation under a wide variety of conditions and the most recent examples also include simulations of repolarization wave fronts and potentials [130].

8.4.4 FitzHugh and Nagumo

The FitzHugh–Nagumo model is a popular method of describing not only cardiac propagation but also other reaction-diffusion systems such as other excitable organs [132], calcium waves, and chemical reactions. Unlike many of the cardiac models that bear the name of their authors, FitzHugh and Nagumo developed their ideas independently and largely concurrently [133, 134].

Given a dimensionless activation variable u and a dimensionless recovery variable v, the FitzHugh–Nagumo model can be written as

$$\frac{du}{dt} = c_1 u \left(u - \alpha \right) \left(1 - u \right) - c_2 v + \nabla \cdot \boldsymbol{D} \nabla u, \tag{8.20}$$

$$\frac{dv}{dt} = b \left(u - dv \right) \tag{8.21}$$

with the boundary condition

$$\frac{du}{d\boldsymbol{n}} = 0 \tag{8.22}$$

Here $\boldsymbol{D}$ is the diffusion tensor, c_1 is an excitation rate constant, c_2 is an excitation decay constant, b is a recovery rate constant, d is a recovery decay constant, α is the dimensionless threshold potential and $\boldsymbol{n}$ is a unit outward normal vector. This system defines a cubic polynomial activation profile while the inclusion of a recovery variable allows the system to return to its initial resting state, thus enabling the simulation of phenomena that depend on repeated activations.

This type of model can be thought of as an oscillator and a careful selection of parameters can form an excitable model with the model equilibrium below α (as is needed for ventricular cells) or a self-exciting oscillator with the model equilibrium above α (as is appropriate for sinoatrial node pacemaker cells). The presence of the Laplacian term means that in most cases, an appropriate numerical solution technique is required, e.g., finite element or finite difference. An omission of the Laplacian term from (8.20) removes the propagation aspect and leaves a single-cell model that can be adjusted to return I_{ion}, which can then feed into the monodomain or bidomain equations. One could also easily think of this model as a nondimensionalized monodomain equation with a simple two-variable cell model. Given a resting membrane potential V_r, a peak membrane potential V_p, and a threshold of V_{th}, the following relationships can be used to convert between the dimensional monodomain equation and the nondimensional form.

$$u = \frac{V_m - V_r}{V_p - V_r}, \tag{8.23}$$

$$\alpha = \frac{V_{th} - V_r}{V_p - V_r}, \tag{8.24}$$

$$I_{ion} = C_m \left(V_p - V_r \right) \frac{du}{dt} \tag{8.25}$$

Rogers and McCulloch made a slight modification to (8.20) in order to provide a more cardiac-like waveform, multiplying the recovery variable by the activation variable [135].

$$\frac{du}{dt} = c_1 u \left(u - \alpha \right) \left(1 - u \right) - c_2 uv + \nabla \cdot \boldsymbol{D} \nabla u \tag{8.26}$$

Their recommended parameter values were $\alpha = 0.13$, $b = 0.013$, $c_1 = 0.26$, $c_2 = 0.1$, and $d = 1.0$. In isotropic simulations, D had the value 1.0 and in anisotropic simulations $\mathbf{D}$ was 4.0 in the direction of the muscle fibers and 1.0 in the transverse direction. Among other results, this parameter set was used to provide a demonstration of the influence wavefront curvature has on propagation velocity.

Although the FitzHugh–Nagumo approach has been used to investigate a number of different phenomena, it is in the simulation of reentrant waves (representing arrhythmias) in which it has proved to be most useful. The popularity of this formalism arises in large part because it is computationally efficient for simulating activation and recovery; modeling reentrant waves requires considerably longer simulations (several to tens of beats) than for a single heart beat. Examples of this type of model appeared in the early 1970s and subsequently focused primarily on two-dimensional tissue blocks [136, 137] but as computational power increased, three-dimensional models appeared, including some based on anatomically realistic geometries [138–140].

8.4.5 Computing Extracardiac Potentials

With a propagation sequence available, either from measurements or from one of the propagation models already described, the second stage of bioelectric source modeling is converting information that is essentially timing into the electric sources – typically currents – that would then generate the potentials measured from the heart or the body surface. The typical approach is to use the activation time and some assumptions about the resulting potential gradients that arise at the spreading wavefront to create some reasonable number of current sources. Because current and current density have direction, it is also necessary to determine the orientation of discrete current sources, which in turn requires knowledge of the spatial orientation of the spreading activation wavefront. The final component required is the amplitude of the current sources, which one can derive naturally from the spatial gradient of the potential in the myocardium.

The typical assumption during the activation phase is that the most significant potential gradients are localized in the region of the spreading wave of excitation so that it is necessary to evaluate only those regions of the heart. One particular simplifying assumption is to assign a fixed potential difference across all regions of the activation wavefront, which assumes that both the extracellular and intracellular potentials are identical for every cell. A more realistic version of this scheme assigns an action potential to each region of the heart, based either on a local implementation of one of the cell simulation models described in ❷ Sect. 8.3.1 or on measurements and taking into account the natural variations in action potential characteristics over the heart.

Mathematically, one can express this approach as computing a current density from Ohm's Law

$$\mathbf{J}_i = -\sigma_i \nabla \Phi_i, \tag{8.27}$$

where $\mathbf{J}_i$ is the current density in some region i, σ_i is the effective intracellular conductivity (which may be a tensor quantity), and $\nabla \Phi_i$ is the potential gradient over the same region. Depending on the model geometry and structure, there is a discrete form of this equation that applies at some appropriate resolution either throughout the heart or in regions of appreciable gradients (defined, for example, by the location of the activation wavefront at any given time).

In some formulations of the extracardiac potential, this expression for current density is enough, while in others, a more discrete form is necessary and one computes a dipole moment by integrating the current density over some region in space,

$$\mathbf{P}_{l,m,n} = -\int \sigma_i \nabla \Phi_i \, dl \, dm \, dn, \tag{8.28}$$

where $dl \, dm \, and \, dn$ describe some region in the (usually discrete) representation of the region collapsed into a single dipole with moment $\mathbf{P}_{l,m,n}$.

8.4.6 Applications

The applications of the bidomain approach and propagation modeling are very numerous and include a wide range of problems. One of the earliest applications of this approach to cardiac propagation was by Henriquez et al., who constructed detailed models of bundles of cardiac tissue and examined the critical values for spread of excitation [93, 94].

A more modern version of this approach has recently appeared in simulations by Stinstra et al., first of the passive electrical characteristics of cardiac tissue [141, 142], and then using those parameters to simulate at unparalleled spatial resolution the effects of cell shape and size on propagation [143]. Henriquez and his various colleagues have published a series of report of applying bidomain approaches to ever more complex slabs of tissue to investigate the role of structure, coupling and especially anisotropy on cardiac excitation in the ventricles [144–148].

Bidomain models have also become tractable enough to simulate some behaviors in whole heart models. For example Fischer et al. used a bidomain model of the heart together with a propagation model to simulate cardiac potentials under realistic conditions of anisotropy [95]. Other studies by Weinstein and Henriquez et al. have described the first computations of cardiac potentials in mice using bidomain models [149, 150]. Hopenfeld et al. also used a realistic, anisotropic dog heart model and the bidomain approach to simulate cardiac potentials from acute ischemia under varying conditions of ischemic zone location and depth [97, 151]. The fact that they simulated an essentially static condition from potentials during the plateau phase of the action potential made these simulations very tractable compared with models with propagation. For that, the model allowed unprecedented examination of the relationship between ischemic border zone shape and alignment with local myocardial fiber structure.

There are some less obvious applications of the bidomain for problems of tissue stimulation that make use of the unique ability of this formulation to capture spatially variable anisotropy. In one such application, Frazier et al. used a bidomain model of heart tissue to investigate the fields that arise during extracellular stimulation of tissue and thus to investigate the role of tissue structure, electrode location, and stimulus strength on stimulation [152]. Using even stronger extracellular fields, Trayanova and her colleagues have published many studies on defibrillation using the bidomain approach [153–157]. Recent studies by Jolley and Triedman et al. have illustrated the feasibility of carrying out simulations of cardiac defibrillation using realistic electrode placements inside the human child thorax [158]. Successful studies such as these will make it possible to simulate intracardiac defibrillator placement in subject-specific models and thus optimize lead placement and defibrillation protocols for each patient.

8.5   Models of Volume Conductor Potentials

In this section we describe the mathematical models and numerical methods required to compute body surface potentials from cardiac bioelectric sources. This is the last of the four components of the complete forward solution introduced in ❷ Sect. 8.1, which, in essence, describes the biophysical characteristics of the volume conductor, a passive medium with heterogeneous electrical conductivity. In practice, however, it is necessary to match the model of the volume conductor to the specific representation of the source and the desired outcome of the forward problem. For example, if one represents the heart as Einthoven did as a single current dipole [6] and seeks to compute the body-surface ECG, the volume conductor model and the associated mathematical formulation will differ from the case of the source described in terms of activation times on the epicardial and endocardial surfaces. Thus any discussion of the volume conductor potentials is closely tied to the source formulation, a fact that we reflect in the organization of this section.

The choice of numerical method is also a product of the type of source model and desired outcome of the simulation, as well as assumptions about the volume conductor itself. For example, a forward problem based on epicardial and endocardial surface activation times and under assumptions of heterogeneous but isotropic torso volume conductor leads naturally to a numerical implementation based on the boundary element method (BEM). By contrast, a solution based, for example, on bidomain computations of cardiac currents embedded in an anisotropic model of the heart and heterogeneous (and possibly anisotropic) torso is better served by an implementation using the finite element method (FEM). Wherever possible, we will indicate the numerical approach best suited for a particular problem formulation and direct the reader to ❷ Sect. 8.6 for details of the associated numerical methods.

This section describes the biophysics and mathematics of volume conductors required to form the bridge between the descriptions of bioelectric sources in the previous sections to the numerical methods that are necessary to implement working solutions to electrocardiographic forward problems. It is impossible in a single chapter to provide comprehensive coverage of all combinations of source models and volume conductors so that we focus here on some of the more frequently studied scenarios and describe at least the main numerical methods in contemporary use.

8.5.1 Biophysical Background

The physics of potential fields describes this component of the forward problem and is also the topic of ❷ Sect. 2.6 of this volume. Here we avoid some of the simplifications of ❷ Sect. 2.6 and arrive at a more general framework, specifically one that supports a wider range of realistic tissue characteristics.

The basic formulation of all such problems leads either to Poisson's or Laplace's equation, i.e.,

$$\nabla \cdot (\sigma \nabla \Phi) = -i_v = \nabla \cdot \vec{J}^i, \tag{8.29}$$

as in (2.87), the general expression that applies to inhomogeneous, anisotropic conductivity. In case the conductivity is anisotropic, σ denotes the tensor character (❷ Chap. 7, "Appendix: The EDL and Bidomain Theory").

Similarly, we can write a Laplace's equation

$$\nabla \cdot (\sigma \nabla \Phi) = 0 \tag{8.30}$$

for any region in which there are no active sources, i.e., $i_v = 0$. To make use of Laplace's equation, the solution domain cannot include the sources, which then appear as imposed boundary conditions of the resulting solution, an approach outlined in ❷ Sect. 2.6.4. These boundary conditions include electric potentials that are known at some subset of the problem domain, typically on or within the heart, and this is known as the "Dirichlet" boundary condition.

The solutions of (8.29) and (8.30) also depend on boundary conditions that arise from the physics of the problem. At the boundary of the outer surface of the torso and air, for example, no current flow leaves the body so that

$$(\sigma \nabla \Phi) \cdot \mathbf{n} = 0, \tag{8.31}$$

where $\mathbf{n}$ is a unit vector pointing in normal direction to the surface. This is known as the "Neumann" boundary condition on the flux through the surface. At the boundaries within the volume conductor there are also boundary conditions dictated by the fact that potentials must be equal on both sides of a shared boundary and normal current flow must therefore also be the same, i.e., for a boundary between compartments p and q

$$\Phi_p = \Phi_q, \tag{8.32}$$

$$(\sigma_p \nabla \Phi_p) \cdot \mathbf{n}_p = (\sigma_q \nabla \Phi_q) \cdot \mathbf{n}_q \tag{8.33}$$

8.5.2 Analytical Models

Under highly simplified conditions, it is possible to formulate closed form or analytical solutions to (8.29) and (8.30) and there is a rich history of applying this approach to the forward problem in electrocardiography. The simplified conditions typically include a source described in terms of a modest number of discrete current dipoles and a volume conductor with a mathematically simple shape, for example a circle, sphere, or cylinder. Examples of this approach include studies from Wilson and Bayley [159] and then Frank [160], who computed body-surface potentials from a single current dipole source located in a spherical surface model of the torso. Burger et al. [161] and Okada [162] carried out similar studies using cylindrical model of the torso and concentric and eccentric dipole sources, which led eventually to the extensive studies based on a model of eccentric spheres developed by Bayley and Berry [163–165]. Rudy et al. later further developed this approach extensively [166–168], and it is still in use, largely as a means of validating solution techniques based on numerical approximations of the sources and volume conductors [43, 169–173] (as we describe in the following sections). It is rare to use analytical models for any realistic solutions to forward (or inverse) problems in electrocardiography, simply because the resulting accuracy is inadequate when compared with measured values in a real subject/patient.

8.5.3 Discrete Source Models

There is a rich history of forward problem formulations based on discrete source models of the heart, the background of which is covered in ❷ Sect. 8.3.2 and ❷ Chaps. 2, ❷ 5, and ❷ 6 of this volume. The underlying notion of all these approaches is that a very simple current source can adequately represent the electrical activity of the heart, at least when viewed from some distance from the heart, e.g., the body surface. The huge advantage of these approaches is the small number of parameters required to describe the sources and the resulting simplicity of the associated forward (and inverse) problems. The most notable disadvantage is that there are no clear physical or physiological links between discrete sources and either the true sources they represent or any directly measurable quantities; there is no way to directly measure dipole locations or amplitudes nor to unambiguously link their parameters to action potentials or spread of activation. Discrete source models nevertheless play important roles in both the analytical approaches already outlined and the numerical approaches described in the following section.

The descriptions of bioelectric fields from discrete sources begin with the expression for the potential from a single dipole in an infinite space, (2.99), rewritten as

$$\Phi(\vec{r'}) = \frac{1}{4\pi\sigma} \frac{\vec{R}}{R^3} \cdot \vec{P}(\vec{r}),\tag{8.34}$$

where $\vec{R}$ is the vector from the location of the dipole to the location $\vec{r'}$ in space where Φ is calculated and $\vec{P}(\vec{r})$ is the srength (dipole moment) of the dipole at location $\vec{r}$, specifying both the direction and the magnitude of the current dipole source.

To compute the potentials from a current dipole located within a finite medium, even one with several regions having different conductivities (σ) is also possible using the equation (derived in ❷ Sect. 2.6.4.4 resulting in (2.17))

$$\Phi(\vec{r'}) = \frac{1}{4\pi\sigma} \frac{\vec{R}}{R^3} \cdot \vec{P}(\vec{r}) - \frac{1}{4\pi} \sum_{l=0}^{N_S} \int_{S_l} (\sigma_l^+ - \sigma_l^-)\Phi(\vec{r}) \, d\Omega_{rr'},\tag{8.35}$$

where σ_l^+ and σ_l^- are the conductivities on either side of the boundary l and $d\Omega_{rr'}$ is the solid angle described in ❷ Sect. 2.2.12 of ❷ Chap. 2. With a numerical implementation of this equation (usually via the boundary element method described in ❷ Sect. 2.6.4 and in the following section) it is then possible to compute the potential at any point provided the dipole location, orientation, and strength and the spatial locations of all boundaries and the conductivities around them are known. It is also possible to extend this approach to other discrete sources, i.e., quadropoles or octopoles, which are capable of representing more complex versions of the cardiac sources at the cost of more parameters but still without a clear link to measurements or physiological sources [1].

8.5.4   Cardiac Surface Potential Models

This form of the forward problem is one of the two dominant approaches in modern applications and is based on a source description of epicardial potentials. More precisely, the potentials on any closed surface that encompasses all active cardiac sources forms a completely equivalent representation of the true cardiac sources. Out of convenience – because it permits direct measurement of the source parameters – one usually selects the enclosing surface to be the epicardium (or pericardium) and the challenge then becomes to derive a mathematical formulation that predicts the potentials throughout the thorax (include the body surface) from this source. Barr and his colleagues solved this problem in the mid-1970s in a way that also provides a natural numerical solution by means of the boundary element method [37, 38, 174].

❷ Figure 8.13 describes schematically the configuration and the associated variables involved in linking the potentials the heart surface S_H and the body surface S_B. In this figure, the region between the heart surface and the body surface is taken to have a uniform conductivity. The derivation of this link as derived from the BEM is described in ❷ Sect. 2.6.4.5. Equation (2.173) implies that inhomogeneities in the region between S_H and S_B, like those of the lungs, can also be treated by means of the BEM.

In its numerical form, the transfer can be described by a matrix A. Any element a_{BH} of this matrix represents the effect of the potential at location P_H on the heart surface S_H to points P_B on the body surface S_B.

The transfer coefficients relate to the specification of the geometry and conductivities of the problem, i.e., it depends only on the volume conductor and not on the time-varying source potentials.

Although the formalities of all the terms of the transfer (2.173) are crucial when carrying out the calculations, it is their qualitative meanings that are fundamental to understanding this entire approach. The equations (and diagrams)

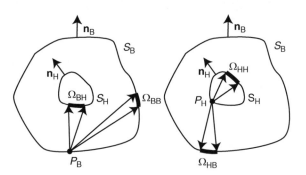

◘ Fig. 8.13
Schematic diagram of the forward problem in terms of surface potentials. (a and b) represent the approach to calculating the potentials on each of the heart (P_B on S_B) and body (P_H on S_H) surfaces respectively. Both surfaces have outward normals (n_H and n_B) and all active sources are contained within S_H. The heavy line segments between the tips of the arrows represent the contribution of a surface element to the potential at the common origin of the arrows and the Ω symbols represent the solid angle that weights each of these contributions

reveal that the potential at any point on the surface of, for example, the body surface is the sum of contributions from the potentials (and perhaps potential gradients) at the other surfaces in the problem.

The full expression of the forward transfer reads

$$\Phi_B = A_{BH}\Phi_H \tag{8.36}$$

The computation of potentials on the heart surface from body surface potentials is based on evaluationg the inverse of the transfer matrix involved, a topic treated in ❷ Sect. 9.3 of ❷ Chap. 9.

One of the essential aspects of this approach to the forward problem is that it is based on epicardial (or pericardial) surface potentials, which are, in principle, measurable quantities. In fact, as we outlined in ❷ Sect. 8.2.2, these quantities are measured in experiments and in clinical practice, because they convey directly information about the electrical state of the heart. This form of the forward solution is also unique in the sense that for any given set of source potentials there is one and only one set of associated body surface potentials (as we shall see in the next chapter, the reverse is also true, at least under assumptions of perfect numerical calculations and noise-free measurements). The information necessary to solve this problem consists of a description of the heart and body surfaces and of any other surfaces that separate regions of differing conductivity along with the tissue conductivities of each of these regions.

8.5.5 Equivalent Double Layer Based Models

A final formulation of the forward problem is based on a representation of the spread of activation and repolarization in the heart and this represents the sources not as variable potential amplitudes but on the timing of activation and repolarization on the epicardial and endocardial surfaces of the heart. ❷ Chapters 6 and ❷ 7 contain descriptions of these sources (the uniform and equivalent double layers) and the resulting forward problem respectively. The ECGSIM software described in ❷ Sect. 8.6.6, is a very user-friendly and powerful implementation of this forward model.

8.6 Numerical Approaches and Computational Aspects

8.6.1 Introduction

This section describes a family of numerical methods that are common to many different types of electrocardiographic forward problems and in some cases, several of them may solve the same problem. Hence they are combined here into one section rather than organized within the previous sections describing the types of problems to which one might apply them. These methods are common not only to forward problems but also to many other applications across the broadest spectrum of engineering and science, which has the considerable advantage that they are well supported with robust theory and easily available implementations as computer programs and libraries. Here we provide only outlines of these methods with emphasis on the intuition that motivates each and the specific applications to the forward problem. We refer the interested reader to other sources through this section.

Please note that in this section the symbol Ω denotes a region in space, rather than a solid angle as used at several other places in this volume, and that Γ denotes its boundary.

To provide a common framework for all these methods, we begin with Laplace's equation (8.30) and note that it is a differential form, also known as a strong form

$$\nabla \cdot (\sigma \nabla \Phi) = 0 \tag{8.37}$$

Numerical solutions to differential equations always involve some degree of approximation and uncertainty. Thus, any numerical solution for (8.37) will also be to some extent approximate. If we use the notation $\hat{\phi}$ to represent the numerical solution, then the substitution of $\hat{\phi}$ into the left hand side of (8.37) will not yield identically 0; there will be some error, or residual, remaining that one would like to minimize, thereby yielding an accurate answer. Different numerical techniques seek to minimize this residual in different ways, typically by trying to force the average (or weighted) error to be zero. The general expression for this is the *weighted residual expression* or "weak form" given by

$$\int_{\Omega} \nabla \cdot (\sigma \nabla \phi) \, \omega \, d\Omega = 0, \tag{8.38}$$

where Ω represents the solution domain whose boundary is denoted Γ and ω is an as-yet-unspecified weighting function. The presence of this weighting function leads to the term weighted residual for this approach. It should be noted that there is nothing inferior or inadequate about the weak form of the equation when compared with the strong form.

In terms of the numerical techniques outlined in the subsequent sections, the finite element method (FEM) and the boundary element method (BEM) both solve the weak form while the finite difference method (FDM) solves the strong form. Consequently the FEM and BEM enforce the governing equation in an integral sense, i.e., the governing equation will be satisfied over each element but not necessarily at any given point. Finite differences, on the other hand, do satisfy the governing equation at the difference points but not necessarily within the space between these points.

The choice of numerical approach is closely tied to the specific forward problem and there is no single best method for all applications [4]. The finite difference method (FDM) is intuitively the most straightforward, because it directly estimates the derivatives explicit in the strong form of the equation (Poisson's or Laplace's). However, the FDM usually requires a regularly sampled, orthogonal grid for the solution domain, which is rarely the most efficient way to describe complex geometries as they arise in the body. The FDM method requires this grid to encompass the entire volume and can represent anisotropic characteristics of this domain. As a result, the FDM approach has seen widespread use in models of regular slabs of myocardium [175, 176] and also to represent the whole torso [117, 177–180]. Recent studies have even suggested a generalized FDM approach suitable for irregular grids applied to the bidomain method [181].

The boundary element method (BEM) is based on a grid of the boundaries of a region, e.g., the surfaces that surround the heart, torso, and internal organs of differing electrical conductivity. The BEM is well suited to inhomogeneous tissues but not to regions with anisotropy. Its major advantage lies in the requirement only for surface descriptions, which is often the first step in creating volume grids and is more flexible and easily adjustable than finite element (or finite volume) methods. A related advantage comes from the fact that the number of nodes – the degrees of freedom – involved in the computation is smaller for BEM than FEM (surface rather than volume). As a result, the matrices involved in solving the forward problem by the BEM are generally much smaller than in the other methods, although, the latter involve sparse matrices so that the overall size of the computation may ultimately be comparable.

Applications of the boundary element method to forward problems in electrocardiography abound and virtually all the early simulation studies (as well as many contemporary studies) have made use of this technique [38, 40, 41, 44, 64, 88, 182–186].

The finite element method (FEM) and the related finite volume method (FVM) have gained broad support in the past decade, in large part for their general utility, their ability to include all forms of tissue conductivity, and the advanced support available in the form of efficient computational implementations. The chief disadvantage of the FEM is the requirement for carefully constructed volumetric meshes of nodes and polygons: a task that is still arguably the largest barrier to practical use of all forms of numerical methods for partial differential equations. Any changes in geometry of the heart or torso also require a reorganization of the mesh, often best achieved by starting again from the beginning (or at least from the adjusted surfaces). Perhaps the first widely published use of the FEM was from Colli-Franzone et al. [187] but many others have also adopted this technique for all types of electrocardiographic field problems [48, 50, 97, 152, 188–197]. A particularly novel approach has been to combine techniques, taking advantage of their relative strengths in appropriate portions of the solution domain [198, 199].

We now provide brief descriptions of the major numerical methods used for electrocardiographic forward problems and refer the reader to more detailed descriptions.

8.6.2 The Finite Difference Method (FDM)

The finite difference method represents arguably the simplest approach to solving the generalized Laplace equation governing the potential fields and current flows within the torso volume conductor. The inherent simplicity of the FDM relies on an underlying mesh that is a grid of evenly spaced solution points distributed along orthogonal axes across the solution domain. Meshes for the FDM are relatively easy to construct, at least for pieces of tissue that represent rectilinear slabs or in cases for which image data with equal sampling in all directions are available. The resulting system of equations has some advantageous structure that can facilitate computational solution approaches.

The FDM solves the strong or differential form of the generalized Laplace equation shown in (8.37) and thus depends on estimates of first and second spatial derivatives of the potential field variable, ϕ, and the conductivity tensor, σ. The method is illustrated here over a two-dimensional domain but easily extends to three dimension. Expanding (8.37) gives

$$
\begin{aligned}
\nabla \cdot (\sigma \nabla \phi) = {} & \frac{\partial \sigma_{11}}{\partial x} \frac{\partial \phi}{\partial x} + \sigma_{11} \frac{\partial^2 \phi}{\partial x^2} + \frac{\partial \sigma_{12}}{\partial x} \frac{\partial \phi}{\partial y} + \sigma_{12} \frac{\partial^2 \phi}{\partial x \partial y} \\
& + \frac{\partial \sigma_{21}}{\partial y} \frac{\partial \phi}{\partial x} + \sigma_{21} \frac{\partial^2 \phi}{\partial x \partial y} + \frac{\partial \sigma_{22}}{\partial y} \frac{\partial \phi}{\partial y} + \sigma_{22} \frac{\partial^2 \phi}{\partial y^2},
\end{aligned}
\tag{8.39}
$$

where the two subscripts on σ indicate the value from the appropriate row and column of the conductivity tensor.

Several simplifications may be possible at this stage. If the principle axes of the conductivity tensor are aligned with the coordinate axes then the terms involving σ_{12} and σ_{21} can be omitted. A further simplification is possible if the conductivity tensor is homogeneous throughout the solution domain, in which case the four terms involving derivatives of σ can be omitted. Here, however, we proceed without a loss of generality.

Each continuous partial derivative in (8.39) may be approximated by a discrete finite difference that is usually formed from a truncated Taylor's series expansion of the dependent variable in terms of values at neighboring points. Given a regular mesh with a constant spacing in the x (i) direction of Δx and a constant y (j) spacing of Δy, it is possible to describe, for example, the point one step away in the negative x direction as $(i-1)(j)$. Similarly, the point located at $(+\Delta x, +\Delta y)$ from the point of interest can be denoted $(i+1)(j+1)$. While a number of formulations are possible using differing numbers of surrounding points to control the accuracy of the approximation, the most common approximation is a second-order, central finite differencing scheme. Using this approach, the second-order partial derivatives from (8.39) can be approximated from a Taylor's series expansion as

$$
\frac{\partial^2 \phi}{\partial x^2} = \frac{\phi_{(i-1)(j)} - 2\phi_{(i)(j)} + \phi_{(i+1)(j)}}{\Delta x^2},
\tag{8.40}
$$

$$
\frac{\partial^2 \phi}{\partial y^2} = \frac{\phi_{(i)(j-1)} - 2\phi_{(i)(j)} + \phi_{(i)(j+1)}}{\Delta y^2},
\tag{8.41}
$$

$$
\frac{\partial^2 \phi}{\partial x \partial y} = \frac{\phi_{(i-1)(j-1)} - \phi_{(i-1)(j+1)} - \phi_{(i+1)(j-1)} + \phi_{(i+1)(j+1)}}{\Delta x \Delta y}
\tag{8.42}
$$

The first-derivatives from (8.39) for a generic variable u can be approximated as

$$\frac{\partial u}{\partial x} = \frac{u_{(i+1)(j)} - u_{(i-1)(j)}}{2\Delta x}, \tag{8.43}$$

$$\frac{\partial u}{\partial y} = \frac{u_{(i)(j+1)} - u_{(i)(j-1)}}{2\Delta y}, \tag{8.44}$$

where u can be substituted for either the potential field, ϕ, or any of the σ_{ij} components as necessary.

The discrete derivative approximations given in Eqs. (8.40)–(8.44) can then be substituted into (8.39) in place of the continuous derivatives. Following this, (8.39) can be rearranged to uncover the weighting coefficients for ϕ at each referenced point resulting in an expression of the form

$$\begin{aligned} k_1 \phi_{(i-1)(j-1)} + k_2 \phi_{(i)(j-1)} + k_3 \phi_{(i+1)(j-1)} + k_4 \phi_{(i-1)(j)} + k_5 \phi_{(i)(j)} \\ + k_6 \phi_{(i+1)(j)} + k_7 \phi_{(i-1)(j+1)} + k_8 \phi_{(i)(j+1)} + k_9 \phi_{(i+1)(j+1)} = 0 \end{aligned} \tag{8.45}$$

One such equation will be generated for each finite difference point that does not lie on the boundary of the domain and the resulting equations then assembled into a matrix system of the form

$$\boldsymbol{K}\boldsymbol{\phi} = \boldsymbol{f}, \tag{8.46}$$

where the right-hand side vector, $\boldsymbol{f}$, will be zero at all internal points.

On the boundary of the solution domain, either a potential (Dirichlet) or a flux (Neumann) boundary condition must be set at every point. Dirichlet boundary conditions are set by directly specifying the value of potential at a given point. In order to preserve the matrix structure, this is often achieved by placing a "1" on the diagonal of the appropriate row and the desired value of the boundary potential in the same row of $\boldsymbol{f}$. For Neumann boundary conditions, a simple one-sided difference is often adequate, e.g.,

$$c = \sigma \frac{\partial \phi}{\partial n} = \sigma \frac{\phi_{(i+1)} - \phi_i}{\Delta x}, \tag{8.47}$$

where c is the magnitude of the flux condition (zero on the surface of the torso). The coefficients of the ϕ terms are assembled into $\boldsymbol{K}$ and c is placed into $\boldsymbol{f}$. Selecting this form of flux boundary condition preserves the symmetry of $\boldsymbol{K}$, which is also highly sparse for large meshes, and the final system can be readily solved by either direct or iterative means.

8.6.3 The Finite Element Method (FEM)

The finite element method has become increasingly pervasive in traditional engineering disciplines and is also becoming a popular solution methodology for problems in cardiac bioelectricity. The starting equation for the finite element method is the weighted residual form of the generalized Laplace equation given in (8.38), to which we apply Green's first formula, which can be thought of as a multidimensional version of integration by parts.

Given scalar fields f and g with a tensor k, Green's first formula can be written as

$$\int_\Omega \left(f\nabla \cdot (k\nabla g) + \nabla f \cdot (k\nabla g) \right) d\Omega = \int_\Gamma fk\nabla g \cdot \boldsymbol{n} \, d\Gamma \tag{8.48}$$

This is also known as the Green–Gauss theorem because the scalar fields must obey the divergence theorem of Gauss. Applying (8.48) to (8.38) yields

$$\int_\Omega \nabla \cdot (\sigma\nabla\phi) \, \omega d\Omega = \int_\Omega (\sigma\nabla\phi) \cdot \nabla\omega d\Omega - \int_\Gamma (\sigma\nabla\phi) \cdot \boldsymbol{n}\omega d\Gamma = 0, \tag{8.49}$$

and from (8.38) we obtain

$$\int_\Omega (\sigma \nabla \phi) \cdot \nabla \omega d\Omega = \int_\Gamma (\sigma \nabla \phi) \cdot \boldsymbol{n} \omega d\Gamma \qquad (8.50)$$

To solve (8.50) using finite elements, as the name suggests, the solution domain is first subdivided into L smaller domains or elements. These elements are nonoverlapping and in combination completely cover Ω. This can be written mathematically as

$$\Omega = \bigcup_{l=1}^{L} \Omega_l \qquad (8.51)$$

Typically the geometry of these elements is defined by a set of nodes which, in the simplest cases, correspond to the vertices of the elements. The set of nodes associated with a particular element are known as *local element nodes*.

Field variables can be interpolated between the local element nodes and hence over an element by what are known as *basis functions*. Instead of performing the interpolation in global space, it is preferable to introduce a local element-based coordinate system referred to here as local element or ξ space. In this space, the axes are orthogonal and the ξ directions are normalized to lie between 0 and 1 in each direction. This approach has the advantage that regardless of their physical geometry, each element in the mesh appears identical in ξ space and thus evaluating (8.50) over one element easily extends to the remaining elements. The relationship between global and local element space is illustrated in ❷ Fig. 8.14.

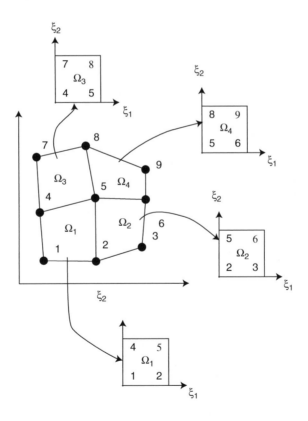

⬛ Fig. 8.14

A two-dimensional example of the mapping between the solution domain Ω and local finite element space. The solution domain is divided into four finite elements, Ω_1, Ω_2, Ω_3 and Ω_4 with nine global nodes. Each of these elements is then mapped to the normalized local ξ space with four local nodes and the geometric basis functions are used to interpolate nodal quantities over these elements

The details of the basis functions required to interpolate among the local element nodes in ξ space largely depend on the shape of each element and the number of nodes it contains (e.g., a triangular element will have three nodes while a hexahedral element will have eight). As an example, the bilinear interpolation of a variable u between the four nodes of a quadrilateral element can be described by

$$u\left(\xi_1, \xi_2\right) = \Psi_1\left(\xi_1, \xi_2\right) u_1 + \Psi_2\left(\xi_1, \xi_2\right) u_2 + \Psi_3\left(\xi_1, \xi_2\right) u_3 + \Psi_4\left(\xi_1, \xi_2\right) u_4, \tag{8.52}$$

where ξ_1 and ξ_2 represent the coordinate axes in local element space and both lie between 0 and 1 inclusive. The terms u_1, u_2, u_3 and u_4 refer to the value of u at each of the four local nodes, and the four basis functions from (8.52) can be written in terms of ξ_1 and ξ_2 as

$$\begin{aligned}
\Psi_1\left(\xi_1, \xi_2\right) &= \left(1 - \xi_1\right)\left(1 - \xi_2\right) \\
\Psi_2\left(\xi_1, \xi_2\right) &= \xi_1\left(1 - \xi_2\right) \\
\Psi_3\left(\xi_1, \xi_2\right) &= \left(1 - \xi_1\right)\xi_2 \\
\Psi_4\left(\xi_1, \xi_2\right) &= \xi_1\xi_2
\end{aligned} \tag{8.53}$$

In general the interpolation of a variable over an element can be written as

$$u\left(\boldsymbol{\xi}\right) = \Psi_n\left(\boldsymbol{\xi}\right) u_n, \tag{8.54}$$

where n represents the appropriate number of local element nodes and noting the vector form of $\boldsymbol{\xi}$ indicating the presence of an appropriate number of ξ coordinates.

Using these ideas we can rewrite the volume integral from (8.50) in terms of individual elements and their local ξ coordinates as

$$\sum_{l=1}^{L} \int_{\Omega_l} \left(\sigma\nabla\phi\right) \cdot \nabla\omega \, d\Omega_l = \sum_{l=1}^{L} \int_0^1 \left(\sigma\nabla\phi\right) \cdot \nabla\omega \left|J\left(\boldsymbol{\xi}\right)\right| d\boldsymbol{\xi}, \tag{8.55}$$

where J is the Jacobian for the transformation from global to local element coordinates and all of the terms inside the resulting integral are expressed in terms of local element space. The emboldened integral notation is used to represent the presence of the appropriate number of integrals – three for a volume integral over a three-dimensional element.

To simplify the expressions in the following step, we make use of the Einstein summation convention, which states that the letter used for an index is arbitrary, a repeated index indicates a summation, and no index may be repeated more than twice. An example of such a summation is as follows.

$$x_i y_i = \sum_{i=1}^{3} x_i y_i = x_1 y_1 + x_2 y_2 + x_3 y_3 \tag{8.56}$$

Within the integral the two gradient terms may be expressed as

$$\nabla\phi = \frac{\partial\phi}{\partial\xi_k}\frac{\partial\xi_k}{\partial x_j}, \tag{8.57}$$

$$\nabla\omega = \frac{\partial\omega}{\partial\xi_h}\frac{\partial\xi_h}{\partial x_j}, \tag{8.58}$$

which is essentially just applying the chain rule for partial derivatives. For a scalar conductivity value the integrand then becomes

$$\left(\sigma\nabla\phi\right) \cdot \nabla\omega = \sigma\frac{\partial\phi}{\partial\xi_k}\frac{\partial\xi_k}{\partial x_j}\frac{\partial\omega}{\partial\xi_h}\frac{\partial\xi_h}{\partial x_j}, \tag{8.59}$$

noting the summations over h, j, and k. For information on the extension of this formula to a general conductivity tensor, please see Pullan et al. [200].

Within each element, the dependent variable to be evaluated (in this case ϕ) can be described via interpolation using basis functions and (8.54), i.e., $\phi = \Psi_n(\xi)\phi_n$. It is now necessary to also choose a set of weighting functions ω and a common choice are the dependent variable basis functions, i.e., $\omega = \Psi_m(\xi)$, yielding what is known as a Galerkin finite element formulation. Equation (8.59) then becomes

$$(\sigma\nabla\phi)\cdot\nabla\omega = \phi_n\,\sigma\frac{\partial\Psi_n(\xi)}{\partial\xi_k}\frac{\partial\xi_k}{\partial x_j}\frac{\partial\Psi_m(\xi)}{\partial\xi_h}\frac{\partial\xi_h}{\partial x_j} \tag{8.60}$$

The ϕ_n terms are now no longer functions of space but instead refer specifically to the value of ϕ at the n local element nodes. Thus, they can be moved outside the integral expression, resulting in

$$\sum_{l=1}^{L}\int_{\Omega_l}(\sigma\nabla\phi)\cdot\nabla\omega d\Omega_l = \sum_{l=1}^{L}\phi_n\int_0^1\sigma\frac{\partial\Psi_n(\xi)}{\partial\xi_k}\frac{\partial\xi_k}{\partial x_j}\frac{\partial\Psi_m(\xi)}{\partial\xi_h}\frac{\partial\xi_h}{\partial x_j}|J(\xi)|d\xi_l \tag{8.61}$$

There is seldom an analytical means of evaluating these integrals so that the numerical integration technique known as quadrature is required. The most efficient quadrature scheme for this integral is Gauss–Legendre quadrature, sometimes referred to as Gaussian quadrature [201]. For a single element, (8.61) describes a total of $m \times n$ integrals as there is no implied summation over either of these indices. In a Galerkin formulation $m = n$ and the evaluated integrals can be assembled into an element stiffness matrix, E_{mn}, that is both square and symmetric, resulting in a set of element equations of the form

$$E_{mn}\phi_n = f_m \tag{8.62}$$

Performing the required summation over all of the elements in the solution domain results in a global system of equations that is sparse and also symmetric.

$$K\phi = f \tag{8.63}$$

A zero entry in f is prescribed for all nodes internal to the mesh, representing a conservation of flux at these points. Unlike the FDM, no special treatment of the boundary nodes is needed in order to construct K. On the domain boundary, the same weighting function, ω, can be used to transform the boundary integral from the right-hand side of (8.50) where the dependent variable is a flux of the form $(q = (\sigma\nabla\phi)\cdot n)$.

$$f = \sum_{l=1}^{L}q_n\int_0^1\Psi_n(\xi)\Psi_m(\xi)|J(\xi)|d\xi \tag{8.64}$$

This gives rise to a matrix system of the form

$$K\phi = f = Nq \tag{8.65}$$

After the application of either potential (Dirichlet) or flux (Neumann) boundary conditions at each boundary node, this system can be solved for ϕ. In practice, the N matrix is rarely constructed and integrated flux values are inserted directly into f.

8.6.4 The Boundary Element Method (BEM)

Like the FEM, the derivation of the boundary element method can begin with the weighted residual form of Laplace's equation, a highly relevant conceptual framework that is given a separate theoretical treatment in ❷ Sect. 2.6.4. Also, like the other numerical approximation methods, the endpoint of the derivation can be cast in the form of a matrix as follows. After discretization of its integrals, Eqn. (2.172) can be expressed as

$$\phi = g - A\phi, \tag{8.66}$$

where ϕ represents the potentials at the nodes of the triangulated boundary surfaces, g are the scaled versions of the same potentials in the virtual, infinite homogeneous medium, and $\mathbf{A}$ is the expression of the inhomogeneities. Recall (❯ Sect. 2.6.4) that in an infinite homogeneous medium the secondary sources vanish ($\sigma^- = \sigma^+$ at all interfaces), and hence, only the first term on the right remains.

Formaly, we may write

$$(\mathbf{I} - \mathbf{A})\phi = g, \tag{8.67}$$

from which the desired potential ϕ can be found as

$$\phi = (\mathbf{I} - \mathbf{A})^{-1}g \tag{8.68}$$

By writing $(\mathbf{I} - \mathbf{A})^{-1} = \mathbf{B}$ we may write

$$\phi = \mathbf{B}g \tag{8.69}$$

and thus express the solution as a simple matrix multiplication. This expression is particularly useful in situations in which the same geometry (and conductivity) apply to a number of sets of potentials, which requires only a change in g as the coefficient matrix, $\mathbf{B}$, remains the same [202].

Until the 1990s, the BEM approach was the dominant method in bioelectric field problems and it still dominates the literature in problems in which current-dipole sources adequately capture the phenomena of interest, most typically in representing discrete sources of bioelectricity in the brain. As we have already seen, in the electrocardiographic forward problem the sources are usually more elaborate, which has led to a wider range of numerical approaches so that today there is a balance between BEM and FEM applications. As already described, the choice of method is multifaceted and depends on both the source formulation and the shape and nature of the volume conductor, and the ultimate goal of the study. Of particular note in the use of the BEM approach are the breakthroughs of Barr et al. in a series of seminal studies leading to the epicardial potential based electrocardiographic forward (and inverse) problem [37, 38, 182, 203]. Solutions using the BEM approach are typically best suited to conditions in which torso conductivities are at least piecewise constant and isotropic.

Of the three numerical approaches, the BEM has the longest history in the field of cardiac bioelectricity.

8.6.5 Geometric Modeling

The three numerical methods already described all assume some form of discrete representation of the geometry of the problem; the creation of these discrete descriptions is what we refer to as geometric modeling. The broader field of geometric modeling contains many additional aspects of computational geometry and computer aided geometry design that seek to capture shape and structure in analytical or statistical form so that its use in the forward problem is just one limited application. In the description to follow, we take a very pragmatic approach and outline the essential requirements for our problem.

Geometric modeling is required whenever a simulation problem has a specific geometric context, i.e., it uses neither a schematic representation of actual shape nor a geometrically simplified model made from simple shapes such as lines (planes), circles (spheres), rectangles (cylinders) in two (and three) dimensions. Instead, the geometric models of interest here describe real anatomy derived from some form of images or otherwise digitized reference points and represented as a set of points joined into polygonal elements. Thus a typical geometric modeling pipeline begins with (1) raw geometric data, often a set of medical image data from magnetic resonance (MR) or computed X-ray tomography (CT) from a particular subject or patient. These images sometimes contain specific markers or anatomical fiducial points that provide a reference frame for additional geometry information either from other discrete sources or other image modalities. The next step in the pipeline is (2) to extract from the image data the points (pixels or voxels) that define surfaces between regions of different conductivity. Obviously, the surfaces of interest include the outer boundary of the torso, the surfaces on or inside the heart, and surfaces that surround any other region whose conductivity is considered relevant to the simulation – a determination that is still the topic of research. From these surface boundaries, the next step in geometric model is usually to (3) define a set of suitable points on these boundaries and then connect them into surface polygons (lines in two dimensions and triangles or quadrilaterals in three dimensions). For methods like the BEM, the geometric model is essentially complete at this point but for FDM and FEM, there is an additional step that (4) adds more points and links them into polygons (typically hexahedra or tetrahedra) to describe the volume of the problem domain, e.g., the heart and/or thorax.

1. Raw geometric data

There are two typical sources of raw information for geometric models: medical imaging data from MR or CT and perhaps ultrasound, and sets of discrete points from some form of digitization, e.g., mechanical or electromagnetic digitizer devices, or with growing frequency, location-sensing systems incorporated into catheter-based electrophysiological mapping systems [3, 204–206]. Image data are sampled at very regular intervals, and assuming the field of view is adequate, covers the entire problem domain, even regions inside the otherwise inaccessible interior of organs and tissues.

Each imaging modality has its own strengths and weaknesses, especially with regard to the types of tissue that appear visible in the images, e.g., CT is an X-ray based system and therefore is especially useful for revealing bone whereas MRI performs much better in differentiating soft tissues. Modern, multiscanner CT systems are very fast whereas MRI is generally slower, a concern of special impact for imaging the heart because it moves and motion artifacts can blur or distort the images and the resulting geometric model. CT, however, presents potential risk to subjects because of its use of ionizing radiation whereas MR imaging has no known risks to subjects–unless they have implanted metal devices, in which case the large magnetic fields of MR devices make this form of imaging impossible. Ultrasound is a widely used modality for medical imaging, especially in cardiac evaluations and presents no known risks to any patients; however, it is a challenging modality for geometric modeling; that quality of individual images is very poor compared with CT or MR, and perhaps more daunting, ultrasound images normally have no fixed reference frame. Instead, the region of view in ultrasound is a wedge-shaped, two-dimensional slice whose orientation depends completely on the location and orientation of a handheld probe. Intracardiac echocardiography (ICE) is a modern version of cardiac ultrasound that addresses both these limitations and has proved suitable for geometric model construction of the ventricular chamber of the heart [207, 208]. Fluoroscopy from a limited set of orientation presents a similar challenge but is constrained enough to be the source of several approaches to creating geometric models of the heart and thorax [209].

Another challenge of using imaging data for geometric models is the sheer volume of data. Image resolution is glowing rapidly so that data sets with 512^3, or over 130 million voxels, are not unusual. Even more modest data sets of $256 \times 256 \times 100$ still represent over 6 million data values to store and manipulate. A further challenge to using imaging data for quantitative geometric models lies in the distortions and errors that are inevitable in three-dimensional modalities. Such distortions are not so relevant in the clinical use of images, much of which is based on qualitative evaluation or uses quantitative measurements only in rather small regions of the field of view, where distortions are limited. Geometric models are based on quantitative information from throughout the field of view so that corrective measures are often required. In MR imaging, for example, variations in the magnetic field strength that are present (and different) in every device require correction before they are suitable to providing accurate geometric information [210–212].

Digitizing devices that provide another source of geometric information for models have certain advantages and disadvantages compared with imaging data. A digitizing device, either as a free standing device or as part of a catheter based mapping system, can allow a great deal of user control of the location and density of sample points. When carefully controlled, direct digitization can generate directly the set of points that are used in the polygonal model, thus omitting the segmentation step already described for image data. At a minimum, some form of resampling of points can replace segmentation at considerable savings in time and technical complexity. Of course, with high levels of user control comes a high cost in user time so that acquiring the digitized points typically takes considerably longer than an imaging scan. As we describe in ❥ Sect. 8.6.6, there are also few standard software tools for acquiring and especially manipulating digitized point sets, compared with software for at least some parts of the image acquisition and processing phase of creating geometric models. However, the single largest disadvantage of acquired geometry by means of a digitizing device is the lack of access to necessary regions of the problem domain. Digitizers can only reach surfaces adjacent to some form of air or liquid spaces as these spaces provide the physical means of access, e.g., the body surface or the inner walls of the heart chambers. Of most relevance to the electrocardiographic forward problem is the lack of access to the epicardial surface of the heart, which is crucial for many forms of the forward problem.

In cases of life-threatening arrhythmias that justify the invasive nature of the measurement, there are now methods of inserting catheters through the thoracic wall and the pericardium to reach the epicardium [213–215] so that this information is at least potentially available.

Not surprisingly, combining image and digitizer systems for generating raw model data has many advantages. One may, for example, take a CT or MR scan from a patient and then augment this with digitized locations of electrodes or sites of functional or clinical interest such as pacing, ablation, or coronary artery lesions. Because such mixed data sets come from separate scans based on their own, local, coordinate systems, it is necessary to carry out alignment or registration in order to merge them. Such registration, in turn, requires that the same points be in some form visible in all data sets. With such common points measured in each coordinate systems, it is possible to apply robust fitting methods to align these systems [216, 217] and thus create a complete data set.

2. **Segmentation**

Segmentation is a process by which, through either manual or automatic means, one extracts from image data the boundaries between regions of interest. In the context of the electrocardiographic forward problem, this step in geometric modeling typically includes identification of body and heart surfaces along with any regions of inhomogeneous electrical conductivity that should be explicitly incorporated into the model. The topic of segmentation is huge and has a substantial place within the field of computer science. Fortunately, in recent years some of the research in biomedical segmentation has resulted in software (see ❯ Sect. 8.6.6) that is useful for electrocardiographic geometry modeling; previously, many geometric models were the product of largely manual tracing of boundaries from individual images [39, 218–220]. While hardly trivial and still not completely automatic, modern segmentation algorithms are capable of identifying most of the bounding surface from which to create geometric models [117, 221–224].

3. **Surface descriptions**

From either a segmented volume or a set of digitized points, it is necessary to next identify a new set of points and polygons linking them that efficiently define the surfaces of the geometric model. The need for identifying a (possible new) set of points may not be altogether clear, especially for the case in which a set of digitized points already exists, but the quality of the resulting model depends on certain features of this point set that are rarely achieved through manual digitization. First, the distance between adjacent points will ultimately determine the size of the surface polygons that one must construct from them. The characteristic size metric for the mesh is a parameter one often wishes to adjust or control at the time of surface model generation and for numerical reasons, this parameter may even vary over the problem domain. Moreover, the selection of high quality point locations and spacing is a function of the underlying surface shape. For example, regions of sharp edges or rapid changes in surface orientation are often captured better when there are points that lie along the edges or at least with relatively higher density than over regions of relatively flat or smooth surface shape.

One common approach to defining surface boundary points is to create from each image (or in each plane in which digitized points lie) parametric descriptions of contours, e.g., B-splines or Bezier curves [225, 226]. To such contours one can then apply variable degrees of smoothing and then compute a new set of points to represent the curves with whatever density is desired. To create surfaces from the contours, one can employ a fairly simple algorithm that will "lace" adjacent sets of nodes into triangular surface elements [227–229]. ❯ Figure 8.15 shows schematically the basic configuration (Panel A) and two conditions that may confound algorithms that do not anticipate and recognize such situations (Panels B and C). The goal of the algorithm is to link points from the upper and lower layers of a pair of contours in a way that minimizes the length of the diagonal connection between opposite nodes in each quadrilateral (Segment 2–11 vs. Segment 1–12 in Panel A).

For a segmented volume data set, the need to create a smoothed boundary surface between regions is more obvious because of the tessellation that is inherent in any set of regularly spaced points. One elegant solution to this problem is the "scanline surfacing" algorithm from Weinstein et al., which even deals with abutting and interpenetrating surfaces and has found application in a variety of biomedical geometric modeling applications [230]. This approach identifies the voxels at boundaries between regions of different extracts and then smoothes not the contours, but entire surfaces. This treatment of the problem in its full three-dimensional extent allows more sophisticated recognition of surfaces and reduces the incidence of many problems (like those in Panels B and C of ❯ Figs. 8.15) that arise in contour-based methods.

Another class of approaches to the problem of creating surfaces from point sets is to fit them to piecewise analytical functions. Such fitting is part of the scanline surface algorithm [230] and others have used, for example, surface

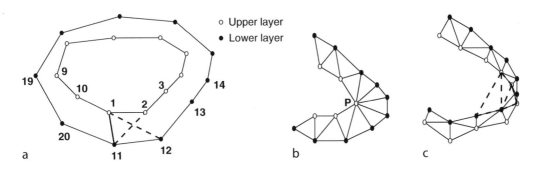

Fig. 8.15

Lacing algorithm to create surfaces from surface contours. (a) shows the basic algorithm for linking nodes in surface contours from adjacent layers of a geometric model derived from segmented image data. (b and c) show two different potentially troublesome conditions that arise in such applications and for which the algorithm has to have robust solutions

harmonics [197, 231] and Hermite polynomials [192, 232] to describe body and or heart surface geometry. Van Oosterom was one of the first to apply such an approach by using Fourier transform to represent the surface shape and then create triangulated surface meshes that are not only smooth but also optimally adjusted to aspects of the boundary element (BEM) solution he then applied to the forward problem [202]. Another approach by Gumhold et al. was to identify local surface features from an existing set of points and then refine the point locations to better represent those features without adding more points (and complexity) to the description [233]. The main advantages of any such representations is the ability from them to create models that have better characteristics in terms of, for example, smoothness, conformity to the original surfaces, and spatial resolution.

4. **Volume mesh generation**

The final step in geometric model construction, required specifically for numerical techniques like the finite difference (FDM) and finite element (FEM) methods already described. This step is known as "mesh generation" in the technical literature and usually starts with a surface representation based on triangles or quadrilaterals and produces a mesh based on tetrahedra and hexahedra respectively [234]. The main challenge of generating such a volume mesh is to introduce additional points within the volume that preserve the quality of the individual mesh elements and also respect the internal boundaries that separate regions of differing characteristics (e.g., electric conductivity). The first, and still challenging, step is to define a metric of quality that an algorithm can apply to evaluate candidate point locations. The most common choice for such a metric is the "Delaunay" criterion, which seeks to maximize the smallest internal angle of a tetrahedron and has led to many useful algorithms [234–239]. Unfortunately, a completely flat tetrahedron can meet Delaunay criteria and yet still be highly unsuitable for numerical calculations so that modifications or additions to the Delaunay criterion are necessary, a recent example of which is from Alliez et al. [240].

In many cases, the mesh that comes from a single application of any set of criteria is not optimal when it forms the basis for a computation of a particular forward problem or when exposed to different boundary conditions. In this case, some sort of adaptive approaches are necessary or at least useful. Adaptive methods seek either to increase the local resolution of a mesh or to otherwise alter it slightly in order to achieve some improvement in simulation efficiency or accuracy. For example, it is easy to imagine that in regions of high amplitude or spatial gradient of the quantity of interest, a higher resolution of the mesh could improve the simulation results. Similarly, in regions of low amplitude or low spatial gradients, it is intuitively apparent that one requires fewer points and larger elements to maintain the same levels of accuracy with reduced numbers of degrees of freedom and hence computational cost. Because full forward problems that go from cells or tissues to the body surface are always computationally daunting, any approaches that reduces degrees of freedom without meaningful loss in accuracy are of interest.

The challenges of all adaptive approaches include defining a good metric by which to determine if adaptation is actually useful and then creating robust and efficient schemes for making appropriate changes to the mesh.

This is an area of research in electrocardiographic problems and there is as yet no single approach that is effective in all cases [196, 237, 238, 241–244].

8.6.6 Software for Electrocardiographic Forward Problems

From a practical perspective, mathematical, and numerical modeling and simulation approaches are only as good as the software that implements them and that is available for scientists to apply to their own problems. As in almost all research environments, most software created in the laboratories of even the most sophisticated and experienced electrocardiographic researchers is used exclusively in those laboratories and is rarely available for other researchers to use or evaluate. Fortunately, in the area of forward simulations, this situation is better than in many other areas, perhaps a reflection of the relative maturity of at least some segments of this research domain.

Software for Cellular Simulations

Software for the simulation of membrane kinetics using the Hodgkin–Huxley formalism described in ❷ Sect. 8.3.1 is relatively widely available, although not always in the flexible, efficient, and simple-to-use form that most serious researchers seek. The simulation approach that is most widely used for cardiac myocytes is probably one of the models from Luo and Rudy [74, 75] and the authors provide a version of the software written in C/C++ at their web site (http://www.case.edu/med/CBRTC/LRdOnline/content.htm). The following is a partial list of software available for download that includes support for cardiac myocyte models.

1. *Cell electrophysiology simulation environment (CESE)*: One of the most flexible, portable, and powerful software systems for membrane modeling is a recent projects of Sergey Missan at Dalhousie University, who has created a comprehensive framework that includes implementations for all the leading forms of membrane model [245]. The software is open source and freely available at http://sourceforge.net/projects/cese/.
2. *E-Cell Project*: is an international, multicenter research project aiming at developing necessary theoretical supports, technologies, and software platforms to allow precise whole cell simulation that has recently added support for the Luo–Rudy model [246].
3. *iCell*: is a web-based program from Semahat Demir et al. at the University of Memphis for carrying out simple simulations of nerve or heart cells. It is very simple to use but there is no access to the source code nor can the application become part of another system, thus it is not useful for research (http://ssd1.bme.memphis.edu/icell/).
4. *LabHEART*: is a model of the myocyte developed by Don Bers and investigators at the Loyola University Physiology Department that includes standard electrophysiological parameters as well as a simulation of calcium concentration in the cell. The application is originally written in LabView but the authors have recently created a new version in MATLAB (http://www.luhs.org/depts/physio/personal_pages/bers_d/index.html).

Software for Tissue Simulations

The availability of software for simulation of cardiac tissue is much more limited than for cardiac myocytes, a reflection of the research state of the field and the technical complexity of especially the bidomain forms of simulation. Perhaps the only generally available software for simulation of propagation in cardiac tissue using the bidomain is Cardiowave from Henriquez et al. at Duke University. Cardiowave is capable of creating high-performance simulation programs for a range of platforms, even some that make use of vectorized and parallel computing (http://cardiowave.duke.edu/pmwiki.php). Programming cellular automata is relatively straightforward so that most researchers have developed their own code. There are numerous sources of general purpose cellular automata software, although most of these feature the Game of Life as the driving application (http://cafaq.com/other_software/index.php).

Software for Volume Conductor Problems

There are many public domain and commercial software packages for the solution of BEM, FEM, and FDM problems but only a small number of dedicated systems have been developed for use in electrocardiographic forward problems. Fortunately, these are some of the best developed and well-supported programs in this application area, providing useful entry points for a range of different types of users.

1. *CMISS*: CMISS stands for *C*ontinuum *M*echanics, *I*mage analysis, *S*ignal processing and *S*ystem Identification and is a massive software system developed by investigators at Auckland University for a broad range of problems, including the electrocardiographic forward problem. The system supports membrane models using the *XML* markup language known as *CellML*, bidomain simulations, and volume conductor simulations using both BEM and FEM techniques. (http://www.cmiss.org)

2. *ECGSIM*: ECGSIM is an interactive program that is very specifically directed at the electrocardiographic forward problem based on the uniform double layer formulation described in ❷ Sect. 8.5.5 and ❷ Chaps. 6 and ❷ 7 of this volume [247]. The user can adjust many parameters of the action potentials and immediately see the resulting changes in all relevant whole heart and body surface parameters (depolarization times, repolarization times, action potential durations and amplitudes, transmembrane potentials, and surface potentials). ❷ Figure 8.16 shows an example of creating a simulation with ECGSIM.

3. *SCIRun/BioPSE*: SCIRun is a large-scale interactive problem-solving environment developed at the University of Utah, Scientific Computing and Imaging (SCI) Institute [248, 249]. Similar to CMISS, the application domain of SCIRun is very broad, although there has always been a special emphasis on bioelectric field problems of the brain and heart [230, 250–252]. SCIRun software has several different forms of user interface including an interactive network editor for data-flow visual programming (as shown in ❷ Fig. 8.17) that allows users to create and modify networks

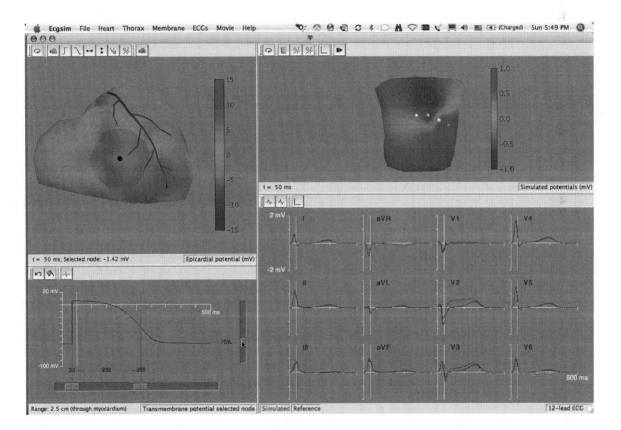

□ Fig. 8.16

User screen for ECGSIM. The user can interact with all panels of the screen to adjust display features, select specific time instants, and adjust action potential parameters. The specific example here shows the effect of elevating the resting potential of action potentials in the anterior right ventricle similar to a local transmural ischemic region. Standard ECG signals show the standard shape (*in blue*) and simulated for this intervention (*in red*). *Yellow vertical lines* in the time signals show the time instant displayed in the spatial distributions of potential on epicardium and body surface

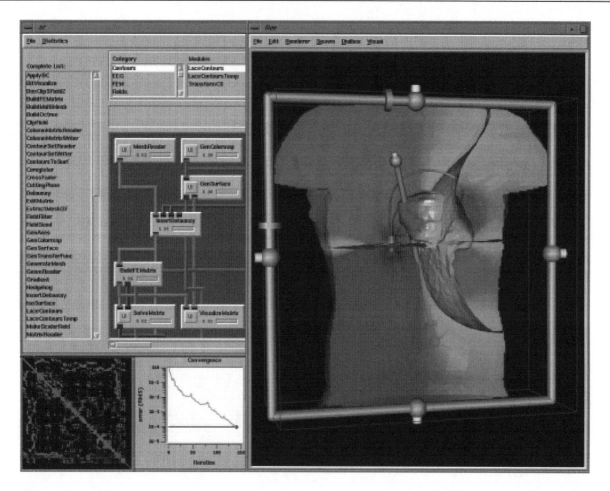

☐ Fig. 8.17

SCIRun problem-solving environment for a cardiac defibrillation forward problem. The *middle pane shows* the network diagram that illustrates the visual programming interface for the program while the *right hand panel* shows the results of a simulation of internal cardiac defibrillation. The *small panels in the lower, left-hand corner* show the structure of the resulting solution matrix along with a graph showing the convergence of the linear system solver over time. The user can interact with the visualization of the results and each of the blocks in the network diagram has its own user interface for control of the simulation. Moreover, the user can interactively add new blocks to the network and thus tailor the simulation to specific needs of the application

from functional modules connected with data pipes. Less flexible but simpler for the user to learn are various forms of "PowerApps," which appear to the user as dedicated applications with a focused set of options and functionality but are actually built on underlying self-modifying networks. The SCIRun/BioPSE suite also includes a dedicated application for segmentation of volume data called Seg3D, which uses core functionality from SCIRun libraries but does not have the data-flow structure of other previous SCIRun software. Finally, the SCI Institute also supports a program called *map3d*, which provides visualization capabilities for the type of surface-based mapping data that is common to many applications of the forward problem and the experimental techniques described in ❯ Sect. 8.2 [253]. All these applications are well documented, under constant development, and freely available for download in open-source form (http://software.sci.utah.edu/scirun.html).

8.7 Outstanding Challenges of the Forward Problem

8.7.1 The Multiscale Challenge

Evidence is emerging that one day forward modeling will begin at the subcellular level and extend to predicting the clinical ECG. Such simulations are already being performed at the single and multiple cell levels, and it seems a natural progression to migrate this further up the size continuum. For example, Clancy et al. placed a Markovian model of the cardiac sodium channel within a cardiac cellular model to predict the mechanisms of early depolarization and the effects of mutations in this channel on action potential behavior [254]. The particular behavior under examination was the inactivation and subsequent reactivation of the L-type calcium channel. The same paper reported findings using a larger spatial scale in which slow conduction in a string of cardiac cells was examined. Here the conduction was slowed by reducing the conductivity of the gap junctions between the cells and not through a loss of cellular excitability. This model provided a quantitative measure of the stability of propagation and produced insights into the mechanisms behind very slow conduction that can be observed under certain conditions experimentally. For example, because of the long time taken before a neighboring cell depolarizes, Clancy et al. showed that it was actually the L-type calcium channel that provided the charge gradient for propagation to continue long after the inward sodium current has ceased. It seems a natural path for these types of simulations to consider increasingly larger tissue blocks, leading ultimately to simulations involving the whole heart and torso. Thus, a gene defect may result in a malfunctioning channel, and then, through the forward modeling, gives rise to macroscopic phenomena such as long QT syndrome.

Forward simulation of cardiac electrophysiology may be poised for a revolution driven by rapid developments in biomedicine, imaging, and computing. The completion of the first draft of the human genome sequence [255] provides fundamental information on the structure of the proteins that determine ion-channel function and transmembrane currents. This landmark event signifies the beginning of comprehensive studies of the relationship between genetic code and channel, cell, tissue, and whole-heart function, developments suggested by the authors of the genome project when they stated "In principle, the string of genetic bits holds long-sought secrets of human development, physiology, and medicine. In practice, our ability to transform such information into understanding remains woefully inadequate." Only through sophisticated use of imaging, modeling, and simulations strategies, based on enhanced computational capabilities, will it be possible to overcome these inadequacies.

The challenge therefore is clear – to integrate this incredible wealth of information to allow the determination of structure and function at all levels of biological organization. One has very little choice but to use computation simulation to help to cope with this explosion in complexity: a fact which has led to the development of the Physiome project (see http://www.physiome.org.nz/, [2, 256, 257]). The International Union of Physiological Sciences has adopted the Physiome as a major focus, with the aim of developing mathematical and computer models to integrate the observations from many laboratories into quantitative, self-consistent, and comprehensive descriptions. The models not only will provide new insights into basic science and biological mechanisms but will also fuel breakthroughs in human health. The forward problem in electrocardiography will feed into and benefit from these developments and the relatively mature simulation approaches that exist for this problem make it a natural candidate for further advances based on novel information and computational capabilities.

8.7.2 Computability

One implicit aspect of the challenge of computing the forward problem over multiple scales is the computational burden of such complexity. Computers – and the software that controls them – have always placed limits on the level of detail that a numerical simulation could feasibly incorporate so that simplification has always been required. In fact, the art of numerical simulation lies mainly in selecting the appropriate simplifications and implementing the essential components in the most efficient way possible. Similarly, computer simulations tend to require more or less fixed amounts of time; when the computers become faster or the numerical methods more efficient, the model simply becomes more detailed or enlarged in scope to incorporate more realism so that the time required is once again set at whatever a researcher considers acceptable.

The electrocardiographic forward problem has just under a century of history [6] and thus has seen many changes in the nature and form of simulations. The first simulations were based on single dipoles and required the solution to simple systems of linear equations expressed in terms of measured body-surface potentials and dipole location and/or strength [27, 161, 258]. As computers became first available to scientists and then ever more powerful, so too did the source models, to the point where we are now able to carry out simulations of both small animal [149, 150] and human ECGs [247]. Some groups have even begun to compute some form of the full forward problem, i.e., from cellular to body-surface ECG [244, 259]. However, it is not currently possible to apply the same level of spatial or temporal detail or level of representation in all these simulations. For example to apply the bidomain equations with a biophysically realistic membrane model, which many consider the minimal acceptable approach for addressing relevant questions in electrophysiology, to a human heart model embedded within a torso model is at or beyond the limit of current computational resources [260]. As a result of this perpetual need for increased complexity, some investigators of the forward model spend significant effort focusing on techniques to improve the efficiency of the calculations [261–263]. Even with such tools, it is necessary to address many of the questions that arise in the electrocardiographic forward problem using lower resolution (and potentially incomplete) models.

8.7.3   Selection of Models/Parameters

There are many sources of variability in the solution methods and parameters for the forward problem, and selecting those most appropriate for a given set of research or clinical goals remains an open challenge. There is a wide range of cell models available for use in the bidomain equations (see, for example, www.cellml.org or ssd1.bme.memphis.edu/icell), all of which give rise to slightly different action potentials. Simulated EG's or ECG's computed using these different cell models generate quantitatively (and possibly qualitatively) different results. Similarly, as described in ❷ Sect. 8.5, there are different numerical approaches to solving the volume conductor equations that relate cardiac sources to body-surface potentials, each of which will give different results.

Even after the choice of numerical method and simulation software, however, there are many decisions related to the parameters settings required to make a working simulation. At the membrane/cellular level, one must first determine the appropriate, species-specific parameters that control the dynamics of the ion channels. To further complicate matters, there are a variety of different cell types within any heart, each of which reflects a different balance of ion-channel densities and thus has different action potential features. It is well known that there is a transition of cellular properties from the ventricular endocardium to the mid-myocardial M-cells and then to the epicardium. The affects of these variations in cell characteristics on the ECG are still under debate but may have potentially profound affects on arrhythmia generation and maintenance. The torso also consists of many tissue types, each of which could play a role in shaping the electric current in the thorax and thus the body-surface potentials. It is not yet clear what level of accuracy or fidelity in the electrical conductivity parameters is required to carry out useful forward simulations – the answer will surely depend on the particular goals of the simulation. And across all scales there are variability and uncertainty in the geometry of the problem that can have consequences on solution accuracy. Although the effects of each of these sources of variability are largely unknown as this point, the efficacy of using detailed forward simulation in the clinical arena over the longer term may depend on our ability to include these small-scale features and to understand the multiple interactions among these parameters that are associated with specific pathologies.

8.7.4   Mechanical and Chemical Interactions

The electrical activity of the heart does not occur in isolation. Many factors can significantly influence cardiac electrical activity, including cardiac mechanics, coronary blood flow, cellular metabolism, and the autonomic nervous system. Mathematical models of many of these factors are being developed, but integrating these within a forward modeling framework is extremely challenging. Such combinations will ultimately help to provide the foundations for models that link cardiac excitation to myocardial mechanics, perfusion, and regulation. This form of comprehensive simulation will ultimately be necessary for in silico study of pathologies such as myocardial ischemia, in which reduced coronary blood flow adversely affects cell and heart function, or heart failure, in which reduced mechanical performance leads to electrical instability.

8.8   Summary

The forward problem in electrocardiography has become very broad and deep in scope in the last decades as mathematical and computational capabilities allow an unparalleled integration of behaviors in the form of simulations. Progress continues at all levels of the problem as researchers uncover the relationships between the genetic code and ion channel structure and function, examine in more and more detail the linking of cells into myocardium, and use advanced imaging and signal acquisition and processing approaches to capture the shape, structure, and bioelectric (and biomagnetic) fields from the body. At every level of this problem, computational and simulation techniques are essential, not just to gather, analyze, and visualize the experimental data but also to begin to test hypotheses about the roles and interactions of all the elements of this problem. Computers are essential to describe and evaluate possible protein structures and to predict the impact of subtle local changes in action potential shape and duration on the resulting body surface ECGs.

The role of the forward problem in cardiac electrocardiography is thus very secure and will provide an intellectual playground for basic questions at all levels of electrophysiology as well as the essential starting point for the inverse problems that we describe in the following chapter.

Acknowledgements

The authors thank their colleagues Drs. Dana Brooks and Andrew Pullan for valuable comments and suggestions for this chapter. We also gratefully acknowledge the support of the Nora Eccles Treadwell Foundation and the National Center for Research Resources (NCRR) at the NIH.

References

1. Gulrajani R.M., Models of the electrical activity of the heart and the computer simulation of the electrocardiogram. *Crit. Rev. Biomed. Eng.*, 1988;**16**: 1–66.

2. Hunter P., P. Robbins, and D. Noble, The iups human physiome project. *Pflugers Arch.*, 2002;**445**(1): 1–9.

3. Beatty G.E., S.C. Remole, M.K. Johnston, J.E. Holte, and D.G. Benditt, Non-contact electrical extrapolation technique to reconstruct endocardial potentials. *PACE*, 1994;**17**(4): 765.

4. Gulrajani R.M., F.A. Roberge, and G.E. Mailloux, The forward problem of electrocardiography, in *Comprehensive Electrocardiology*, P.W. Macfarlane and T.D. Veitch Lawrie, Editors. Pergamon Press, Oxford, England, 1989, pp. 197–236.

5. Waller A.D., A demonstration on man of electromotive changes accompanying the heart's beat. *J. Physiol.*, 1887;**8**: 229–234.

6. Einthoven W., G. Fahr, and A. de Waart, Über die Richting und manifest Grösse der Potentialschwankungen im menschlichen Herzen und über den Einfluss der Herzlage auf die Form des Elektrokardiograms. *Pflügers Arch. ges. Physiol.*, 1913;**150**:275–315.

7. Hodgkin A.L. and A.F. Huxley, Resting and action potentials in single nerve fibres. *J. Physiol.*, 1945;**10**: 176–195.

8. Neher E., B. Sakmann, and J.H. Steinbach, The extracellular patch clamp: A method for resolving currents through individual open channels in biological membranes. *Pflügers Arch. ges. Physiol.*, 1978;**37**: 219–228.

9. Ling G. and R.W. Gerard, The normal membrane potential of frog sartorius fibers. *J. Cell Physiol.*, 1949;**34**: 383–396.

10. Smith T.G., J.L. Barker, B.M. Smith, and T.R. Colburn, Voltage clamping with microelectrodes. *J. Neurosci. Methods*, 1980;**3**: 105–128.

11. Hodgkin A.L. and A.F. Huxley, A quantitative description of membrane current and its application to conduction and excitation in nerve. *J. Physiol.*, 1952;**11**: 500–544.

12. Hodgkin A.L. and A.F. Huxley, The components of membrane conductance in the giant axon of loligo. *J. Physiol.*, 1952;**11**: 473–496.

13. Li R.A., M. Leppo, T. Miki, S. Seino, and E. Marban, Molecular basis of electrocardiographic ST-segment elevation. *Circ. Res.*, 2000;**87**(10): 837–909.

14. Lux R.L., M. Akhtar, and R.S. MacLeod, Mapping and invasive analysis, in *Foundations of Cardiac Arrhythmias: Basic Concepts and Clinical Approaches*, chapter 15, P.M. Spooner and M.R. Rosen, Editors. Marcel Dekker, New York, 2001, pp. 393–424.

15. Lux P.R. and P.R. Ershler, Reducing uncertainty in the measures of cardiac activation and recovery. in *Proceedings of the IEEE Engineering in Medicine and Biology Society 9th Annual International Conference*. IEEE Press, New York, 1987, pp. 1871–1872.

16. Ndrepepa G., E.B. Caref, H Yin, N. El-Sherif, and M. Restivo, Activation time determination by high-resolution unipolar and bipolar extracellulcar electrograms. *J. Cardiovasc. Electrophysiol.*, 1995;**6**(3): 174–188.

17. Macleod R.S., R.O. Kuenzler, B. Taccardi, and R.L. Lux, Estimation of epicardial activation maps from multielectrode venous catheter measurements. *PACE*, 1998;**21**(4): 595.

18. Ni Q., R.S. MacLeod, and R.L. Lux, Three-dimensional activation mapping in canine ventricles: Interpolation and approximation of activation times. *Ann. Biomed. Eng.*, 1999;**27**(5): 617–626.

19. Punske B.P., Q. Ni, R.L. Lux, R.S. MacLeod, P.R. Ershler, T.J. Dustman, Y. Vyhmeister, and B. Taccardi, Alternative methods of excitation time determination on the epicardial surface. In *Proceedings of the IEEE Engineering in Medicine and Biology Society 22nd Annual International Conference*, 2000.

20. Pieper C.F. and A. Pacifico, The epicardial field potential in dog: Implications for recording site density during epicardial mapping. *PACE*, 1993;**16**: 1263–1274.

21. Ni Q., R.S. MacLeod, R.L. Lux, and B. Taccardi, Interpolation of cardiac electric potentials. *Ann. Biomed. Eng.*, **1997**, 25(Suppl): 61. Biomed. Eng. Soc. Annual Fall Meeting.

22. Ni Q., R.S. MacLeod, R.L. Lux, and B. Taccardi, A novel interpolation method for electric potential fields in the heart during excitation. *Ann. Biomed. Eng.*, 1998;**26**(4): 597–607.

23. Yılmaz B., R.S. MacLeod, B.B. Punske, B. Taccardi, and D.H. Brooks, Training set selection for statistical estimation of epicardial activation mapping from intravenous multielectrode catheters. *IEEE Trans. Biomed. Eng.*, 2005;**52**(11): 1823–1831.

24. Yılmaz B., R.S. MacLeod, B.B. Punske, B. Taccardi, and D.H. Brooks, Venous catheter mapping of epicardial ectopic activation: Leadset analysis for statistical estimation. *Comp. in Biol. & Med.*, (in press), 2006.

25. Pullan A.J. and M.P. Nash, Challenges facing validation of noninvasive electrical imaging of the heart. *Ann. Noninvasive Electrocardiol.*, 2005;**10**(1): 73–82.

26. MacLeod R.S. and D.H. Brooks, Validation approaches for electrocardiographic inverse problems, in *Computational Inverse Problems in Electrocardiography* Peter Johnston, Editor. WIT Press, Ashurst, UK, 2001, pp. 229–268.

27. Burger H.C. and J.B. van Milaan, Heart-vector and leads. Part II. *Br. Heart J.*, 1947;**9**: 154–160.

28. Burger H.C. and J.B. van Milaan, Heart-vector and leads. Part III: Geometrical representation. *Br. Heart J.*, 1948;**10**: 229–333.

29. Grayzel J. and F. Lizzi, The combined influence of inhomogeneities and dipole location. *Am. Heart J.*, 1967;**74**: 503–512.

30. Grayzel J. and F. Lizzi, The performance of VCG leads in homogenous and heterogenous torsos. *J. Electrocardiol.*, 1969;**2**(1): 17–26.

31. Nagata Y., The electrocardiographic leads for telemetering as evaluated from the view point of the transfer impedance vector. *Jap. Heart J.*, 1970;**11**(2): 183–194.

32. Nagata Y., The influence of the inhomogeneities of electrical conductance within the torso on the electrocardiogram as evaluated from the view point of the transfer impedance vector. *Jap. Heart J.*, 1970;**11**(5): 489–505.

33. De Ambroggi L. and B. Taccardi, Current and potential fields generated by two dipoles. *Circ. Res.*, 1970;**27**: 910–911.

34. Mirvis D.M., F.W. Keller, R.E. Ideker, J.W. Cox, R.F. Dowdie, and D.G. Zettergren, Detection and localization of a multiple epicardial electrical generator by a two dipole ranging technique. *Circ. Res.*, 1977;**41**: 551.

35. Mirvis D.M., F.W. Keller, R.E. Ideker, D.G. Zettergren, and R.F. Dowdie, Equivalent generator properties of acute ischemic lesions in the isolated rabbit heart. *Circ. Res.*, 1978;**42**: 676–685.

36. Mirvis D.M., Electrocardiographic QRS changes induced by acute coronary ligation in the isolated rabbit heart. *J. Electrocardiol.*, 1979;**12**: 141–150.

37. Barr R.C. and M.S. Spach, Inverse solutions directly in terms of potentials, in *The Theoretical Basis of Electrocardiography*, C.V. Nelson and D.B. Geselowitz, Editors.. Clarendon Press, Oxford, 1976, pp. 294–304.

38. Barr R.C., M. Ramsey, and M.S. Spach, Relating epicardial to body surface potential distributions by means of transfer coefficients based on geometry measurements. *IEEE Trans. Biomed. Eng.*, 1977;**24**: 1–11.

39. Barr R.C. and M.S. Spach, A comparison of measured epicardial potentials with epicardial potentials computed from body surface measurements in the intact dog. *Adv. Cardiol.*, 1978;**21**: 19–22.

40. Pilkington T.C., M.N. Morrow, and P.C. Stanley, A comparison of finite element and integral equation formulations for the calculation of electrocardiographic potentials. *IEEE Trans. Biomed. Eng.*, 1985;**32**: 166–173.

41. Pilkington T.C., M.N. Morrow, and P.C. Stanley, A comparison of finite element and integral equation formulations for the calculation of electrocardiographic potentials – II. *IEEE Trans. Biomed. Eng.*, 1987;**34**: 258–260.

42. Bradley C.P., M.P. Nash and D.J. Paterson, Imaging electrocardiographic dispersion of depolarization and repolarization during ischemia: simultaneous body surface and epicardial mapping. *Circ.*, 2003.

43. Oster H.S., B. Taccardi, R.L. Lux, P.R. Ershler, and Y. Rudy, Noninvasive electrocardiographic imaging: Reconstruction of epicardial potentials, electrograms, and isochrones and localization of single and multiple electrocardiac events. *Circ.*, 1997;**96**(3): 1012–1024.

44. Messinger-Rapport B.J. and Y. Rudy, Noninvasive recovery of epicardial potentials in a realistic heart-torso geometry. *Circ. Res.*, 1990;**66**(4): 1023–1039.

45. Ahmad G.F., D. H Brooks, and R.S. MacLeod, An admissible solution approach to inverse electrocardiography. *Ann. Biomed. Eng.*, 1998;**26**: 278–292.

46. Brooks D.H., G.F. Ahmad, R.S. MacLeod, and G.M. Maratos,. Inverse electrocardiography by simultaneous imposition of multiple constraints. *IEEE Trans. Biomed. Eng.*, 1999;**46**(1):3–18.

47. Burns J.E., B. Taccardi, R.S. MacLeod, and Y. Rudy, Noninvasive electrocardiographic imaging of electrophysiologically abnormal substrates in infarcted hearts: A model study. *Circ.*, 2000;**101**: 533–540.

48. Colli Franzone P., L. Guerri, B. Taccardi, and C. Viganotti, The direct and inverse problems in electrocardiology. Numerical aspects of some regularization methods and applications to data collected in isolated dog heart experiments. *Lab. Anal. Numerica C.N.R.*, Pub. N:222, 1979.

49. Colli Franzone P., G. Gassaniga, L. Guerri, B. Taccardi, and C. Viganotti, Accuracy evaluation in direct and inverse electrocardiology, In *Progress in Electrocardiography*, P.W. Macfarlane, Editor. Pitman Medical, 1979, pp. 83–87.

50. Colli Franzone P., L. Guerri, B. Taccardi, and C. Viganotti, Finite element approximation of regularized solution of the inverse potential problem of electrocardiography and application to experimental data. *Calcolo*, 1985;**22**: 91.

51. Colli Franzone P., L. Guerri, S. Tentonia, C. Viganotti, S. Spaggiari, and B. Taccardi, A numerical procedure for solving the inverse problem of electrocardiography. Analysis of the

time-space accuracy from *in vitro* experimental data. *Math. Biosci.*, 1985;**77**: 353–396.

52. Soucy B., R.M. Gulrajani, and R. Cardinal, Inverse epicardial potential solutions with an isolated heart preparation, in *Proceedings of the IEEE Engineering in Medicine and Biology Society 11th Annual International Conference*. IEEE Press, New York, 1989, pp. 193–194.

53. Oster H. and Y. Rudy, The use of temporal information in the regularization of the inverse problem of electrocardiography, in *Proceedings of the IEEE Engineering in Medicine and Biology Society 12th Annual International Conference*. IEEE Press, New York, 1990, pp. 599–600.

54. Rudy Y. and Oster H. The electrocardiographic inverse problem. *Crit. Rev. Biomed. Eng.*, 1992;**20**: 22–45.

55. MacLeod R.S., B. Taccardi, and R.L. Lux, The influence of torso inhomogeneities on epicardial potentials, in *IEEE Comput. Cardiol.*. IEEE Computer Society, 1994, pp. 793–796.

56. Brooks D.H. and R.S. MacLeod, Imaging the electrical activity of the heart: Direct and inverse approaches, in *IEEE International Conference on Image Processing*. IEEE Computer Society, 1994, pp. 548–552.

57. Brooks D.H., H. On, and R.S. MacLeod, Multidimensional multiresolution analysis of array ECG signals during PTCA procedures, in *IEEE Symposium on Time-Frequency and Time-Scale*. IEEE Computer Society, 1994, pp. 552–555.

58. Brooks D.H., G. Ahmad, and R.S. MacLeod, Multiply constrained inverse electrocardiology: Combining temporal, multiple spatial, and iterative regularization, in *Proceedings of the IEEE Engineering in Medicine and Biology Society 16th Annual International Conference*. IEEE Computer Society, 1994, pp. 137–138.

59. MacLeod R.S., B. Taccardi, and R.L. Lux, Electrocardiographic mapping in a realistic torso tank preparation, in *Proceedings of the IEEE Engineering in Medicine and Biology Society 17th Annual International Conference*. IEEE Press, New York, 1995, pp. 245–246.

60. Oster H.S., B. Taccardi, R.L. Lux, P.R. Ershler, and Y. Rudy, Electrocardiographic imaging: Noninvasive characterization of intramural myocardial activation from inverse-reconstructed epicardial potentials and electrograms. *Circ.*, 1997;**96**:1496–1507.

61. MacLeod R.S., Q. Ni, B. Punske, P.R. Ershler, B. Yilmaz, and B. Taccardi, Effects of heart position on the body-surface ECG. *J. Electrocardiol.*, 2000, **33**(Suppl): 229–238.

62. MacLeod R.S., B. Punske, S. Shome, B. Yilmaz, and B. Taccardi, The role of heart rate and coronary flow during myocardial ischemia. *J. Electrocardiol.*, 2001: 43–51.

63. MacLeod R.S., S. Shome, J.G. Stinstra, B.B. Punske, and B. Hopenfeld, Mechanisms of ischemia-induced ST-segment changes. *J. Electrocardiol.*, 2005;**38**(Suppl): 8–13.

64. Khoury D.S. and Y. Rudy, A model study of volume conductor effects on endocardial and intracavitary potentials. *Circ. Res.*, 1992;**71**(3): 511–525.

65. Khoury D.S. and Y. Rudy, Reconstruction of endocardial potentials from intracavitary probe potentials: a model study. *IEEE Comput. Cardiol.*, 1992: 9–12.

66. Lui Z.W., P.R. Ershler, B. Taccardi, R.L. Lux, D.S. Khoury, and Y. Rudy, Noncontact endocardial mapping: Reconstruction of electrocardiograms and isochrones from intracavitary probe potentials. *J. Cardiovasc. Electrophysiol.*, 1997;**8**:415–431.

67. MacLeod R.S., B. Taccardi, and R.L. Lux, Mapping of cardiac ischemia in a realistic torso tank preparation. In *Building*

Bridges: International Congress on Electrocardiology International Meeting*, 1995, pp. 76–77.

68. MacLeod R.S., R.L. Lux, M.S. Fuller, and B. Taccardi, Evaluation of novel measurement methods for detecting heterogeneous repolarization. *J. Electrocardiol.*, 1996;**29**(Suppl): 145–153.

69. MacLeod R.S., R.L. Lux, and B. Taccardi, A possible mechanism for electrocardiographically silent changes in cardiac repolarization. *J. Electrocardiol.*, 1997;**30**(Suppl): 114–121.

70. Hodgkin A.L. and A.F. Huxley, The dual effect of membrane potential on sodium conductance in the giant axon of loligo. *J. Physiol.*, 1952;**11**: 497–506.

71. Plonsey R. and R.C. Barr, *Bioelectricity: A Quantitative Approach*. Plenum Publishing, New York, London, 1988.

72. Keener J. and J. Sneyd, *Mathematical Physiology*. Springer, Berlin, 1998.

73. Sachse F.B., *Computational Cardiology: Modeling of anatomy, electrophysiology, and mechanics*. Springer, Berlin, 2004.

74. Luo C.H. and Y. Rudy, A model of the ventricular cardiac action potential. *Circ. Res.*, 1991;**68**(6): 1501–1526.

75. Luo C.H. and Y. Rudy, A dynamic model of the cardiac ventricular action potential: I. Simulations of ionic currents and concentration changes. *Circ. Res.*, 1994;**74**(6): 1071–1096.

76. Einthoven W., Le telecardiogramme. *Arch. Int. de Physiol.*, 1906;**4**: 132–164.

77. Goldberger A.L. and E. Goldberger, *Clinical Electrocardiography*. C.V. Mosby, 1986.

78. Taccardi B., Distribution of heart potentials on the thoracic surface of normal human subjects. *Circ. Res.*, 1963;**1**: 341–351.

79. Macchi E., G. Arisi, and B. Taccardi, Identification of ectopic ventricular foci by means of intracavity potential mapping: A proposed method. *Acta Cardiol.*, 1992;**XLVII**(5): 421–433.

80. Cobb F.R., S.D. Blumenschein, and W.C. Sealy, Successful surgical interruption of the bundle of Kent in a patient with Wolff–Parkinson–White syndrome. *Circ.*, 1968;**38**: 1016.

81. De Ambroggi L., B. Taccardi, and E. Macchi, Body surface maps of heart potential: Tentative localization of preexcited area of forty-two Wolff–Parkinson–White patients. *Circ.*, 1976;**54**: 251.

82. Lux R.L., P.R. Ershler, K.P. Anderson, and J.W. Mason, Rapid localization of accessory pathways in WPW syndrome using unipolar potential mapping, in *Proceedings of the IEEE Engineering in Medicine and Biology Society 11th Annual International Conference*. IEEE Press, New York, 1989, pp. 195–196.

83. Shenasa M., R. Cardinal, P. Savard, M. Dubac, P. Page, and R. Nadeau, Cardiac mapping. part I: Wolff-Parkison-White syndrome. *PACE*, 1990;**13**: 223–230.

84. Shahidi A.V., P. Savard, and R. Nadeau, Forward and inverse problems of electrocardiography: Modeling and recovery of epicardial potentials in humans. *IEEE Trans. Biomed. Eng.*, 1994;**41**(3): 249–256.

85. Penney C.J., J.C. Clements, M.J. Gardner, L. Sterns, and B.M. Horáček, The inverse problem of electrocardiography: Application to localization of Wolff-Parkinson-White pre-excitation sites, in *Proceedings of the IEEE Engineering in Medicine and Biology Society 17th Annual International Conference*. IEEE Press, New York, 1995, pp. 215–216.

86. Yee R., G.J. Klein, and G.M. Guiraudon, The Wolff–Parkinson–White syndrome, in *Cardiac Electrophysiology, From Cell to Bedside*, D.P. Zipes and J. Jalife, Editors. W.B. Saunders Co., London, 1995, pp. 1199–1214.

87. Gallagher J.J., M. Gilbert, R.H. Svenson, W.C. Sealy, J. Kasell, and A.G. Wallace, Wolff–Parkinson–White syndrome: The problem, evaluation, and surgical correction. *Circ.*, 1975;**5**: 767–785.

88. Barr R.C. and T.C. Pilkington, Computing inverse solutions for an on-off heart model. *IEEE Trans. Biomed. Eng.*, 1969;**16**: 205–214.

89. Schmitt O.H., Biological information processing using the concept of interpenetrating domains, in *Information Processing in the Nervous System*, K.N. Leibovic, Editor. Springer, New York, 1969.

90. Miller W.T. and D.B. Geselowitz, Simulation studies of the electrocardiogram: I The normal heart and II Ischemia and infarction. *Circ. Res.*, 1978;**4**: 301–323.

91. Tung L., *A Bidomain Model for describing ischemic myocardial DC potentials*. PhD thesis, M.I.T., 1978.

92. Roth B.J. and J.P. Wikswo, A bidomain model for the extracellular potential and magnetic field of the cardiac tissue. *IEEE Trans. Biomed. Eng.*, 1986;**33**: 467–469.

93. Henriquez C.S. and R. Plonsey, Simulation of propagation along a cylindrical bundle of cardiac tissue–I: Mathematical formulation. *IEEE Trans. Biomed. Eng.*, 1990;**37**: 850–860.

94. Henriquez C.S. and R. Plonsey, Simulation of propagation along a cylindrical bundle of cardiac tissue–II: Results of simulation. *IEEE Trans. Biomed. Eng.*, 1990;**37**: 861–875.

95. Fischer G., B. Tilg, R. Moore, G.J.M. Huiskamp, J. Fetzer, W. Rucker, and P. Wach, A bidomain model based BEM-FEM coupling formulation for anisotropic cardiac tissue. *Ann. Biomed. Eng.*, 2000;**28**: 1228–1243.

96. Lines G., J. Sundnes, and A. Tveito, A domain embedding strategy for solving the bidomain equations on complicated geometries. *Int. J. Bioelectromagn.*, 2002;**4**(2): 53–54.

97. Hopenfeld B., Stinstra J.G., and MacLeod R.S., Mechanism for ST depression associated with contiguous subendocardial ischemia. *J. Cardiovasc. Electrophysiol.*, 2004;**15**(10):1200–1206.

98. Henriquez C.S., Simulating the electrical behavior of cardiac tissue using the bidomain model. *Crit. Rev. Biomed. Eng.*, 1993;**21**(1): 1–77.

99. Gardner M., Mathematical games. *Scient. Amer.*, October 1970: 120–123.

100. Moe G.K., W.C. Rheinboldt, and J.A. Abildskov, A computer model of fibrillation. *Am. Heart J.*, 1964;**67**: 200–220.

101. Abildskov J.A., Mechanism of the vulnerable period in a model of cardiac fibrillation. *J. Cardiovasc. Electrophysiol.*, 1990;**1**:303–308.

102. Restivo M., W. Craelius, W.B. Gough, and N. El-Sherif, A logical state model of reentrant ventricular activation. *IEEE Trans. Biomed. Eng.*, 1990;**37**: 344–353.

103. Leon L.J. and B.M. Horáček, Computer model of excitation and recovery in the anisotropic myocardium: I Rectangular and cubic arrays of excitable elements. *J. Electrocardiol.*, 1991;**24**: 1–15.

104. Grogin H.R., M.L. Stanley, S. Eisenberg, B.M. Horáček, and M.D. Lesh, Body surface mapping for localization of accessory pathways in WPW syndrome, in *IEEE Comput. Cardiol.*. IEEE Computer Society, 1992, p. 255.

105. Gharpure P.B. and C.R. Johnson, A 3-dimensional cellular automation model of the heart, in *Proceedings of the IEEE Engineering in Medicine and Biology Society 15th Annual International Conference*. IEEE Press, New York, 1993, pp. 752–753.

106. Hren R. and Punske B.B., A comparison of simulated QRS isointegral maps resulting from pacing at adjacent sites: Implications for the spatial resolution of pace mapping using body surface potentials. *J. Electrocardiol.*, 1998;**31**(Suppl): 135.

107. Hren R., J. Nenonen, and B.M. Horacek, Simulated epicardial potential maps during paced activation reflect myocardial fibrous structure. *Ann. Biomed. Eng.* 1998;**26**(6): 1022.

108. Bailie A.H., R.H. Mithchell, and J. McCanderson, A computer model of re-entry in cardiac tissue. *Comp. in Biol. & Med.* 1990, **20**: 47–54.

109. Saxberg B.E. and R.J. Cohen, Cellular automata models for reentrant arrhythmias. *J. Electrocardiol.*, 1990**23**(Suppl): 95.

110. Leon L.J. and Horáček B.M., Computer model of excitation and recovery in the anisotropic myocardium: II Excitation in the simplified left ventricle. *J. Electrocardiol.*, 1991;**24**: 17–31.

111. Leon L.J. and B.M. Horáček, Computer model of excitation and recovery in the anisotropic myocardium: III Arrhythmogenic conditions in the simplified left ventricle. *J. Electrocardiol.*, 1991;**24**: 33–41.

112. Wei D., O. Okazaki, K. Harumi, E. Harasawa, and H. Hosaka, Comparative simulation of excitation and body surface electrocardiogram with isotropic and anisotropic computer heart models. *IEEE Trans. Biomed. Eng.*, 1995;**42**(4): 343–357.

113. Weixue L. and X. Ling, Computer simulation of epicardial potentials using a heart-torso model with realistic geometry. *IEEE Trans. Biomed. Eng.*, 1996;**43**(2): 211–217.

114. Hren R., R.S. MacLeod, G. Stroink, and B.M. Horáček, Assessment of spatial resolution of body surface potentials maps in localizing ventricular tachycardia foci. *Biomed. Technik*, 1997;**42**(Suppl): 41–44.

115. Hren R. and B.M. Horacek, Value of simulated body surface potential maps as templates in localizing sites of ectopic activation for radiofrequency ablation. *Physiol. Measur.*, 1997;**18**(4): 373.

116. Spitzer V., M.J. Ackerman, A.L. Scherzinger, and D. Whitlock, The visible human male: a technical report. *J Am Med Inform Assoc*, 1996;**3**(2): 118–130.

117. Sachse F.B., C.D. Werner, K. Meyer-Waarden, and O. Dossel, Development of a human body model for numerical calculation of electrical fields. *Comput Med Imaging Graph*, 2000;**24**(3): 165–171.

118. Freudenberg J., T. Schiemann, U. Tiede, and K.H. Hohne, Simulation of cardiac excitation patterns in a three-dimensional anatomical heart atlas. *Comput Biol Med*, 2000;**30**(4): 191–205.

119. Okajima M., T. Fujino, T. Kobayashi, and K. Yamada, Computer simulation of the propagation process in excitation of the ventricles. *Circ. Res.*, 1968;**23**(2): 203–211.

120. Solomon J.C. and R.H. Selvester, Simulation of measured activation sequence in the human heart. *Am Heart J*, 1973;**85**(4): 518–524.

121. Lorange M. and Gulrajani R.M., Computer simulation of the Wolff–Parkinson–White preexcitation syndrome with a modified miller-geselowitz heart model. *IEEE Trans. Biomed. Eng.*, 1986;**33**: 862–873.

122. Saxberg B.E., M.P. Grumbach, and R.J. Cohen, A time dependent anatomically detailed model of cardiac conduction. *Comput Cardiol*, 1985;**12**: 401–404.

123. Plonsey R. and R.C. Barr, Mathematical modeling of electrical activity of the heart. *J. Electrocardiol.*, 1987;**20**: 219–226.

124. Keener J.P., An eikonal-curvature equation for action potential propagation in myocardium. *J Math Biol*, 1991;**29**(7): 629–651.

125. Hooks D.A., K.A. Tomlinson, S.G. Marsden, I.J. LeGrice, B.H. Smaill, A.J. Pullan, and P.J. Hunter, Cardiac microstructure: implications for electrical propagation and defibrillation in the heart. *Circ. Res.*, 2002;**91**(4): 331–338.

126. Colli Franzone P., L. Guerri, and B. Taccardi, Potential distributions generated by point stimulation in a myocardial volume: Simulation studies in a model of anisotropic ventricular muscle. *J. Cardiovasc. Electrophysiol.*, 1993;**4**: 438–458.

127. Colli Franzone P., L. Guerri, and B. Taccardi, Spread of excitation in a myocardial volume: Simulation studies in a model of anisotropic ventricular muscle activated by point stimulation. *J. Cardiovasc. Electrophysiol.*, 1993;**4**: 144–160.

128. Colli Franzone P., L. Guerri, M. Pennacchio, and B. Taccardi, Spread of excitation in 3-d models of the anisotropic cardiac tissue. iii. effects of ventricular geometry and fiber structure on the potential distribution. *Math Biosci*, 1998;**151**(1): 51–98.

129. Colli-Franzone P., L. Guerri, and B. Taccardi, Modeling ventricular excitation: axial and orthotropic anisotropy effects on wavefronts and potentials. *Math Biosci*, 2004;**188**: 191–205.

130. Colli Franzone P., L.F. Pavarino, and B. Taccardi, Simulating patterns of excitation, repolarization and action potential duration with cardiac bidomain and monodomain models. *Math Biosci*, 2005;**197**(1): 35–66.

131. Taccardi B., B.B. Punske, F. Sachse, X. Tricoche, P. Colli-Franzone, L.F. Pavarino, and C. Zabawa, Intramural activation and repolarization sequences in canine ventricles. experimental and simulation studies. *J. Electrocardiol.*, Oct 2005;**38**(4 Suppl): 131–137.

132. Pullan A., L. Cheng, R. Yassi, and M. Buist, Modelling gastrointestinal bioelectric activity. *Prog. Biophys. Mol. Biol.*, 2004;**85**(2–3): 523–550.

133. Fitzhugh R., Impulses and physiological states in theoretical models of nerve membranes. *Biophys. J.*, 1961;**1**: 445–466.

134. Nagumo J., S. Arimoto, and S. Yoshizawa, An active pulse transmission line simulating nerve axons. *Proc. IRL*, 1960;**50**: 2061–2070.

135. Rogers J.M. and A.D. McCulloch, A collocation–galerkin finite element model of cardiac action potential propagation. *IEEE Trans. Biomed. Eng.*, 1994;**41**(8): 743–757.

136. Pertsov A.M., J.M. Davidenko, R. Salomonsz, W.T. Baxter, and J. Jalife, Spiral waves of excitation underlie reentrant activity in isolated cardiac muscle. *Circ. Res.*, 1993;**72**(3): 631–650.

137. Starmer C.F., D.N. Romashko, R.S. Reddy, Y.I. Zilberter, J. Starobin, A.O. Grant, and V.I. Krinsky, Proarrhythmic response to potassium channel blockade. numerical studies of polymorphic tachyarrhythmias. *Circ.*, 1995;**92**(3): 595–605.

138. Karma A., Electrical alternans and spiral wave breakup in cardiac tissue. *CHAOS*, 1994;**4**(3): 461–472.

139. Aliev R.R. and A.V. Panfilov, Modeling of heart excitation patterns caused by a local inhomogeneity. *J Theor Biol*, 1996;**181**(1): 33–40.

140. Fenton F. and A. Karma, Vortex dynamics in three-dimensional continuous myocardium with fiber rotation: Filament instability and fibrillation. *Chaos*, 1998;**8**(1): 20–47.

141. Stinstra J.G., B. Hopenfeld, and R.S. MacLeod, On the passive cardiac conductivity. *Ann. Biomed. Eng.*, 2005;**33**: 1743–1751.

142. Stinstra J.G. , S. Shome, B. Hopenfeld, C.S. Henriquez, and R.S. MacLeod, Modeling the passive cardiac conductivity during ischemia. *Comp. in Biol. & Med.*, 2005;**43**(6): 776–782.

143. Shome S., J.G. Stinstra, B. Hopenfeld, B.B. Punske, and R.S. MacLeod, A study of the dynamics of cardiac ischemia using

experimental and modeling approaches, in *Proceedings of the IEEE Engineering in Medicine and Biology Society 26th Annual International Conference.* IEEE EMBS, IEEE Press, New York, 2004.

144. Muzikant A.L. and C.S. Henriquez, Paced activation mapping reveals organization of myocardial fibers: A simulation study. *J. Cardiovasc. Electrophysiol.*, 1997;**8**: 281–294.

145. Muzikant A.L. and C.S. Henriquez, Bipolar stimulation of a three-dimensional bidomain incorporating rotational anisotropy. *IEEE Trans. Biomed. Eng.*, 1998;**45**(4): 449–462.

146. Harrild D.M., R.C. Penland, and C.S. Henriquez, A flexible method for simulating cardiac conduction in three-dimensional complex geometries. *J. Electrocardiol.*, 2000;**33**(3): 241–251.

147. Tranquillo J.V., M.R. Franz, B.C. Knollmann, A.P. Henriquez, D.A. Taylor, and C.S. Henriquez, Genesis of the monophasic action potential: role of interstitial resistance and boundary gradients. *Am. J. Physiol.*, Apr 2004;**286**(4): H1370–H1381.

148. Tranquillo J.V., D.O. Burwell, and C.S. Henriquez, Analytical model of extracellular potentials in a tissue slab with a finite bath. *IEEE Trans. Biomed. Eng.*, Feb 2005;**52**(2): 334–338.

149. Weinstein D.M., C.R. Johnson, J. Tranquillo, C. Henriquez, R.S. MacLeod, and C.R. Johnson, BioPSE case study: Modeling, simulation, and visualization of three dimensional mouse heart propagation. *Int. J. Bioelectromagnet.*, 2003;**5**(1):(in press).

150. Sampson K.J. and C.S. Henriquez, Electrotonic influences on action potential duration dispersion in small hearts: a simulation study. *Am. J. Physiol.*, 2005;**289**(1): H350–H360.

151. Hopenfeld B., J.G. Stinstra, and R.S. MacLeod, The effect of conductivity on ST segment epicardial potentials arising from subendocardial ischemia. *Ann. Biomed. Eng.*, 2005;**33**(6): 751–763.

152. Frazier D.W., W. Krassowska, P.S. Chen, P.D. Wolf, E.G. Dixon, W.M. Smith, and R.E. Ideker, Extracellular field required for excitation in three-dimensional anisotropic canine myocardium. *Circ. Res.*, 1988;**63**: 147–164.

153. Trayanova N., K. Skouibine, and F. Aguel, The role of cardiac tissue structure in defibrillation. *Chaos*, 1998;**8**(1): 221–233.

154. Trayanova N. and J. Eason, Shock-induced arrhythmogenesis in the myocardium. *Chaos*, 2002;**12**(3): 962–972.

155. Trayanova N.A., R.A. Gray, D.W. Bourn, and J.C. Eason, Virtual electrode-induced positive and negative graded responses: new insights into fibrillation induction and defibrillation. *J. Cardiovasc. Electrophysiol.*, Jul 2003;**14**(7): 756–763.

156. Rodriguez B., L. Li, J.C. Eason, I.R. Efimov, and N.A. Trayanova, Differences between left and right ventricular chamber geometry affect cardiac vulnerability to electric shocks. *Circ. Res.*, Jul 2005;**97**(2): 168–175.

157. Trayanova N., Defibrillation of the heart: insights into mechanisms from modelling studies. *Exp Physiol*, 2006;**91**(2): 323–337.

158. Jolley M., J. Triedman, C.F. Westin, D.M. Weinstein, R.S. Macleod, and D.H. Brooks, Image based modeling of defibrillation in children, in *Proceedings of the IEEE Engineering in Medicine and Biology Society 28th Annual International Conference.* IEEE, IEEE Press, New York, 2006, pp. 2564–2567.

159. Wilson F.N. and R.H. Bayley, The electric field of an eccentric dipole in a homogeneous spherical conducting medium. *Circ.*, 1950;**1**: 84–92.

160. Frank E., Electric potential produced by two point current sources in homogeneous conducting sphere. *J. Appl. Phys.*, 1952;**23**: 1225–1228.

161. Burger H.C., H.A. Tolhoek, and F.G. Backbier, The potential distribution on the body surface caused by a heart vector. calculations on some simple models. *Am. Heart J.*, 1954;**48**: 249–263.

162. Okada R.H., Potentials produced by an eccentric current dipole in a finite-length circular conducting cylinder. *IRE Trans. Med. Electron.*, 1956;**7**: 14–19.

163. Bayley R.H. and P.M. Berry, The electrical field produced by the eccentric current dipole in the nonhomogeneous conductor. *Am. Heart J.*, 1962;**63**: 808–820.

164. Bayley R.H. and P.M. Berry, The arbitrary electromotive double layer in the eccentric "heart" of the nonhomogeneous circular lamina. *IEEE Trans. Biomed. Eng.*, 1964;**11**.

165. Bayley R.H., J.M. Kalbfleisch, and P.M. Berry, Changes in the body's QRS surface potentials produced by alterations in certain compartments of the nonhomogeneous conducting model. *Am. Heart J.*, 1969;**77**.

166. Rudy Y. and R. Plonsey, The eccentric spheres model as the basis for a study of the role of geometry and inhomogeneities in electrocardiography. *IEEE Trans. Biomed. Eng.*, 1979;**26**:392–399.

167. Rudy Y. and R. Plonsey, The effects of variations in conductivity and geometrical parameters on the electrocardiogram, using an eccentric spheres model. *Circ. Res.*, 1979;**44**(1):104–111.

168. Rudy Y. and R. Plonsey, A comparison of volume conductor and source geometry effects on body surface and epicardial potentials. *Circ. Res.*, 1980;**46**: 283–291.

169. Throne R.D., L.G. Olson, T.J. Hrabik, and J.R. Windle, Generalized eigensystem techniques for the inverse problem of electrocardiography applied to a realistic heart-torso geometry. *IEEE Trans. Biomed. Eng.*, 1997;**44**(6): 447.

170. Iakovidis I. and R.M. Gulrajani, Regularization of the inverse epicardial solution using linearly constrained optimization, in *Proceedings of the IEEE Engineering in Medicine and Biology Society 13th Annual International Conference*. IEEE Press, New York, 1991, pp. 698–699.

171. Throne R. and L. Olsen, A generalized eigensystem approach to the inverse problem of electrocardiography. *IEEE Trans. Biomed. Eng.*, 1994;**41**: 592–600.

172. Throne R. and L. Olsen, The effect of errors in assumed conductivities and geometry on numerical solutions to the inverse problem of electrocardiography. *IEEE Trans. Biomed. Eng.*, 1995;**42**: 1192–1200.

173. He S., Frequency series expansion of an explicit solution for a dipole inside a conducting sphere at low frequencies. *IEEE Trans. Biomed. Eng.*, 1998;**45**(10): 1249–1258.

174. Barr R.C. and M.S. Spachm Inverse calculation of QRS-T epicardial potentials from body surface potential distributions for normal and ectopic beats in the intact dog. *Circ. Res.*, 1978;**42**: 661–675.

175. Pollard A. and Barr R.C. Computer simulations in an anatomically based model of the human ventricular conduction system. *IEEE Trans. Biomed. Eng.*, 1991;**38**: 982.

176. Pollard A.E., M.J. Burgess, and K.W. Spitzer, Computer simulations of three-dimensional propagation in ventricular myocardium. Effects of intramural fiber rotation and inhomogeneous conductivity on epicardial activation. *Circ. Res.*, 1993;**72**(4): 744–756.

177. Budgett D.M., D.M. Monro, S.W. Edwards, and R.D. Stanbridge, Comparison of measured and computed epicardial potentials from a patient-specific inverse model. *J. Electrocardiol.*, 1993;**26**(Suppl): 165–173.

178. Sachse F.B., C. Werner, K. Meyer-Waarden, and O. Dössel, Comparison of solution to the forward problem in electrophysiology with homogeneous, heterogeneous and anisotropic impedance models. *Biomed. Technik*, 1997;**42**(Suppl): 277–280.

179. Geselowitz D.B. and J.E. Ferrara, Is accurate recording of the ECG surface laplacian feasible? *IEEE Trans. Biomed. Eng.*, April 1999**46**(4): 377–381.

180. Wu D., H.C. Tsai, and B. He, On the estimation of the laplacian electrocardiogram during ventricular activation. *Ann. Biomed. Eng.*, 1999;**27**(6): 731–745.

181. Trew M., I. Le Grice, B. Smaill, and A. Pullan, A finite volume method for modeling discontinuous electrical activation in cardiac tissue. *Ann. Biomed. Eng.*, 2005;**33**(5):590–602.

182. Barr R.C., T.C. Pilkington, J.P. Boineau, and M.S. Spach, Determining surface potentials from current dipoles, with application to electrocardiography. *IEEE Trans. Biomed. Eng.*, 1966;**13**: 88–92.

183. Messinger-Rapport B.J. and Y. Rudy, The inverse problem in electrocardiography: A model study of the effects of geometry and conductivity parameters on the reconstruction of epicardial potentials. *IEEE Trans. Biomed. Eng.*, 1986;**33**: 667–676.

184. Rudy Y. and B.J. Messinger-Rapport, The inverse solution in electrocardiography: Solutions in terms of epicardial potentials. *Crit. Rev. Biomed. Eng.*, 1988;**16**: 215–268.

185. Derfus D.L., T.C. Pilkington, and R.E. Ideker, Calculating intracavitary potentials from measured endocardial potentials, in *Proceedings of the IEEE Engineering in Medicine and Biology Society 12th Annual International Conference*. IEEE Press, New York. 1990, p. 635.

186. Charulatha R. and Y. Rudy, Electrocardiographic imaging:I. effect of torso inhomgeneities on body surface electrocardiographic potentials. *J. Cardiovasc. Electrophysiol.*, 2001;**12**: 229–240.

187. Colli Franzone P., B. Taccardi, and C. Viganotti, An approach to inverse calculation of epicardial potentials from body surface maps. *Adv. Cardiol.*, 1978;**21**: 50–54.

188. Colli Franzone P., L. Guerri, C. Viganotti, E. Macchi, S. Baruffi, S. Spaggiari, and B. Taccardi, Potential fields generated by oblique layers modeling excitation wavefronts in the anisotropic myocardium. *Circ. Res.*, 1982;**51**: 330–346.

189. Yamashita Y. and T. Takahashi, Use of the finite element method to determine epicardial from body surface potentials under a realistic torso model. *IEEE Trans. Biomed. Eng.*, 1984;**31**: 611–621.

190. Hunter P.J., A.D. McCulloch, P.M.F. Nielsen, and B.H. Smaill, A finite element model of passive ventricular mechanics. *ASME BED*, 1988;**9**: 387–397.

191. Sepulveda N.G., J.P. Wikswo, and D.S. Echt, Finite element analysis of cardiac defibrillation current distributions. *IEEE Trans. Biomed. Eng.*, 1990;**37**: 354–365.

192. Nielsen P.M.F., I.J. Le Grice, B.H. Smaill, and P.J. Hunter, Mathematical model of geometry and fibrous structure of the heart. *Am. J. Physiol.*, 1991;**260**: H1365–H1378.

193. Panfilov A.V. and J.P. Keener, Modelling re-entry in a finite element model of the heart. *J. Physiol.*, 1993;**467**: 152.

194. Hunter P.J., P.M.F. Nielsen, B.H. Smaill, and I.J. LeGrice, An anatomical heart model with application in myocardial activation and ventricular mechanics, in *High Performance Computing in Biomedical Research*, chapter 1, T.C. Pilkington, B. Loftis, J. F. Thompson, S. L-Y Woo, T.C. Palmer, and T.F. Budinger, Editors. CRC Press, Boca Raton, 1993, pp. 3–26.

195. Klepfer R.N., C.R. Johnson, and R.S. MacLeod, The effects of inhomogeneities and anisotropies on electrocardiographic fields: A three-dimensional finite element study. *IEEE Trans. Biomed. Eng.*, 1997;**44**(8): 706–719.

196. Ramon C., Y. Wang, J. Haueisen, P. Schimpf, S. Jaruvatanadilok, and A. Ishimaru, Effect of myocardial anisotropy on the torso current flow patterns, potentials and magnetic fields. *Phys Med Biol*, 2000;**45**(5): 1141–1150.

197. Hopenfeld B., Spherical harmonic-based finite element meshing scheme for modelling current flow within the heart. *Med. & Biol. Eng. & Comp.*, 2004;**42**(6): 847–851.

198. Stanley P.C. and T.C. Pilkington, The combination method: A numerical technique for electrocardiographic calculations. *IEEE Trans. Biomed. Eng.*, 1989;**36**: 456–461.

199. Pullan A., A high-order coupled finite/boundary element torso model. *IEEE Trans. Biomed. Eng.*, 1996;**43**(3):292–298.

200. Pullan A., M.L. Buist, and L.K. Cheng, *Mathematically Modeling the electrical activity of the heart.* World Scientific Co, Singapore, 2005.

201. Phillips G.M., Numerical integration in two and three dimensions. *Comput. J.*, 1967;**10**(2): 202–204.

202. Oostendorp T.F. and A. van Oosterom, Source parameter estimation in inhomogeneous volume conductors of arbitrary shape. *IEEE Trans. Biomed. Eng.*, 1989;**36**: 382–391.

203. Barr R.C., T.C. Pilkington, J.P. Boineau, and C.L. Rogers, An inverse electrocardiographic solution with an on-off model. *IEEE Trans. Biomed. Eng.*, 1970;**17**: 49–57.

204. Zickler P., Cardiac mapping. *Biomed Instrum Technol (BTI)*, 1997;**31**(2): 173–175.

205. Smeets J., S. Ben Haim, L. Rodriguez, C. Timmermans, and H. Wellens, New method for nonfluoroscopic endocardial mapping in humans. *Circ.*, 1998;**97**: 2426–2432

206. Callans D.J., J.F. Ren, J. Michele, F.E. Marchlinski, and S.M. Dillon, Electroanatomic left ventricular mapping in the porcine model of healed anterior myocardial infarction. correlation with intracardiac echocardiography and pathological analysis. *Circ.*, 1999;**100**: 1744–1750.

207. Rao L., C. Ding, and D.S. Khoury, Nonfluoroscopic localization of intracardiac electrode-catheters combined with noncontact electrical-anatomical imaging. *Ann. Biomed. Eng.*, 2004;**32**(12): 1654–1661.

208. Ding C., L. Rao, S.F. Nagueh, and D.S. Khoury, Dynamic three-dimensional visualization of the left ventricle by intracardiac echocardiography. *Ultrasound Med. Biol.*, 2005;**31**(1): 15–21.

209. Ghanem R.N., C. Ramanathan, P. Jia, and Y. Rudy, Heart-surface reconstruction and ECG electrodes localization using fluoroscopy, epipolar geometry and stereovision: application to noninvasive imaging of cardiac electrical activity. *IEEE Trans. Med. Imaging*, 2003;**22**(10): 1307–1318.

210. Jezzard P. and R.S. Balaban, Correction for geometric distortion in echo planar images from B0 field variations. *Mag. Res. Med.*, 1995;**34**(1): 65–73.

211. Ernst T., O. Speck, L. Ittl, and L. Chang, Simultaneous correction for interdscan patient motion and geometric distortion in echoplanar imaging. *Mag. Res. Med.*, 1999;**42**: 201–205.

212. Studholme C., T. Constable, and J.S. Duncan, A phantom based investigation of non-rigid registration constraints in mapping fMRI to anatomical MRI, in *Medical Imaging 2000: Image Processing, 2000*, 2000.

213. Sosa E., M. Scanavacca, A. D'avila, and F. Pilleggi, A new technique to perform epicardial mapping in the electrophysiology laboratory. *J. Cardiovasc. Electrophysiol.*, 1996;**7**: 531–536.

214. Sosa E., M. Scanavacca, A. D'avila, J. Piccioni, O. Sanchez, J.L. Velarde, M. Silva, and B. Reolao, Endocardial and epicardial ablation guided by nonsurgical transthoracic epicardial mapping to treat recurrent of ventricular tachycardia. *J. Cardiovasc. Electrophysiol.*, 1998;**9**: 229–239.

215. Sosa E., M. Scanavacca, A. D'Avila, F. Oliviera, and J.A.F Ramires, Nonsurgical transthoracic epicardial ablation to treat recurrent of ventricular tachycardia. *J. Am. Coll. Cardiol.*, 2000;**35**(1): 1442–1449.

216. Spoor C.W. and F.E. Veldpaus, Rigid body motion calculated from spatial co-ordinates of markers. *J. Biomech.*, 1980;**13**:391–393.

217. Challis J.H., A procedure for determining rigid body transformation parameters. *J. Biomechanics*, 1995;**28**(6): 733–737.

218. Horáček B.M., *The Effect on Electrocardiographic Lead Vectors of Conductivity Inhomogeneities in the Human Torso.* PhD thesis, Dalhousie University, Halifax, N.S., Canada, 1971.

219. MacLeod R.S., C.R. Johnson, and P.R. Ershler, Construction of an inhomogeneous model of the human torso for use in computational electrocardiography, in *Proceedings of the IEEE Engineering in Medicine and Biology Society 13th Annual International Conference.* IEEE Press, New York, 1991, pp. 688–689.

220. MacLeod R.S., R.M. Miller, M.J. Gardner, and B.M. Horáček, Application of an electrocardiographic inverse solution to localize myocardial ischemia during percutaneous transluminal coronary angioplasty. *J. Cardiovasc. Electrophysiol.*, 1995;**6**: 2–18.

221. Modre R., B. Tilg, G. Fischer, F. Hanser, B. Messnarz, F.X. Roithinger, and F. Hintringer, A clinical pilot study on the accessory pathway localization accuracy applying ECG mapping, in *Proceedings of the IEEE Engineering in Medicine and Biology Society 24th Annual International Conference*, vol. 2, 2002, pp. 1381–1382.

222. Fischer G., B. Pfeifer, M. Seger, C. Hintermuller, F. Hanser, R. Modre, B. Tilg, T. Trieb, C. Kremser, F.X. Roithinger, and F. Hintringer, Computationally efficient noninvasive cardiac activation time imaging. *Methods Inf. Med.*, 2005;**44**(5): 674–686.

223. Fischer G., F. Hanser, B. Pfeifer, M. Seger, C. Hintermuller, R. Modre, B. Tilg, T. Trieb, T. Berger, F.X. Roithinger, and F. Hintringer, A signal processing pipeline for noninvasive imaging of ventricular preexcitation. *Methods Inf. Med.*, 2005;**44**(4): 508–515.

224. Pfeifer B., G. Fischer, F. Hanser, M. Seger, C. Hintermuller, R. Modre-Osprian, T. Trieb, and B. Tilg, Atrial and ventricular myocardium extraction using model-based techniques. *Methods Inf. Med.*, 2006;**45**(1): 19–26.

225. Patterson R.R., Projective transformations of the parameter of a Bernstein-Bézier curve. *ACM Trans. Graph.*, 1985;**4**(4): 276–290.

226. Robeson S.M., Spherical methods for spatial interpolation: Review and evaluation. *Cartog. Geog. Inf. Sys.*, 1997;**24**(1): 3–20.

227. Mercer R.R., G.M. McCauley, and S. Anjilvel, Approximation of surfaces in a quantitative 3-D reconstruction system. *IEEE Trans. Biomed. Eng.*, 1990;**37**: 1136–1146.

228. Vesely I., B. Eickmeier, and G. Campbell, Automated 3-D reconstruction of vascular structures from high definition casts. *IEEE Trans. Biomed. Eng.*, 1991;**38**: 1123–1129.

229. MacLeod R.S., C.R. Johnson, and M.A. Matheson, Visualization tools for computational electrocardiography. In *Visualization in Biomedical Computing*, Bellingham, Wash., 1992. Proceedings of the SPIE #1808, pp. 433–444.

230. Weinstein D., Scanline surfacing: Building separating surfaces from planar contours, in *Proceeding of IEEE Visualization 2000*, 2000, pp. 283–289.

231. Hren R. and G. Stroink, Application of the surface harmonic expansions for modeling the human torso. *IEEE Trans. Biomed. Eng.*, 1995;**42**(5): 521.

232. Bradley C.P., A.J. Pullan, and P.J. Hunter, Geometric modeling of the human torso using cubic hermite elements. *Ann. Biomed. Eng.*, 1997;**25**: 96–111.

233. Gumhold S., X. Wang, and R.S. MacLeod, Feature extraction from point clouds, in *Proceedings, 10th International Meshing Roundtable*. Sandia National Laboratories, 2001, pp. 293–305.

234. Bern M. and D. Eppstein, Mesh generation and optimal triangulation, in *Computing in Euclidean Geometry*, F.K. Hwang and D.Z. Du, Editors. World Scientific, Singapore, 1992.

235. Lee D.T. and B.J. Schachter, Two algorithms for constructing a Delaunay triangulation. *Int. J. Comp. Inf. Sci.*, 1980;**9**: 219–242.

236. Schumaker L.L., Triangularization methods, in *Topics in Multivariate Analysis*. Academic Press, London, 1987, pp. 219–232.

237. Schmidt J.A., C.R. Johnson, J.A. Eason, and R.S. MacLeod, Applications of automatic mesh generation and adaptive methods in computational medicine, in *Modeling, Mesh Generation, and Adaptive Methods for Partial Differential Equations*, J. Flaherty and I. Babuska, Editors. Springer, Berlin, 1994, pp. 367–394.

238. Schimpf P.H., D.R. Haynor, and Y. Kim, Object-free adaptive meshing in highly heterogeneous 3-D domains. *Int. J. Biomed. Comput.*, 1996;**40**(3): 209–225.

239. Peraire J. and K. Morgan, Unstructured mesh generation including directional refinement for aerodynamic flow simulation. *Finite Elements Anal. Design*, 1997;**25**: 343.

240. Alliez P., D. Cohen-Steiner, M. Yvinec, and M. Desbrun, Variational tetrahedral meshing, in *International Conference on Computer Graphics and Interactive Techniques*. ACM Press, New York, NY, USA, 2005, pp. 617–625.

241. Yu F. and C. R. Johnson, An automatic adaptive refinement and derefinement method, in *Proceedings of the 14th IMACS World Congress*, 1944, pp. 1555–1557.

242. Livnat Y. and Johnson C.R., The effects of adaptive refinement on ill-posed inverse problems. Personal communication, 1997.

243. Schimpf P.H., Y. Wang, D.R. Haynor, and Y. Kim, Sensitivity of transvenous defibrillation models to adaptive mesh density and resolution: the potential for interactive solution times. *Int. J. Med. Inf.*, 1997;**45**(3): 193–207.

244. Lines G., P. Grottum, and A. Tveito, Modeling the electrical activity of the heart –A bidomain model of the ventricles embedded in a torso. *Comput. & Vis. Sci.*, 2003;**5**(4): 195–213.

245. Missan S. and T. F. McDonald, CESE: Cell Electrophysiology Simulation Environment. *Appl. Bioinformat.*, 2005;**4**(2): 155–156.

246. Tomita M., K. Hashimoto, K. Takahashi, T.S. Shimizu, Y. Matsuzaki, F. Miyoshi, K. Saito, S. Tanida, K. Yugi, J.C. Venter, and C.A. Hutchison. E-CELL: software environment for whole-cell simulation. *Bioinformatics*, 1999;**15**(1): 72–84.

247. van Oosterom A. and T.F. Oostendorp, ECGSIM: an interactive tool for studying the genesis of QRST waveforms. *Heart*, 2004;**90**(2): 165–168.

248. SCIRun: A Scientific Computing Problem Solving Environment, Scientific Computing and Imaging Institute (SCI), 2006.

249. BioPSE: Problem Solving Environment for modeling, simulation, image processing, and visualization for biomedical computing applications. Scientific Computing and Imaging Institute (SCI), 2006.

250. Weinstein D.M., S.G. Parker, and C.R. Johnson, A physically based mesh generation algorithm: Applications in computational medicine, in *IEEE Engineering in Medicine and Biology Society 16th Annual International Conference*. IEEE Press, New York,1994, pp. 718–719.

251. Weinstein D.M., L. Zhukov, and C.R. Johnson, Lead-field bases for EEG source imaging. *Ann. Biomed. Eng.*, 2000;**28**(9): 1059–1065.

252. Weinstein D.M., L. Zhukov, and C.R. Johnson, An inverse EEG problem solving environment and its applications to EEG source localization. *NeuroImage (suppl.)*, 2000: 921.

253. MacLeod R.S. and C.R. Johnson, Map3d: Interactive scientific visualization for bioengineering data, in *Proceedings of the IEEE Engineering in Medicine and Biology Society 15th Annual International Conference*. IEEE Press, New York, 1993, pp. 30–31. http://software.sci.utah.edu/map3d.html.

254. Clancy C.E. and Y. Rudy, Linking a genetic defect to its cellular phenotype in a cardiac arrhythmia. *Nature*, 1999**400**(6744): 566–509.

255. Venter J.C., M.D. Adams, E.W. Myers, and P.W. Li, The sequence of the human genome. *Science*, 2001**291**(5507): 1304–1351.

256. Hunter P.J. and T.K. Borg, Integration from proteins to organs: the physiome project. *Nat. Rev. Mol. Cell. Biol.*, 2003;**4**(3): 237–243.

257. Hunter P.J., The iups physiome project: a framework for computational physiology. *Prog. Biophys. Mol. Biol.*, 2004;**85**(2–3): 551–569.

258. H.C. Burger and van Milaan J.B., Heart-vector and leads. Part I. *Br. Heart J.*, 1946;**8**: 157–61.

259. Sundnes J., G.T. Lines, X. Cai, B.F. Nielsen, K.A. Mardal, and A. Tveito, *Computing the Electrical Activity in the Heart*. Spinger, Berlin, 2006.

260. Potse M., B. Dube, J. Richer, A. Vinet, and R.M. Gulrajani, A comparison of monodomain and bidomain reaction-diffusion models for action potential propagation in the human heart. *IEEE Trans. Biomed. Eng.*, 2006;**53**(12): 2425–2435.

261. Austin T.M., M.L. Trew, and A.J. Pullan, Solving the cardiac bidomain equations for discontinuous conductivities. *IEEE Trans. Biomed. Eng.*, 2006;**53**(7): 1265–1272.

262. Austin T., D. Hooks, P. Hunter, D. Nickerson, A.J. Pullan, G. Sands, B. Maaill, and M. Trew, Modelling cardiac electrical activity at the cell and tissue levels, in *Interactive and Integrative Cardiology*, vol. 1080, S. Sideman, R. Beyar, and A. Landesberg, Editors. Annals of NY Academy of Sciences, 2006;**1080**: 334–347.

263. Trew M.L., B.J. Caldwell, G.B. Sands, D.A. Hooks, D.C. Tai, T.M. Austin, I.J. LeGrice, A.J. Pullan, and B.H. Smaill, Cardiac electrophysiology and tissue structure: bridging the scale gap with a joint measurement and modelling paradigm. *Exp Physiol*, 2006;**91**(2): 355–370.

9 The Inverse Problem of Electrocardiography

Andrew J. Pullan · Leo K. Cheng · Martyn P. Nash · Alireza Ghodrati ·
Rob MacLeod · Dana H. Brooks

P. W. Macfarlane et al. (eds.), *Basic Electrocardiology*, DOI 10.1007/978-0-85729-871-3_9,

9.1   Introduction

In very broad terms, the inverse problem of electrocardiography may be defined as the determination of the electrical function of the heart from a number of remote recordings of potentials on some noninvasive or minimally invasive surface. In this sense, even clinical electrocardiographic or vectorcardiographic diagnosis is an inverse problem solved on an empirical basis by using previously cataloged information. In this chapter, the phrase "inverse problem of electrocardiography" is used in its more formal sense to mean the deduction of electrical information about the heart by mathematical manipulation of the measured potentials on the body surface (or from inside the cavities of the heart). The description of this inverse problem and various forms of its solution forms the principal subject matter of this chapter. We consider the clinical interpretation of the calculated electrical information only briefly, since clinical deduction may be viewed as subsequent to the solution of the mathematical inverse problem.

In contrast to the forward problem, which can be solved uniquely to within a constant for the zero of potential, the inverse problem does not possess a complete solution that is mathematically unique. By this we mean that it is not possible to identify unique cardiac sources within the heart as long as the active region is inaccessible, because the electric field that they generate outside any closed surface enclosing them may be duplicated by equivalent single- or double-layer sources on the closed surface itself [1]. This difficulty is usually circumvented by using simplified models for the cardiac sources; in this case, the parameters of these models may be uniquely determined from the surface potentials with additional assumptions regarding the intervening volume conductor. (We note that if one takes into account the physiological constraints of cardiac bioelectricity, most notably the electrical anisotropy of cardiac tissue and the wavefront behavior of activation (or the quasi-wavefront behavior of recovery), and one considers measurements at multiple time instants, it is less clear to what extent intramural activity may indeed be imaged. This may seem contradictory to the previous statement; certainly, at any single time instant the "internal" sources are not unique. However, by considering multiple temporal measurements *as a whole*, many solutions which might well be mathematically valid on a time-instant-by-time-instant basis will now be invalid, because they represent source behavior that is nonphysiological. Thus, the spatio-temporal behavior of reasonable solutions, that is, of cardiac sources, can be used to make the space of feasible solutions smaller (in the mathematical sense) and thus make the solution closer to being unique. In summary, it is not yet clear what the limits are on the degree to which one can image intramural activity from body surface or intracavitary measurements, nor how reliable such imaging may be. We discuss in some detail in the following section how to use temporal behavior to improve inverse solutions for surface models, as well as some recent, initial attempts to reconstruct intramural activity.)

A simple description of a parametric model for the inverse problem is the vectorcardiogram (VCG), which assumes that the heart's electrical activity may be approximated by a fixed-location, variable-amplitude, variable-orientation current dipole within a finite homogeneous torso. More sophisticated inverse solutions upgrade the heart source model by using a more realistic description of cardiac depolarization/repolarization. Along with these upgraded heart models, most contemporary simulations include a realistically shaped and often patient-specific geometric model of the torso, as illustrated in ❷ Chap. 8. We note that the inverse solution cannot, in general, be obtained unless the corresponding forward problem, using the assumed heart and torso models, is solved first.

Early formulations of the inverse problem in electrocardiography treated it as a kind of extension of the traditional electrocardiogram (ECG), based on measurements made on the body surface. With the advent of intracavitary catheter-based probes for clinical electrophysiology (EP) procedures, researchers also began to use measurements from multielectrode noncontact probes, located inside one of the heart chambers, in an inverse solution to reconstruct the electric potential on the inner wall of the chamber. In the literature, this has been called the "endocardial inverse problem." However, a number of inverse solutions using body surface measurements can reconstruct parameters of electrical activity on the endocardium, and indeed, as we discuss a little later in this section, the surface upon which the measurements are made is not uniquely tied to the location of the sources to be reconstructed. Thus, it is perhaps more accurate to distinguish between measurement surface (body surface or intracavitary) and source locations (discussed in the next paragraph).

The first edition of this chapter dealt almost exclusively with inverse solutions in terms of discrete, equivalent bioelectric sources, i.e., simple-dipole, moving-dipole, multipole-series, or multiple-dipole heart models, and there is no need to repeat that excellent treatment. Here, we have chosen to describe the progression to solutions based on more realistic sources. Thus, we concentrate on source models that capture electrophysiological parameters that one can physically measure, specifically surface potentials (epicardial and/or endocardial), transmembrane potentials on the epicardial and/or endocardial surfaces or even in the myocardium itself (Transmembrane potentials can be measured as monophasic action potentials, using floating glass microelectrodes, or optically using voltage sensitive dyes; we note, however, that these technologies are not yet suitable for the verification of inverse solutions), or that directly represent fiducial-time parameters such as activation or repolarization times (usually derived from measurements of potentials). The fact that these formulations are based on measurable quantities has opened the possibility of direct validation of the solution, a facet of all approaches that is of fundamental importance. With any discrete source approach (dipole or multipole), such direct validation is not possible because of the difficulty of relating measured activation times or potentials to equivalent dipoles. We note that the term "equivalent sources" can be somewhat ambiguous, since in some sense any source model that does not start with the true cardiac sources at the microscopic scale must use equivalent sources. Indeed, the term appears at times in the literature to mean source models such as the epicardial potential distribution. However, we use it here in the same sense as in the first edition of this book, to mean a small set of discrete dipole or multipole sources that do not attempt to closely mimic any physiological phenomenon.

As described in some detail in ➋ Chap. 8, the surface upon which these potential or temporal parameters are reconstructed is somewhat independent of the source model itself. Traditionally, potential-type sources have used a *single-surface* model (the epicardium for body-surface measurements, the endocardium for intracavitary measurements), while fiducial-time based approaches have by necessity used a combined endocardial/epicardial surface. However, as mentioned earlier, since any surface which encloses all the sources is a valid surface on which to model the sources, potential-based methods can also use a combined surface, and indeed at least one recent report [2] described such an approach. Here, to keep an appropriate level of generality, we adopt at times the convention of Messnarz et al. in [2] and use the term "heart surface potentials" (HSP) to include any relevant surface model; when needed, we will use specific variants such as epicardial, endocardial, and combined epi/endocardial potentials.

As in the first edition, any coverage of this vast topic will be incomplete and we apologize in advance for any omissions or oversights. The references cited here are representative and by no means comprehensive. An additional technical note is that we will use the terms "electrocardiology" and "electrocardiography" interchangeably in the context of this inverse problem despite possible differentiations [3].

A final introductory note before addressing the details is the importance of understanding and appreciating from the outset the difficult nature of the inverse problem. Keener and Sneyd summarized the forward/inverse problem relationship well in a recent book [4]:

- "... If the exact location and strength of this dipole surface and the conductivity tensor for the entire body were known, then we could in principle solve the Poisson equation to find the body surface potential at all times during the cardiac cycle."

- This problem is known as the forward problem of electrocardiography.
  "Even more useful ... one could determine the sources by inverting the forward problem. This problem, known as the inverse problem of electrocardiography, is even harder to solve than the forward problem ..."

Despite the conceptual simplicity of this so-called forward problem, as Keener and Sneyd point out, its solution is far from trivial. The major utility of a forward solution is that it provides a means of probing the fundamental relationships between bioelectrical sources and electrocardiographic potentials; it serves as a tool for both learning and experimenting with those relationships. This tool has clinically oriented uses (for instance, design of defibrillators [5] or mapping systems) and forward models are also needed for inverse solutions. By contrast, the most common goal of inverse solutions is to evaluate the state of the heart from remote measurements, and thus it has an explicitly clinical context. We note, however, that results of a forward solution describe *possible* pathways for source-measurement relationships, but by themselves they do not show *causality* – one can easily imagine different parameters in forward models, or even different models, leading to similar predictions of measurements. To establish causality one wants to also show *uniqueness*, or perhaps to quantify the uncertainty in the forward predictions, and this requires an inverse solution.

To appreciate the source of difficulty in the inverse problem, one must examine the extent to which it allows a unique solution, and even when it is unique, whether the problem is sufficiently constrained to actually solve in practice. Simply put, in the inverse problem one would like to *invert* the forward model, or equivalently solve for the source parameters which, together with the forward model, explain or predict the measurements. However, a naive attempt at this is doomed to failure. As already noted, it is impossible to recreate the electrical state of each cell in the heart (or even each small cluster of cells) from surface or intracavitary electrical recordings, no matter how many recordings are available. Some of the reasons for this are described in previous chapters or will become apparent in the following sections. However, the impossibility of this reconstruction is a mathematical certainty – perhaps most simply explained by the fact that multiple configurations of cellular activity can give rise to the same measurements (that is to say, the problem is not unique). If, however, attention is restricted to finding some alternative parameters to represent the electrical activity of the heart (for instance the epicardial potential distribution), then it is possible to construct an inverse problem with a mathematically unique solution. Unfortunately, unless this problem is appropriately constrained, in all likelihood it will be ill-posed in the sense of Hadamard [6] – the solution will not depend continuously on the data, meaning that small perturbations in the input data will result in disproportionately large changes in the computed solution. This is illustrated in ❷ Fig. 9.1c, which shows computed epicardial potentials that best match the measured body surface potentials in a least-squares sense; with no constraints the results are completely erroneous. An important consequence of nonuniqueness and ill-posedness is that the level of detail that one can reconstruct from body surface electrical recordings is significantly lower than that which can be simulated with a similarly resolved forward solution.

Why does ill-posedness arise? We can consider the difficulty and the effects of ill-posedness in an electrocardiographic inverse problem as an imaging problem. The goal in this case is to reconstruct the electrical state of the heart

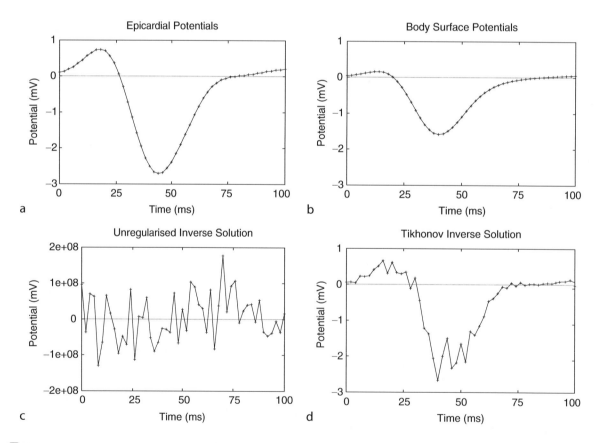

❏ Fig. 9.1

An illustration of ill-posedness. Shown are (a) epicardial and (b) body surface signals generated in a forward simulation. Also shown are resultant inverse solutions for (c) an unconstrained inverse solution taken from the data in (b); and (d) a Tikhonov regularized inverse also using data in (b) (see ❷ Sect. 9.3.1). The unconstrained epicardial signals are clearly erroneous, highlighting the ill-posedness of such an inverse problem

just as anatomy is reconstructed using an inverse solution in the more widely known imaging modalities of magnetic resonance imaging (MRI) or computed tomography (CT). In MRI, the forward model is a (discrete) Fourier transform, and thus, there is no difficulty inverting it reliably to create an image. However, for the inverse ECG problem, the forward solution includes attenuation that is of different degrees for different spatial scales (technically, at different spatial frequencies). In particular, higher spatial frequencies (smaller-scale phenomena) are attenuated more than those with lower frequencies. As a consequence, trying to invert the forward solution directly (or solve for the "best-fit-to-data" solution) leads to the amplification of high-frequency components. Of course, any noise in the measurements and any error in the forward model will contain such high-frequency components which will then dominate unconstrained solutions, as seen in ❷ Fig. 9.1; the effects of these components on the solution must be constrained if the result is to be useful.

Put more formally, the source/data relationship is subject to the inverse square law inherent in Laplace's and Poisson's equations, while the superposition of currents that takes place in the torso volume means that each measurement is a combination of the entire set of sources – thus the measured body surface potentials are, at best, a highly blurred and attenuated version of the intracardiac sources. Deblurring (inverting) is a tractable mathematical problem only after the application of auxiliary constraints. In the absence of such constraints, the effective nonuniqueness means that there is no unique *deblurred* solution. In other words, there are many equally valid candidates for the electrical image and no way to determine which one actually represents reality. This nonuniqueness implies that one can be completely misled if the wrong solution is chosen, is clearly unacceptable for scientific or clinical applications.

Thus, the great difficulty in solving the inverse ECG problem is the identification and application of appropriate physiological and mathematically tractable constraints so that the nonuniqueness is resolved in a clinically appropriate manner, yielding a physically and physiologically meaningful image of cardiac electrical activity. Indeed, it is the design and application of such constraints as will occupy most of the rest of this chapter.

In the appendix to ❷ Chap. 2 a brief introduction is given to the matrix and vector notations used, as well as to some of the basic concepts taken from the field of linear algebra.

9.2 Inverse Problem Formulation

In this section we describe in general terms a formulation of the inverse problem that encompasses all the variants we will then describe in more detail. We will then discuss, again in general terms, solution strategies that address the ill-posedness explained in the previous section.

Two requirements for solving an electrocardiographic inverse problem are: (1) a mathematical (geometric) description of the region through which the electrical currents generated within the heart flow to the recording sensors, whether they are on the torso surface or in the intracavitary blood volume and (2) recordings of those electrical signals themselves, sampled at tens to perhaps two hundred known locations, at typically between 500 and 2,000 samples per second, using lead systems described elsewhere in this book.

❷ Figure 9.2 illustrates the various types of inverse solutions we consider here. As the figure shows, measurements of body surface potentials can be used in one of two ways depending on the source and forward model to which they are applied: either to reconstruct potentials (surface or transmembrane) or to reconstruct fiducial times such as timing of wavefront arrivals on the epicardial and endocardial surfaces (activation times). Measurements of intracavitary potentials can be used to reconstruct surface or even transmembrane potentials as well, although to date this technique has usually been applied to reconstruct endocardial potentials.

To formalize this setting, we first summarize in a general form the results of a solution to the forward problem (note that we use general notation here, leaving more specific notation as appropriate for specific classes of formulations):

$$b = A(x) + n, \tag{9.1}$$

where A is a (possibly nonlinear) forward operator which incorporates a parameterized model of the cardiac sources and produces a prediction of the measured potentials, x holds the solution of interest (e.g., epicardial potentials or activation isochrones), b holds the measurements (whether body-surface or intracavitary), and n represents the measurement noise. For linear forward operators, A becomes a matrix A and measurements, solution and noise can be denoted as column vectors: b, x, and n respectively. In this situation the forward model becomes

$$b = Ax + n \tag{9.2}$$

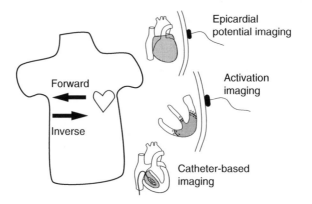

○ Fig. 9.2

There are three basic types of inverse problems treated in this chapter, as illustrated here: in two of them, body surface measurements are used to reconstruct potentials (surface or transmembrane) or activation wavefront locations (isochrones), and in the third intracavitary potentials are used to reconstruct surface potentials

Although we have written the forward operator A above as free of error, it is important to recognize that generally none of the components of (9.1) or (9.2) are exact – in addition to measurement noise the forward operator is corrupted to some degree by the geometric noise arising from many sources: inaccuracies in developing the geometric model, errors associated with the numerical solution of the forward problem, errors in conductivities, etc. Moreover, the measured signals have errors in the recording of the positions of the electrodes. Errors may be considered small (e.g., signal noise below 10 microvolts, submillimeter MRI or CT image accuracy) but such errors can and do become greatly amplified in an inverse calculation, especially without careful treatment, due to the ill-posed nature of the problem.

9.2.1 Including Time in the Formulation

There are a number of ways that temporal aspects of the inverse problem can be formulated. We can consider x, b, and n as representing an entire temporal sequence of the relevant parameters in the case of potential sources. Alternatively, b and n could contain temporal sequences, while x could be the relevant fiducial timings for activation or recovery time source models. An alternative formulation for potential models could be to consider x, b, and n as spatial samples at a given time instant, and then write a temporal sequence of equations of the form of (9.1), one for each sample instant.

In the context of a linear model, x, b, and n in (9.2) would be block vectors formed by concatenations of the different time instants, and the matrix A would then be a large block diagonal matrix, with the forward matrix repeated in each of the diagonal blocks. Written explicitly, then, the vector x becomes

$$x = \left[x(t_0)^{\mathrm{T}} \; x(t_0 + 1)^{\mathrm{T}} \cdots x(t_n)^{\mathrm{T}} \right]^{\mathrm{T}}, \tag{9.3}$$

where $x(t_i)$ is the vector formed by stacking the potentials over the solution surface at time t_i and the time instants taken into consideration range from t_0 to t_n. The block vectors for b and n would be written similarly, and then A would have the form (where here we use $\widetilde{A}$ to represent the single time-instant forward matrix):

$$A = \begin{bmatrix} \widetilde{A} & 0 & \cdots & 0 \\ 0 & \widetilde{A} & \cdots & 0 \\ \vdots & \ddots & \ddots & \vdots \\ 0 & \cdots & 0 & \widetilde{A} \end{bmatrix} \tag{9.4}$$

Another useful formulation is to simply stack each time sample as one column of a matrix and then re-write the forward solution over the entire time sequence as

$$B = AX + N, \tag{9.5}$$

where the matrices B, X, and N have columns b, x, and n, which are spatial vectors at discrete locations, and each row is a time series at a given spatial position. We note that the block vector/matrix formulation and the matrix/matrix formulations can be formally equated with the use of vectorization and Kronecker product operators.

We point out that there is no explicit time dependence in the forward operator A in any of the above equations. Indeed, in the inverse problem, A is generally taken to be temporally invariant, defined using the geometry of the heart in diastasis without consideration of the dynamic variation of that geometry. One could certainly argue that ignoring the dynamic nature of A (which arises as a result of heart motion, among other sources of physiological motion) is a possibly meaningful source of error. However, there are a number of justifications that support this static assumption. First, because of the delay between excitation and contraction in cardiac myocytes, significant contraction does not occur until after the QRS complex. As a result, ignoring contraction should be a reasonable approximation for imaging the depolarization of the heart. This argument is, of course, not valid for imaging repolarization, and the importance of this additional error source in repolarization imaging has yet to be determined. However, perhaps the strongest reasons for treating A as a static matrix are pragmatic ones. It is already difficult enough to obtain and use image data (e.g., MRI or CT) to create a mesh of the heart and surrounding torso volume of a specific patient at one time instance; repeating this process to construct multiple transfer operators would be prohibitive, given the present state of model-creation technology. One recent attempt to mitigate this problem has been the suggestion to use electrical impedance tomography, which may allow one to image changes in the geometry in a time-resolved fashion [7, 8]. Perhaps most important, to date, no evidence has been presented that indicates that the error incurred by assuming a fixed ventricular geometry during depolarization is as large as that arising from the many other approximations and error sources common to inverse problems.

9.2.2 The Inverse Problem

With the notation mentioned in the previous section, the inverse problem can be stated very succinctly as finding a solution x which (1) matches the measurements that the model A would predict for that particular solution to the actual measurements b and (2) also is indeed a reasonable solution for parameters of cardiac electrical activity. One can think of this as "inverting" the operator in (9.1) (although, as discussed in the following section, there are iterative approaches to finding x that do not explicitly compute an inverse, for either algorithmic or computational reasons). As we have already stated, even with a linear forward matrix and x representing a vector of epicardial potentials ϕ, the inverse problem is ill-posed. This ill-posedness manifests itself in the severe ill-conditioning of the matrix A. There is no reason to expect A to be square, and therefore, it is typically not invertible. The usual solution in such cases, at least if the number of measurements is greater than the number of potentials to be solved for on the solution surface (so that A is over-determined, that is, it has more rows than columns), is to solve for the least-squares solution. This is the solution which minimizes the (Euclidean) magnitude of the residual error $\|A\phi - \phi_B\|_2$ (where ϕ represents the solution x for the specific case of heart surface potentials, and ϕ_B represents b for the specific case of body surface measurements). The resulting solution solves the square matrix equation

$$\phi = (A^\mathrm{T} A)^{-1} A^\mathrm{T} \phi_B \tag{9.6}$$

This equation, in theory, has a unique solution if the columns of A are linearly independent (in effect, if the vectors which describe how each source location is related to all the measurement locations are not redundant). However, even in this case, $A^\mathrm{T} A$ is even more poorly conditioned than A, meaning that its inverse is even more challenging to obtain reliably. In the case that the number of measurements is less than the number of cardiac locations at which one desires to estimate the relevant parameters, (i.e., the matrix A is under-determined) there can be no unique solution. The most common strategy in this case is to find a solution that minimizes the Euclidean magnitude of the residual and is itself the shortest (in Euclidean length) of the infinite number of vectors that will achieve this minimum error. The "formula" for finding the solution is similar in spirit to (9.6). It too requires solving a very badly conditioned system of equations, which leads to the same problem as discussed in the framework of (9.6).

Thus, since the forward operator is ill-posed, a simple data fit by the minimization of the residual norm $\|A(x) - b\|_2^2$, for any of these formulations, leads to a (almost certainly) wildly erroneous inverse solution, with unrealistically large magnitudes, as illustrated in ❷ Fig. 9.1. To obtain a reasonable inverse solution, prior knowledge about the solution needs to be added to the problem formulation as a constraint or set of constraints. The difficulties in accomplishing this goal include identification of physiologically useful descriptions of such prior knowledge, of mathematically tractable ways of including them into the inverse problem, and of practical algorithmic approaches to solving the resulting constrained optimization problem.

The problem of determining x in (9.2) is an example of a rather general type of "inverse problem" that arises frequently in science and engineering. (For a more general treatment of inverse problems see one of the many good textbooks on the subject, for instance, Hansen [9] or Kaipio and Somersalo [10].) In inverse electrocardiography, as in other such inverse problems, common formulations fall into two categories. One is a deterministic framework, generally referred to as "regularization," in which an objective function to be minimized or a constraint function to be satisfied is composed of a combination of the norm of the residual error and some norm of a constraint function (or multiple constraint functions). The other category of formulation is a statistical framework, in which the solution is treated as random with an appropriate probability model, and a probabilistic error measure is minimized to find a likely solution.

Conceptually, deterministic regularization approaches can be summarized by two different ideas:

1. *Approximate the best-fit-to-data solution.* One or more spatial penalty functions acting on a candidate solution are defined, and then a weighted sum of these functions plus the residual norm is minimized. This approach is generally called Tikhonov regularization [9, 11, 12]. The penalty functions generally used constrain the magnitude of the inverse solution or its high spatial frequency content (often formulated via a first or second order spatial derivative). One can summarize the resulting formulation as:

$$\widehat{x}_\lambda = \operatorname{argmin}\{\|A(x) - b\|_2^2 + \lambda^2\|R(x)\|\}, \tag{9.7}$$

where R represents a "regularization operator" and λ is the regularization parameter whose value controls the level of regularization (i.e., the balance between the data fit and the amount of regularization). For a nonlinear operator A or nonlinear regularization operator R, nonlinear optimization methods are used to obtain the solution. For the linear cases, A and R become matrices and the Tikhonov solution simplifies to:

$$\widehat{x}_\lambda = (A^{\mathrm{T}}A + \lambda^2 R^{\mathrm{T}}R)^{-1}A^{\mathrm{T}}b \tag{9.8}$$

(or equivalently solving $(A^{\mathrm{T}}A + \lambda^2 R^{\mathrm{T}}R)x_\lambda = A^{\mathrm{T}}b$ by any appropriate algorithm).

2. *Approximate the forward operator.* In this approach, the forward operator A is approximated with an operator A_r that is "similar" to A in some well-defined sense, but much better conditioned. Formally, given A_r as some well-behaved approximation of A, one solves

$$\widehat{x}_r = \operatorname{argmin}\{\|A_r(x) - b\|_2^2\} \tag{9.9}$$

In the discrete linear case, the most common version of this approach is called the Truncated Singular Value Decomposition (TSVD) [9] (see the Appendix to ❷ Chap. 2 for a discussion of the Singular Value Decomposition)), and A_r is A_r, a well-conditioned low-rank least squares approximation to A.

We note that under quite general conditions the linear versions of these two approaches can be shown to be closely related, somewhat surprising given the difference in their conceptual underpinnings. We discuss this in more detail in what follows.

In statistical approaches x and n are considered as random vectors with given probability models. In particular, the probability model for x encodes our belief about how a reasonable, or physiological, solution should behave. The optimum Bayesian solution is the posterior mean of x [13], meaning that it is the statistical average, or expected value, of the random solution given the data and the probability models. Applications of this approach to inverse electrocardiography to date have tended to use a simplified version of this general model with the following assumptions:

1. A linear forward matrix A
2. Gaussian statistical models for both x and n

Under these assumptions, the Bayesian solution becomes identical to the maximum of the posterior probability distribution of x, given the measurements b, and this solution is commonly called the Maximum a Posteriori (MAP) solution. With non-Gaussian models, the MAP solution is the best linear mean square error solution for x, but not necessarily the optimum Bayesian solution [13].

Independent of the assumption of probability models, there are a number of ways one can treat the temporal variation of x statistically. For simplicity, we discuss the possibilities in the context of Gaussian distributions for both the unknowns and the noise, which means that we need only specify the mean and the covariance. The simplest and most widely used model assumes that each time instant is a vector drawn from a (second-order) stationary distribution; in the case of a Gaussian model, this means that a constant mean (almost always taken to be zero) and a fixed covariance matrix determine the model. One can also assume the covariance matrix to be fixed over time but let the mean be time-varying, or one can assume a constant mean but a general spatio-temporal covariance matrix, or one can let the mean vary in time and have a spatial-temporal covariance matrix as well. In any of the zero-mean cases, the MAP solution can be written as:

$$\widehat{x}_{\text{MAP}} = (A^{\text{T}} C_n^{-1} A + C_x^{-1})^{-1} A^{\text{T}} C_n^{-1} b, \tag{9.10}$$

where C_x and C_n are appropriate solution and noise covariance matrices, respectively.

If n is assumed to be white noise $(C_n = \sigma_n^2 I)$, the solution becomes:

$$\widehat{x}_{\text{MAP}} = (A^{\text{T}} A + \sigma_n^2 C_x^{-1})^{-1} A^{\text{T}} b \tag{9.11}$$

Comparing this result with (9.8), we note a parallel structure; the inverse of the solution covariance matrix plays the role of the regularization term $R^{\text{T}} R$ in the Tikhonov solution and the noise variance plays the role of the regularization parameter.

The relative strengths of the deterministic and statistical formulations lie in the ability to specify constraint functions R or statistical priors as determined by the covariance matrix C_x. We will see examples of how each has been used to capture and formulate relevant assumptions about realistic solutions and to then solve the resulting version of the inverse problem.

In the following sections we explicitly deal with the various types of inverse methods that arise from different measurement locations and source assumptions. We note that several acronyms have been presented in the contemporary literature to describe some of these methods, including NICE (Noninvasive functional source imaging [14, 15]), ECGI (electrocardiographic imaging [16, 17]) and 3DEIT (three-dimensional electrocardiography imaging technique [18]).

We also note that the previous edition of this chapter [19] described in excellent detail inverse approaches based on equivalent source models, and therefore we omit coverage of these methods. They are of limited relevance to current practical applications in the heart, although they remain the topic of great attention in the localization of focal electrical activity in the brain [20].

9.3   Potential-Based Inverse Solutions from Body Surface Measurements

In this section, we describe the conceptually most straightforward version of the inverse ECG problem – reconstructing potentials on the heart surface (denoted HSP in what follows) from measurements on the body surface. As is shown in ❷ Sect. 8.54, the forward transfer between these potentials can be expressed by a matrix equation (8.36). As already discussed, the nature of the matrix involved demands a more elaborate treatment than just an inversion.

We begin with the most common variant – reconstruction of epicardial potentials – and explain in more detail the two standard deterministic approaches outlined earlier: Tikhonov regularization and TSVD. We then describe some recent efforts to achieve more reliable and accurate solutions by incorporating more prior information through use of truncation of iterative matrix equation solutions, more complicated statistical models, multiple spatial regularization constraints, and constraints on temporal behavior. We then discuss two other potential-based source models to which inverse solutions have recently been applied: transmembrane potentials and then transmural potentials. From here on, we will use $\phi_H(x, t)$ to represent HSPs at positions x on the heart surface at time t, and similarly, $\phi_B(y, t)$ to represent the potential at positions y on the body surface.

By posing the inverse problem in terms of reconstructing heart surface potentials, the problem is linear and the resulting solution is theoretically unique [21]. However, as already noted, because the inverse problem is ill-posed, such a formulation is inherently unstable; even extremely low levels of signal noise or very small geometric errors can result in an unbounded solution. Hence, in order to stabilize the problem and to obtain a reasonable solution, it is necessary to incorporate further constraints before attempting to solve the equations. The need for constraints in epicardial solutions, graphically illustrated in ❯ Fig. 9.1, was first demonstrated by Martin and Pilkington [22] and later via singular-value decompositions of A [23, 24]. As discussed above, the most common and straightforward approach to this problem is via regularization of the inverse problem. A successful regularization procedure will yield a feasible solution that has useful properties in common with the exact solution of the underlying unperturbed problem. The main challenges in applying this approach are to determine both the type and the amount of regularization required to produce the desired solution. Regularization can be viewed as a procedure that imposes constraints on the solution, typically on its magnitude or smoothness. The goal is that these constraints relate to the underlying physiology or other known information about the solution.

Treating every individual column of the system in (9.5) independently and solving for each column, ϕ_B, to obtain the regularized solution, ϕ of (9.6), i.e., the heart potential $\phi_H(t)$

$$\phi_H = A_{\lambda_t}^{\dagger} \phi_B, \tag{9.12}$$

where $A_{\lambda_t}^{\dagger}$ is the regularized inverse matrix at time t (although the matrix A itself is time-invariant, its regularized inverse need not be). Next we describe in detail two of the most common specific approaches to generating the pseudo-inverse, both of which are widely used in cardiac applications.

9.3.1   Tikhonov Regularization

As stated earlier, the Tikhonov regularized solution is obtained by minimizing an appropriate objective function, i.e.,

$$\phi_H = \min \left[\|A\phi_H - \phi_B\|_2^2 + \lambda_t^2 \|R\phi_H\|_2^2 \right], \tag{9.13}$$

where R is an $N \times N$ constraint matrix and $\| \cdot \|_2$ is the Euclidean norm. The R term in (9.13) helps to constrain (or regularize) the inverse solution.

The first term in (9.13) represents the least-squares solution to each column of (9.5), while the second term constrains, in the spatial domain, the amplitude of the solution according to the choice of the particular constraint matrix R [25]. The constant λ_t is the *regularization parameter* at each time, t, which controls the weight given to the residual and solution norm and hence controls the degree of smoothing. The full solution is then a balance between the unconstrained least-squares solution and a set of constraints that in some way encapsulates a priori knowledge of a physiologically realistic solution.

There are three Tikhonov regularization constraints typically used in inverse electrocardiography, known in that literature as zero-order, first-order, and second-order Tikhonov regularization. Zero-order Tikhonov regularization uses $R = I$, the identity matrix, which effectively limits the total magnitude of the solution; first-order Tikhonov regularization uses $R = G$, a discrete approximation to the surface gradient operator, and limits the steepness of the solution; and the second-order Tikhonov method uses $R = L$, a discrete approximation to the surface Laplacian operator, to restrict the rate of change of the steepness, i.e., the overall nonsmoothness of the solution.

With the Tikhonov approach we can write a closed form solution for (9.13) that leads to an expression for the pseudo-inverse [26]

$$A_{\lambda_t}^{\dagger} = (A^{\mathrm{T}} A + \lambda_t^2 R^{\mathrm{T}} R)^{-1} A^{\mathrm{T}} \tag{9.14}$$

Messinger-Rapport and Rudy [27] studied regularizations of different orders by comparing analytic solutions in a spherical model [27]. Their results suggested that zero-order Tikhonov regularization performed as well as the higher-order schemes. Others have carried out similar studies comparing regularization on realistic geometries with dipole sources and found that second order Tikhonov performed best [28, 29]. It may be that the choice of the best Tikhonov regularizing function depends on the particular case and conditions.

Substituting (9.14) into (9.12), the solution for zero-order Tikhonov regularization becomes

$$\boldsymbol{\phi}_H = (\boldsymbol{A}^\mathrm{T}\boldsymbol{A} + \lambda_t^2 \boldsymbol{I})^{-1}\boldsymbol{A}^\mathrm{T}\boldsymbol{\phi}_B \tag{9.15}$$

9.3.2   Truncated SVD (TSVD)

As already described, another method of treating the ill-conditioned nature of the transfer matrix A is to derive a new problem with a well-conditioned *rank deficient* transfer matrix [26]. A common approach is to use the singular value decomposition (SVD) [30], a matrix factorization technique that is introduced in the Appendix of ❷ Chap. 2. From a singular value decomposition, one can determine the *principal components* of the information contained within a matrix [31]. If an SVD is applied to a transfer matrix A, then the transfer matrix can be written in the form

$$
\begin{aligned}
\boldsymbol{A} &= \boldsymbol{U}_A \boldsymbol{\Sigma}_A \boldsymbol{V}_A^\mathrm{T} \\
&= \sum_{i=1}^N \sigma_i \boldsymbol{u}_i \boldsymbol{v}_i^\mathrm{T}\text{,}
\end{aligned}
\tag{9.16}
$$

where $\boldsymbol{U}_A$ and $\boldsymbol{V}_A$ are orthogonal matrices (their columns are orthonormal) and diagonal matrix $\boldsymbol{\Sigma}_A$ contains as its diagonal entries the *singular values*, while $\boldsymbol{u}_i$ and $\boldsymbol{v}_i$ are the column vectors forming these orthogonal matrices and σ_i are the singular values for $i = 1, \ldots, N$. We assume in this case that the number of measurements, or the row-size of A, M is larger than the number of HSP reconstruction sites, or the column size of A, N. If $M < N$ some details change but the results are substantially the same. The singular values are greater than or equal to zero and are typically sorted in order of decreasing size. For a matrix representing an ill-posed process (as is the case here) the range of nonzero singular values covers many orders of magnitude. This large range of singular values is directly related to the noise amplification properties of the direct least squares solution.

The smaller singular values, the reciprocals of which are used in the least-squares inverse, will tend to magnify components in the data which lie in the subspace of their corresponding left singular vectors, while data components in the subspace of the singular vectors corresponding to the larger singular values are not amplified that dramatically. Thus, these "low singular value" components dominate the solution. Moreover, for forward solutions that smooth high frequencies, as in electrocardiography, those same singular vectors will also represent high frequencies and thus contain only highly attenuated information about the sources. As a consequence, the *relative* contribution of the noise to those components will be very large. The result is extreme noise amplification, as seen in our original example in ❷ Fig. 9.1.

To overcome this problem, the truncated SVD (TSVD) solution proposes to substitute for A a low rank approximation, which simply leaves out the modes with unstably small singular values, i.e., we replace A with

$$\boldsymbol{A}_{\lambda_t} = \sum_{n=1}^{\lambda_t} \sigma_{A(n)} \boldsymbol{u}_{A(n)}^\mathrm{T} \boldsymbol{v}_{A(n)} \qquad \lambda_t \le N, \tag{9.17}$$

where $\boldsymbol{u}_{A(n)}$ and $\boldsymbol{v}_{A(n)}$ are the nth vectors from the SVD of A, $\sigma_{A(n)}$ are their corresponding singular values, and N is the full rank of the matrix. The size of λ_t determines the level of regularization for time t (where λ_t is a positive integer). In the notation of (9.17), we wish to emphasize that the right singular vectors have the dimension of, and indeed are a basis for, the "data space," while the left singular vaectors have the dimension of, and indeed are a basis for, the "solution space." Thus below we denote the former as functions of $\boldsymbol{y}$ and the latter as functions of $\boldsymbol{x}$.

The TSVD solution is obtained by minimizing the objective function

$$\boldsymbol{\phi}_H = \min \|\boldsymbol{A}_{\lambda_t}\boldsymbol{\phi}_H - \boldsymbol{\phi}_B\| \tag{9.18}$$

The solution to this can be computed by means of the pseudo-inverse [26]

$$A^{\dagger}_{\lambda_t} = (A^{\mathrm{T}}_{\lambda_t} A_{\lambda_t})^{-1} A^{\mathrm{T}}_{\lambda_t} \tag{9.19}$$

The pseudo-inverse can be found easily from the SVD of A as

$$A^{\dagger}_{\lambda_t} = \tilde{V}_A \tilde{\Sigma}^{-1}_A \tilde{U}^{\mathrm{T}}_A, \tag{9.20}$$

where $\tilde{U}_A$ and $\tilde{V}_A$ contain the first λ_t columns of U_A and V_A respectively, and $\tilde{\Sigma}_A$ is a $\lambda_t \times \lambda_t$ diagonal submatrix of Σ_A. Substituting (9.20) into (9.12), the TSVD solution is

$$
\begin{aligned}
\phi_H &= \tilde{V}_A \tilde{\Sigma}^{-1}_A \tilde{U}^{\mathrm{T}}_A \, \phi_B \\
&= \sum_{n=1}^{\lambda_t} \frac{u^{\mathrm{T}}_{A(n)} \, \phi_B}{\sigma_{A(n)}} v_{A(n)}(x)
\end{aligned} \tag{9.21}
$$

It is useful to compare this TSVD solution with the zero-order Tikhonov solution given in (9.15). Expressing (9.15) in terms of the u and v components from the SVD of A we can write

$$
\begin{aligned}
\phi_H &= (A^{\mathrm{T}} A + \lambda_t^2 I)^{-1} A^{\mathrm{T}} \phi_B \\
&= \sum_{n=1}^{N} f_n(t) \frac{u^{\mathrm{T}}_{A(n)} \, \phi_B}{\sigma_{A(n)}} v_{A(n)}(t),
\end{aligned} \tag{9.22}
$$

where $f_n(t)$ are the Tikhonov *filter factors* given by

$$f_n(t) = \frac{\sigma^2_{A(n)}}{\sigma^2_{A(n)} + \lambda_t^2} \begin{cases} 1 & \sigma_{A(n)} \gg \lambda_t \\ \sigma^2_{A(n)}/\lambda_t^2 & \sigma_{A(n)} \ll \lambda_t \end{cases} \tag{9.23}$$

These filter factors have the effect of filtering out contributions to the reconstructed ϕ_H that correspond to the small singular values while leaving the SVD components corresponding to large singular values almost unaffected. Equation (9.21) is identical to (9.22) with the corresponding filter factors being equal to zero or one; the terms up to and including λ_t are included in the summation and have a filter factor of one while the remaining terms are zero. In other words, we use an effective λ which is zero for the singular vectors we retain and infinity for those we reject. In practice, the performance of TSVD regularization is often indistinguishable from that of zeroth-order Tikhonov regularization [32]. Thus, as mentioned above, despite the different conceptual basis for the two approaches, the resulting equations are closely connected. For higher-order Tikhonov regularization, and indeed for general regularization matrices, a similar analysis can be made via what is known as the Generalized SVD (GSVD); details can be found in Hansen [9].

9.3.3   Truncated Iterative Approaches

Truncated iterative methods are another deterministic approach to solving the inverse problem. In these methods, a sequence of candidate solutions is produced and each one is evaluated according to a "goodness" criterion: if the solution meets some threshold of accuracy, the iterations stop and otherwise they continue with additional candidate solutions. These approaches draw on the standard techniques for solving large linear systems of equations [30]. However, because such methods, like the unconstrained least-squares methods already described, will converge to unreliable solutions, the regularization approach is to truncate the iterations *before* convergence [9]. In this case, the number of iterations plays the role of a regularization parameter.

Iterative methods are especially favorable for large-scale problems for which direct regularization methods are computationally expensive, and in problems in which a matrix representation of the forward operator or an explicit representation of the inverse solution are not available. However, their use is not limited to these cases; they can be used as an alternative approach to direct regularization approaches. Most iterative methods can be represented in terms of filter factors such as those already discussed for Tikhonov and TSVD approaches [9], which demonstrates the similarity between iterative methods and direct methods in their filtering of the small singular values of the forward matrix. In regularized iterative methods, the solution converges to the lower frequency modes of the right singular vectors of A in the earlier iterations, and thus stopping the iteration filters out the effect of the otherwise amplified higher frequency modes.

The most commonly used iterative methods in this context are in the class of Krylov subspace methods, for which the connection between iteration number and modes of A is most clear. Brooks et al. [33] reported an early attempt to use this approach, in which the Conjugate Gradient (CG) iterative method was combined with regularization constraints. More recently, Ramanathan et al. [34] have reported using another Krylov subspace method, the Generalized Minimum Residual (GMRes) method, with significant success.

Reports suggest that the inverse solution reconstructed by the GMRes method was more accurate than the Tikhonov solution in terms of the pattern and localization of epicardial potentials [34]. No comparison was reported between the GMRes and CG methods. Also it was reported that in some cases the L-curve criterion, based on the condition number of a particular matrix, reflected a clear location at which to specify the regularization parameter, while the appropriate point on the L-curve for the Tikhonov approach was difficult to determine [34]. However, despite the strong empirical evidence supporting the GMRes approach, as well as the success of other initial results [33], as yet there is no theoretical justification to explain why this method reconstructs a localized solution better than Tikhonov regularization. We note that in both approaches, Tikhonov-type regularization was *combined* with the iterative regularization, either by iterating on a regularized (albeit under-regularized) set of equations [33] or by using the Tikhonov solution as the starting point for the iterative regularization [34].

9.3.4 Statistical Approaches

Although some of the original reports on inverse electrocardiography for epicardial potentials [35] were based on the statistical model in (9.10), the main challenge of this approach remains specifying the model (i.e., determining appropriate parameters of the mean and covariance of the desired solution and the noise). The simplest technique, which was adopted by these early investigators, is to assume that not only is the noise white and uncorrelated, as in (9.11), but that the *solution* has the same structure, with zero mean and variance σ_x^2. In this case the relevant equation becomes

$$\widehat{\boldsymbol{x}}_{\mathrm{MAP}} = \left(A^{\mathrm{T}} A + \frac{\sigma_n^2}{\sigma_x^2} I \right)^{-1} A^{\mathrm{T}} \boldsymbol{b} \tag{9.24}$$

This is the same as Tikhonov regularization with an identity matrix as the regularizer (i.e., Tikhonov zero-order) and with a statistical model for picking the regularization parameter. Since a good model for the variance of the unknown solution is hard to specify a priori, most of the research that followed these early reports concentrated on the deterministic regularization approaches described above.

However, in the late 1990s, van Oosterom, in a series of publications [36–38], re-introduced the idea of using this model with a more complicated and realistic covariance matrix. He showed that if one can in fact obtain even a reasonable approximation of the true covariance matrix (and assuming the time-invariant, statistically stationary, zero-mean model is valid), one can recover detail about the surface potentials more reliably and one is less sensitive to errors introduced by internal inhomogeneities such as the lungs. The key problem, of course, is how to obtain a useful, valid, and reasonably accurate statistical model of the cardiac sources. One approach, introduced in the context of estimation of activation times all over the heart from sparse catheter-based measurements [39], and then extended to the inverse problem [40–42], is to use previously recorded data to determine such a model. One version of this idea uses a "training database" of prior recordings of the sources, where available, to estimate a covariance matrix to be applied in the inverse solution. An additional enhancement is to use sparse catheter measurements to "tailor" this statistically derived result to an individual subject. The results, based on simulations using canine epicardial recordings, indicated that improvements in the inverse solutions are indeed possible using such an approach, if the necessary prior and catheter measurements can be acquired.

9.3.5 Multiple Spatial Regularization Operators

All of the traditional methods – Tikhonov regularization, TSVD, and the Tikhonov-equivalent "white Gaussian source" statistical model – have produced results that showed that it is indeed possible to recover meaningful information about cardiac surface potentials from body surface measurements. However, these results were neither precise nor reliable enough to be really attractive for potential clinical or even scientific use. An example of these limitations can be seen in ❯ Fig. 9.1; the Tikhonov solution shown there, although certainly orders of magnitude improved over the unconstrained solution, is both rather noisy and overly smooth, in the sense that it cannot match the rapid downward deflection of activation in the original electrogram. The next few subsections discuss various ideas introduced to try to improve the accuracy and reliability of inverse reconstructions. One approach that has shown some success is to combine two distinct types of regularization. For instance, TSVD and Tikhonov regularization were used together in Shahidi et al. [43], and we have already mentioned two approaches which combined Tikhonov-type regularization with truncated iterative regularization.

Another approach starts from the observation that if the problem is that we need constraints to improve inverse solutions because the measurements contain insufficient information in themselves, one can consider the possibility of using more than one constraint at the same time. This approach, in the context of simply extending the Tikhonov formalism to more than one constraint, has been applied to inverse electrocardiography using both Tikhonov zero-order and Tikhonov second-order regularizers [44]. The results were reported to be somewhat improved, and in particular were more robust to the exact choice of regularization parameters. (Here, with multiple constraints, one needs multiple regularization parameters as well.) This approach had its difficulties, however, in particular in picking a good set of regularization parameters without undue computational burden, and this problem gets dramatically worse if the number of constraints increases beyond two. At the same time, it was not clear that any particular pair of constraints contained the most useful information for reconstructions.

Ahmad et al. [45] proposed a method that flexibly allows the inclusion of more than two constraints, as well as constraints that do not lend themselves mathematically to easy treatment in the Tikhonov framework. This approach, which had seen significant use in the formally related problem of image restoration, consists in considering the desired solution as a single "point" in some space of possible inverse solutions. Then each constraint, including the constraint that the solution must correspond reasonably well to the measurement data after application of the forward model, can be treated as a constraint set in this solution space. Reasonable – technically, feasible or admissible – solutions would lie inside each constraint set, and only infeasible solutions lie outside it. For example, if we believe that a good solution should have a residual error below some reasonable value, then the corresponding "constraint set" is all solutions that indeed have a residual error less than that value. If the constraint is that the 2-norm of the solution, or its gradient, is below some value, then the constraint set is all solutions for which this is true.

One can easily devise constraints that are somewhat less mathematically simple, for instance bounds on the maximum, or minimum, or some norm other than 2, of the solution or of some spatial derivative of the solution, or even any such constraint applied only to one or several subregions. Moreover, given any number of such constraints, all admissible solutions will lie in the *intersection* of all the constraint sets. It turns out that, if the constraints can all be described by convex functions (a class that includes all the examples given above), one can apply any of a large number of convex optimization algorithms to find a feasible solution. Note that in this approach, the optimization algorithm is stopped as soon as one finds a solution that matches all the constraints, before converging to an "optimal" solution – similar in spirit to the way in which the iterative Krylov-subspace linear system solvers like CG or GMRes are truncated when dealing with ill-posed problems. The application of this approach to inverse electrocardiography, using one such convex optimization algorithm called the ellipsoid algorithm, has shown encouraging results [45]. However, again there was no clear set of constraints on the potentials that emerged as giving the level of accuracy and reliability required.

9.3.6 Spatio-Temporal Approaches

As mentioned in the introduction to this chapter, the temporal behavior of cardiac electrical signals is known to have a strong deterministic, hence at least partially predictable, component. It would make sense to make use of this strong prior knowledge to constrain solutions over multiple time instants. One approach along these lines involves parameterizing the sources by means of fiducial time parameters, and we discuss such approaches at some length in the following section. With potential-based methods, the temporal behavior of the source, if it can be effectively captured in a constraint, would also seem to be a powerful tool in the inverse solution toolbox.

In fact, from a statistical standpoint, it is commonplace in the fields of statistical signal processing and estimation theory that, if the quantities in (9.10) are taken as potentials at single time instants, the solution is optimal only if the desired heart surface potentials are temporally uncorrelated [46]; otherwise their temporal correlation must be included in the estimation equation. In fact, algorithms commonly used in devices such as modems and cell phones make use of the so-called Viterbi algorithm for Maximum-Likelihood Sequence Estimation that exploits exactly this fact. It should be clear from the earlier chapters in this book that any reasonable model for cardiac sources will be far from temporally uncorrelated, and thus it is not surprising that inverse electrocardiography algorithms have been introduced to take advantage of models of expected temporal behavior.

We first treat extensions of the heart surface potential (HSP) inverse solution formulation described earlier to include temporal or spatio-temporal constraints. We then discuss a relatively new approach that replaces the heart surface model with a transmembrane potential (TMP) model. Based on this model, temporal constraints that are a reasonable approximation of TMP temporal behavior can be applied; the hoped-for advantage is that TMP temporal behavior may lend itself to simpler, more effective and useful, constraints.

9.3.6.1   Spatio-Temporal Constraints with Heart Surface Potential Models

Some of the earliest work in this field used a simple On–Off model to incorporate temporal information [47], but this was not pursued as the importance of various factors such as regularization constraints and parameters and the development of appropriate validation models took precedence. In the late 1980s researchers began to consider again the use of temporal behavior, first in the sense of temporal correlation via a frequency-domain approach [48], and then, in research that had significant historical impact on the field, in a direct regularization framework, by simply adding a temporal constraint after an initial Tikhonov solution [49]. This latter method penalized subsequent time instants for changing too dramatically from the preceding one, by constraining the Euclidean norm of the difference between them as a regularization (generally referred to in the inverse electrocardiography literature as Twomey regularization). Formally, (9.8), with a linear model and linear regularization constraint, becomes:

$$\widehat{\boldsymbol{x}}_\lambda = \operatorname{argmin}\{\|\boldsymbol{Ax} - \boldsymbol{b}\|_2^2 + \lambda^2 \|\boldsymbol{R}(\boldsymbol{x} - \boldsymbol{x}_0)\|\}, \tag{9.25}$$

where $\boldsymbol{x}_0$ represents an initial estimate of the solution, as for instance the estimated value of $\boldsymbol{x}$ at a previous time instant. Thus this approach requires an initial estimate of the solution; the quality of the resulting inverse solution was shown to depend on the quality of this estimate, and the final solution is therefore biased towards it [49].

Starting from this approach, several alternative methods were introduced that attempted to *combine* spatial and temporal constraints into a true spatio-temporal regularization method. The three methods that had the most success were:

1. A method that added a temporal constraint to one (or more) spatial constraint(s) [44],
2. A method that added an equation containing an explicit model of temporal evolution of the potentials to the standard forward problem equation (which models the spatial relation between potentials on two different surfaces), with the pair of equations formulated as a state-space model and solved via a Kalman filter or smoother [50, 51], and
3. A method introduced and developed primarily by Greensite and Huiskamp which attempted to simultaneously regularize in time and space by finding a temporal whitening transform according to a statistically informed assumption [52, 53].

The initial version of the method was presented in a specific variant with a heuristic justification that Greensite has since developed into a more general and theoretically based formulation using an assumption he called "isotropy"; here we start with the latter and then include a detailed description of the specific earlier implementation, which has seen the most use in practice. Indeed this earlier method has become perhaps the most widely accepted for reconstruction of potentials by inverse electrocardiography, used, for example, by groups such as those in Innsbruck and Auckland, who have reported significant success with it [54–56].

Initially, it appeared that these were three distinct methods with no clear connection or comparison among them except in terms of exemplary results. We note that the paper describing the first method did show that the method in Oster and Rudy [49] was a one-step simplified version of an iterative solution to the full multiple regularization method. However, recently it has been shown that in fact all the three of these methods can be cast into the same statistical framework [57]. We outline this framework here, leaving the details to the literature, and then proceed to describe in some detail the popular implementation of Greensite's method. The key to unifying these approaches is to consider (9.11) with the quantities defined as in (9.3) and (9.4); the vectors are all block vectors concatenating the spatial distribution of the potentials across all time instants, and A is a block diagonal matrix with the forward solution matrix repeated on the diagonal blocks. We employ the statistical model described earlier in which both the noise and the unknown signals are assumed to be zero-mean, and the noise is assumed to be white as noted, here in both space and time. In this case the key quantity that governs the solution is the spatio-temporal covariance matrix C_x, or equivalently, its inverse:

$$C_x = E\{xx^T\} = E\left\{ \begin{bmatrix} x(t_0) \\ x(t_0+1) \\ \vdots \\ x(t_n) \end{bmatrix} \begin{bmatrix} x(t_0)^T & x(t_0+1)^T & \cdots & x(t_n^T) \end{bmatrix} \right\}, \tag{9.26}$$

where $E\{\cdot\}$ represents statistical expectation. Thus, in the spatio-temporal formulation, C_x is a *spatio-temporal* covariance matrix which can be divided into blocks of the form $E\{x(t_i)x(t_j)^T\}$; the dimension of each block is the number of nodes used on the heart surface; the number of blocks (in both directions) is equal to the number of time instants; and each block is a spatial cross-covariance matrix at different time instants (except for the diagonal blocks which are spatial covariances at the same time instant). The temporal covariance is embedded in the variation from block to block across the matrix, as indexed by the difference (or time lag) between t_i and t_j.

Considering this formulation, two significant problems arise:

1. How can one derive or estimate the parameters required to populate this matrix (or its inverse, since the inverse covariance plays the role of regularization constraint matrix)?
2. How can one handle the dramatic increase in computational requirements stemming from the fact that the matrices now have dimensions on each side that are equal to the number of spatial nodes on the relevant surface multiplied by the number of time instants considered?

Each of the three methods introduced separately – multiple regularization, Kalman filtering, and isotropy – solves exactly this same pair of problems, but in different ways, based on different assumptions. Each assumption, and its resulting formulation, turns out to impose a particular structure on C_x or its inverse, which then leads to a specific algorithm or set of algorithms. Here we briefly describe the simplest form of the approach taken in each method; for details see Zhang et al. [57].

1. *Multiple regularization.* In this approach one assumes that we can build separate constraints for the spatial behavior (typically a standard constraint on the norm of the solution or its derivative, effectively a spatial high-pass filter) and for the temporal behavior (again typically a high-pass temporal filter, based on the idea that potentials do not change dramatically from one sample time instant to the next). When formulated in terms of statistical regularization, such assumptions impose a particular structure on the inverse of the spatio-temporal covariance matrix, as the sum of two block matrices; one is a block diagonal matrix, which contains the spatial regularization constraints, and the other is a block matrix that has all its blocks restricted to be themselves diagonal matrices, and that enforces the temporal regularization constraint. A consequence of this structure is that fast algorithms can be developed which reduce the computational complexity down to the order of the number of nodes in the heart surface model [44].
2. *State-space model.* In this approach, the spatial distribution of potentials at each time instant is modeled by a prediction or temporal evolution equation, in which the potentials from each time instant evolve from the previous time by applying a known prediction matrix plus a random perturbation. For example, imposing an identity prediction matrix assumes that the potentials do not change rapidly from one time sample to the next (a random walk model). More general models, which take into account, for instance, the behavior of neighboring nodes, can easily be employed.

One consequence of these assumptions is that the resulting structure of the spatio-temporal covariance matrix shows a kind of block exponential decay (for a stable model) across the blocks. More importantly, the *inverse* covariance matrix has a block tri-diagonal structure; in other words, regularization is applied only between adjacent time instants in this model. The computational consequence of this simple structure is in fact the Kalman filter/smoother algorithm, and thus, a reduction in computational complexity is achieved.

3. *Isotropy model.* One consequence of the assumption of isotropy, which Greensite frames as a kind of invariance to unknown prior information for the case in which one has no useful model of the temporal behavior, is what in statistical terms is known as *separability* between the spatial and temporal correlation. The effect on the structure of the inverse covariance matrix is that all blocks (that is, the spatial cross-covariance matrices) are exactly the same except for a scalar multiplication; the set of scalars needed to relate all the blocks contains the information about the temporal covariance. Mathematically, this assumption means that the spatio-temporal covariance matrix can be factored as the Kronecker product of a single spatial covariance matrix by a single temporal covariance matrix. As a further consequence of this assumption, the temporal covariance of the *heart* surface potentials is identical to within a scalar to that of the *body* surface potentials. This assumption suggests the following algorithm:

(a) Estimate the temporal covariance matrix of the body surface potentials directly from the data.
(b) Find the SVD of this matrix; its right singular vectors can be used to decorrelate, or whiten, the entire problem, by a simple matrix multiplication.
(c) Once the problem has been so whitened, it is optimal to solve it column by column (in effect, "time-instant" by "time-instant" in the new "temporal" coordinate system induced by the decorrelation). Spatial regularization is still required and can be done by any relevant method, including Tikhonov regularization or TSVD. We discuss this last point in more detail in the following section.
(d) Once the column-by-column solutions are complete, "re-correlate" by multiplying by the transpose of the decorrelating matrix. Since this matrix comes from the SVD and is therefore orthogonal, the optimality of the solution is preserved.

As should be clear, this algorithm, since it does its primary work on a column-by-column basis, again reduces the computational complexity to the order of the spatial dimension.

As discussed in Zhang et al. [57], each of these methods has its advantages and limitations. The multiple regularization approach gives the designer great freedom in choosing regularizers, but requires considerable prior knowledge to make good choices. Moreover, one cannot consider nearby (or, in fact, any other) spatial nodes when regularizing in time without incurring a dramatic increase in computational complexity. The state-space model gives even more flexibility in the design of the temporal model, and indeed, this model has a very direct physical or physiological interpretation as the expected temporal progression of the solution. Moreover it opens access to a truly vast literature of modeling and solution methods – the literature on Kalman estimation algorithms [e.g. 46, 58, 59]. However, it does depend on an effective prior knowledge of this evolution, and most applications of this method to inverse electrocardiography have simply used the random walk approach. In addition, it does not allow one to directly consider more than one previous time instant in predicting the next time instant, again unless one is willing to increase the computational order and the modeling complexity.

The isotropy/separability method has the significant attraction that one does not need to model or make any further explicit assumptions on the temporal behavior; the required parameters are in the temporal correlation matrix of the body surface potentials, which can be directly estimated out of the measurements. However, the underlying assumption of isotropy, or separability, is difficult to interpret in physical or physiological terms, and it is not yet clear how one can verify or test its accuracy. Moreover, the assumption rests on the idea that one knows nothing about the expected temporal behavior of the solution. If, in fact, one has some prior knowledge, it is not clear if or how one might incorporate that knowledge into this approach. Nonetheless, as already noted, not only the original authors of this method but also independent groups have reported success with it in several settings.

There is one key aspect of the isotropy method, which is critical to its performance, and which indeed was incorporated explicitly in the original, less general, version of the method in Greensite [60]. After the decorrelating transform achieved by multiplication of the data by the right singular vectors of the data matrix, one has exchanged the original set of L equations, where L is the number of time instants used, for a new set of L equations. As mentioned earlier, each of these equations still involves the badly conditioned forward matrix A and thus still needs to be (spatially) regularized. If one uses a standard method to find an appropriate regularization parameter for each equation, as for instance the L-curve method described in the following section, and then solves all L equations, the results are dominated by noise and are not useful. This is true because the new set of equations has its own set of "singular values" in the transformed domain, which are unknown even under the isotropy assumption (in effect, they are known for the data matrix but not for the "solution matrix," and these two sets of singular values differ). Therefore, one must find a way to "truncate" this process, only solving the set of equations that contain reliable information, because they correspond to the relatively large singular values of the unknown solution matrix. As we describe in the following section, the original version of this spatio-temporal approach, as introduced by Greensite [60] before the isotropy theory was developed, included an ad hoc method for exactly this truncation, via a kind of "double TSVD," which uses an SVD of the data matrix to determine which equations to solve, and an SVD of A to regularize each of those solutions.

We now proceed to a detailed description of the version of the isotropy method generally used in practice. One starts by performing an SVD of the torso surface signal data matrix Φ_B, where Φ_B is a specific variant of the matrix B in (9.5) which stores the signal information in its rows and the potentials at each time instant in its columns, to determine its principal components. The result of this process is a factorization of Φ_B into a matrix of spatial singular vectors (U_B) and temporal singular vectors (V_B). The idea that will be exploited here is that, because of the spatial smoothing and attenuation, only a relatively small number of time signals can represent almost all the information in this data matrix; the rest of these components are dominated by noise.

Indeed, one could, "filter" the data matrix to remove the noise-dominated components before attempting an inversion – even if one ignored any other spatio-temporal constraints, this might improve the results. We note that this relatively low-dimensionality of the torso data has been known, and used, for a long time – in the early 1980s Lux et al. published a series of papers on the use of the principal component method, or Karhunen-Loeve transform, for compression and data reduction of body surface potential maps [61, 62], which indeed used exactly the same principle for temporal compression as the one described here.

Specifically, the columns of U_B and V_B corresponding to small singular values are assumed to correspond to noise-dominated signals and are typically removed [63]. A determination of which singular values correspond to this "noise subspace" can be estimated in a somewhat ad hoc fashion by plotting the log of the ordered singular values against the rank of the matrix obtained from the appropriate subsets of these singular values [64]. This typically results in a characteristic 'L' shaped curve as shown in ❯ Fig. 9.3. It has been postulated that the singular values below the point at which the curve

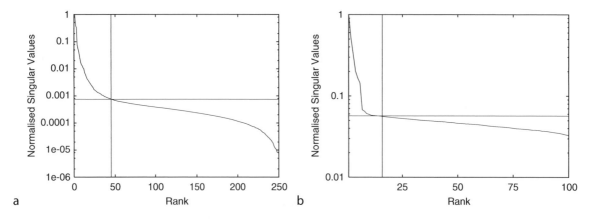

a   b

◼ **Fig. 9.3**

Singular value spectra of two different torso surface signal matrices. In panel (a) are the singular values from a signal matrix recorded from a normal male volunteer and in (b) signals from a simulated cardiac source. The singular values have been normalized and plotted on a log scale to emphasize the curvature in their values. The lower right quadrant (as defined by the *vertical and horizontal lines*) corresponds to the ranks and singular values which have been considered to correspond to noise, and the upper left quadrant those which have been considered as "signal"

levels off correspond to the noise subspace [63]. A number of different methods have been used for determining the best place to locate this leveling off point, including the Akaike Information Criterion [65] and the point of steepest curvature. However, none of these has been found to be truly reliable in practice [66].

The key idea of this version of the isotropy method is not to simply filter the data, as shown, but rather to combine this filtering with regularization. To start, we write the SVD expansion of the matrix of torso potentials matrix as

$$\boldsymbol{\Phi}_B = \boldsymbol{U}_B \boldsymbol{\Sigma}_B \boldsymbol{V}_B^\mathsf{T}, \tag{9.27}$$

where $\boldsymbol{U}_B$ is an $M \times N_e$ matrix that represents the spatial basis, $\boldsymbol{\Sigma}_B$ is an $N_e \times N_e$ matrix with the singular values stored on the diagonal, $\boldsymbol{V}_B$ is an $N_e \times N_e$ matrix that represents the temporal basis, and $N_e = \min(M, L)$ where M is the number of recording electrodes on the body surface and L is the number of time samples recorded. We assume once more that the number of measurement locations is greater than the number of nodes on the HSP model, that is, that $M \geq N$. If this is not the case, once again minor changes are required but the procedure is essentially the same. Inserting (9.27) into (9.12) leads to

$$\boldsymbol{\Phi}_H = \boldsymbol{A}_{\lambda_t}^\dagger \boldsymbol{\Phi}_B$$
$$= \boldsymbol{A}_{\lambda_t}^\dagger \boldsymbol{U}_B \boldsymbol{\Sigma}_B \boldsymbol{V}_B^\mathsf{T} \tag{9.28}$$

Multiplying on the right by $\boldsymbol{V}_B$, which is what the isotropy assumption would lead to as the optimal decorrelating transform, leads to

$$\boldsymbol{\Phi}_H \boldsymbol{V}_B = \boldsymbol{A}_{\lambda_t}^\dagger \boldsymbol{\Phi}_B \boldsymbol{V}_B$$
$$= \boldsymbol{A}_{\lambda_t}^\dagger \boldsymbol{U}_B \boldsymbol{\Sigma}_B \boldsymbol{V}_B^\mathsf{T} \boldsymbol{V}_B = \boldsymbol{A}_{\lambda_t}^\dagger \boldsymbol{U}_B \boldsymbol{\Sigma}_B \tag{9.29}$$

because of the orthogonality of the matrix $\boldsymbol{V}_B$.

Next, we define

$$\boldsymbol{\Gamma} = \boldsymbol{\Phi}_H \boldsymbol{V}_B \tag{9.30}$$

and proceed by solving $\boldsymbol{\Gamma}$ from

$$\boldsymbol{\Gamma} = \boldsymbol{A}_{\lambda_t}^\dagger \boldsymbol{U}_B \boldsymbol{\Sigma}_B \tag{9.31}$$

This problem is tackled for each column vector $\boldsymbol{\gamma}_i$ of $\boldsymbol{\Gamma}$, paired to each column vector i of matrix $[\boldsymbol{U}_B \boldsymbol{\Sigma}_B]$, with $i = 1, \cdots, N_e$.

We use the "noise subspace" method already described, which permits the selection of regularization parameters for each value of i in any type of pseudo-inverse (e.g., Tikhonov or TSVD) selected. The amount of regularization used for each of the paired columns can be determined using the methods described in ❷ Sect. 9.6.

The solution to (9.27) is then found from

$$\boldsymbol{\Phi}_H = \boldsymbol{\Gamma} \boldsymbol{V}_B^\mathsf{T} \tag{9.32}$$

Note that only the columns of $\boldsymbol{\Gamma}$ deemed significant by testing the singular values of the data matrix are used.

Two recent attempts to incorporate spatio-temporal constraints in the context of wavefront propagation were reported in Ghodrati [67]. The first used the Kalman state-estimation formalism in the context of a constraint based on wavefront propagation. This work, which in principle is like the activation-based methods in that it considers the arrival time of the wavefront at each point on the surface as the unknown values to reconstruct, uses a nonlinear state evolution model built on phenomenological study of canine epicardial data, along with fiber directions drawn from the Auckland heart, to propagate the wavefront on the epicardial surface. A second model, also built from a study of canine epicardial data [189], maps the wavefront location to a potential distribution; the latter is then used with a standard forward matrix to relate the wavefront location at any time instant to the body surface potential measurements. The second approach uses a regularization constraint based on a nonlinear mapping of the previous time instant solution to a wavefront-based model; this constraint is then used in a standard Tikhonov solution to calculate the solution at the current time instant. Both methods were reported to show a significantly improved localization and extent of reconstructed wavefronts in simulations with cardiac data.

9.3.6.2   Spatio-Temporal Constraints with Surface Transmembrane Potential Models

As described in ❯ Chap. 7, transmembrane potentials can also be used as the source strength of a double layer (EDL) upon which an appropriate forward model, and thus a corresponding inverse model, can be formulated. As discussed there, the tractability of this model is greatly improved if one makes simplifying assumptions about homogeneity and isotropy of cardiac conduction. These assumptions are the basis for most activation-based inverse solutions, as described below in ❯ Sect. 9.4, which have been under development since the 1980s. However, more recently there has been interest in the development of *potential-based* TMP models. In these models, the forward solution employed is one that maps the TMPs directly to the body surface potentials. TMPs have some conceptual and practical disadvantages compared with HSPs; for example, they require additional isotropy and homogeneity assumptions, and are only guaranteed to be unique (even in theory) if these assumptions hold. In addition, TMPs are more difficult to measure directly in experimental settings, especially for purposes of validation of inverse solutions. In the context of activation-based solutions, as we will see, they have the very important advantage of directly imposing the dominating spatio-temporal constraint, and of the propagating nature of the activation wavefront for QRS reconstructions. These advantages also apply to the reconstruction of repolarization activity.

One effect of the constraints used in activation-based methods is that the height of the jump and the shape of the profile across the wavefront must be constant across the surface, which translates to constant height and constant shape of the action potential, and in particular, of the "phase 0" transition. In an attempt to relax this restriction, Messnarz et al. [54] recently introduced a TMP-based inverse solution. The goal was to achieve some of the flexibility of HSP-based solutions while imposing a physiologically-based constraint based on expected TMP behavior. The specific formulation they employed constrained the TMPs to become progressively more positive over time – i.e., be monotonically nondecreasing, or equivalently have a nonnegative temporal derivative – during the activation (QRS) interval. From a potential-based inverse problem point of view, the idea is that the shape of the TMP is generally much simpler than that of an electrogram and thus lends itself to a simple yet powerful (and physiologically meaningful) constraint such as the one just described.

The formulation of the inverse problem in Messnarz et al. [54] was quite similar to that for the other spatio-temporal models described earlier; the time samples of interest were concatenated into block vectors and the forward matrix became a block diagonal matrix with A on all its blocks (as per (9.4) and (9.5)). A spatial regularization term was used with a Laplacian regularizer, the same way that spatial regularization was accomplished by Brooks et al. [44] in the multiple regularization context, which fits perfectly into the block structure. Imposing the temporal constraint, however, required a matrix inequality constraint, in which the temporal derivative of the solution was approximated via a simple difference operator written as a large, sparse matrix (again similar to the way Brooks et al. [44] applied a high-pass temporal filter). However, instead of simply adding this as a second regularization constraint, it was necessary to enforce the condition that all elements of the vector of temporal derivatives, over all time instants, were nonnegative. Thus, the problem became one of minimizing the spatially regularized residual error, subject to the constraint that the side term, the temporal derivative vector, had all nonnegative elements. This problem falls into the class of convex optimization problems, in which the *forward problem* is linear and the constraint imposed in the inverse problem is nonlinear but convex. Given the relatively simple form of this convex optimization, Messnarz et al. were able to employ a standard version of the interior point optimization approach, an algorithm known as MOSEK [68], rather than the more general ellipsoid algorithm used previously in the truncated convex optimization approach [45] described above. To validate their approach, Messnarz et al. [54] used simulations of normal and abnormal hearts and compared results with standard Tikhonov spatial regularization of the single time instant TMP problem. No attempt was made to use spatiotemporal regularization of any kind with the Tikhonov method, although the authors did impose minimum and maximum amplitude constraints (−90 and +10 mV) on the reconstructed potentials. Results indicated that the method was able to recover important aspects of propagation for both the normal and abnormal hearts more accurately than single-time instant reconstruction of the TMPs.

In a second report, Messnarz et al. [2] explored from both a mathematical and (numerical) experimental viewpoint a direct comparison between the HSP model (using a combined epi/endocardial surface) and their TMP model. The mathematical approach involved examining the numerical null-spaces of the forward problems for the two methods. The numerical null-space is the space of possible source behaviors that are seen so weakly in the body surface potentials that they are below the measurement noise level. There is a nontrivial null-space of this sort for all complete inverse electrocardiography formulations because of the attenuation and smoothing that makes the problem ill-posed. Messnarz et al. [2] compared the null-spaces and their complements, and the signal-spaces (technically the row spaces), of their implementation of the two (HSP and TMP) forward problems. They showed that the information present in the measurements was insufficient to reconstruct the HSPs or TMPs accurately, confirming the need, widely accepted in the field, to find regularization methods that can "restore" the null-space components. Note that Tikhonov methods do reconstruct some null-space components, while TSVD methods do not. Interestingly, the HSP forward model was somewhat better conditioned than the TMP forward model. The authors suggested that this was due to differences in the uniqueness properties of the HSPs compared with the TMPs. An alternative explanation might be that the HSPs are simply smoother than the TMPs; thus the forward problem from HSP to body surface involves less (additional) smoothing than the forward problem from TMPs to body surface, and hence may be better conditioned. Numerical experiments carried out using the same simulated measurement data for both methods showed that the TMP model produced more accurate reconstructions of activation times, especially on the endocardium. The HSP reconstruction method used was the "truncated isotropy" spatio-temporal regularization method introduced by Greensite and Huiskamp described in detail earlier. The authors attribute the superiority of the TMP reconstructions to what they hypothesize is the ability of the TMP non-decreasing-in-time constraint to better add physiologically correct null-space components to the reconstruction, compared with the isotropy/separability assumption used in the HSP reconstruction. No results were included on the actual null-space components of the HSPs or TMPs themselves, and thus no direct evaluation and analysis of the presumed better reconstruction of these null-space components were reported.

9.3.7   Imaging Transmural Potentials

The inverse methods described earlier attempt to reconstruct electrical activity on the epi- and/or endocardial surfaces of the heart. There have also been a few recent attempts to noninvasively image cardiac electrical activity *within* the myocardial wall [55, 69]. This problem is even more difficult than that of imaging surface electrical activity, as it is less constrained and hence more likely to yield nonunique solutions.

The basic approach used in this type of inverse problem starts with a forward model that incorporates a description of the three-dimensional myocardium. These forward models are designed to simulate surface electrograms that originate from within the myocardium. As discussed earlier, on a time-instant by time-instant basis such models are clearly not unique, and even with temporal constraints included a reasonable question to ask is whether such source models result in a unique inverse solutions for the myocardium. To our knowledge, this question has not been addressed in the literature.

In one approach, He et al. [69] proposed a cellular automata solution procedure based on predefined transmembrane potential descriptions (❷ Sect. 8.4.2). This model required only an initial site (or sites) of activity to be specified to generate a full potential description on the torso surface. The inverse problem was then formulated as an optimization problem in which one minimizes the average correlation covariance between the measured and simulated body surface potentials by altering the initial site (or sites) of myocardial electrical activity used in the forward model. The solution must also satisfy two heuristically designed constraints based on the position of the minima of the body surface potentials and the number of body recording leads whose potentials are less than a certain negative threshold. These extra constraints are justified by the presumed relation of the position of the minima on the body surface with the origin of the activation in the heart (in recent work from the same group [70], these two constraints were replaced by the averaged relative error between the measured and simulated body surface potentials). For this procedure to be computationally feasible, the size of the initial activation sites are generally taken to be significantly larger than the elements of the computational mesh. Once the optimization process has converged, one obtains a representation of the transmembrane potentials everywhere within and on the myocardium. However, we note that these transmembrane potentials are obtained by using a model with predetermined parameters and might not present a good estimate of the true transmembrane potentials; thus, this approach in some senses is more similar to a fiducial-time based imaging method than to a potential-based one.

We also note that this approach applies a very strict spatial-temporal constraint on the solution behavior, since the cellular automata model parameters depend on the physiological properties of the heart. However, these parameters may vary from one heart to another, and from a normal heart to a diseased one. Therefore, these predefined parameters of the cellular automata model may produce a model error whose effect has not yet been addressed in the literature. A possible solution to this problem might be to reconstruct more parameters of the cellular automata model from the body surface measurements rather than just reconstructing the site of origin of activation.

Skipa et al. [55] reported on another approach to reconstructing the transmural activity of the heart, in which they described the electrical sources in the heart by three-dimensional patches of transmembrane voltage. A linear forward model, obtained by using FEM, related the transmembrane voltages in the heart volume to the body surface potentials, taking into consideration the anisotropic properties of the myocardium. For the inverse problem, Tikhonov zero and second order regularization were used while temporal information was incorporated using the Greensite method. However, the simulation results obtained by this approach did not deliver a meaningful solution for the nodes inside the cardiac wall, while the transmembrane voltages on the epicardial surface were comparable to reconstructions obtained using an epicardial potential source model [71]. We emphasize again that to our knowledge, no discussion about the uniqueness of the myocardial inverse solution has been offered for this approach.

9.4   Fiducial-Time Based Inverse Algorithms

In HSP and TMP methods, the potentials at each point in space and time are essentially free variables in the reconstruction; thus, strong explicit constraints are required to achieve useful solutions, and as we have seen, it is not a trivial matter to find constraints that both capture relevant physiology (and thus produce physiologically accurate, meaningful, and reliable solutions) and are mathematically tractable. Another general approach to the inverse electrocardiography problem starts from almost the other extreme; it imposes very strong physiologically based constraints in the source model itself and reduces the number of free parameters. The basic idea is to focus on reconstructing the time of activation at each point in space on the epicardial and endocardial surfaces (a complementary formulation also exists for finding recovery time). A separate benefit of this approach is that from a physiological standpoint, activation times are the most clinically relevant aspect of cardiac electrical activity; although they can be derived from a potential-based reconstruction (e.g., by finding extrema of temporal derivatives), it is simpler to reconstruct them directly. But perhaps more importantly, from an inverse problems perspective, this formulation becomes much better constrained; instead of needing to reconstruct an entire time series at each surface location, we only need to reconstruct one number at each location to capture the entire heartbeat. Of course, if there is relevant information in other aspects of electrical activity (for example, variation in the height of the wavefront or the location and behavior of the maxima that typically precede it early in activation and that are related to depth in the wall of an ectopic focus [72]), we cannot reconstruct it with such a restricted source model. But the advantage of greatly reduced complexity on the source model, especially when achieved with such a physiologically motivated parameterization, holds great promise for a more robust, accurate, and meaningful solution. One particular advantage that one could hope for from such an approach is greater robustness to errors in the geometry of the forward model; put simply, because the space of the solution is so much smaller, the effects of ill-conditioning are lessened and we can consequently expect to be less sensitive to model error in particular. In addition, from a physiological perspective, the potentials are sensitive to loading effects of the torso volume conductivities, while the activation sequence is not; this adds even greater robustness to this approach.

The main drawback of the activation time imaging formulation is that the forward problem, which now maps activation times to body surface potentials, is nonlinear. For example, adding two vectors of activation times together (for example simply delaying activation in time by making one of the vectors have identical elements) will not produce the sum of the body surface potentials due to each of these sets of activation times. Hence, nonlinear optimization algorithms must be used to solve the inverse problem for the set of activation times that best fits the body surface data. Although somewhat more robust to errors in the input, the problem is still ill-posed and requires regularization. Nonlinear, ill-posed problems are notoriously difficult to solve in general and the same has proved true in this case. In particular, experience has shown that results can be very sensitive to the starting point for these nonlinear optimizations; presumably there are multiple minima in the objective function, even with a regularization term added.

The original papers in this area came from a group in Nijmegen, The Netherlands, in the 1980s [73–76]. In these papers, the starting point for the nonlinear search was found by integrating in time over the entire QRS interval, then using a

Newton-type nonlinear optimization to find an improved estimate. However, this approach was somewhat heuristic and without any particular physiological motivation.

More recently a powerful algorithm by Huiskamp and Greensite [63] based on this activation imaging approach has re-invigorated this area of investigation. This activation-based inverse algorithm is centered around the identification of what are known as "critical points" and associated times in the surface activation function (i.e., epi- and endocardial breakthrough/termination points and times), which are found using a modified MUltiple SIgnal Classification (MUSIC) algorithm [77]. Closely related approaches have been used for the EEG and MEG inverse problems since the early 1990s, presented primarily in a series of papers from Richard Leahy and coworkers, starting from Mosher et al. [78]. Examples of critical points in a cardiac excitation wavefront are shown in ❷ Fig. 9.4. The key idea behind this critical-point approach stems from the observation that when an evolving cardiac excitation wavefront intersects the epicardial surface, a *hole* develops in the wavefront. This is a significant change to the topology of the wavefront, which generates a sudden alteration in the surface potential recordings. If $\tau(x)$ is defined to be the activation time on the surface of the heart (note that in this formulation, x is a location parameter on the heart surface, and $\tau(\cdot)$ has units of time, measured with respect to some arbitrary $t = 0$), then these breakthrough points are critical points of $\tau(x)$; that is, $\nabla\tau(x') = 0$, where x' is the location of the breakthrough point (note that if we use V_m to represent the TMPs, the nonlinearity is in the transfer from $\tau(x)$ to V_m; given V_m we can define a forward matrix A that predicts the body surface potentials just as in TMP potential-based formulations):

This critical point observation leads, after much mathematical derivation [81], to the two following important results:

1. x' is a critical point of $\tau(x)$ with critical time $\tau(x') \iff a$ is in the space spanned by the spatial singular functions of Φ_B, where a is the column of the V_m to ϕ_B transfer matrix A corresponding to x', and
2. with all critical points of $\tau(x)$ determined, the computation of $\tau(x)$ (on both the epicardial and endocardial surfaces) is a well-posed problem.

The key assumption required to prove the first point is that V_m is modeled as a uniform step jump across the wavefront; i.e.,

$$V_m = a + bH(t - \tau(x)), \tag{9.33}$$

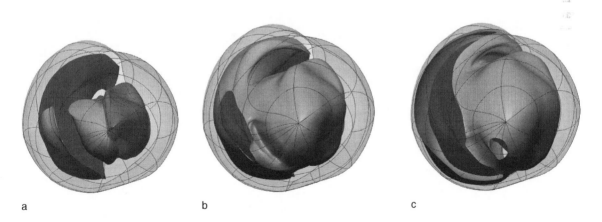

a   b   c

❏ **Fig. 9.4**
The formation of critical points and their associated critical times as an excitation wavefront (*gold surfaces*), derived from a simulation based on an eikonal model, collides with the heart walls [79]. Panel (a) shows the initial excitation sites near the endocardial surfaces. Panels (b) and (c) show critical points as the excitation wavefront (*gold surface*) collides with the epicardial surface and a hole is formed in the wavefront. The heart is viewed from the apex with the epicardium shown as a transparent surface, the left ventricular surface in *green* and the right ventricular surface in *blue* (Figure reproduced from Pullan et al. [80] with permission)

where a is a constant offset value, b controls the height of the step jump of the action potential, H is the Heaviside step function, and $t \in [0, T]$.

The Heaviside step function models an elementary source at a point on the heart surface x, excited at time $\tau(x)$, which remains excited until the entire domain has been excited. Equation (9.33) represents only phase 0 of the action potential and hence the inverse algorithm derived from the two results just shown is specific to the intervals occupied by the P wave (atrial depolarization) and the QRS complex (ventricular depolarization) of the ECG. If, instead of (9.33), one assumed

$$V_m = a + b - bH(t - \tau(x)),\qquad(9.34)$$

(i.e., a step jump down) and we now considered $\tau(x)$ to be a time corresponding to the phase 3 (repolarization) of the action potential, then results similar to the two listed earlier could be obtained. Thus, any inverse algorithm derived from those two results for imaging depolarization could, in theory, be used to image repolarization, and thus this approach is a means of complete fiducial-time based imaging. However, imaging repolarization is complicated by a number of its unique features. As shown in ❯ Fig. 5.3, repolarization occurs over a relatively long time period, and therefore, it is difficult to define a distinct recovery time (compared with the activation time), which means that (9.34) is a more severe approximation than (9.33). Moreover, since it is the change in time of the TMP that produces the "source" in this model, the effective signal-to-noise ratio is considerably reduced. Also, repolarization occurs during the mechanical motion of the heart, meaning that the transfer matrix may contain substantially more geometric error in the repolarization phase compared with the depolarization phase.

The use of the critical-point method to locate breakthroughs suggests a two-step approach for fiducial-time based imaging:

1. Find the critical points and times using the theory above, using, for example, the algorithm described in some detail below, and then
2. Obtain the entire activation sequence by solving a non-linear minimization problem in which the objective is to minimize the difference between the calculated torso potentials $\hat{\phi}_B$, and the measured potentials, ϕ_B (where $\hat{\phi}_B$ is calculated using $A(x, y)$ and any estimate of $\tau(x)$), starting from an initial estimate found n the first step.

During this optimization process, the critical points and times that have been identified can either be fixed or be constrained to remain local extrema of $\tau(x)$. Additional constraints on the optimization process can be imposed, such as the surface Laplacian of $\tau(x)$ [82],

$$E(\tau(x)) = \min \left\{ \left\| \phi_B - \hat{\phi}_B \right\|_2 + \lambda \cdot L\tau(x) \right\},\qquad(9.35)$$

where E is the objective function being minimized with respect to the activation times on the heart ($\tau(x)$), λ is a parameter controlling the degree of regularization imposed on the objective function and L is a discrete approximation of the Laplacian of the excitation field. We return to a discussion of this second optimization step in the following section, but first we describe how the "critical times" can be found computationally.

The following algorithm computes the critical points and times. First, the signal matrix, Φ_H, recorded from surface electrodes, and $A(x, y)$ mapping from V_m to ϕ_B, are required. The spatial singular functions of $\Phi_B(y, t)$ are computed using the singular value decomposition

$$\Phi_B = U_B \Sigma_B V_B^{\mathrm{T}} \quad \text{with an effective rank } R\qquad(9.36)$$

As already described, singular vectors corresponding to small singular values are discarded. Noting that each column of A corresponds to the map from a particular node x on the heart surface to all the body surface nodes, the following function can be defined for each x for all values of $t \in [t_0, t_1]$,

$$M_{t_0}^{t_1}(x) = \left(1 - \sum_{r=1}^{R} [\tilde{a}(y) \cdot u_r(x)]^2 \right)^{-1},\qquad(9.37)$$

where $\tilde{a}(y) = \dfrac{a(y)}{\|a(y)\|}$ is the unit (Euclidean) normalized column of the transfer matrix $A(x, y)$ which corresponds to x, and $u_r(x)$ is the rth column of the spatial (left) singular matrix U and R is the number of singular values retained, as just described. The summation term in (9.37) is the projection of the normalized vector $\tilde{a}(y)$ onto the vector space spanned by the spatial singular vectors $u_r(x)$. With the normalization in $\tilde{a}$ and the fact that the singular vectors are also unit norms, if $\tilde{a}(y)$ is contained in this space then the summation will yield 1 (and hence $M_{t_0}^{t_1}(x)$ will be infinite), while if no component of $\tilde{a}(y)$ is contained in this space, the summation will yield 0. This is the principle behind the well-known MUSIC method for spectral estimation and array processing [83]. Hence, (9.37) can be thought of as a measure of the distance of $\tilde{a}(y)$ from the space spanned by the set $u_r(x)$, which we can think of as the "signal space." This distance measure greatly exaggerates points x that are close to this space. In theory, $M_{t_0}^{t_1}(x)$ is singular at critical points $\in [t_0, t_1]$, although, in practice, there are no singularities, due to noise and other errors associated with Φ and A.

To find the activation times corresponding to these critical points, the following matrices are constructed,

$$M_{xt}^{\oplus} = M_0^t(x), \tag{9.38}$$

$$M_{xt}^{\ominus} = M_t^T(x) \tag{9.39}$$

Each row of both matrices corresponds to a particular node x, while each element of that row is the value of the function defined in (9.37) for the appropriate interval at a time t in the measurement time series which corresponds to its column index. Thus, these two functions describe the distance from signal space, where the two signal spaces are restricted to $[0, t]$ and $[t, T]$ respectively. From these matrices, a zero-crossing matrix is created, defined by

$$Z_{xt} = M_{xt}^{\oplus} - M_{xt}^{\ominus}, \tag{9.40}$$

which enhances the difference in behavior between $M_{xt}^{\oplus}$ and $M_{xt}^{\ominus}$ at each time t. Each row of this zero-crossing matrix corresponds to the distance from signal space at a particular location on the heart as a function of time.

In ❷ Fig. 9.5, we show sample functions defined by the rows of Z_{xt} (called the critical point functions); one observes that they are similar to step functions in the sense that they have high gradients at the point at which the horizontal axis is crossed. Theoretically, the critical point function corresponding to a critical point crosses zero at the critical time. In practice, the distinction between critical points on the one hand, and activation times that occur in regions where the activation surface is continuous, on the other, is not as clear, due to noise and errors. Thus, there are several alternative ways to use the rows of Z_{xt}. One could, for instance, define a threshold on the height of the jumps (which can differ dramatically, as seen in the right-hand column of ❷ Fig. 9.5), consider those jumps that are above the threshold as detected critical points, and run the optimization algorithm initializing it by fixing or restricting its ability to change the detected critical times. Another alternative is to use the zero-crossing of each critical point function to obtain an initial estimate of the activation time at each location. With critical points and times, or activation times, thus identified, the process of determining $\tau(x)$ everywhere is, theoretically, a well-posed problem and in practice can be solved via the optimization process described next.

Once the critical points or initial activation times, or other results of the application of the critical point theorem, are found, we are left with a nonlinear optimization problem such as the one in (9.35), with the critical points serving either simply as a starting point for the optimization or also as an additional constraint throughout the procedure. We note again that this problem is nonlinear because $\hat{\phi}_B$ depends on the fiducial times in a highly nonlinear manner, in contrast to its dependence on the HSP or TMP values. We also note that many optimization algorithms run better if one can compute the appropriate Jacobians. However, if the sources are simply switched on at discrete locations on the heart surface (i.e., the nodal positions) according to (9.33), the resultant simulated potentials $\hat{\phi}_B$ are discontinuous, which in fact gives rise to body surface potentials that are not continuous with respect to the activation times. For use in the optimization phase of the activation inverse procedure, it is more desirable to deal with functions that are continuous; moreover, the speed of convergence is greatly aided by having continuous derivatives [82].

Thus, alternatives to (9.33) have been used by various investigators. The purpose of these alternatives it to generate values of V_m that are smooth and continuous but still contain the general features of the activation phase of a ventricular action potential. One such alternative is the sigmoid function $S(t - \tau)$, as shown in ❷ Fig. 9.6 and described in

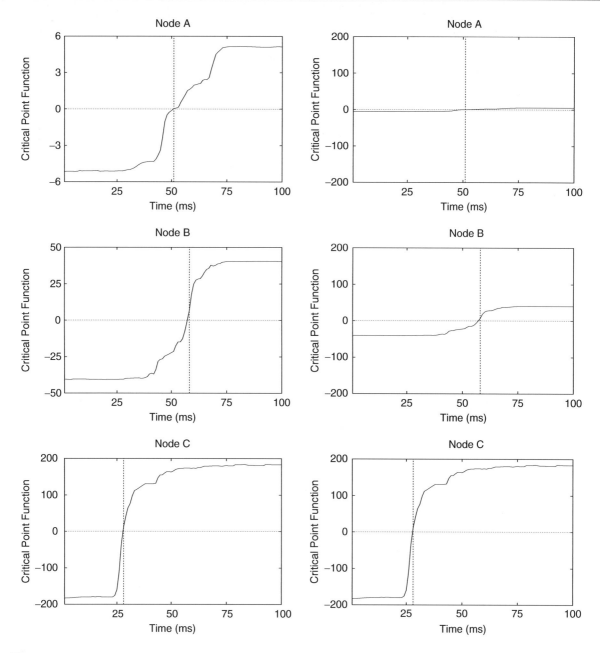

◼ Fig. 9.5

Comparison of critical point functions between critical and noncritical points. The *left column* shows the three functions and their corresponding ranges. The *right column* re-plots all the functions scaled to the same range. The larger jump in the critical point function for node C indicates that it corresponds to a critical point. The *vertical line* marks the points at which the functions cross the *horizontal axis* (critical times) and provides an estimate of the activation time at each location

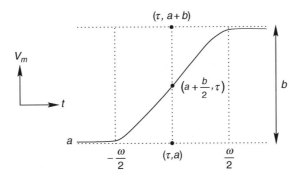

◻ Fig. 9.6
Approximation of the Heaviside step function by a sigmoidal function. This function contains the parameters ω and b to determine its shape. The ω parameter controls the width or window of the activation upstroke (i.e., the duration of the depolarization), while the b parameter controls the height of the transmembrane jump, i.e., the difference between the resting potential (a) and the peak of the action potential upstroke. Time is shown on the horizontal axis and the transmembrane potential on the vertical axis

the following section in (9.41), and another is the arctangent function, as used by Tilg et al. [84]. Like the Heaviside step transition, all these functions rely on assumptions about the shape of the action potential that are likely not a practical restriction for normal hearts, but do provide a measure of the expected spatial resolution of this activation-inverse approach. Moreover, abnormal hearts may provide a more serious problem, a fact that, as noted earlier, motivated the introduction of the surface TMP imaging method described in ❷ Sect. 9.3.6.2.

When specifying the sigmoid function as follows, the a and b parameters again represent the transmembrane resting potential and the transmembrane jump respectively. The smooth function is created by gradually activating the sources over a time-span of ω. If u is defined as $t - \tau(x)$, the smooth activation function can be represented mathematically by the function

$$S(u) = \begin{cases} a & u \le -\dfrac{\omega}{2} \\[2mm] a + \dfrac{b}{2}\left(\dfrac{2}{\omega}u + 1\right)^2 & -\dfrac{\omega}{2} < u \le 0 \\[2mm] b - \dfrac{b}{2}\left(\dfrac{2}{\omega}u - 1\right)^2 & 0 < u < \dfrac{\omega}{2} \\[2mm] a + b & u \ge \dfrac{\omega}{2} \end{cases} \tag{9.41}$$

The derivatives of the torso surface potential with respect to the activation times for use in the optimization phase are then given by

$$\frac{\partial \hat{\phi}_B}{\partial \tau} = A \cdot (-1) \begin{cases} 0 & u \le -\dfrac{\omega}{2} \\[2mm] b\left(\dfrac{2}{\omega}u + 1\right)\dfrac{2}{w} & -\dfrac{\omega}{2} < u \le 0 \\[2mm] -b\left(\dfrac{2}{\omega}u - 1\right)\dfrac{2}{\omega} & 0 < u < \dfrac{\omega}{2} \\[2mm] 0 & u \ge \dfrac{\omega}{2} \end{cases} \tag{9.42}$$

A recent addition to the literature on activation-time imaging has suggested an alternative way to solve the nonlinear regularized optimization [85]. This approach, based on a method suggested for general nonlinear inverse problems [86], replaces the iterative gradient descent approach used in Newton methods with iterations using a sequence of linearizations around the current solution. The key benefit claimed for this method is that, for the case of regularized ill-posed problems, it allows one to use a standard regularization parameter determination method (such as the *L*-curve) on the *linear* update optimization that needs to be solved on each iteration. Thus, one solves a sequence of linear regularizations, each with its own regularization parameter. Results indicate that this method leads to *L*-curves that are much better defined than the single *L*-curve obtained using a standard Gauss–Newton technique [85], especially when applied to clinical data.

An alternative method for both initializing and regularizing the activation (and recovery) time algorithms has recently been introduced by van Oosterom and coworkers, who report improved results with it over standard initializations and Laplacian-based regularization [87]. The basic idea is to compute a set of simplified propagation patterns, initialized in turn from all of the nodes on the HSP geometry. This pattern is computed by finding the lengths of shortest paths from each node to all other nodes, the paths following straight line segments that lie entirely inside the myocardium. The shortest route is found by using an optimization method called the "shortest path algorithm." Applying an assumed constant propagation velocity to the resulting distances leads to an activation pattern for each node on the surface. The body surface potentials predicted by the forward model based on each of these activation patterns are compared with the measured potentials and the best fit pattern is chosen to initialize the nonlinear optimization as described earlier. The same distance function has also been used to regularize the nonlinear optimization. It is interesting to note that the underlying principle seems to have something in common with the wavefront-based methods for curve and potential reconstruction of Ghodrati et al. [67] described earlier, in that the idea is to impose a propagating wavefront behavior on the reconstruction, although the specifics of both the formulation and the method are quite different.

9.5   Inverse Solutions from Intracavitary Measurements

Another method of inverse electrocardiography is to measure the potentials within a chamber of the heart by means of a noncontact, multielectrode catheter array and then to estimate the endocardial surface potentials from them. The forward model of this approach has a similar form to other potential-based approaches and relates the potentials on the endocardial surface to the measurement leads inside the cavity. Since the measurements are recorded relatively close to the endocardial surface, the corresponding forward matrix is generally less ill-conditioned than the epicardial potential forward matrix. On the other hand, obtaining accurate geometrical data from which to construct the transfer matrix is challenging, because it requires medical imaging [88–90] and because the probe moves due to blood flow in the chamber. Overcoming this challenge is critical, because the accuracy of the computed inverse solutions is highly sensitive to errors in the geometry [91]. The only currently available commercial device based on inverse electrocardiography, the Ensite system produced by St. Jude Medical [90], obtains the geometry of the endocardial surface point by point using a catheter navigating on the endocardial surface. The sampled points are then fitted to a bicubic spline surface to improve the estimate of the actual chamber.

Due to the similarity of the forward model of this approach to the potential-based approach, all inverse methods mentioned in ❷ Sect. 9.3 apply to this problem as well. Khoury et al. have tested and reported several inverse methods for the endocardial inverse problem [88, 92, 93] and here we describe briefly two approaches that are slightly different from those covered in ❷ Sect. 9.3. While initially developed for the endocardial problem, there is no reason why these approaches could not be used for other potential-based formulations.

1. The first approach, developed by Khoury [92], uses the first order Tikhonov regularization method and the BEM method to define the regularization matrix as the derivative of the endocardial potentials in the normal direction to the surface rather than tangential to the surface. This means that the regularization term constrains the magnitude of the normal current density on the endocardial surface, a strategy that lacks a solid theoretical justification, but nonetheless appears to work. Khoury et al. reported improved accuracy with this approach compared with simple zero-order Tikhonov regularization.
2. The second approach, also from Khoury and his colleagues, is again in the framework of Tikhonov regularization, but tries to define a regularization matrix that will satisfy the discrete Picard condition [93]. The regularization matrix in this approach has the same right and left singular vectors as the forward matrix, but its singular values are determined from the energy spectrum of the data. Therefore, the singular values of the regularization matrix and the particular measured data directly affect the filter factors of the inverse solution. The inverse solution obtained by this method produces superior results than the zero order Tikhonov solution [93].

9.6 Determining the Regularization Parameters

There are many a posteriori methods for determining the appropriate levels of regularization required for virtually all forms of inverse problem. (By a posteriori here we mean that these methods try many regularization parameters, test the results of each trial, and pick one of these based on some criterion. This is in contrast to a priori methods, which rely on the knowledge of noise statistics or other prior knowledge.) Each of these regularization parameter estimation methods attempts to provide a balance between the solution and regularization norm. Commonly accepted methods, which we discuss briefly here, include: the L-curve [94], the CRESO criterion [95], the zero-crossing criterion [96], and generalized cross-validation [97]. We briefly explain these methods here with reference to the HSP inverses given in ❷ Sect. 9.3. In addition, we first describe the *optimal criterion method*, by which we mean picking the regularization parameter using the knowledge of the true solution – clearly not a practical approach, but useful for simulation studies and in exploring the best case behavior of various inverse methods. For the optimal method, we illustrate the procedure using both the Greensite potential-based inverse and the Tikhonov and TSVD inverses. We explain the other methods described in the following section with reference only to the Tikhonov and TSVD inverses.

9.6.1 Optimal Criterion

The optimal criterion solution, although clinically not feasible because it requires a priori the knowledge of the epicardial potential distribution, places a lower bound on the accuracy of a given regularization scheme and thus leads to a valid comparison measure between relative regularization inverse approaches.

The optimal solution for Tikhonov and TSVD regularization schemes can be obtained by choosing the value of the regularization parameter λ_t at each time t that leads to the best solution to (9.12), i.e., that minimizes

$$\|\hat{\boldsymbol{\phi}}_{H(i)} - \boldsymbol{\phi}_{H(i)}\|_2, \tag{9.43}$$

where $\hat{\boldsymbol{\phi}}_{H(i)}$ is the ith regularized solution and $\boldsymbol{\phi}_{H(i)}$ is the exact solution on the heart. Note that, of course, one could define a different measure of optimality instead of the Euclidean norm of the reconstruction error, but to the best of our knowledge, this one has enjoyed universal support in the field. The optimally regularized solution to Greensite's epicardial potential method can be obtained via regularizing every ith equation individually if the isotropy condition truly holds; since the columns of $\boldsymbol{U}_B$ are orthogonal, they are linearly independent. Thus, for every solution $\boldsymbol{y}_i(\boldsymbol{x})$ to (9.31), the optimal regularization parameter is the value which minimizes

$$\|\sigma_{B(i)}\boldsymbol{y}_i(\boldsymbol{x})\boldsymbol{v}_{B(i)} - \boldsymbol{\Phi}_H\|_F, \tag{9.44}$$

where $\|\cdot\|_F$ denotes the *Frobenius* norm. We note that in practice one does not usually find a true optimal point, but rather tests over a dense grid of regularization parameters to locate the best value.

9.6.2 *L*-Curve Criterion

The L-curve method uses a parametric plot of the regularization objective function $\|\boldsymbol{R}\hat{\boldsymbol{\phi}}_H\|_2$ against the corresponding residual objective function $\|\boldsymbol{A}\hat{\boldsymbol{\phi}}_H - \boldsymbol{\phi}_B\|_2$ for a wide range of regularization parameters (λ). For discrete ill-posed problems, this curve, when plotted on a log-log scale, often has a characteristic L-shaped appearance with a corner separating the vertical and horizontal components of the curve, as shown in ❷ Fig. 9.7. The regularization parameter increases as the curve moves from the upper left to the lower right portions of the graph. The "corner" identifies a value of λ that provides an ideal (in some sense) balance between the two components that are minimized in (9.13). Regularization parameters that correspond to the upper left part of the curve produce results dominated by high regularization error and tend to be overly responsive to the noise and error (under-regularized). Regularization parameters that correspond to the lower right part of the curve produce results dominated by high residual error and tend to be overly insensitive to the measurements (over-regularized). The point for which any change in regularization parameter causes a large increase in one of the two

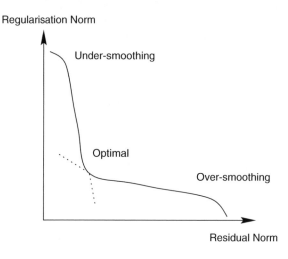

■ Fig. 9.7

The *L*-curve is a log–log plot of the residual norm, $\|A\hat{\phi}_H - \phi_B\|_2$, against the regularization norm, $\|R\hat{\phi}_H\|_2$. This plot is typically of the form of an "L." The corner of the "L" strikes a balance between the residual of the solution and the regularization norm

terms with little decrease in the other is considered to be a good choice; this occurs at the corner. The corner of the *L*-curve is also the point of maximum curvature, which provides the basis of a number of automatic methods that can detect this point, either through careful search techniques or using interpolants such as splines.

9.6.3 CRESO Criterion

The Composite REsidual and Smoothing Operator (CRESO) criterion chooses the regularization parameter for which the difference between the derivative of the residual term and the derivative of the smoothing term is maximized [95]. The CRESO regularization parameter is chosen to be the smallest value of λ_t^2 that results in a local maximum of the function

$$C(\lambda_t) = \|\phi_H(\boldsymbol{x}, \lambda_t)\|_2^2 + 2\lambda_t^2 \frac{\mathrm{d}}{\mathrm{d}\lambda_t} \|\phi_H(\boldsymbol{x}, \lambda_t)\|_2^2, \tag{9.45}$$

where $\phi_H(\boldsymbol{x}, \lambda_t)$ are the potentials on the heart regularized by the parameter λ_t. The function $C(\lambda_t)$ is the derivative of the function $B(\lambda_t)$, where

$$B(\lambda_t) = \lambda_t^2 \|\phi_H(\boldsymbol{x}, \lambda_t)\|_2^2 - \|A\phi_H(\boldsymbol{x}, \lambda_t) - \phi_B(\boldsymbol{y}, t)\|_2^2 \tag{9.46}$$

Strictly, the CRESO function is defined only for a continuous regularization parameter and hence cannot be used for the discrete TSVD approximation [98].

9.6.4 Zero-Crossing Criterion

The zero-crossing criterion aims to find the regularization parameter by solving the function $B(\lambda_t) = 0$ in (9.46). If more than one value of λ_t satisfies this condition, then the smallest value is chosen. Thus is essentially the minimum-product criterion proposed by Lian et al. [98] as another approach to locating the corner from the *L*-curve [99].

9.6.5 Generalized Cross Validation (GCV)

The generalized Cross Validation (GCV) method [97], like the L-curve, estimates a regularization parameter as a result of a trade off between minimization of the residual norm (data misfit) and the level of regularization. For this purpose the GCV function is defined as follows:

$$G = \frac{\|A\phi_H - \phi_B\|_2^2}{\text{trace}(I - AA_\lambda^{\overset{\circ}{}})}, \tag{9.47}$$

where I is the identity matrix and $A_\lambda^{\overset{\circ}{}}$ is the regularized inverse matrix for regularization parameter, λ. The numerator of the GCV function represents the data misfit and the denominator the level of regularization. The minimum of the GCV function for a range of regularization parameters determines the GCV regularization parameter; therefore, this method chooses a regularization parameter that results in a minimum misfit while regularizing sufficiently. The denominator of the GCV function can be shown to be related to the filter factors, for details see Hansen [9].

9.7 Validation and the Effect of Error

An essential component of any simulation approach is thorough validation of its results; in the case of a technique that aims to provide diagnostic information, validation must also include a careful evaluation of the relationship between error and uncertainty in the model and its ultimate diagnostic accuracy. Hence, it is necessary not only to show that electrocardiographic inverse solutions can provide credible images of cardiac electrical activity but also to establish the limits on the accuracy of the results and determine how errors in all components of the model effect the overall accuracy of the inverse solution. There are two basic approaches that are common to this type of validation, one based on computing the inverse solutions from the results of computed forward solutions (simulation studies) and one based on comparing measured results from experiments or clinical measurements with expectations from simulations of the same conditions (experimental studies). We describe both approaches below and then discuss some of the still unresolved questions about the effects of model components on accuracy.

9.7.1 Simulation Studies

The goal of simulation studies is to generate both source and remote data with a high degree of accuracy and then let the inverse method(s) under examination use only the remote data and seek to predict the sources. Ideally, the method used to generate the simulated test data should be independent of the inverse solution, i.e., use different geometric models and mathematical formulations. Otherwise, the inverse solution is likely to be overly optimistic, since solutions to ill-posed problems tend to magnify all error sources, including modeling error. This type of error is inevitable in practice but in such a validation model will be suppressed. For example, a forward transfer coefficient matrix, A, used to generate test data is not the ideal basis of an associated inverse solution because that inverse was specifically created to match the effect of A on the sources. Validation may then indicate how various parameters affect the inverse solution, and perhaps even how different inverse algorithms compare with each other, but not necessarily how well any particular method will work at finding sources from measured remote potentials. One can mitigate the inherent bias of this approach by adding known quantities of random noise to the forward-computed potentials; however, it is generally advisable to maintain independence between the forward solutions used to generate simulated test data and the inverse solutions under evaluation.

Another essential feature of a robust validation scheme is that it includes a wide range of test data. An inverse solution that is very accurate with one type of data or in one specific case (e.g., for a particular geometric model) may perform poorly for a different set of conditions. There is no known comprehensive approach to determining robustness; hence, there is no substitute for testing over a wide range of parameter space.

9.7.1.1   Analytical Solutions

The most straightforward form of simulation to use for validation is one that employs an analytical expression to generate the test data, which then forms the input to a numerical (discrete) inverse solution. This tests all aspects of the inverse solution, including the mathematical formulation and the numerical and computational implementation. Such solutions also allow for a great deal of variation of at least some parameters so that it is possible to compute test data under a wide range of conditions. Unfortunately, for electrocardiographic inverse problems there are relatively few geometries that contain sufficient symmetry and simplicity that an analytical expression is possible.

The best-known analytically tractable validation models in electrocardiology are those based on concentric and eccentric spheres proposed by Bayley and Berry [100–102] developed extensively by Rudy et al. [103–105] and still in use today [106–108]. Rudy et al. used these models not only for validating their numerical solution; by varying source types and locations and geometric model eccentricity, error, and conductivity, as well as regularization functionals used for the inverse solutions, they developed several fundamental hypotheses about the effect of each of these factors on inverse solution accuracy. One of these ideas that has subsequently been validated by physical models and human clinical studies is the relative insensitivity of the inverse solution to variations in thorax conductivity. These studies did indicate, in contrast, a strong sensitivity of the solution accuracy on knowledge of the true heart position; unaccounted shifts of only a few centimeters could result in substantial errors in recovered epicardial potentials [105]. However, the intrinsic limitation of analytical models based on simple geometries is their inability to capture the influence of realistic anatomical structures, which are both complex and asymmetric. This, in turn, means that conclusions drawn from such studies cannot readily be applied to physiologic situations.

Throne et al. also used the layered inhomogeneous eccentric spheres system to evaluate the effect of errors in geometry and conductivity on solutions to the inverse problem of electrocardiology [106]. They compared the abilities of four different numerical methods to solve the inverse problem, two of which used regularization, and found that, although the regularized methods performed better in the presence of geometric errors, small errors in heart size and position still had a significant effect on the resulting solution. Such results are evidence that analytical validation approaches, even under highly simplified conditions, can reveal fundamental insights into the important aspects of the behavior of inverse solutions.

9.7.1.2   Numerical Solutions

An implicit assumption of most simulation-based validation schemes is that the inverse solution is inherently much less accurate than the associated forward solution. This discrepancy comes from the ill-posed nature of the problem; one consequence is that it may be acceptable to treat a numerically computed forward solution as being almost as accurate as one calculated from an analytical solution, at least compared with the associated inverse solution. This observation provides justification for the use of numerical forward solutions to generate test data for the associated inverse problem. The motivation for such an approach is the much broader range of variation that is possible, compared with analytical models, when the constraint of simplified geometry is removed. Thus numerical solutions have become the dominant approach in simulation-based validation schemes.

In order to address the problem of testing an inverse solution using test data from the same forward solution, one can use different simulation methods to create test data. For example, it is possible to use dipole sources to calculate both epicardial and torso surface potentials directly based on a realistic geometry, which are then available to test an explicit torso-to-epicardial-surface inverse solution [28, 109]. Because the two formulations are different, the dipole source forward model does not match exactly the surface-to-surface model. This is one example of cross validation, in which one compares the directly computed epicardial potentials against those inversely computed from the torso potentials.

Hren et al. proposed a valuable extension of this approach by means of a more realistic cross-validation approach, in which the source was not a dipole, but a cellular automata model of cardiac propagation [110–112]. Cellular automata models represent cardiac tissue as a regular mesh of "cells," each representing a region of approximately 0.5–1 mm^3 and use simplified cell-to-cell coupling and state transition rules to determine the activation sequence. Although not as detailed as the monodomain and bidomain models that are based on descriptions of membrane kinetics, cellular automata models have a long history in simulations of normal and abnormal cardiac activation [113–116] (❯ Sect. 8.4.2). In order to apply cellular automata models to the validation of electrocardiographic inverse solutions, Hren et al. developed a method by which they assigned electrical source strength to the activation wavefront, and were thus able to compute epicardial and torso potentials from the cellular automata model for realistic geometric models of the human torso [110, 117]. They used this technique both to validate inverse solutions [111] and to examine the spatial resolution of body surface mapping [118, 119]. The major weaknesses of this form of validation is inherent to the underlying assumptions of the cellular automata approach, i.e., the limited ability to mimic myocardial sources, especially for pathological conditions such as ischemia or complex ion channel disorders.

Messnarz et al. have reported perhaps the most elaborate example of this approach by using a realistic, anisotropic, finite element model of the heart as the basis for a cellular automata simulation of the activation sequence [2]. The anatomical model also contained lungs and thorax and the simulation assumed unequal anisotropy ratios in the cardiac intracellular and extracellular spaces. From the resulting activation time simulations, they assigned an action potential shape and from these time signals then computed both heart surface and torso potentials.

The most common contemporary approach to validation of inverse problems is to compute remote (e.g., torso surface) potentials from known sources (e.g., epicardial potentials or activation sequences) and then add noise to the results before computing the source using the inverse solution under evaluation. Most often, the scientific focus of these studies is to determine the sensitivity of the inverse solution to variations in model parameters, some of which may be unaccounted for in the inverse formulation. One example would be to study the sensitivity of epicardial potential reconstruction to (unaccounted) shifts or errors in the heart location or to the number of body-surface measurement electrodes.

For example, Modre [120] conducted investigations to determine the effect of varying both the number of torso residuals in the activation inverse and the complexity of the torso model. In that study, the investigators varied the number of body-surface electrodes from 21 to 41 to 62 and used models with and without lungs, and that included unaccounted alterations in geometry. Little variation was seen with the electrode arrangements containing 41 and 62 electrodes, whereas results were significantly poorer when using 21 electrodes and either correct or incorrect geometry.

In a study reminiscent of earlier reports from Rudy et al. using analytical solutions, Ramanathan and Rudy [121] studied the effects of inhomogeneities in tissue conductivity on the reconstruction of epicardial potentials using zero-order Tikhonov regularization. By solving the inverse problem with different torso configurations, they found that spatial variations in conductivity had a minimal effect on the inverse solutions. The resulting assumption that a homogeneous geometric model can perform adequately received further support when they added Gaussian signal noise and electrode location error to the input data and found even less dependence on tissue conductivity.

Cheng et al. reported a comprehensive and systematic simulation-based validation studies [66, 122] that used a framework established by Pullan et al. [123]. These studies compared both epicardial potential- and activation-based inverse procedures, using different cardiac sources, with regularization parameters calculated according to the different methods described in ❿ Sect. 9.6 under a variety of both Gaussian and correlated noise conditions. Their results illustrated that the activation-based inverse method produced the most stable solutions in the presence of geometric uncertainty. However, when no geometric error was present in the system (something not achievable in practice), the potential-based approaches performed marginally better. As an example of another parameter important in implementing an inverse solution, their studies also included a comparison of different methods of determining regularization parameters (see ❿ Sect. 9.6 for a discussion).

Using the optimal criterion already described for setting regularization levels, all of the potential-based methods in the study by [122] provided similar results. However, this method of selecting the regularization parameter is not usually feasible. Of all the potential-based inverse methods considered in that study, the most favorable results come from using the Greensite potential-based inverse method with the rank of each equation determined by the maximum curvature of the singular values, and using Tikhonov with CRESO or L-curve regularization for each equation. This was the case whether the solutions were compared with the original epicardial potential solutions or with the original activation times.

9.7.2 Experimental Validation

By far the oldest approaches to validating both forward and inverse solutions in electrocardiography have been based on experiments with physical analogs of the torso and cardiac sources. For example, the studies by Burger and Van Milaan [124, 125] employed a shell molded on a statue of a supine human into which they inserted a set of copper disks oriented along one of the body axes and adjustable from outside the tank by means of a rod. More modern variation of this scheme employ more elaborate electrolytic tanks and measuring systems and some have used anesthetized, instrumented animals to record both source and remote data simultaneously. We present here a few examples of the current state of the art and refer to other sources for more detail (e.g., MacLeod and Brooks [126] and Nash and Pullan [127]).

Spach and Barr carried out the earliest studies that included simultaneously recordings from dense arrays of torso and heart electrodes from experimental chimpanzees [128] and dogs [129]. The relative lack of spatiotemporal resolution and the fact that these studies were published prior to the major theoretical developments in ECG inverse techniques have resulted in a somewhat limited interpretation of the results. Neither of these data sets is currently available in electronic form, and this further limits their use in contemporary validation studies. These landmark studies, did, however, allow the first detailed qualitative comparison of heart and body-surface potentials and showed that spatial information is maintained on the body surface. These findings also provided great motivation for the subsequent growth in the field of electrocardiographic imaging.

Simultaneous recording of epicardial and body surface potentials in the closed chest of animals have been attempted by at least two other research groups. At Oxford University, pigs were the animal of choice [130], while Zhang et al. [131] used rabbits. The protocal of the Oxford experiments (shown in ❯ Fig. 9.8) involved placing multiple electrodes on the heart and torso of the animal and simultaneously recording the potentials at all electrode locations during normal and abnormal rhythms, as well as recording the geometrical locations of the recording sites [132]. To position the heart

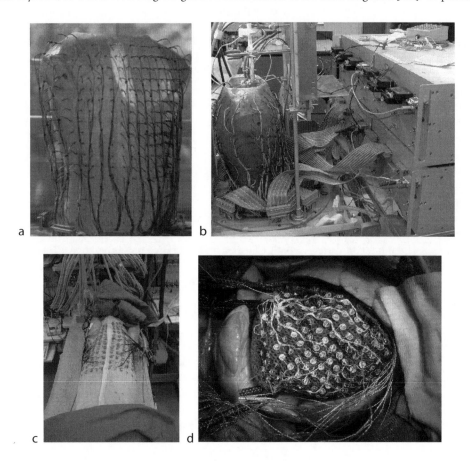

a   b   c   d

◨ Fig. 9.8

Panel (a) shows the torso tank of the Cardiovascular and Research Training Institute, University of Utah, used to collect simultaneous epicardial and body surface electrocardiograms. In panel (b) a perfused heart is suspended within the torso tank which is filled with a saline solution. Panels (c) and (d) show the experimental setup at Oxford University. In panel (c) is the vest of electrodes on the body surface and in (d) the sock of electrodes around the heart

electrodes, the pigs were thoracotomised and an epicardial electrode sock (containing 256 electrodes) was placed inside the pericardium. Upon successful placement of the sock (as verified by successful recordings from the electrodes) the chest was reclosed, leaving in place a suction line to drain any excess air and fluid to re-establish intrathoracic pressure. A body surface suit, consisting of 256 unipolar electrodes was then placed around the pig, and simultaneous recordings commenced. A variety of abnormal beats were initiated, either by pacing down any of the epicardial electrodes, via the injection of various drugs, or by the closing and opening of ligatures around the left anterior descending coronary artery. Geometrical information was obtained using a mechanical digitiser. These data have proved useful for a variety of studies (e.g., [130, 132, 133]), but unfortunately the lack of a complete accurate geometrical data set has limited the use of these data for quantitative inverse validation work.

In the recent work of Zhang et al. [131] body surface potential maps were used together with their previously described inverse procedure [69] to reconstruct the cardiac activation sequence in rabbits. To validate these results, experimental studies were performed on rabbits. First, the animals were subjected to an ultrafast CT scan to obtain the necessary geometrical data. Three-dimensional intracardiac recordings (up to 200 intramural sites) using specially designed plunge needle electrodes in the (eventually) closed-chested rabbit were made. These data are the first of their kind ever reported in the literature. Estimated activation times were found to be in good agreement with those measured experimentally during left and right ventricular pacing.

In a parallel development over the past 40 years, Taccardi and his colleagues have developed a series of realistically shaped electrolytic tanks and the experimental techniques to suspend isolated, instrumented animal hearts into these tanks. The first studies used a cylindrical tank and a frog heart to study the shape of the bioelectric field from a beating heart [134] and then an isolated, perfused, dog heart in which they occluded a coronary artery to study the effects of injury current [135]. The first studies that generated quantitative validation data for inverse solutions were from Colli-Franzone and Taccardi et al. using the first of a series of human-shaped torso tanks with hearts suspended in an instrumented cage [136, 137]. Data from these experiments have been the subject of subsequent validation studies [25, 138–140] that have greatly advanced the field of electrocardiographic imaging. Subsequent generations of the torso-tank model (as shown in ❷ Fig. 9.8) have continued to provide insights and support the advancement of the field through improved instrumentation and a wider variety of interventions and experiments. Data from these preparations have validated not only inverse solutions [34, 141, 142] but also novel interpolation [143, 144] and estimation techniques [39, 145]. They have also supported the study of qualitative and quantitative features of electrocardiology, such as myocardial ischemia [146, 147] and repolarization abnormalities [148, 149].

This experimental model is very well suited to quantitative analysis, because it provides relatively tight control of the size, shape, and orientations of the heart within a known torso geometry, together with locations of the concurrent epicardial and tank surface potential recordings. The weaknesses of this preparation includes the typically homogeneous volume and the unphysiological condition of the heart perfused by retrograde flow through the aorta. For example, the isolated heart does not perform mechanical work and hence presumably responds somewhat differently to stresses that lead to contraction failure, such as ischemia or infarction. Similarly, the autonomic nervous system is absent in this preparation, making it difficult to study, for example, the role of sympathetic stimulation on the genesis and maintenance of arrhythmias. Finally, although it would, in principle, be possible to study human hearts in such a preparation (as Durrer et al. [150] did for their landmark study published in 1970), the lack of availability of human hearts has precluded such studies.

9.7.3   Clinical Validation

9.7.3.1   Inverse Solutions Computed from Body Surface Potentials

The target application of electrocardiographic imaging is, of course, diagnostics and monitoring in humans, so that ultimately, clinical validation is essential. For any inverse algorithm to be accepted as a standard procedure when diagnosing a patient with a cardiac condition, its merit must be justified in the mind of the clinician. It is necessary to prove beyond all reasonable doubt that the inverse results are accurate and robustly reproducible. Because direct, controlled experiments are often ethically unacceptable in humans, investigators have found numerous ways to carry out studies in humans both to validate inverse solutions and to determine their parameter sensitivity. Such approaches are often based on indirect evidence or make use of information available through invasive procedures or other imaging modalities that are clinically justified.

An excellent early example of a clinical validation strategy is the series of studies that Huiskamp et al. performed to evaluate the role of torso geometry on inversely computed activation times [75, 76]. As an absolute indicator of accuracy, they compared their solutions with the human activation data available from the classic experiments of Durrer et al. [150] under the assumption that key features of the order of activation would be preserved across individual subjects. To determine the role of error in the geometric model, they compared solutions using a standard realistic torso geometry with those from the actual geometry of the subjects and even exchanged geometric models among the subjects while keeping the same body-surface data. The results of these tests suggested that a fixed standard torso model gave unreliable results when used to solve the inverse problem; thus, it was necessary to create a specific model for each subject incorporating at least an accurate torso shape and heart orientation and position with respect to the ECG lead positions. Johnston et al. reported similar findings from a comparable study using 16 realistic torsos with varying sizes and positions of the heart [151].

Although clinical validations seldom offer complete source data, there are a number of investigators who have used indirect methods or methods based on other modalities to identify features that can become the basis for the validation of an electrocardiographic inverse solution. One example from MacLeod et al. [29] used fluoroscopic data from patients undergoing coronary angioplasty (PTCA) to identify the region likely to be at risk from acute ischemia during the angioplasty balloon inflation. They then compared the locations of these regions with those predicted from the inverse solutions on the basis of elevated ST-segment potentials, a typical marker of ischemia.

A clinical modality that provides very useful validation information is catheter-based mapping of endocardial activation by means of one of several available systems [152–154]. These systems allow for electro-anatomical mapping of the heart, often through fusion of measurements from many individual beats and for at least the endocardium, one can compare their results with those from almost simultaneous body surface recordings and activation time based inverse solutions. Tilg and his colleagues have carried out one of the most quantitative clinical ECG inverse validation studies to date using this approach [84, 155, 156]. They created patient specific geometric models based on MR images from each case and then localized an inverse-computed focal site of activation that they compared directly with catheter-based measurements from the patients. Localization of initial activation sites showed good agreement with data measured using the catheter based CARTO system for paced hearts, for patients with Wolff–Parkinson–White syndrome, and in patients with atrial arrhythmias. These are some of the first clinical ECG imaging studies to validate the ECG inverse techniques using concurrent in vivo cardiac and body surface ECGs from humans.

An example of the type of results obtained using such data is shown in ❯ Fig. 9.9. The torso model constructed from one particular set of MR images in shown in panel (a) of that figure. The model contains surfaces representing the skin, lungs, epicardium, and left and right endocardial boundaries. Using electrocardiograms recorded at the 51 sites shown on the torso model, an activation time-based inverse method was used to construct the image shown in panel (b). The initial site of excitation is shown in red together with the site of the pacing tip of the catheter.

A recent breakthrough study by Ramanathan et al. [157] used a much expanded form of this approach by evaluating data from patients showing a range of clinical conditions, including right bundle branch block, left and right ventricular pacing from known sites, and chronic atrial flutter. They based their inverse solution on patient-specific geometric models from CT imaging, generating both epicardial potentials and activation and recovery times (extracted from the potential time signals). Evaluation of their results was qualitative, as they were able to show in each case the presence of the abnormality; for the case of single-site pacing they could compare known and predicted sites of earliest activation and found at least qualitative agreement. Further work on validating the inverse results using human data from this group has recently appeared [158, 159]. More directly than any previous studies, research from the Rudy lab provides strong evidence for the clinical potential of inverse cardiac bioelectric imaging.

9.7.3.2   Validation of Endocardial Solutions

The most frequent forms of validation for the endocardial inverse solution are either to measure intracavitary and endocardial potentials from animal preparations or to evaluate somewhat indirectly the accuracy of derived information in human studies. Khoury et al. have reported several studies on validation of the endocardial inverse solution using animal

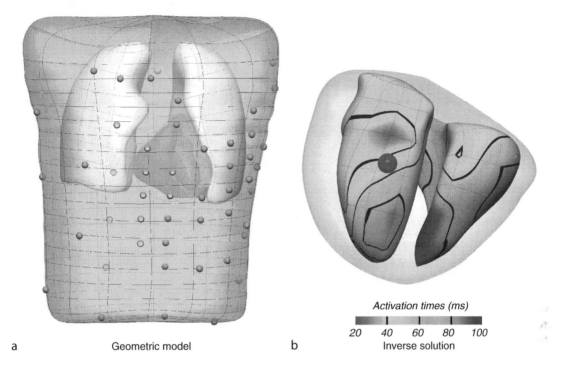

a   Geometric model   b   Inverse solution

Activation times (ms)

20   40   60   80   100

⬛ Fig. 9.9

Results from clinical inverse solutions. Panel (a) shows the geometric torso model comprised of skin, lungs, epicardium and left and right endocardial surfaces constructed from MRI images. The *gold spheres* represent the 51 body surface potential recording sites. In panel (b) is an anterior view of the heart with inversely computed activation times displayed on the endocardial surfaces. The *purple sphere* (10 mm in diameter) indicates the site of pacing from the catheter tip. This correlates well with the site of initial excitation (colored *red*) on the anterior left ventricular surface. The model and inverse result were computed by the first two authors of this chapter using data supplied by Tilg and coworkers (Reproduced from Pullan et al. [80] with permission)

models with simultaneously recorded chamber and endocardial surface potentials. In their earlier approach [93], they used a multielectrode basket-catheter in which expanding the basket inside the heart provided direct contact with the endocardium. However, the most challenging part of this approach was to obtain an accurate geometrical description of the basket (or the endocardium) [91, 160]. In more recent studies [161], they have reported using a recording electrode catheter that navigates the endocardial surface while a low-current locator signal is emitted from the tip electrode to determine its position. To generate accurate endocardial data, they have also used intracardiac echocardiography. Jia et al. also carried out validation studies from a spiral shaped endocardial probe introduced into the left ventricle of an isolated canine heart, which they compared with measurements from transmural needles [162].

The St Jude Medical Ensite catheter mapping system [163] has also been the subject of many validation studies in phantom, canine, and human experiments. As an example, Gornick et al. localized electrodes within an electrolytic tank, compared computed with measured canine endocardial potentials, and marked predicted sites of endocardial pacing all based on the Ensite technology [164]. Kadish et al. applied the same technology to mapping the right atrium in dogs, again comparing computed with directly measured endocardial potentials [165]. Clinical validation of endocardial inverse solutions is challenging because of limited access to complete measured potentials and has often been more qualitative in nature than animal studies. A study by Peters et al. is typical in which the authors documented reentrant endocardial potential patterns characteristic of fascicular tachycardia in a patient known to have this condition [166]. Other studies have validated the accuracy of the endocardial potential solutions according to the clinically relevant criteria of localizing sites of focal activity and treating them with catheter ablation [167]. One recent study applied the Ensite system for the first time to the determination of repolarization characteristics of the endocardium and compared computed results with directly measured monophasic action potentials [168]. They concluded that computed endocardial potentials could accurately determine activation recovery intervals in humans.

A recent study by Thiagalingam et al. [169] has provided unique quantitative information about the accuracy of the Ensite system and suggested some limitations on its ability to localize myocardial activity. Their results come from extensive comparison of over 32,000 electrograms computed using the Ensite system and measured from sheep hearts in which they located endocardial, midmyocardial, and epicardial myocardial needle electrodes. They found good accuracy of reconstruction of electrograms for sites located within 40 mm of the Ensite catheter but a sharp reduction in accuracy beyond this distance. They also suggested that computed potentials represent a summation of transmural activity, i.e., not simply endocardial or subendocardial activity. Ultimately, the fact that this system has found widespread – though not universal – acceptance in clinical practice, the only device based on an electrocardiographic inverse solution to date, is perhaps the most compelling form of validation.

9.8 Current Status and Futures Direction

The solution to the electrocardiographic inverse problems is motivated largely by the potential for clinical applications, specifically for methods that can determine the state of the heart from painless, noninvasive, ideally cheap, external measurements. Thus, to evaluate the present state of the art, there are a set of questions one must address. First, is there actually a clinical need for such a system? What are the shortcomings of other imaging modalities and what additional information might we expect to gain from electrocardiographic inverse imaging? Second, how close is the field to addressing some of the needs? We have discussed the approaches to validation of inverse problems, and hence, how good are the best systems? Finally, what are the most important remaining hurdles that prohibit successful deployment of inverse technologies and what must occur to overcome them? And is the result (a limited resolution image of the electrical activity of the heart) worth all the extra work compared with a standard 12-lead ECG?

The basis for clinical need lies primarily in the fact the inverse electrocardiographic imaging is a *functional* modality. That is, it generates not anatomical images but images of the spatial distribution of electrical information, clearly very relevant and valuable in the evaluation of the electrophysiological state of the heart. The standard ECG is also a functional measurement, but it lacks the spatial coverage and resolution to be considered an imaging modality. However, although many studies have described the additional information that body surface potential mapping provides [170–175] (see also ❯ Chaps. 9 and ❯ 10 of *Cardiac Arrhythmias and Mapping Techniques*), there are few such systems in clinical use today because there has not yet been enough value in that additional information to warrant the additional expense of carrying out the measurements. One reason why physicians are willing to forego this additional source of information is that other modalities, most notably echocardiography, provide complementary functional images of the beating heart – in real time and at a reasonable expense. Another reason to avoid this additional complexity is that the standard ECG already provides a cheap, painless, real-time way to monitor at least some aspects of cardiac activity.

The prime clinical application of electrocardiographic mapping is likely to lie in diseases that are essentially electrical in nature and that may not have an anatomical, mechanical, or biochemical counterpart, at least not one that is easily monitored in real time. Moreover, the motivation for applying mapping techniques, i.e., employing enough electrodes to gather spatial as well as temporal information, is strongest in diseases that reflect spatial inhomogeneity or in which distributions over the heart are meaningful. These have, not coincidently, also been the areas of primary interest and success in inverse electrocardiography.

The most common and potentially useful target application domain for inverse electrocardiography has been the study of cardiac arrhythmias, currently carried out by means of multiple catheter-based electrodes introduced into the heart chambers. As already noted, the most successful application of this approach has been by means of the endocardial surface inverse problem [176] and through the use of the Ensite system [163]. Detection of arrhythmias has also been the application in which several contemporary inverse solutions based on body-surface potentials have also shown promising success [155–157, 177]. There are also examples of using inverse solutions to guide interventions, for example, catheter ablation or drug therapy [178, 179]. In ablation procedures, noninvasive determination of the arrhythmogenic focus from body surface ECG recordings would certainly be advantageous; however, achieving this goal may be very challenging in situations of deeply placed focus, e.g., within the ventricular septum. Another potential application is to localize and document electrophysiological changes that arise during cardiac stress tests with more precision than is currently available with the 12-lead ECG.

And thus, one comes to the second question of how effective current inverse solution technology has become. As we have already described, there are a number of recent reports that suggest promising accuracy in the electrocardiographic inverse problem. The success of the Ensite system [163] and that of Khoury et al. [176] in the endocardial inverse are the most advanced, perhaps because of the inherently better conditions of this inverse problem formulation. The notable success of Rudy and coworkers [157] and Tilg and coworkers [84, 155, 156] also indicate that with enough attention to the details of the geometric model and appropriate application of constraints, it is possible to generate clinically relevant maps of heart surface activation and epicardial potentials. However, it is clear that quantitative clinical validation of inverse ECG methods remains an elusive challenge [127].

This discussion of requirements for an accurate inverse solution leads naturally to the hurdles before this imaging approach can become a useful and ubiquitous technique. The first step in an inverse solution is to create the associated forward solution; many aspects of computing the transfer matrices or the predictive function for the forward problem are very straightforward. However, a substantial and only partially resolved component of this task is creating an accurate, well-structured geometric model. Although modern imaging based on computed tomography or MRI provides excellent raw data for making models, the task of determining boundaries between tissues (segmentation) and creating a computational mesh from these data still involves considerable human guidance and hence time and expertise. For a recent exposition of one of the most current approaches see Pfeifer et al. [180]. Open questions related to this phase of the problem include the relationship between simulation accuracy and the level of model resolution, the set of included inhomogeneous regions, and the level of geometric fidelity, especially the size, shape, and the location of the heart. Most inverse solutions also assume a static geometry, even though the contraction of the heart will affect at least the repolarization phase of the cardiac electric cycle; at present, it is not clear how large the effect of this discrepancy might be nor how to deal with it in practical terms. One technology that may, at least partially, address this concern is electrical impedance tomography (EIT), which may have the potential to allow direct measurement of the actual conductivity profile, in the same sessions as the electrical mapping, and with relatively good temporal resolution [181, 182].

There are several other unresolved practical hurdles to a practical electrocardiographic inverse solution that deserve mention. One open question that is related to the body surface mapping, which is the input of many inverse solutions, is the determination of how many electrodes are required and where they might best be located. A related question is how to resolve the often-dramatic difference between the number of measurement electrodes and the number of nodes on the surface of the geometric model; is it best to interpolate the potential or remove the associated rows or columns from the forward or inverse solutions [183]? It is also necessary to determine where the electrodes lie in space relative to the nodes of the geometric model.

An additional set of open questions involves the choice of the problem formulation and the method of regularization. Some experimental studies suggest that the pattern of cardiac excitation is a more stable parameter than the epicardial potentials in the face of variations of geometric factors or torso conductivities [184, 185], implying that activation-based imaging may be more stable than potential-based imaging. (A relatively recent addition to this set of questions is the possibility of direct imaging of model TMPs [2, 54]). At least some modeling studies have confirmed this suggestion [66, 186]. However, fiducial time formulations of the problem have their own limitations. Implicit in fiducial formulations are assumptions about the electrical anisotropy of the heart; the influence of any weaknesses in these assumptions is still unknown. Also, although the same approaches can predict both activation and recovery times, they cannot at this stage deal appropriately with re-entrant phenomena. They will also fail in the case of myocardial infarction unless the location and the extent of the infarcted region are known a priori [187]. More generally, fiducial time approaches will be unsatisfactory for any pathology or condition that alters potentials without a concomitant change in the timing of fiducials, most notably alterations in ST-segment potentials that are the well-known hallmarks of acute ischemia. The two approaches also differ in their computational complexity; however, with the constant improvements in performance, the additional computing time required for fiducial-based approaches is of ever diminishing importance [188].

Perhaps the most active area of research and controversy in electrocardiographic inverse problems lies in the approaches and tuning of regularization. As we have already discussed, there are a substantial number of different approaches, each of which performs better or worse under different conditions. Moreover, within each approach, there are different ways to determine optimal regularization parameters. The resulting complexity and confusion provide a daunting hurdle to a practical clinical implementation of any of these approaches.

Will electrocardiographic inverse technology eventually take an equal place among the imaging modalities available for diagnosing and treating cardiac abnormalities? As we have discussed, there is clearly a need for imaging the electrical activity of the heart for which there is simply no other direct measurement modality; functional diseases that affect only or primarily cardiac electrophysiology will appear only indirectly in any images that are not electrical (or magnetic) in origin. Other compelling advantages of electrical vs. other forms of imaging include the reduced cost of a system and the relatively small size of the equipment, which enable long-term monitoring of patients and thus capture dynamic aspects of their disease. Compared with ultrasound, the technical skill required to acquire data is also minimal. There are no size constraints or problems with existing implantible devices such as those that arise with MRI. Measuring body-surface potentials has absolutely no risk and includes virtually no discomfort to the subject so that, unlike with, for example, CT, serial scanning and even routine screening are very feasible. Recent results suggest that with enough care and attention to detail, it is already possible to resolve many features of normal and abnormal cardiac activity; one type of inverse solution is already implemented in a clinical device and is in widespread use. Thus the major problem yet to be resolved is creating the necessary tools (some of which require additional research) in order to achieve the required efficiency and ease of use for clinical practice. There is some irony also in the fact that improvements in anatomical imaging of heart will also enhance the usability of electrocardiographic imaging, nominally a competing – but more sensibly a complementary – technology.

In summary, although there are still several hurdles to jump before quantitative noninvasive electrical imaging of the heart becomes a routine tool in cardiovascular research or clinical practice, the benefits of the technology remain extremely compelling and its successful implementation is within reach.

References

1. Yamashita Y., Theoretical studies on the inverse problem in electrocardiography and the uniqueness of the solution. *IEEE Trans. Biomed. Eng.*, November 1982;**29**(11): 719–725.

2. Messnarz B., M. Seger, R. Modre, G. Fischer, F. Hanser, and B. Tilg, A comparison of noninvasive reconstruction of epicardial versus transmembrane potentials in consideration of the null space. *IEEE Trans Biomed. Eng.*, Sept. 2004;**51**(9): 1609–1618.

3. Titomir L.I., The remote past and near future of electrocardiology – view point of a biomedical engineer. *Bratisl Lek Listy*, 2000;**101**(5): 272–279.

4. Keener and Sneyd, *Mathematical Physiology*, volume 8 of *Interdisciplinary Applied Mathematics*, 1st ed. Springer, Berlin, 1998.

5. Schmidt J., C. Johnson, and R. MacLeod, An interactive computer model for defibrillation device design, in *Building Bridges: International Congress on Electrocardiology International Meeting*, T. Oostendorp and G. Oiju, Editors, 1995, pp. 160–161.

6. Hadamard J., *Lectures on Cauchy's Problems in Linear Partial Differential Equations.* Yale University Press, New Haven, CT, 1923.

7. Babaeizadeh S., D.H. Brooks, D. Isaacson, and J. Newell, Electrode boundary conditions and experimental validation for BEM-based EIT forward and inverse solutions. *IEEE Trans. Med. Imag.*, September 2006;**25**(9): 1180–1188.

8. Babaeizadeh S., D.H. Brooks, and D. Isaacson, 3-D Electrical Impedance Tomography for piecewise constant domains with known internal boundaries. *IEEE Trans. Biomed. Eng.*, January 2007;**54**(1): 2–10.

9. Hansen P., *Rank-Deficient and Discrete Ill-Posed Problems: Numerical Aspects of Linear Inversion.* SIAM, Philadelphia, 1998.

10. Kaipio J. and E. Somersalo, *Statistical and Computational Inverse Problems.* Applied Mathematical Sciences, vol. 160. Springer, Berlin, 2005.

11. Tikhonov A. and V. Arsenin, *Solution of Ill-posed Problems.* Winston, Washington, DC, 1977.

12. Hansen P., *Rank-Deficient and Discrete Ill-Posed Problems: Numerical aspects of linear inversion.* PhD thesis, Technical University of Denmark, 1996.

13. Berger J., *Statistical Decision Theory and Bayesian Analysis.* Springer, Berlin, 1988.

14. Greensite F., Cardiac electromagnetic imaging as an inverse problem. *Electromagnetics*, September 2001;**21**(7–8): 559–577.

15. Pullan A.J., Paterson, and Greensite, Noninvasive imaging of cardiac electrophysiology. *Phil. Trans. R. Soc. Lond. A*, June 2001;**359**(1783): 1277–1286.

16. Greensite F., Well-posed formulation of the inverse problem of electrodiography. *Ann. Biomed. Eng.*, 1994;**22**: 172–183.

17. Oster H., B. Taccardi, R. Lux, P. Ershler, and Y. Rudy, Noninvasive electrocardiographic imaging: Reconstruction of epicardial potentials, electrograms, and isochrones and localization of single and multiple electrocardiac events. *Circulation*, 1997;**96**: 1012–1024.

18. Li G. and B. He, Localization of sites of origins of cardiac activation by means of a new heart-model-based electrocardiographic imaging approach. *IEEE Trans. Biomed. Eng.*, June 2001;**48**(6): 660–669.

19. Gulrajani R.M., F.A. Roberge, and G.E. Mailloux, The forward problem of electrocardiography/The inverse problem of electrocardiography, in *Comprehensive Electrocardiography*, P. Macfarlane and T.V. Lawrie, Editors. Pergamon Press, New York, 1989, pp. 197–288.

20. da Silva F.L., Functional localization of brain sources using EEG and/or MEG data: Volume conductor and source models. *Magn. Reson. Imaging*, December 2004;**22**(10): 1533–1538.

21. Yamashita Y., Theoretical studies on the inverse problem in electrocardiography and the uniqueness of the solution. *IEEE Trans, Biomed. Eng.*, 1982;**29**: 719–725.

22. Martin R.O. and T.C. Pilkington, Unconstrained inverse electrocardiography: Epicardial potentials. *IEEE Trans. Biomed. Eng.*, July 1972;**19**(4): 276–285.

23. Damen A.A. and J. van der Kam, The use of the Singular Value Decomposition in electrocardiographs. *Med. Biol. Eng. Comput.*, July 1982;**20**(4): 473–482.

24. Okamoto Y., Y. Teramachi, and T. Musha, Limitation of the inverse problem in body surface potential mapping. *IEEE Trans. Biomed. Eng.*, November 1983;**30**(11): 749–754.

25. Rudy Y. and B. Messinger-Rapport, The inverse solution in electrocardiography: Solutions in terms of epicardial potentials. *Crit. Rev. Biomed. Eng.*, 1988;**16**: 215–268.

26. Hansen P.C., *Rank-Deficient and Discrete Ill-Posed Problems: Numerical Aspects of Linear Inversion*. Society for Industrial and Applied Mathematics, Philadelphia, 1998.

27. Messinger-Rapport B.J. and Y. Rudy, Regularization of the inverse problem of electrocardiology: A model study. *Math. Biosci.*, 1988;**89**: 79–118.

28. MacLeod R., *Percutaneous Transluminal Coronary Angioplasty as a Model of Cardiac Ischemia: Clinical and Modelling Studies*. PhD thesis, Dalhousie University, Halifax, N.S., Canada, 1990.

29. MacLeod R., R. Miller, M. Gardner, and B. Horacek, Application of an electrocardiographic inverse solution to localize myocardial ischemia during percutaneous transluminal coronary angioplasty. *J. Cardiovasc. Electrophysiol.*, 1995;**6**: 2–18.

30. Golub G. and C.V. Loan, *Matrix Computations*. Johns Hopkins, Baltimore, 1989.

31. Press W.H., S.A. Teukolsky, W.T. Vetterling, and B.P. Flannery, *Numerical recipies in FORTRAN, the art of scientific computing*, 2nd ed. Cambridge University Press, Cambridge, 1992.

32. Hansen P.C., Analysis of discrete ill-posed problems by means of the L-curve. *SIAM Review*, December 1992;**34**(4): 561–580.

33. Brooks D., G. Ahmad, and R. MacLeod, Multiply constrained inverse electrocardiology: Combining temporal, multiple spatial, and iterative regularization, in *Proceedings of the IEEE Engineering in Medicine and Biology Society 16th Annual International Conference*. IEEE Computer Society, 1994, pp. 137–138.

34. Ramanathan C., P. Jia, R. Ghanem, D. Calvetti, and Y. Rudy, Noninvasive electrocardiographic imaging (ECGI): application of the generalized minimal residual (GMRes) method. *Ann. Biomed. Eng.*, September 2003;**31**(8): 981–994.

35. Barr R. and M. Spach, A comparison of measured epicardial potentials with epicardial potentials computed from body surface measurements in the intact dog. *Adv. Cardiol.*, 1978;**21**: 19–22.

36. van Oosterom A., Incorporation of the spatial covariance in the inverse problem. *Biomed. Technik*, 1997;**42**(Suppl): 43–52.

37. van Oosterom A., The use of spatial covariance in computing pericardial potentials. *IEEE Trans Biomed. Eng.*, 1999;**46**(7): 778–787.

38. van Oosterom A., The spatial covariance used in computing the pericardial potential distribution, in *Computational Inverse Problems in Electrocardiography*, P.R. Johnston, Editor. WIT Press, Southampton, UK, 2001, pp. 1–50.

39. Yılmaz B., R. MacLeod, B. Punske, B. Taccardi, and D. Brooks, Training set selection for statistical estimation of epicardial activation mapping from intravenous multielectrode catheters. *IEEE Trans Biomed. Eng.*, November 2005;**52**(11): 1823–1831.

40. Serinagaoglu Y., R. MacLeod, and D. Brooks, A Bayesian approach to inclusion and performance analysis of using extra information in bioelectric inverse problems, in *International Conference on Image Processing*. IEEE Press, New York, 2003.

41. Serinagaoglu Y., D. Brooks, and R. MacLeod, Bayesian solutions and performance analysis in bioelectric inverse problems. *IEEE Trans. Biomed. Eng.*, 2005;**52**(6): 1009–1020.

42. Serinagaoglu Y., D.H. Brooks, and R.S. MacLeod, Improved performance of Bayesian solutions for inverse electrocardiography using multiple information sources. *IEEE Trans. Biomed. Eng.*, October 2006;**53**(10): 2024–2034.

43. Shahidi A., P. Savard, and R. Nadeau, Forward and inverse problems of electrocardiography: Modeling and recovery of epicardial potentials in humans. *IEEE Trans Biomed. Eng.*, 1994;**41**(3): 249–256.

44. Brooks D., G. Ahmad, R. MacLeod, and G. Maratos, Inverse electrocardiography by simultaneous imposition of multiple constraints. *IEEE Trans. Biomed. Eng.*, 1999;**46**(1): 3–18.

45. Ahmad G., D.H. Brooks, and R. MacLeod, An admissible solution approach to inverse electrocardiography. *Ann. Biomed. Eng.*, 1998;**26**: 278–292.

46. Kay S.M., *Fundamentals Of Statistical Signal Processing: Estimation Theory*. Prentice-Hall, Englewood Cliffs, NJ, 1993.

47. Barr R. and T. Pilkington, Computing inverse solutions for an on-off heart model. *IEEE Trans Biomed. Eng.*, 1969;**16**: 205–214.

48. Brooks D., C.L. Nikias, and J. Siegel, An inverse solution in electrocardiography in the frequency domain, in *Proceedings of the IEEE Engineering in Medicine and Biology Society 10th Annual International Conference*, 1988, pp. 970–971.

49. Oster H. and Y. Rudy, The use of temporal information in the regularization of the inverse problem of electrocardiography. *IEEE Trans. Biomed. Eng.*, 1992;**39**(1): 65–75.

50. Joly D., Y. Goussard, and P. Savard, Time-recursive solution to the inverse problem of electrocardiography: A model-based approach. In *Proc. 15th Annual IEEE-EMBS Conf.*, 1993, pp. 767–768.

51. El-Jakl J., F. Champagnat, and Y. Goussard, Time-space regularization of the inverse problem of electrocardiography. In *Proc. 17th Annual IEEE-EMBS Conf.*, 1995, pp. 213–214.

52. Greensite F., A new treatment of the inverse problem of multivariate analysis. *Inverse Problems*, 2002;**18**: 363–379.

53. Greensite F., The temporal prior in bioelectromagnetic source imaging problems. *IEEE Trans. Biomed. Eng.*, 2003;**50**: 1152–1159.

54. Messnarz B., B. Tilg, R. Modre, G. Fischer, and F. Hanser, A new spatiotemporal regularization approach for reconstruction of cardiac transmembrane potential patterns. *IEEE Trans. Biomed. Eng.*, Feb. 2004;**51**(2): 273–281.

55. Skipa O., M. Nalbach, F. Sachse, C. Werner, and O. Dossel, Transmembrane potential reconstruction in anisotropic heart model. *Intl. J. Bioelectromagnet.*, 2002;**4**(2): 17–18.

56. Cheng L.K., G.B. Sands, R.A. French, S.J. Withy, S.P. Wong, M.E. Legget, W.M. Smith, and A.J. Pullan, Rapid construction of a patient specific torso model from 3D ultrasound for noninvasive imaging of cardiac electrophysiology. *Med. Biol. Eng. Comput.*, 2005;**43**(3): 325–330.

57. Zhang Y., A. Ghodrati, and D.H. Brooks, An analytical comparison of three spatio-temporal regularization methods for dynamic linear inverse problems in a common statistical framework. *Inverse Problems*, 2005;**21**: 357–382.

58. Anderson B. and J. Moore, *Optimal Filtering*. Prentice-Hall, Englewood Cliffs, NJ, 1979.

59. Kailath T., A.H. Sayed, and B. Hassibi, *Linear Estimation*. Prentice-Hall, Englewood Cliffs, NJ, 2000.

60. Greensite F., Second-order approximation of the pseudoinverse for operator deconvolutions and families of ill-posed problems. *SIAM J. Appl. Math.*, 1998;**59**(1): 1–16.

61. Lux R., K. Evans, M. Burgess, R. Wyatt, and J. Abildskov, Redundancy reduction for improved display and analysis of body surface potential maps: I. Spatial compression. *Circ. Res.*, 1981;**49**: 186–196.

62. Evans K., R. Lux, M. Burgess, R. Wyatt, and J. Abildskov, Redundancy reduction for improved display and analysis of body surface potential maps: II. Temporal compression. *Circ. Res.*, 1981;**49**: 197–203.

63. Huiskamp G. and F. Greensite, A new method for myocardial activation imaging. *IEEE Trans. Biomed. Eng.*, 1997;**44**: 433–446.

64. Hansen P., Analysis of discrete ill-posed problems by means of the L-curve. *SIAM Rev.*, 1992;**34**(4): 561–580.

65. Akaike H., A new look at the statistical model identification. *IEEE Trans. Automat. Contr.*, December 1974;**19**(6): 716–723.

66. Cheng L.K., J.M. Bodley, and A.J. Pullan, Comparison of potential and activation based formulations for the inverse problem of electrocardiology. *IEEE Trans. Biomed. Eng.*, January 2003;**50**(1): 11–22.

67. Ghodrati A., D. Brooks, G. Tadmor, and R. MacLeod, Wavefront-based models for inverse electrocardiography, September 2006; **53**(9): 1821–1831.

68. Andersen E. and K. Andersen, *High Performance Optimization*, chapter The MOSEK interior point optimizer for linear programming: an implementation of the homogeneous algorithm. Kluwer, Dordrecht, the Netherlands, 2000.

69. He B., G. Li, and X. Zhang, Noninvasive imaging of cardiac transmembrane potentials within three-dimensional myocardium by means of a realistic geometry anisotropic heart model. *IEEE Trans. Biomed. Eng.*, October 2003;**50**(10): 1190–1202.

70. Liu C., G. Li, and B. He, Localization of the site of origin of reentrant arrhythmia from body surface potential maps: a model study. *Phys. Med. Biol.*, 2005;**50**(7): 1421–1432.

71. Skipa O., *Linear inverse problem of electrocardiography: Epicardial potentials and Transmembrane voltages*. PhD thesis, University Karlsruhe, 2004.

72. Taccardi B., E. Macchi, R. Lux, P. Ershler, S. Spaggiari, S. Baruffi, and Y. Vyhmeister, Effect of myocardial fiber direction on epicardial potentials. *Circ.*, 1994;**90**: 3076–3090.

73. Cuppen J. and A. van Oosterom, Model studies with the inversely calculated isochrones of ventricular depolarization. *IEEE Trans. Biomed. Eng.*, 1984;**31**: 652–659.

74. Cuppen J., Calculating the isochrones of ventricular depolarization. *SIAM J. Sci. Statist. Comp.*, 1984;**5**: 105–120.

75. Huiskamp G. and A. van Oosterom, The depolarization sequence of the human heart surface computed from measured body surface potentials. *IEEE Trans. Biomed. Eng.*, 1989;**35**: 1047–1059.

76. Huiskamp G. and A. van Oosterom, Tailored versus standard geometry in the inverse problem of electrocardiography. *IEEE Trans. Biomed. Eng.*, 1989;**36**: 827–835.

77. Schmidt R.O., Multiple emitter location and signal parameter estimation. *IEEE Trans. Antennas Propagat.*, March 1986;**34**(3): 276–280.

78. Mosher J.C., P.S. Lewis, and R.M. Leahy, Multiple dipole modeling and localization from spatio-temporal MEG data. *IEEE Trans. Biomed. Eng.*, 1992;**39**(6): 541–557.

79. Tomlinson K.A., *Finite Element Solution of an Eikonal Equation For Excitation Wavefront Propagation in Ventricular Myocardium*. PhD thesis, The University of Auckland, New Zealand, 2000.

80. Pullan A.J., M.L. Buist, and L.K. Cheng, *Mathematically Modelling the Electrical Activity of the Heart: From Cell to Body Surface and Back Again*. World Scientific Publishing Company, Singapore, 2005.

81. Greensite F., Remote reconstruction of confined wavefront propagation. *Inverse Problems*, 1995;**11**: 361–370.

82. Huiskamp G. and A. van Oosterom, The depolarization sequence of the human heart surface computed from measured body surface potentials. *IEEE Trans. Biomed. Eng.*, December 1988;**35**(12): 1047–1059.

83. Stoica P. and R. Moses, *Spectral Analysis of Signals*. Prentice-Hall, Englewood Cliffs, NJ, 2005.

84. Tilg B., G. Fischer, R. Modre, F. Hanser, B. Messnarz, M. Schocke, C. Kremser, T. Berger, F. Hintringer, and F.X. Roithinger, Model-based imaging of cardiac electrical excitation in humans. *IEEE Trans. Med. Imag.*, September 2002;**21**(9): 1031–1039.

85. Modre R., B. Tilg, G. Fischer, and P. Wach, Noninvasive myocardial activation time imaging: a novel inverse algorithm applied to clinical ECG mapping data. *IEEE Trans. Biomed. Eng.*, October 2002;**49**(10): 1153–1161.

86. Tautenhahn U., On a general regularization scheme for nonlinear illposed problems: Ii. regularization in hilbert scales. *Inverse Problems*, 1998;**14**: 1607–1616.

87. van Oosterom A. and P. van Dam, The intra-myocardial distance function used in inverse computations of the timing of depolarization and repolarization, in *Computers in Cardiology '05*, vol. 32, Murray A, Editor. IEEE Computer Society Press, Piscataway, 2005, pp. 567–570.

88. Berrier K.L., D.C. Sorensen, and D.S. Khoury, Solving the inverse problem of electrocardiography using a Duncan and Horn formulation of the Kalman filter. *IEEE Trans. Biomed. Eng.*, 2004;**51**(3): 507–515.

89. Rao L., C. Ding, and D.S., Nonfluoroscopic localization of intracardiac electrode-catheters combined with noncontact electrical-anatomical imaging. *Ann. Biomed. Eng.*, 2004;**32**: 1654–1661.

90. Voth E., The inverse problem of electrocardiography: industrial solutions and simulations. *Int. J. Bioelectromag.*, 2005;**7**(2): 191–194.

91. Khoury D., Importance of geometry in reconstructing endocardial electrograms from noncontact multielectrode cavitary probe data, in *Proceedings of the IEEE Engineering in Medicine and Biology Society 19th Annual International Conference*, vol. 1, 1997, pp. 188–190.

92. Khoury D., Use of current density in the regularization of the inverse problem of electrocardiography, in *Proceedings of the IEEE Engineering in Medicine and Biology Society 16th*

Annual International Conference. IEEE Press, New York, 1994, pp. 133–134.

93. Velipasaoglu E., H. Sun, F. Zhang, K. Berrier, and D. Khoury, Spatial regularization of the electrocardiographic inverse problem and its application to endocardial mapping. *IEEE Trans. Biomed. Eng.*, March 2000;**47**(3): 327–337.

94. Hansen P.C. and D.P. O'Leary, The use of the L-curve in the regularisation of discrete ill-posed problems. *SIAM J. Sci. Comput.*, November 1993;**14**(6): 1487–1503.

95. Colli Franzone P., L. Guerri, B. Taccardi, and C. Viganotti, Finite element approximation of regularised solutions of the inverse potential problem of electrocardiography and applications to experimental data. *Calcolo*, 1985;**22**(1): 91–186.

96. Johnston P.R. and R.M. Gulrajani, A new method for regularization parameter determination in the inverse problem of electrocardiography. *IEEE Trans. Biomed. Eng.*, January 1997;**44**(1): 19–39.

97. Golub G.H., M.T. Heath, and G. Wahba, Generalized cross-validation as a method for choosing a good ridge parameter. *Technometrics*, 1979;**21**: 215–223.

98. Lian J., D. Yao, and B. He, A new method for implementation of regularization in cortical potential imaging, in *Proceedings of the 20th Annual International Conference of the IEEE Engineering in Medicine and Biology Society*, vol. 20, Hong Kong, China, 1998. IEEE Computer Society Press, 1988, pp. 2155–2158.

99. Johnston P.R. and R.M. Gulrajani, Selecting the corner of the L-curve approach to Tikhonov regularisation. *IEEE Trans. Biomed. Eng.*, September 2000;**47**(2): 1293–1296.

100. Bayley R. and P. Berry, The electrical field produced by the eccentric current dipole in the nonhomogeneous conductor. *Am. Heart J.*, 1962;**63**: 808–820.

101. Bayley R. and P. Berry, The arbitrary electromotive double layer in the eccentric "heart" of the nonhomogeneous circular lamina. *IEEE Trans. Biomed. Eng.*, 1964;**11**(4): 137–147.

102. Bayley R., J. Kalbfleisch, and P. Berry, Changes in the body's QRS surface potentials produced by alterations in certain compartments of the nonhomogeneous conducting model. *Am. Heart J.*, 1969;**77**(4): 517–528.

103. Rudy Y. and R. Plonsey, The eccentric spheres model as the basis for a study of the role of geometry and inhomogeneities in electrocardiography. *IEEE Trans. Biomed. Eng.*, 1979;**26**: 392–399.

104. Rudy Y. and R. Plonsey, The effects of variations in conductivity and geometrical parameters on the electrocardiogram, using an eccentric spheres model. *Circ. Res.*, 1979;**44**(1): 104–111.

105. Rudy Y. and R. Plonsey, A comparison of volume conductor and source geometry effects on body surface and epicardial potentials. *Circ. Res.*, 1980;**46**: 283–291.

106. Throne R. and L. Olson, The effect of errors in assumed conductivities and geometry on numerical solutions to the inverse problem of electrocardiography. *IEEE Trans. Biomed. Eng.*, 1995;**42**: 1192–1200.

107. Oster H., B. Taccardi, R. Lux, P. Ershler, and Y. Rudy, Noninvasive electrocardiographic imaging: Reconstruction of epicardial potentials, electrograms, and isochrones and localization of single and multiple electrocardiac events. *Circ.*, 1997;**96**(3): 1012–1024.

108. He S., Frequency series expansion of an explicit solution for a dipole inside a conducting sphere at low frequencies. *IEEE Trans. Biomed. Eng.*, 1998;**45**(10): 1249–1258.

109. Brooks D. and R. MacLeod, Electrical imaging of the heart: Electrophysical underpinnings and signal processing opportunities. *IEEE Sign. Proc. Mag.*, 1997;**14**(1): 24–42.

110. Hren R., *A Realistic Model of the Human Ventricular Myocardium: Application to the Study of Ectopic Activation*. PhD thesis, Dalhousie University, Halifax, Nova Scotia, 1996.

111. Hren R., X. Zhang, and G. Stroink, Comparison between electrocardiographic and magnetocardiographic inverse solutions using the boundary element method. *Med. & Biol. Eng. & Comp.*, 1996;**34**(2): 110.

112. Hren R., R. MacLeod, G. Stroink, and B. Horacek, Assessment of spatial resolution of body surface potentials maps in localizing ventricular tachycardia foci. *Biomed. Technik*, 1997;**42**(Suppl): 41–44.

113. Moe G., W. Rheinboldt, and J. Abildskov, A computer model of fibrillation. *Am. Heart J.*, 1964;**67**: 200–220.

114. Okajima M., T. Fujinaa, T. Kobayashi, and K. Yamada, Computer simulation of the propagation process in excitation of the ventricles. *Circ. Res.*, 1968;**23**: 203–211.

115. Abildskov J., Mechanism of the vulnerable period in a model of cardiac fibrillation. *J. Cardiovasc. Electrophysiol.*, 1990;**1**: 303–308.

116. Gharpure P. and C. Johnson, A 3-dimensional cellular automation model of the heart, in *Proceedings of the IEEE Engineering in Medicine and Biology Society 15th Annual International Conference*. IEEE Press, New York, 1993, pp. 752–753.

117. Hren R., J. Nenonen, and B. Horacek, Simulated epicardial potential maps during paced activation reflect myocardial fibrous structure. *Ann. Biomed. Eng.*, 1998;**26**(6): 1022.

118. Hren R. and B. Punske, A comparison of simulated QRS isointegral maps resulting from pacing at adjacent sites: Implications for the spatial resolution of pace mapping using body surface potentials. *J. Electrocardiol.*, 1998;**31**(Suppl): 135.

119. Hren R., B. Punske, and G. Stroink, Assessment of spatial resolution of cardiac pace mapping when using body surface potentials. *Med. & Biol. Eng. & Comp.*, 1999;**37**(4): 477.

120. Modre R., *A Regularization Technique for Nonlinear Ill-Posed Problems Applied to Myocardial Activation Time Imaging*. PhD thesis, Department of Biophysics, Institute of Biomedical Engineering, Technical University Graz, Austria, February 2000.

121. Ramanathan C. and Y. Rudy, Electrocardiographic imaging: II. Effects of torso inhomogeneities on noninvasive reconstruction of epicardial potentials, electrograms, and isochrones. *J. Cardiovasc. Electrophysiol.*, February 2001;**12**(2): 241–252.

122. Cheng L.K., J.M. Bodley, and A.J. Pullan, Effects of experimental and modeling errors on electrocardiographic inverse problems. *IEEE Trans. Biomed. Eng.*, January 2003;**50**(1): 23–32.

123. Pullan A.J., L.K. Cheng, M.P. Nash, C.P. Bradley, and D.J. Paterson, Noninvasive electrical imaging of the heart: Theory and model development. *Ann. Biomed. Eng.*, October 2001;**29**(10): 817–836.

124. Burger H. and J. van Milaan, Heart-vector and leads. Part II. *Br. Heart J.*, 1947;**9**: 154–160.

125. Burger H. and J. van Milaan, Heart-vector and leads. Part III: Geometrical representation. *Br. Heart J.*, 1948;**10**: 229–233.

126. MacLeod R. and D. Brooks, Validation approaches for electrocardiographic inverse problems, in *Computational Inverse Problems in Electrocardiography*, P. Johnston, Editor. WIT Press, Ashurst, UK, 2001, pp. 229–268.

127. Nash M.P. and A.J. Pullan, Challenges facing validation of noninvasive electrical imaging of the heart. *Ann. Noninvasive Electrocardiol.*, January 2005;**10**(1): 73–82.

128. Spach M.S., R.C. Barr, C.F. Lanning, and P.C. Tucek, Origin of body surface QTS and the T wave potentials from epicardial potential distributions in the intact chimpanzee. *Circulation*, February 1977;**55**(2): 268–288.

129. Barr R.C. and M.S. Spach, Inverse calculation of QRS-T epicardial potentials from body surface potential distributions for normal and ectopic beats in the intact dog. *Circ. Res.*, 1978;**42**: 661–675.

130. Nash M.P., C.P. Bradley, and D.J. Paterson, Imaging electrocardiographic dispersion of depolarization and repolarization during ischemia: Simultaneous body surface and epicardial mapping. *Circulation*, April 2003;**107**(17): 2257–2263.

131. Zhang X., I. Ramachandra, Z. Liu, B. Muneer, S.M. Pogwizd, and B. He, Noninvasive three-dimensional electrocardiographic imaging of ventricular activation sequence. *Am. J. Physiol. Heart Circ. Phyiol.*, 2005;**289**(6): H2724–H2732.

132. Nash M.P., C.P. Bradley, A. Kardos, A.J. Pullan, and D.J. Paterson, An experimental model to correlate simultaneous body surface and epicardial electropotential recordings *in-vivo*. *Chaos, Solitons & Fractals*, 2002;**13**(8): 1735–1742.

133. Nash M.P., C.P. Bradley, L.K. Cheng, A.J. Pullan, and D.J. Paterson, Electrocardiographic inverse validation study: *in-vivo* mapping and analysis. *FASEB J.*, April 2000;**14**(4): A442.

134. Taccardi B. and G. Marchetti, Distribution of heart potentials on the body surface and in artificial conducting media, in *International symposium on the electrophysiology of the heart*, B. Taccardi and G. Marchetti, Editors. Pergamon Press, New York, 1965, pp. 257–280.

135. Taccardi B., Changes in cardiac electrogenesis following coronary occlusion, in *Coronary Circulation and Energetics of the Myocardium*. S. Karger, Basel/New York, 1966, pp. 259–267.

136. Franzone P.C., L. Guerri, B. Taccardi, and C. Viganotti, The direct and inverse problems in electrocardiology. Numerical aspects of some regularization methods and applications to data collected in isolated dog heart experiments. *Lab. Anal. Numerica C.N.R.*, 1979, Pub. N:222.

137. Franzone P.C., G. Gassaniga, L. Guerri, B. Taccardi, and C. Viganotti, Accuracy evaluation in direct and inverse electrocardiology, in *Progress in Electrocardiography*, P. Macfarlane, Editor. Pitman Medical, London, 1979, pp. 83–87.

138. Messinger-Rapport B. and Y. Rudy, The inverse problem in electrocardiography: A model study of the effects of geometry and conductivity parameters on the reconstruction of epicardial potentials. *IEEE Trans. Biomed. Eng.*, 1986;**33**: 667–676.

139. Rudy Y. and H. Oster, The electrocardiographic inverse problem. *Crit. Rev. Biomed. Eng.*, 1992;**20**: 22–45.

140. Throne R., L. Olson, T. Hrabik, and J. Windle, Generalized eigensystem techniques for the inverse problem of electrocardiography applied to a realistic heart-torso geometry. *IEEE Trans. Biomed. Eng.*, 1997;**44**(6): 447.

141. Brooks D. and R. MacLeod, Imaging the electrical activity of the heart: Direct and inverse approaches, in *IEEE International Conference on Image Processing*. IEEE Computer Society, 1994, pp. 548–552.

142. MacLeod R., B. Yilmaz, B. Taccardi, B. Punske, Y. Serinagaoglu, and D. Brooks, Direct and inverse methods for cardiac mapping using multielectrode catheter measurements. *Biomed. Technik*, 2001;**46**(Suppl): 207–209.

143. Ni Q., R. MacLeod, R. Lux, and B. Taccardi, Interpolation of cardiac electric potentials. *Ann. Biomed. Eng.*, 1997;**25**(Suppl): 61. Biomed. Eng. Soc. Annual Fall Meeting.

144. Burnes J., D. Kaelber, B. Taccardi, R. Lux, P. Ershler, and Y. Rudy, A field-compatible method for interpolating biopotentials. *Ann. Biomed. Eng.*, 1998;**26**(1): 37–47.

145. Yilmaz B., R. MacLeod, S. Shome, B. Punkse, and B. Taccardi, Minimally invasive epicardial activation mapping from multielectrode catheters, in *Proceedings of the IEEE Engineering in Medicine and Biology Society 23rd Annual International Conference*. IEEE EMBS, IEEE Press, New York, 2001.

146. MacLeod R., B. Taccardi, and R. Lux, Mapping of cardiac ischemia in a realistic torso tank preparation, in *Building Bridges: International Congress on Electrocardioloegy International Meeting*, 1995, pp. 76–77.

147. MacLeod R., S. Shome, J. Stinstra, B. Punske, and B. Hopenfeld, Mechanisms of ischemia-induced ST-segment changes. *J. Electrocardiol.*, 2005, vol 38, pp. 8–13.

148. MacLeod R., R. Lux, M. Fuller, and B. Taccardi, Evaluation of novel measurement methods for detecting heterogeneous repolarization. *J. Electrocardiol.*, 1996;**29**(Suppl): 145–153.

149. Punske B., R. Lux, R. MacLeod, M. Fuller, P. Ershler, T. Dustman, Y. Vyhmeister, and B. Taccardi, Mechanisms of the spatial distribution of QT intervals on the epicardial and body surfaces. *J. Cardiovasc. Electrophysiol.*, 1999;**10**(12): 1605–1618.

150. Durrer D., R. van Dam, G. Freud, M. Janse, F. Meijler, and R. Arzbaecher, Total excitation of the isolated human heart. *Circ.*, 1970;**41**: 899–912.

151. Johnston P.R. and D. Kilpatrick, The inverse problem of electrocardiology: The performance of inversion techniques as a function of patient anatomy. *Math. Biosci.*, April 1995;**126**(2): 125–146.

152. Jenkins K., E. Walsh, S. Colan, D. Bergau, P. Saul, and J. Lock, Multipolar endocardial mapping of the right atrium during cardiac catheterization: Description of a new technique. *J. Am. Coll. Cardiol.*, 1993;**22**: 1105–1110.

153. Fitzpatrick A., M. Chin, C. Stillson, and M. Lesh, Successful percutaneous deployment, pacing and recording from a 64-polar, multi-strut "basket" catheter in the swine left ventricle. *PACE*, 1994;**17**:482.

154. Smeets J., S.B. Haim, L. Rodriguez, C. Timmermans, and H. Wellens, New method for nonfluoroscopic endocardial mapping in humans. *Circ.*, 1998;**97**: 2426–2432.

155. Modre R., B. Tilg, G. Fischer, F. Hanser, B. Messnarz, M. Seger, M.F. Schocke, T. Berger, F. Hintringer, and F.X. Roithinger, Atrial noninvasive activation mapping of paced rhythm data. *J. Cardiovasc. Electrophysiol.*, 2003;**14**(7): 712–719.

156. Fischer G., F. Hanser, C. Hintermuller, M. Seger, B. Pfeifer, R. Modre, L. Wieser, B. Tilg, S. Egger, T. Berger, F. Roithinger, and F. Hinteringer, A signal processing pipeline for noninvasive imaging of ventricular preexcitation. *Meth. Inf. Med.*, 2005;**44**(4).

157. Ramanathan C., R. Ghanem, P. Jia, K. Ryu, and Y. Rudy, Noninvasive electrocardiographic imaging for cardiac electrophysiology and arrhythmia. *Nat Med*, April 2004;**10**(4): 422–428.

158. Intini A., R.N. Goldstein, P. Jia, C. Ramanathan, K. Ryu, B. Giannattasio, R. Gilkeson, B.S. Stambler, P. Brugada, W.G. Stevenson, Y. Rudy, and A.L. Waldo, Electrocardiographic imaging (ECGI), a novel diagnostic modality used for mapping of focal left ventricular tachycardia in a young athlete. *Hear. Res.*, 2005;**2**(11): 1250–1252.

159. Jia P., C. Ramanathan, R.N. Ghanem, K. Ryu, N. Varma, and Y. Rudy, Electrocardiographic imaging of cardiac resynchronization therapy in heart failure: Observation of variable electrophysiologic responses. *Hear. Res.*, 2006;**3**(3): 296–310.

160. Velipasaoglu E., H. Sun, L. Rao, and D. Khoury, Role of geometry in the endocardial electrocardiographic inverse problem, in *Proceedings of the IEEE Engineering in Medicine and Biology Society 22nd Annual International Conference*, vol. 2, 2000, pp. 902–903.

161. Rao L., R. He, C. Ding, and D.S. Khoury, Novel noncontact catheter system for endocardial electrical and anatomical imaging. *Ann. Biomed. Eng.*, 2004;**32**: 573–584.

162. Jia P., B. Punske, B. Taccardi, and Y. Rudy, Electrophysiologic endocardial mapping from a noncontact nonexpandable catheter: a validation study of a geometry-based concept. *J Cardiovasc Electrophysiol*, Nov 2000;**11**(11): 1238–1251.

163. Beatty G., S. Remole, M. Johnston, J. Holte, and D. Benditt, Non-contact electrical extrapolation technique to reconstruct endocardial potentials. *PACE*, 1994;**17**(4): 765.

164. Gornick C., S. Adler, B. Pederson, J. Hauck, J. Budd, and J. Schweitzer, Validation of a new noncontact catheter system for electroanatomic mapping of left ventricular endocardium. *Circ.*, Feb 1999;**99**(6): 829–835.

165. Kadish A., J. Hauck, B. Pederson, G. Beatty, and C. Gornick, Mapping of atrial activation with a noncontact, multielectrode catheter in dogs. *Circ.*, Apr 1999;**99**(14): 1906–1913.

166. Peters N., W. Jackman, R. Schilling, and D. Divies, Human left ventricular endocardial activation mapping using a novel noncontact catheter. *Circ.*, 1998;**9**: 887–898.

167. Paul T., B. Windhagen-Mahnert, T. Kriebel, H. Bertram, R. Kaulitz, T. Korte, M. Niehaus, and J. Tebbenjohanns, Atrial reentrant tachycardia after surgery for congenital heart disease: endocardial mapping and radiofrequency catheter ablation using a novel, noncontact mapping system. *Circ.*, May 2001;**103**(18): 2266–2271.

168. Yue A., J. Paisey, S. Robinson, T. Betts, P. Roberts, and J. Morgan, Determination of human ventricular repolarization by noncontact mapping: validation with monophasic action potential recordings. *Circ.*, Sep 2004;**110**(11): 1343–1350.

169. Thiagalingam A., E. Wallace, A. Boyd, V. Eipper, C. Campbell, K. Byth, D. Ross, and P. Kovoor, Noncontact mapping of the left ventricle: insights from validation with transmural contact mapping. *Pacing Clin. Electrophysiol.*, May 2004;**27**(5): 570–578.

170. Ambroggi L.D., B. Taccardi, and E. Macchi, Body surface maps of heart potential: Tentative localization of preexcited area of forty-two Wolff–Parkinson–White patients. *Circ.*, 1976;**54**: 251.

171. Essen R.V., R. Hinsen, R. Louis, W. Merx, J. Silny, G. Rau, and S. Effert, On-line monitoring of multiple precordial leads in high risk patients with coronary artery disease – a pilot study. *Eur. Heart J.*, 1985;**5**: 203–209.

172. Green L., R. Lux, and C. Haws, Detection and localization of coronary artery disease with body surface mapping in patients with normal electrocardiograms. *Circ.*, 1987;**76**: 1290–1297.

173. Ambroggi L.D., T. Bertoni, M. Breghi, M. Marconi, and M. Mosca, Diagnostic value of body surface potential mapping in old anterior non-Q myocardial infarction. *J. Electrocardiol.*, 1988;**21**(4): 321–329.

174. Bell A., M. Loughhead, S. Walker, and D. Kilpatrick, Prognostic significance of ST potentials determined by body surface mapping in inferior wall acute myocardial infarction. *Am. J. Cardiol.*, 1989;**64**: 319–323.

175. Anderson J., G. Dempsey, G. Wright, C. Cullen, M. Crawley, E. McAdams, J. McLaughlin, G. MacKenzie, and A. Adgey, Portable cardiac mapping assessment of acute ischaemic injury. *Methods Inf. Med. (MVI)*, 1994;**33**(1): 72–75.

176. Khoury D., K. Berrier, S. Badruddin, and W. Zoghbi, Three-dimensional electrophysiological imaging of the intact canine left ventricle using a noncontact multielectrode cavitary probe: study of sinus, paced, and spontaneous premature beats. *Circ.*, 1998;**97**(4): 399–409.

177. Tilg B., P. Wach, A. Sippensgroenewegen, G. Fischer, R. Modre, F. Roithinger, M. Mlynash, G. Reddy, T. Roberts, M. Lesh, and P. Steiner, Closed chest validation of source imaging from human ECG and MCG mapping, in *Proceedings of The First Joint BMES/EMBS Conference*. IEEE Press, New York, 1999, p. 275.

178. Potse M., R. Hoekema, A.C. Linnenbank, A. Sippens-Groenewegen, J. Strackee, J.M.T. de Bakker, and C.A. Grimbergen, Conversion of left ventricular endocardial positions from patient-independent co-ordinates into biplane fluoroscopic projections. *Med. Biol. Eng. Comput.*, January 2002;**40**(1): 41–46.

179. Tilg B., G. Fischer, R. Modre, F. FH, B. Messnarz, and F.X. Roithinger, Electrocardiographic imaging of atrial and ventricular electrical activation. *Med. Image Anal.*, September 2003;**7**(3): 391–398.

180. Pfeifer B., F. Hanser, and C.H. Modre-Osprian, G. Fischer, M. Seger, H. Mühlthaler, T. TT, and B. Tilg, Cardiac modeling using active appearance models and morphological operators. medical imaging: Visualization, image-guided procedures, and display, in *Proceedings of the SPIE*, 2005.

181. Cheney M., D. Isaacson, and J. Newell, Electrical Impedance Tomography. *SIAM Rev.*, 1999;**41**(1): 85–101.

182. Saulnier G.J., R.S. Blue, J.C. Newell, D. Isaacson, and P.M. Edic, Electrical Impedance Tomography. *IEEE Signal Process. Mag.*, 2001;**18**(6): 31–43.

183. A. Ghodrati, D. Brooks, and R. MacLeod, Methods of solving reduced lead systems for inverse electrocardiography. *IEEE Trans. Biomed. Eng.*, Feb 2007;**54**(2): 339–343.

184. Green L.S., B. Taccardi, P.R. Ershler, and R.L. Lux, Effects of conducting media on isopotential and isochrone distributions. *Circulation*, 1991;**84**(6): 2513–2521.

185. Bradley C.P., M.P. Nash, L.K. Cheng, A.J. Pullan, and D.J. Paterson, Electrocardiographic inverse validation study: Model development and methodology. *FASEB J.*, April 2000;**14**(4): A442.

186. Messnarz B., M. Seger, R. Modre, G. Fischer, F. Hanser, and B. Tilg, A comparison of noninvasive reconstruction of epicardial versus transmembrane potentials in consideration of the null space. *IEEE Trans. Biomed. Eng.*, September 2004;**51**(9): 1609–1618.

187. Oostendorp T., J. Nenonen, and P. Korhonen, Noninvasive determination of the activation sequence of the heart: application to patients with previous myocardial infarctions. *J. Electrocardiol.*, 2002;**35**(Suppl): 75–80.

188. Fischer G., B. Pfeifer, M. Seger, C. Hintermuller, F. Hanser, R. Modre, B. Tilg, T. Trieb, C. Kremser, F. Roithinger, and F. Hintringer, Computationally efficient noninvasive cardiac activation time imaging. *Methods Inf Med*, 2005;**44**(5): 674–686.

189. Nielsen P.M., I.J. LeGrice, B.H. Smaill, and P.J. Hunter, Mathematical model of geometry and fibrous structure of the heart. *Am. J. Physiol.*, 1991;**260**(4 Pt 2): H1365–H1378.

Part IV

Electrocardiographic Lead Systems and Recording Techniques

10 Lead Theory

B. Milan Horáček

P. W. Macfarlane et al. (eds.), *Basic Electrocardiology*, DOI 10.1007/978-0-85729-871-3_10,

© Springer-Verlag London Limited 2012

10.1   Introduction

The bioelectric sources arising during the heart's electrical excitation process produce a flow of electric current in the surrounding tissues. It is therefore possible to detect, with a pair of electrodes external to the heart, time-varying potential differences known as electrocardiograms. The pair of electrodes constitutes an electrocardiographic lead in its simplest form.

Lead theory deals with the relationship between cardiac electric sources and the potential differences they generate in electrocardiographic leads. Two components can be considered separately in studying this relationship: the active cardiac electric sources (❯ Chaps. 6 and ❯ 7), which are distributed in and restricted to the heart region, and the passive aggregate of electrically conductive extracardiac tissues of the body (the volume conductor), which provides an electric load for cardiac sources and makes the external measurement of cardiac electric activity possible. Lead theory provides a method for visualizing the relationship between cardiac sources and voltages in electrocardiographic leads. This relationship can be studied by performing specific solutions to the volume conductor problem, which consists of evaluating an electric field produced in the bounded volume conductor by a given electric source (❯ Chaps. 2 and ❯ 8).

10.1.1   Classical Theory of Electrocardiographic Leads

Classical lead theory – introduced by Einthoven and coworkers and described in every textbook of electrocardiography – assumes that the human body is part of an infinite, homogeneous conductor in which the heart's electric sources are represented by a single, time-varying current dipole (depicted as a two-dimensional heart vector) at a fixed location. Einthoven's leads (designated lead I, lead II, and lead III) use electrodes at three extremities (❯ Chap. 11). Since such electrodes are relatively remote from the cardiac source, Einthoven felt he could define the relationship between the heart vector and the electrocardiographic potentials observed in these leads in very simple terms: he postulated that the potentials at the three extremities as generated by the heart vector were the same as those generated at the vertices of an equilateral triangle in an infinite, homogeneous, two-dimensional conductor with the dipole source located at the triangle's centroid.

The Wilson central terminal with unipolar limb leads, and augmented leads, were later readily incorporated into Einthoven's theory. However, for interpreting potentials in unipolar precordial leads, a more general solid-angle theory (❯ Chaps. 2, ❯ 5 and ❯ 6) was introduced into electrocardiography by Wilson and coworkers. This theory introduces a double-layer source instead of a single, fixed-location dipole.

10.1.2   Volume Conductor Theory of Electrocardiographic Leads

A more appropriate lead theory, often referred to as the volume-conductor theory, evolved in the 1940s and 1950s. First, Burger and van Milaan took into consideration the fact that the human body is a three-dimensional, bounded, irregularly shaped and inhomogeneous volume conductor. Second, McFee and Johnston, and independently Schmitt, considered the distributed character of cardiac sources. Although Burger's theory is quite general with regard to volume-conductor characteristics, it rests on the fixed-dipole hypothesis; that is, it assumes that at a given instant the potentials anywhere on the body surface can be derived from the projection of a heart vector in 3D space (thought to account for all cardiac sources) into an appropriate spatial lead vector (characterizing lead properties under the assumption that the location of the heart vector is fixed).

The fixed-dipole hypothesis is no longer acceptable, as body-surface potential mapping studies have established (❯ Chap. 5 of *Cardiac Arrhythmias and Mapping Techniques*) that the electrocardiographic body-surface potential distributions exhibit features that cannot be accounted for by a single, fixed-location dipole source. McFee and Johnston's lead theory, by taking into account the distributed nature of cardiac electric sources, overcomes the limitations of the fixed-dipole hypothesis; it generalizes the lead vector into the lead-field concept and defines the source-lead relationship for every element of the distributed cardiac source. Schmitt coined the appropriate term "transfer impedance" for the vector field representing the lead field.

The aim of this chapter is to provide an elementary introduction to modern lead theory. The cornerstones of this theory are the superposition and reciprocity theorems of Helmholz, upon which rest, respectively, the lead-vector concept of Burger and van Milaan and the lead-field concept of McFee and Johnston. The classical concepts of Einthoven and Wilson fit into this lead theory as a special case.

10.1.3 Bibliographic Notes

The equilateral triangle diagram for interpreting limb-lead electrocardiograms was introduced by Einthoven and coworkers [1, 2]. This diagram is described in every text of electrocardiography (❷ Chap. 11), as are the conventions of the Wilson central terminal with the unipolar limb leads [3], augmented leads [4], and unipolar precordial leads [5–7]. Solid-angle theory was introduced into electrocardiography by Wilson et al. [8]; this theory is described in texts, such as Plonsey [9], Plonsey and Barr [10], Malmivuo and Plonsey [11], and in articles [12]. Burger and van Milaan [13–15] took into consideration the fact that the human body is a three-dimensional, inhomogeneous volume conductor. McFee and Johnston [16–18], and Schmitt [19], considered the distributed character of cardiac sources. Reviews of lead theory have been written by Burger [20], Frank [21], McFee and Johnston [16], Schmitt [19], Schaefer and Haas [22], Geselowitz and Schmitt [23], McFee and Baule [24], Geselowitz [25], and Malmivuo and Plonsey [11].

10.2 Prerequisites

The assumptions that underlie electrocardiographic lead theory (as presented in this chapter) are not very restrictive; they allow the theory to be formulated for distributed cardiac sources, for a body of irregular shape and inhomogeneous composition, and for any conceivable electrocardiographic lead. The lead-vector concept requires that only one dipolar source be considered at a time; however, this restriction can be relaxed when the lead vector is interpreted more generally as a local value of the lead field.

10.2.1 Assumptions Concerning Cardiac Bioelectric Sources

Bioelectric sources arising during cardiac activation and repolarization are distributed throughout the heart and are proportional everywhere to the spatial gradient of the transmembrane potential ((7.21) and (8.8)). Such sources can be described as a volume distribution of impressed current density $\vec{J}^i$ (current dipole moment per unit volume, i.e., current per unit area), and $\vec{J}^i dv$ (current dipole moment) may be thought of as an elemental current dipole in a small region of the heart.

Multiple Dipoles

A rigorous but impractical description of cardiac electric sources by a continuous distribution of impressed current density $\vec{J}^i$ can be approximated to any desired degree of accuracy by a finite number of appropriately placed current dipoles; such a source is called a multiple-dipole source. Constituent dipoles of the multiple-dipole source can be obtained by dividing the myocardium into subregions and assigning a local, lumped current dipole to the centroid of each region, i.e.,

$$\vec{p}_k = \int_{\Delta V_k} \vec{J}^i \, dv, \tag{10.1}$$

where the integration is over the volume ΔV_k of the kth region. The dimension of the vector quantity $\vec{p}_k$ is current times length; thus $\vec{p}_k$ can be approximated by a current dipole (❷ Sect. 2.5.1.2).

Heart Vector

The region for which a lumped current dipole is determined can be chosen arbitrarily; as a special case, it can encompass an entire heart. A dipole so obtained is referred to as a heart vector $\vec{H}$. Thus

$$\vec{H} = \int_{V_H} \vec{J}^i \, dv, \tag{10.2}$$

where the integration is over the entire heart volume V_H. The heart vector thus represents the vectorial sum of all elemental current dipoles and is usually placed at the centroid of the heart region. (The position of $\vec{H}$ can be chosen rigorously so that it satisfies certain criteria of optimality, e.g., minimal content of the quadrupolar component [26].)

The concept of the heart vector can be developed from the analysis of the electric field produced in an infinite homogeneous medium at a sufficient distance from the cluster of dipolar sources. In the immediate vicinity of such a cluster, a complete specification of all constituent dipoles, consisting of the location and moment $\vec{p}_k$ for each, is necessary to determine the field potential accurately. However, at a large distance from the source, the field potential converges to that produced by a single equivalent dipole located at the centroid of the cluster. In physics, this equivalent dipole is known as the dipole moment of the cluster.

Potential Field of a Single Dipole

As shown in ❯ Sect. 2.5.1.2 (2.99), the electric field $\Phi(\vec{r}')$ at field point $\vec{r}'$, produced by a single current dipole with moment $\vec{p}$ and location $\vec{r}$ in an infinite homogeneous medium of conductivity σ, is

$$\Phi(\vec{r}') = \frac{1}{4\pi\sigma} \frac{\vec{p}(\vec{r}) \cdot \vec{R}}{R^3} + c \tag{10.3}$$

R is the length of the vector $\vec{R} = \vec{r}' - \vec{r}$ pointing from dipole source location to field point, and c is the arbitrary integration constant. By defining the potential at infinity as zero, we have $c = 0$.

An equivalent variant of (10.3) is

$$\Phi(\vec{r}') = \frac{1}{4\pi\sigma} \frac{p \cos\theta}{R^2} + c, \tag{10.4}$$

with p the magnitude (strength) of the dipole vector and θ the angle between vectors $\vec{p}$ and $\vec{R}$ (2.100).

Potential Field of a Double Layer

A dipolar double layer is an arbitrary surface with which are associated sources of electric current on one (positive) side and sinks of current on the other (negative) side; it is an excellent approximation of electric primary sources at the activation wave front in the heart (❯ Chap. 6). A double layer can be thought of as a set of dipoles, each representing an element (patch) of double-layer surface (❯ Chap. 2). For field points at a large distance from a double layer the potential field can be approximated by field generated by the dipole that is the vectorial sum of these elemental dipoles representing the source strength of the individual patches.

10.2.2 Assumptions Concerning the Human Torso

The volume-conductor problem in electrocardiology involves the determination of an extracardiac electric field produced in the body and on its surface by the distributed and time-varying electric sources of the heart. To solve this problem it is necessary to apply appropriately electromagnetic theory. The problem has two important features that make it amenable to solution: it is quasistatic and linear.

The term "quasistatic" implies that the extracardiac electric field throughout the body is at every instant in equilibrium with the sources in the heart, and thus, for a given distribution of sources at a given instant a corresponding extracardiac field can be determined without any regard to the source distribution at previous instants.

Another important feature of the volume-conductor problem in electrocardiology is that, at the low current densities that are involved, the body can be considered to be a linear physical system. Capacitive and inductive effects can be neglected, and thus, the term linearity refers to the resistive properties (❯ Sect. 2.4). Consequently, as discussed in ❯ Sect. 2.4.3, the relationship between heart-produced current flow and the electric field can be expressed by a vector form of Ohm's law: $\vec{J} = \sigma\vec{E}$, where $\vec{J}$ is a vector of current density, $\vec{E}$ is a vector of electric field intensity and σ, is the conductivity of the extracardiac medium. Associated with the electric field is the electric potential Φ, a scalar function defined from the expression $\vec{E} = -\nabla\Phi$. Since Φ is defined indirectly, i.e., through its gradient (❯ Sect. 2.4), the potential field is always specified from its sources up to an arbitrary constant. However, by considering the difference of the potential between any two points in space, this common constant drops out of the equation and the resulting potential difference has a unique interpretation: it is a scalar quantity defined as the work required to move a unit positive charge from one of the field points to the other (❯ Sect. 2.4.3). When denoting the two field points as A and B, we have

$$V_{AB} = \Phi_A - \Phi_B = -\int_B^A \vec{E} \cdot d\vec{l} \tag{10.5}$$

In the following ❯ Sect. 10.3 the notation Φ is used for the potential field, and V denotes potential differences between two field points and/or two artificially constructed terminals.

Helmholtz stated the three fundamental principles that govern linear physical systems:

1. The principle of superposition
2. The principle of reciprocity
3. The principle of the equivalent double layer

All three principles have a fundamental importance for the theoretical basis of electrocardiography; the first two constitute a foundation of lead theory. The principle of superposition states that an electric field arising from several sources is the sum of the fields that would be present for each source acting separately. Burger and van Milaan made this principle the basis of the lead-vector concept (❯ Sect. 10.3). The reciprocity theorem was applied to electrocardiography by McFee and Johnston, who introduced the lead-field concept (❯ Sect. 10.5).

Finally, a few words about another prerequisite of the electrocardiographic lead theory – Kirchhoff's laws. In electrical network theory, a current and voltage are associated with each branch of the network. Since energy is neither stored nor dissipated in any junction of the network, the electric current must obey a local conservation law. This is expressed by Kirchhoff's current law, which states that the total current leaving any junction must equal the current entering the junction. Since energy is conserved, a series of elements in a closed-loop has a single flow of current, and hence, the sum of voltage differences around the loop equals zero because the potential must be unique at each node of the network; this is Kirchhoff's voltage law.

10.2.3   Definition of Electrocardiographic Lead

Originally, the term "electrocardiographic lead" referred strictly to the configuration (location on the thorax) of two electrodes attached directly to the body for the purposes of recording electrocardiographic signal. This notion had to be later extended to accommodate other recording practices in electrocardiography that produced potential differences between two terminals as weighted sums (linear combinations) of the potentials at multiple electrode sites. The weighting of the surface potentials at the electrode sites was originally performed by using resistive networks (❯ Fig. 10.1). Modern circuitry with operational amplifiers allows the addition/subtraction of voltages from as many recording sites as are deemed necessary. Therefore, the following definition will be adopted:

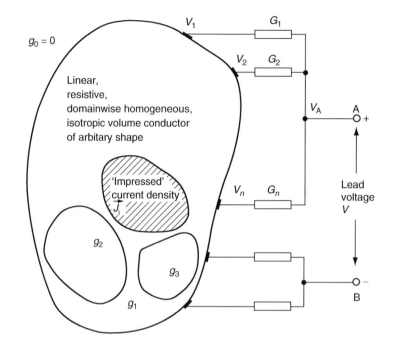

◘ Fig. 10.1

Cardiac sources in the abstracted torso and an electrocardiographic lead. A good approximation of the human torso is a bounded, linear, resistive, domainwise homogeneous and isotropic volume conductor, with electric sources in the heart region represented by a volume distribution of "impressed" current density $\vec{J}^i$, which can be in turn approximated to any desired degree of accuracy by a finite number of elemental current dipoles distributed throughout the heart region. Real constants $g_0, g_1, g_2, \ldots, g_n$ denote conductivities of different regions. The electrocardiogram is a time-dependent voltage between two terminals A and B of an electrocardiographic lead; each terminal can be connected either to a single electrode or, via weighting resistors, to several electrodes. Variables V_1 to V_n are potentials at the electrode sites; V_A is a potential at terminal A; G_1 to G_n are conductances of weighting resistors R_1 to R_n ($G_i = 1/R_i$); the lead voltage can be considered an "open-circuit voltage" because the input impedance of modern ECG amplifiers is very high

The electrocardiographic lead is a pair of terminals with designated polarity, each connected either directly or via a passive/active network to recording electrodes sampling the cardiac potential field on the thorax; the observed potential difference between the two terminals is called the lead voltage.

A lead specification consists of electrode-placement and polarity conventions, and of the diagram of the network; this diagram can be translated into numerical weights for the potentials at all constituent electrodes. The term "composite lead" is sometimes used in this chapter for those leads that include passive/active networks weighting the potentials at one or both lead terminals (❷ Fig. 10.1); the word "composite" emphasizes that the lead is made up of a number of constituent voltages. A well-known composite terminal is Wilson central terminal (WCT), which is formed by taking the mean of the potentials at left arm, right arm, and left foot. WCT was proposed as "indifferent" lead terminal, which approximates for arbitrary cardiac sources the potential that would exist at large distance from these sources (see, however, ❷ Sect. 5.4.1).

Note that, somewhat confusingly, the term "lead" is frequently used as a shorthand for time-varying "lead voltage" recorded by means of the physical lead arrangement. A few additional comments on lead/electrode nomenclature are needed:

1. The term "unipolar lead" is a misnomer: measuring potential differences always requires two terminals.
2. The term "bipolar lead" refers to the situation where measured potential differences are derived directly from two electrodes serving as the lead terminals.

3. The term "sensing electrode" for one of the terminals of a bipolar lead only makes sense if the other electrode/terminal can be considered as "indifferent" (see ❷ Sect. 5.4.1).

10.2.4 Bibliographic Notes

Any text on electromagnetic theory (e.g., [27, 28]) will cover the material on the field of the dipole and the double layer, as well as on the dipole moment of a cluster of sources. Courant and Hilbert [29] deal with the derivation of basic theorems concerning potential of the dipole and double stratum/layer in two and three dimensions (see also Guillemin [30]). Plonsey [9] and Geselowitz and Schmitt [23] justify the quasistatic assumption. Plonsey and Heppner [31] document the absence of capacitive and inductive effects. In 1853, Hermann von Helmholtz [32] was the first to realize that the correct interpretation of bioelectric measurements requires an understanding of the electric field in a volume conductor; he stated the three fundamental principles that govern linear physical systems. Geselowitz and Schmitt [23] and Geselowitz [25] cover Helmholtz' theorems, including derivations. Oster et al. [33] show the fundamental significance of Kirchhoff's laws in biological systems. One of many texts dealing with electric circuit theory is Desoer and Kuh [34].

The experimental evidence needed to support the assumptions stated in this section was gathered over a long period. The first tissue measurements made specifically with electrocardiographic effects in mind were carried out by Kaufman and Johnston [35]; they showed that substantial differences in resistivity existed between different tissues of the body. Schwan and Kay [36] showed that the phase shift can be ignored for the electrocardiographic frequencies. Accurate resistivity measurements were made by Burger and van Dongen [37], Rush et al. [38] and others. Studies of tissue resistivity have been reviewed by Geddes and Baker [39].

10.3 Lead Vector

Provided the assumptions stated in ❷ Sect. 10.2 are satisfied, the relationship between dipolar sources and lead voltages is conceptually very simple. This was first shown by Burger and van Milaan.

10.3.1 Definition

A current dipole with moment $\vec{p}$ can be resolved into three orthogonal components

$$\vec{p} = \vec{e}_x p_x + \vec{e}_y p_y + \vec{e}_z p_z, \tag{10.6}$$

where p_x, p_y, and p_z are the magnitudes of the components and $\vec{e}_x, \vec{e}_y$, and $\vec{e}_z$ are unit vectors along the axes of the Cartesian coordinate system (❷ Sect. 2.2.3). The vector $\vec{p}$ represents the lumped cardiac electric sources of a chosen cardiac region (10.1); when an entire heart region is chosen, $\vec{p}$ becomes the heart vector $\vec{H}$ (10.2). In electrocardiography, it is customary to choose a right-handed coordinate system with x, y, and z axes as shown in ❷ Fig. 10.9; the x axis is directed from the right to the left of the torso, the y axis from head to feet, and the z axis from front to back.

If the dipole is embedded in an arbitrary volume conductor, bounded or unbounded, the amount that each component of vector $\vec{p}$ contributes to any lead voltage V is directly proportional (as a consequence of the linearity assumption) to that component's magnitude, and all three contributions can be added by virtue of the superposition theorem, i.e.,

$$V = c_x p_x + c_y p_y + c_z p_z, \tag{10.7}$$

where c_x, c_y and c_z are scalar constants. This is Burger's equation, a cornerstone of lead theory.

Based on (2.11), Burger"s equation can be interpreted as the scalar product of two vectors

$$V = \vec{c} \cdot \vec{p}, \tag{10.8}$$

where $\vec{c} = \vec{e}_x c_x + \vec{e}_y c_y + \vec{e}_z c_z$ is a vector that specifies the relationship between the dipolar source at a given location $\vec{r}$ and the voltage V in a given lead. The vector $\vec{c}$ is called the lead vector of a given electrocardiographic lead. It depends on the location $\vec{r}$ of the source, the locations of lead electrodes, and – for a bounded volume conductor – on the shape of the torso and the inhomogeneities of the electric conductivities of the torso as a volume conductor.

The units of the lead vector are ohms per meter, since the units of $\vec{p}$ are ampere × meter and voltage V is measured in volts. If a volume conductor's shape and electric properties do not change, the components of the lead vector will stay constant; since the medium is assumed to be resistive, these constants are real numbers.

Although the relationship between cardiac sources and lead voltages as defined by Burger's equation (10.8) is conceptually simple, the scalar coefficients c_x, c_y, and c_z are not easy to determine except in very simplified cases. To estimate lead vectors of the limb leads, Burger constructed a body-shaped tank, filled it with an electrolyte, and inserted a cork "spine" and sand-bag "lungs." His results indicated that the classical lead theory, embodied in the Einthoven triangle diagram, required revision.

10.3.2   Scalar Product and its Geometrical Interpretation

The scalar product (inner product, dot product) of two vectors $\vec{c}$ and $\vec{p}$ is a scalar quantity

$$\vec{c} \cdot \vec{p} = cp \cos \theta,$$

where θ is the angle between the vectors when they are placed with a common origin (❯ Sect. 2.2.4). As seen in ❯ Fig. 10.2, the scalar product has a simple geometrical interpretation: it is the length of one vector multiplied by the length of the projection of the other onto it. Thus, from Burger's equation (10.8), the contribution of a current dipole $\vec{p}$ to the voltage V in any particular lead equals the length of the projection of $\vec{p}$ on the appropriate lead vector $\vec{c}$ times the length of $\vec{c}$. If $\vec{p}$ is orthogonal to $\vec{c}$, $\vec{p} \cdot \vec{c} = 0$; if $\vec{p}$ is parallel/antiparallel to $\vec{c}$, $\vec{p} \cdot \vec{c} = \pm p\, c$.

The scalar product is commutative and distributive:

$$\vec{p} \cdot \vec{c} = \vec{c} \cdot \vec{p},$$

and

$$(\vec{c}_1 + \vec{c}_2) \cdot \vec{p} = \vec{c}_1 \cdot \vec{p} + \vec{c}_2 \cdot \vec{p}$$

These as well as other basic properties of the scalar product are discussed in ❯ Chap. 2.

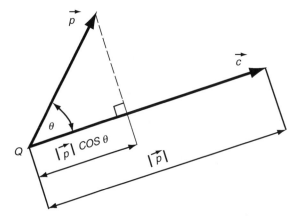

◻ Fig. 10.2

Lead-vector projection. According to Burger's equation (10.8), a current dipole $\vec{p}$ produces the voltage $V = \vec{p} \cdot \vec{c}$ in an electrocardiographic lead, where $\vec{c}$ is a lead vector characterizing the lead. This scalar product of two vectors has a simple geometrical interpretation: it is the length of the projection of $\vec{p}$ on the lead vector $\vec{c}$ multiplied by the lead vector's length $|\vec{c}|$

10.3.3 Lead Vectors and Limb Leads

We consider first the lead vectors associated with the limb leads. There are six limb leads in the set of 12 standard leads; these limb leads are derived from only three independent extremity potentials, and thus only two independent potential differences can be obtained. Even though some limb leads are redundant, they were adopted in the set of 12 standard leads to facilitate the visual interpretation of electrocardiograms.

According to Burger's equation (10.8), any current dipole $\vec{p}$ embedded in any volume conductor of arbitrary shape and extent will produce the following three potential differences at the limb-electrode sites *against any arbitrary reference*.

$$V_R = \vec{c}_R \cdot \vec{p}, \tag{10.9}$$

$$V_L = \vec{c}_L \cdot \vec{p}, \tag{10.10}$$

$$V_F = \vec{c}_F \cdot \vec{p}, \tag{10.11}$$

where $\vec{c}$ denotes a lead vector and the subscripts R, L, and F refer to the right arm, left arm, and the left leg respectively. In the human torso, which is irregularly shaped, the lead vectors $\vec{c}_R$, $\vec{c}_L$, and $\vec{c}_F$ are independent and thus the sum of $V_R + V_L + V_F$ will not necessarily be zero. (However, if WCT is the reference used then $V_R + V_L + V_F = 0$.)

10.3.4 Bipolar Limb Leads

Einthoven introduced bipolar limb leads denoted I, II, and III that yield potential differences V_I, V_{II}, and V_{III} between three limbs:

$$V_I = V_L - V_R, \tag{10.12}$$

$$V_{II} = V_F - V_R, \tag{10.13}$$

$$V_{III} = V_F - V_L, \tag{10.14}$$

Expressed in terms of Burger's equation (10.8), and using (10.9)–(10.14)

$$V_I = \vec{c}_I \cdot \vec{p} = \vec{c}_L \cdot \vec{p} - \vec{c}_R \cdot \vec{p}, \tag{10.15}$$

$$V_{II} = \vec{c}_{II} \cdot \vec{p} = \vec{c}_F \cdot \vec{p} - \vec{c}_R \cdot \vec{p}, \tag{10.16}$$

$$V_{III} = \vec{c}_{III} \cdot \vec{p} = \vec{c}_F \cdot \vec{p} - \vec{c}_L \cdot \vec{p} \tag{10.17}$$

Since scalar multiplication is distributive, the lead vectors of bipolar limb leads can be defined in terms of lead vectors for unipolar limb leads:

$$\vec{c}_I = \vec{c}_L - \vec{c}_R, \tag{10.18}$$

$$\vec{c}_{II} = \vec{c}_F - \vec{c}_R, \tag{10.19}$$

$$\vec{c}_{III} = \vec{c}_F - \vec{c}_L \tag{10.20}$$

10.3.5 Burger Triangle

From the definitions of the bipolar limb-lead voltages (and their designated polarity) it follows that

$$V_I + V_{III} = V_{II}, \tag{10.21}$$

that is, the sum of the lead voltages if leads I and III at any time instant equals the lead voltage of lead II. In electrocardiography this property is known as Einthoven's law; it is a specific application of Kirchhoff's voltage law for a closed circuit. By substituting the expressions shown in the previous subsection it is found that

$$\vec{c}_I + \vec{c}_{III} = \vec{c}_{II} \tag{10.22}$$

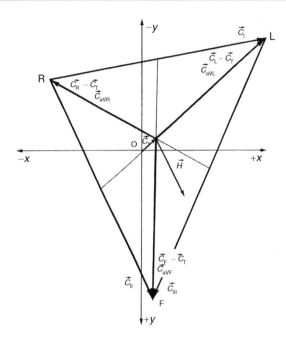

◘ Fig. 10.3

Burger triangle: frontal plane projection. Lead vectors of bipolar limb leads I, II and III satisfy the constraint $\vec{c}_I + \vec{c}_{III} = \vec{c}_{II}$, and thus they form a triangle (the Burger triangle), which does not necessarily lie in the frontal plane. Lead vectors $\vec{c}_R - \vec{c}_T$, $\vec{c}_L - \vec{c}_T$, $\vec{c}_F - \vec{c}_T$ of unipolar extremity leads originate at the median point of this triangle, as can be seen from the definition of the Wilson central terminal (❷ Sect. 10.3.4). Lead vectors $\vec{c}_{aVR}$, $\vec{c}_{aVL}$ and $\vec{c}_{aVF}$ of augmented leads start, respectively, at the midpoints of $\vec{c}_{III}$, $\vec{c}_{II}$ and $\vec{c}_I$, and terminate at the opposite vertex of the Burger triangle; therefore, these lead vectors are concurrent at the median point and are 3/2 of the length of the lead vectors of the corresponding unipolar extremity leads. A heart vector $\vec{H}$ can be placed at the median point, and, in accordance with Burger's equation, its projection on the appropriate lead vector multiplied by that lead vector's length defines the lead voltage. The points R, L, F depicted here are denoted R', L', F' in image space (❷ Fig. 10.8)

This shows that Einthoven's law for the bipolar limb lead potentials has a similar formulation in the corresponding lead vectors. It holds true for an arbitrary cardiac source in any volume conductor that satisfies the linearity assumption. In ❷ Fig. 10.3 the lead vectors of leads I, II, and II are depicted as the edges of a scalene triangle: Burger's triangle. This geometrical interpretation is justified by (10.22). The triangle does not necessarily lie in the frontal plane. In the next subsection it is shown that the Einthoven equilateral triangle is a special case of Burger's scalene triangle.

10.3.6   Einthoven's Triangle

In contrast to Burger's triangle, classical Einthoven's triangle diagram is based on a much more simplified representation of cardiac sources and of extracardiac volume conductor.

1. Three field points R, L, and F, corresponding to right arm, left arm, and left leg are located in the frontal plane; they are the vertices of an equilateral triangle (❷ Fig. 10.4).
2. The position of the source dipole $\vec{p}$ is at the centroid of the triangle and its direction is confined to the triangle's plane.
3. The volume conductor involved may be considered to be either two- or three-dimensional; it may be taken to be of infinite extent, or bounded by a circle (2D space) or a sphere (3D space).

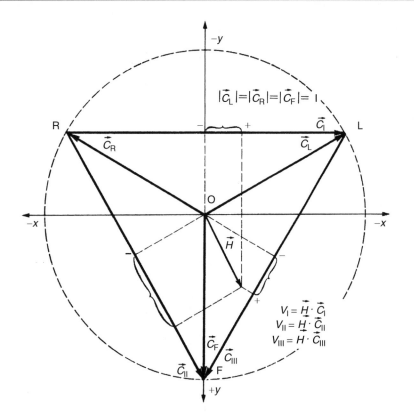

◘ Fig. 10.4
Einthoven triangle in terms of lead vectors. The lead vectors implicitly assumed by Einthoven for limb leads I, II and III lie in the frontal plane and are of equal length, thus forming an equilateral triangle. The projection of the heart vector $\vec{H}$ on sides I, II and III of the Einthoven triangle is equivalent to the scaled scalar product of the heart vector $\vec{H}$ with lead vectors $\vec{c}_\text{I}$, $\vec{c}_\text{II}$ and $\vec{c}_\text{III}$, respectively; this is Burger's equation

For all volume conductor configurations already mentioned the potentials at field points R, L, and F can be shown to be

$$\Phi = \alpha \, \vec{e} \cdot \vec{p} + c, \tag{10.23}$$

where $\vec{e}$ represents the unit vector directed from the dipole location to the respective field point (R, L, or F). The factor α is a proportionality constant depending on the particular volume conductor configuration. For a bounded sphere with unit radius its value is $3/(4\pi\sigma)$ (2.153). The constant C specifies the potential at an arbitrary common reference. It drops out of the equation when considering lead voltages, since the term is common for both terminals of any lead considered.

By choosing the WCT as the common reference, for which $V_R + V_L + V_F = 0$, we find for any of the lead potentials V_R, V_L, and V_F,

$$V(\vec{e}) = \alpha \, \vec{e} \cdot \vec{p} \tag{10.24}$$

A comparison of (10.24) with Burger's equation (10.8) identifies the vectors $\alpha \, \vec{e}$ as lead vectors. Thus, after normalization by taking $\alpha = 1$, the radius vectors of R, L, and F are the lead vectors $\vec{c}_R$, $\vec{c}_L$, and $\vec{c}_F$ respectively. Because of the symmetry of the assumed source-volume conductor configuration we have $\vec{c}_R + \vec{c}_L + \vec{c}_F = 0$, which now – in contrast to the more general situation of Burger's triangle – is as in $V_R + V_L + V_F = 0$. Recall that the latter property always holds true when using Wilson's central terminal.

10.3.7   Composite Leads with Passive Networks

We now consider a lead terminal, e.g., terminal A in ❯ Fig. 10.1, joining n electrodes via conductances $G_1, G_2, \ldots, G_n$. In the past, networks of resistors in electrocardiographic leads had to be designed so that their resistances, $R_i = 1/G_i$, were larger than the impedance of the skin-electrode interface, yet smaller than the input impedance of an amplifier; this problem is now largely irrelevant with the use of operational amplifiers in the lead networks.

Let V_A designate a potential difference *against an arbitrary reference* at junction A and $V_1, V_2, \ldots, V_n$ the potential differences (against the same reference) at the electrode sites connected to terminal A. According to Kirchhoff's current law,

$$(V_A - V_1)G_1 + \ldots + (V_A - V_n)G_n = 0, \tag{10.25}$$

and a potential at terminal A under open-circuit conditions is

$$V_A = \frac{\Sigma G_i V_i}{\Sigma G_i} \tag{10.26}$$

From (10.26) and from Burger's equation (10.8), the potential difference V_A at terminal A is

$$V_A = \frac{\Sigma G_i \vec{c}_i \cdot \vec{p}}{\Sigma G_i}, \tag{10.27}$$

and therefore, because the scalar product is distributive, the following lead vector can be associated with terminal A:

$$\vec{c}_A = \frac{\Sigma G_i \vec{c}_i}{\Sigma G_i} \tag{10.28}$$

This means that the lead vector $\vec{c}_A$ is a linear combination of lead vectors corresponding to all constituent electrode sites.

The Wilson central terminal is defined as the junction of three equal resistors connected to the electrodes with potential differences V_R, V_L, and V_F at the three limbs. It follows from ((10.9)–(10.11), (10.26), and (10.28)) that the potential V_T at the Wilson central terminal (relative to the arbitrary common reference) is

$$V_T = \frac{V_R + V_L + V_F}{3}, \tag{10.29}$$

and

$$\vec{c}_T = \frac{\vec{c}_R + \vec{c}_L + \vec{c}_F}{3}, \tag{10.30}$$

Since the final points of lead vectors $\vec{c}_R$, $\vec{c}_L$, and $\vec{c}_F$ may be viewed as lying at the vertices of the Burger triangle, it follows from (10.30) that the final point of lead vector $\vec{c}_T$ is at the median point of the Burger triangle (❯ Fig. 10.3). The potential of the Wilson central terminal can be zero for an arbitrary source only if the vectorial sum of the three lead vectors $\vec{c}_R$, $\vec{c}_L$, and $\vec{c}_F$ (based on the arbitrary common reference) is zero. Since these vectors are independent, this is not necessarily the case.

By using (10.30), it can be seen that for potentials recorded against an arbitrary reference we have

$$V_R - V_T = \frac{2V_R - V_L - V_F}{3}, \tag{10.31}$$

$$V_L - V_T = \frac{2V_L - V_R - V_F}{3}, \tag{10.32}$$

and

$$V_F - V_T = \frac{2V_F - V_L - V_R}{3} \tag{10.33}$$

In this application, the lead vectors to be used are $\vec{c}_R$, $\vec{c}_L$, $\vec{c}_F$, and $\vec{c}_T$, also with respect to the arbitrary common reference. Note from (10.29), (10.31), (10.32), and (10.33) that the sum of such unipolar limb-lead voltages is zero as is the sum of corresponding lead vectors. If the arbitrary common reference is in fact WCT, the term V_T in the three equations is zero.

The set of three limb leads, known as augmented unipolar limb leads (designated aVR, aVL, and aVF) produces 50% higher voltages than unipolar limb leads. Each augmented lead is defined by two terminals; the positive terminal is at one of the three limbs (left arm, right arm, left leg) and the negative terminal is at the junction of two equal resistors connected to the remaining two limbs. Consider the lead vectors associated with these leads. It follows from (10.28) that when lead terminal A is connected via resistors to just two constituent electrode sites, the final point A of the terminal's lead vector $\vec{c}_A$ lies on the line joining the final points of lead vectors corresponding to the constituent electrode sites, dividing this line into segments whose lengths are in the same ratio as the resistances between A and the electrodes; for augmented leads these resistances are equal, and therefore their corresponding segments are of equal length. This lead arrangement produces the following voltages:

$$V_{aVR} = \frac{2V_R - V_L - V_F}{2} = \frac{3(V_R - V_T)}{2}, \tag{10.34}$$

$$V_{aVL} = \frac{2V_L - V_R - V_F}{2} = \frac{3(V_L - V_T)}{2} \tag{10.35}$$

and

$$V_{aVF} = \frac{2V_F - V_L - V_R}{2} = \frac{3(V_F - V_T)}{2}, \tag{10.36}$$

Since these are merely scaled up versions of the extremity lead potentials their lead vectors are similarly scaled and $V_{aVR} + V_{aVL} + V_{aVF} = 0$ as well as $\vec{c}_{aVR} + \vec{c}_{aVL} + \vec{c}_{aVF} = 0$.

10.3.8 Composite Leads with Active Networks

The specification of the potential at a terminal of a composite lead depicted in ❯ Fig. 10.1, given by the (10.28), involves a weighted sum of the potentials at the electrodes connected to the terminal by means of conductances. The individual values of these conductances are positive, and as a consequence, all weights $G_i/\Sigma G_i$ are nonnegative and not greater than one.

The application of active networks with operational amplifiers permits the construction of arbitrary weights, with unrestricted sign and magnitude. As an example, consider the following summation/subtraction of voltages of Einthoven's bipolar limb leads that produces three new voltages V_{SR}, V_{SL}, and V_{SF}:

$$V_{SR} = V_I + V_{II}, \tag{10.37}$$
$$V_{SL} = V_I - V_{III}, \tag{10.38}$$

and

$$V_{SF} = V_{II} + V_{III}, \tag{10.39}$$

These voltages can be again expressed in the form of Burger's equation (10.8), and because the scalar multiplication is distributive, the lead vectors of the leads SR, SL, and SF (which are created by summation of bipolar limb leads and therefore may be called "sigma leads" [40]) can be defined in terms of lead vectors for unipolar limb leads:

$$-\vec{c}_{SR} = 2\vec{c}_R - \vec{c}_L - \vec{c}_F = 3(\vec{c}_R - \vec{c}_T), \tag{10.40}$$
$$\vec{c}_{SL} = 2\vec{c}_L - \vec{c}_R - \vec{c}_F = 3(\vec{c}_L - \vec{c}_T), \tag{10.41}$$

and

$$\vec{c}_{SF} = 2\vec{c}_F - \vec{c}_L - \vec{c}_R = 3(\vec{c}_F - \vec{c}_T) \tag{10.42}$$

For this particular lead system, it follows from (10.40) to (10.42) that its lead vectors are collinear with the respective lead vectors of unipolar extremity leads and augmented leads; their magnitude is three times as large as the magnitude of lead vectors of unipolar extremity leads and twice as large as the magnitude of the lead vectors of augmented leads, as can be seen from the Burger triangle (❯ Fig. 10.3).

10.3.9   Bibliographic Notes

The reader will find most of the references pertinent to this section in ❷ Sect. 10.1.3. The article by Schaefer and Haas in the Handbook of Physiology [22] reviews the properties of the electrocardiogram and gives an account of elementary electrocardiographic theory. Geselowitz and Schmitt [23], Plonsey [9], and Plonsey and Barr [10] provide a comprehensive review of modern electrocardiographic theory, including the derivation of formulae for lead vectors of composite leads. The text by Malmivuo and Plonsey [11] is richly illustrated and is accessible via Internet.

10.4   Image Surface

The Einthoven triangle and the Burger triangle provide heart-vector projection diagrams for interpreting voltages in the leads that use extremities for electrode sites. This geometric approach can be generalized so that it applies to any electrocardiographic lead. This section will introduce an experimental method of lead-vector construction applicable in an arbitrarily shaped linear volume conductor, and develop a notion of the three-dimensional image surface as a set of lead vectors for all possible body-surface leads. With no loss in generality, the method will be first illustrated in the two-dimensional case, where the image contour will assume the place of the image surface.

10.4.1   Image Surface of Bounded Two-Dimensional Conductor

Imagine a conductive sheet with a body-shaped boundary (❷ Fig. 10.5) and at point Q, somewhere in the "heart region" on this sheet, a dipolar source with moment $\vec{p}$.

The potential difference between any point k on the boundary and an arbitrarily selected point of reference potential (e.g., point 0 on the boundary) is related to the dipole $\vec{p}$ through Burger's equation (10.7):

$$V_k = c_{kx}p_x + c_{ky}p_y \tag{10.43}$$

If the source dipole $\vec{p}$ becomes a unit dipole oriented along the x axis, then $p_x = 1$, $p_y = 0$, and (10.43) becomes

$$V_k = c_{kx} \tag{10.44}$$

Similarly, if $\vec{p}$ is oriented along the y axis, $V_k = c_{ky}$. Having determined c_{kx} and c_{ky} from voltage responses to unit dipoles oriented along the x and y axes, it is possible to construct the lead vector $\vec{c} = \vec{e}_x c_{kx} + \vec{e}_y c_{ky}$ (as defined by (10.8)). For this, a system of coordinates can be assumed where the potential at the reference point maps into the origin (❷ Fig. 10.5). The same procedure can be repeated for as many points on the boundary as necessary; when the final points of the resulting lead vectors are connected, a contour is formed that will be termed the image contour (❷ Fig. 10.5).

Several investigators who attempted to estimate the properties of electrocardiographic leads under realistic boundary conditions constructed two-dimensional scaled models of the torso from semiconducting (Teledeltos) paper. Grayzel and Lizzi determined image contours for both homogeneous and inhomogeneous two-dimensional torso models, and for several dipole-source locations. They cut torso forms from Teledeltos paper and simulated conductivity inhomogeneities caused by lungs and intracavitary blood masses by punching holes or painting silver disks to decrease or increase the conductivity. Unit dipoles along the x and y axes were approximated by a pair of closely spaced pinpoint probes, one of which fed current and the other of which withdrew current, and the voltage V_k at boundary points was measured with respect to the model's right "leg." Image contours obtained by means of a numerical replica of Grayzel and Lizzi's torso (❷ Fig. 10.6) closely resemble those obtained using the Teledeltos paper model (❷ Fig. 10.7). The computational method was analogous to that introduced by Barnard et al. [41] for the three-dimensional inhomogeneous torso; the differences were only in the formulae for the field potential of a dipole and a dipolar double layer (❷ Sect. 10.2.1). The image contours are shown, with inscribed Burger triangle, for four selected locations of the dipole source and three different compositions of the torso. Even a casual examination of these

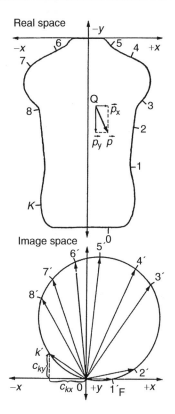

■ Fig. 10.5

Two-dimensional image contour construction. For a conductive sheet with an arbitrary boundary and a dipolar source $\vec{p}$, the potential difference between any point k on the boundary and an arbitrarily selected point of reference potential (e.g. point 0 on the boundary) is related to the dipole $\vec{p}$ through Burger's equation $V_k = c_{kx}p_x + c_{ky}p_y$. If the unit dipole is oriented along the x axis, $V_k = c_{kx}$. Similarly, by setting $p_x = 0$ and $p_y = 1$, it is possible to obtain a value of c_{ky}. With both components determined, the lead vector can be constructed; for this a system of coordinates is assumed where potential at the reference point maps into the origin. This procedure can be repeated for as many points on the boundary as necessary; when the terminal points of their lead vectors are connected, a contour (termed the "image contour") is formed

image contours reveals a striking effect of dipole-source location and boundaries. This two-dimensional modeling gives valuable insight into lead-vector determination in the arbitrarily shaped inhomogeneous conductor; however, it is not quite sufficient for assessing the effect of torso shape and inhomogeneities in the real, three-dimensional setting.

10.4.2   Image Surface of Bounded Volume Conductor

To extend the method of lead-vector determination into three dimensions, let us consider an experimental study performed by Frank, in which the torso-shaped electrolytic tank was used as a substitute for the human torso and the bipolar electrodes located in the model's heart region provided "dipolar" current sources. Frank's method of lead-vector determination was in principle identical to that already described for the two-dimensional case. Frank determined, for an array of pick-up electrodes on the surface of the torso model, the three components of the lead vector $\vec{c}$ by energizing, in turn, bipoles oriented along the x, y, and z axes and measuring for each bipole potential differences between torso-surface electrodes and a reference terminal.

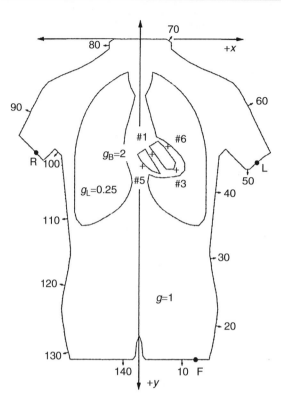

◻ Fig. 10.6

Two-dimensional numerical replica of an inhomogeneous model of a torso constructed from conductive Teledeltos paper by Grayzel and Lizzi [55]. The "lungs" were assigned conductivity g_L = 0.25, "blood masses" had conductivity g_B = 2.0 (in accordance with Grayzel and Lizzi), and the rest of "body tissues" had conductivity g = 1.0. Unit dipoles along the x and y axes were approximated by bipoles. These sources were placed at dipole-source locations marked by numbers

By using this experimental technique (or its numerical alternative), the Burger triangle diagram can be extended as follows. Consider the three-dimensional torso model with three electrodes R, L, and F attached to it at the two "arms" and the left "leg"; in addition, let there be an electrode B attached, for instance, on the back. Thus, beside Einthoven's bipolar limb leads I, II, and III, three new leads can be formed, each obtained by pairing one limb electrode with B; these leads will each be characterized by a lead vector originating at some common image point B′ (determined by Frank's method) and terminating on one of the vertices of the Burger triangle (❯ Fig. 10.8). The six lead vectors connecting image points R′, L′, F′, and B′ will form a tetrahedron the four faces of which will be lead triangles; it is called the Wilson tetrahedron (❯ Sect. 10.4.4). In the Wilson tetrahedron as in the Burger triangle, the potential difference in a lead is determined by multiplying the length of the appropriate lead vector, which forms one of the six connecting sides, by the projection of the dipole-source vector on that side.

The Wilson tetrahedron is a three-dimensional counterpart of the limb-lead triangle. Using the tetrahedron, from any three independent lead voltages that exist between four electrode sites, it is possible to determine all the three components of an arbitrary spatial dipole source (the Einthoven triangle and the Burger triangle, by contrast, permit determination of only two components of a planar dipole source, since only two independent voltages are provided by the set of three electrodes).

Note that in the Wilson tetrahedron, the real space, in which the relationship between points R, L, F, and B is given by vectors of directed distance $\vec{r}$, is replaced by the space in which the relationship between image points R′, L′, F′, and B′ (that correspond to real points R, L, F and B) is given by lead vectors $\vec{c}$.

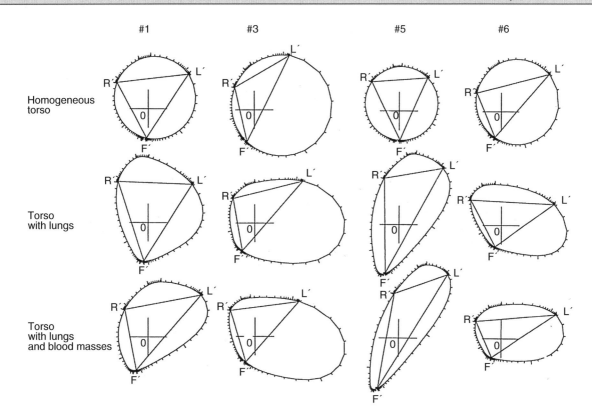

#1   #3   #5   #6

Homogeneous torso

Torso with lungs

Torso with lungs and blood masses

⬛ Fig. 10.7
Image contours of the two-dimensional torso with inscribed Burger triangle for the torso model shown in Fig. 10.6, for four different locations of the source dipole (*columns*) and three different configurations (*rows*): the homogeneous model (*top*); the inhomogeneous model with lungs (*middle*) and the inhomogeneous model with lungs and intracavitary blood masses (*bottom*). Boundary points are marked in accordance with ❷ Fig. 10.6

It is possible to continue this generalization of Burger triangle by considering the fifth, sixth, . . . , nth electrode sites on the surface of Frank's torso model (these sites should preferably form a regular grid that completely covers the torso surface) and determining the lead vector for each. The final points of these lead vectors (image points) define the image surface in the image space (❷ Fig. 10.8). For every point P in the real space there is a point P′ in the image space whose vector from the origin (the origin of the image space corresponds to the reference terminal in the real space) is a lead vector of an electrocardiographic lead formed by an electrode at P and the reference terminal. The same image space is applicable to any dipole at the same dipole-source location Q for which this image space was derived; this follows from the principle of superposition. The lead vector associated with any pair of points on the body may be found by connecting corresponding points on the image surface; this is how the Burger triangle and the Wilson tetrahedron are constructed (❷ Fig. 10.8). Image points corresponding to the lead terminals with passive networks are all enclosed by the image surface; conversely, image points of the lead terminals with active networks and image points of measurement sites that are inside the torso are all outside the image surface.

Numerical models of the human torso currently provide the most convenient method for determining image surfaces; such models can be three-dimensional, realistically shaped, and inhomogeneous. Consider the features of the computed image surface for the dipole-source location Q at the centroid of the heart region; the image surface is displayed in projections into three principal planes in ❷ Fig. 10.9. This image surface can be compared with Frank's image surface which was drawn from data obtained in the electrolytic tank. Care was taken to make the dipole-source location Q similar to that of Frank; also, the coordinate system and labeling of grid- points are compatible.

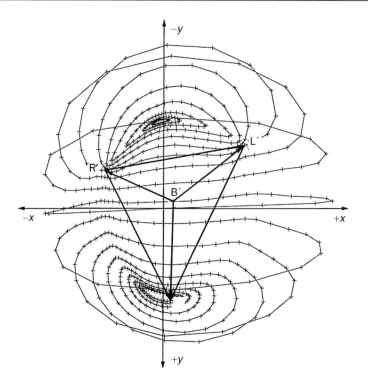

◘ Fig. 10.8
Wilson tetrahedron: frontal plane projection. The figure illustrates the construction of an image surface, where R′, L′, F′ and B′ are image points corresponding to R, L, F, B, respectively. In addition to limb leads three new leads can be obtained by pairing each of the three limb electrodes R, L and F with a fourth electrode B, attached, for instance, on the back. (B is placed in the left midscapular region [52].) These leads are each characterized by a lead vector originating at B′ and terminating on one of the vertices of the Burger triangle R′, L′, F′. The six lead vectors connecting points R′, L′, F′ and B′ form a tetrahedron in which, as in the Burger triangle, the potential difference in a lead is determined by multiplying the length of the appropriate lead vector by the projection of the source-dipole vector on that lead vector. If the reference point is fixed while point B is allowed to sweep over the entire surface of the torso, then the final points of all corresponding lead vectors will sweep out a surface in the three-dimensional image space

Protruding parts of the torso, such as the neck and shoulders, map into areas the relative size of which is diminished on the image surface because the potential gradient in these remote areas is small. In short, the protruding parts of the body "shrink" in the image space. This justifies the use of the human torso (i.e., a body without extremities and head) as a volume-conductor model of the human body. Conversely, the image surface bulges where the torso-surface points P are proximal to the dipole-source location Q. For the source location Q used to compute the image surface in ❷ Fig. 10.9, any area on the left anterior chest maps into an area the relative size of which is increased on the image surface. In short, the regions proximal to the source location are "blown up" in the image space. The parallels on the image surface (corresponding to the transverse sections of the torso surface) do not lie in parallel planes; they form spatial loops. Similarly, meridians on the image surface (corresponding to the sections of the torso surface with equiangular planes through the cranio-caudal axis of the torso) do not lie in planes; the spacing between them is magnified for points proximal to the source location Q and diminished for points remote from it.

The image surfaces for the same outer surface of the torso and the same dipole-source location, but with the torso's internal composition altered by conductivity inhomogeneities, change their shape as is evident in ❷ Fig. 10.10, which depicts an image surface of the homogeneous torso side-by-side with image surfaces of the torso with inhomogeneities.

For this particular (septal) dipole-source location, the lungs increase the y and z components of many lead vectors and attenuate their x component, while intracavitary blood masses tend to counteract the effect of the lungs. Changes of

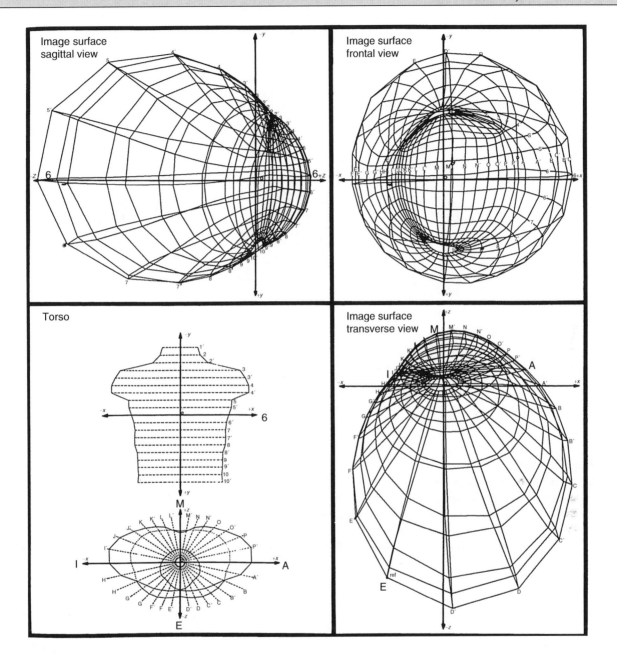

◻ **Fig. 10.9**

Image surface of a homogeneous torso with a coordinate system and a grid. The grid is established by body-surface points at the intersection between transverse planes and equiangular half-planes. The x axis runs from the right to left of the torso, the y axis from head to foot, and the z axis from front to back. The xy plane is the frontal plane, the yz plane is the sagittal plane and the xz plane is the transverse plane. The image surface was computed for the dipole-source location at the centroid of the heart region (level 6, 2.5 cm from the sagittal plane and −4 cm from the frontal plane). Computed lead vectors for all grid points are displayed as three projections of the image surface. Image points corresponding to levels 2–10 on the torso surface form parallels; image points corresponding to torso-surface points in the angular half-planes form meridians (Horáček and Ritsema van Eck [72]. © Presses Académiques Européennes, Brussels. Reproduced with permission)

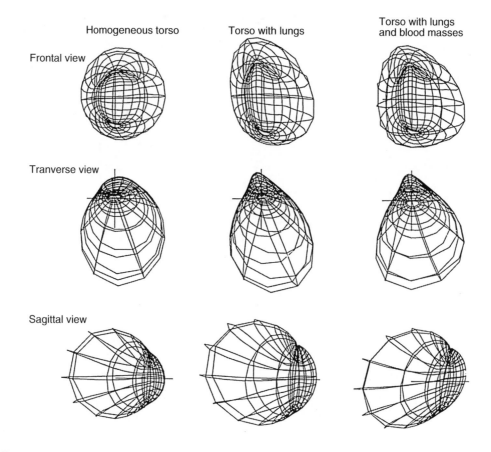

Frontal view — Homogeneous torso — Torso with lungs — Torso with lungs and blood masses

Tranverse view

Sagittal view

☑ Fig. 10.10
The effect of torso inhomogeneities is seen in three image surfaces computed for the dipole-source location at the centroid of the heart region. The projections of the image surface in the *first column* correspond to the homogeneous torso (conductivity $g = 1$; this image surface is identical to the one in ❷ Fig. 10.9 except only 16 of 32 meridians are plotted); the *second column* shows an image surface of the torso with lungs of low conductivity ($g_L = 0.25$); the *third column* shows an image surface of the torso with lungs and highly conductive intracavitary blood masses ($g_B = 3$) (Horáček [67]. © Karger, Basel. Reproduced with permission)

shape in the image surface owing to intracavitary blood masses can be attributed to the Brody effect (❷ Sect. 6.4.2.2): the x component of an arbitrarily oriented dipole is enhanced, because it is approximately normal to the surfaces of both intraventricular blood masses, while the y and z components are attenuated because they are approximately tangential to these surfaces. The effect of the lungs on lead vectors for the same dipole-source location can be described as a "channelling" effect: the z and y components of lead vectors are increased because the dipoles oriented in the z and y directions are approximately tangential to the surface of the poorly conducting lungs. Shifting the dipole-source location considerably changes the resultant image surfaces.

10.4.3   Image-Surface Definitions

The relationship between an arbitrary dipole source at a fixed location Q and electric potentials on the surface of the torso the shape and composition of which are specified can be displayed by means of the image surface; this geometric concept was introduced by Burger and van Milaan.

The concept of the image space and of the image surface can be formalized as follows. Consider a certain bounded linear volume conductor in which one internal point, to be called Q, is designated as a dipole-source location; let the field point P (at a finite distance from Q) be either inside the volume conductor, or on its outer boundary or at the node of a resistor network that extends beyond this boundary. For this volume conductor with the designated Q there is a corresponding image space with the following properties.

1. Every field point P can be mapped into the image space so that there is a unique corresponding image point P'; this mapping defines the electric potential produced at P by a fixed-location dipole of arbitrary moment embedded in the volume conductor.
2. The origin of the image space corresponds to the arbitrary reference point; with a different choice of reference, all points of the image space undergo translation, but their mutual relationship remains unaffected. The ideal reference is a zero potential at a terminal infinitely remote from Q (or at source dipole's midpoint).
3. In the image space, the vector pointing from one image point B' to another image point A' is a lead vector of the lead the positive terminal of which is A and negative (reference) terminal is B. Thus, the Burger triangle, for instance, is constructed in the image space by connecting points R', L', and F'.
4. The set of points on the outer boundary of the volume conductor maps into the image surface.
5. The set of points that is inside the volume conductor maps into image points that are outside the image surface.
6. The nodes of the resistor network connected at discrete points to the outer surface of the volume-conductor map into image points inside the image surface; the latter image points are defined by their lead vectors as in (10.28).

The properties of any conceivable lead can be assessed from the image surface. It should be reiterated, however, that each image surface pertains only to one particular torso and one particular dipole-source location.

10.4.4 Bibliographic Notes

Analytical calculations have been performed with various mathematical models. Wilson and Bayley [42], Frank [43], and Geselowitz and Ishiwatari [44] studied the effect of the eccentric location of the heart in the torso by analyzing the case of a dipole in a sphere. Okada [45, 46] and more recently Cornelis and Nyssen [47] have extended this analysis to a cylinder. Plonsey [48] used the method of images to show the effect of the planar insulating boundary near sources. Brody [49] studied the effect of highly conductive intraventricular blood masses and concluded that blood masses emphasize the radial component of source dipoles in the heart (perpendicular to the ventricular wall) and attenuate the tangential component. Mathematical studies of Bayley et al. [50] on the field of a double layer in a system of nested spheres (later redone by Rudy and Plonsey [51]) have yielded the same results.

Wilson et al. [52] suggested substituting a regular tetrahedron for the Einthoven triangle; Burger and van Milaan [15] thought of this tetrahedron as composed of lead vectors obtained in a realistic model of the torso.

An experimental approach to the investigation of the effect of the body shape and conductivity inhomogeneities on lead vectors was employed in numerous studies. Two-dimensional models included fluid mappers used by McFee et al. [53], and Teledeltos mannequins used by Brody and Romans [54], Grayzel and Lizzi [55], and others. Electrolytic-tank models were used by Burger and van Milaan [13], Frank [56], Schmitt [19], Nagata [57], Rush [58] (the latter article contains a review of experimental studies) and others. The idea of an image surface was conceived by Burger and van Milaan [13]; the first experimental determination of the image surface was performed by Frank [56]. The concept of an image surface was used to design the well-known Frank's lead system [59].

Numerical models of the torso were pioneered by Gelernter and Swihart [60], Barr et al. [61], and Barnard et al. [41]. The mathematical methodology of dealing with general inhomogeneous volume conductors was outlined by Geselowitz [62]. An article by Swihart [63] provides an overview of numerical methods for solving the forward problem of electrocardiography (❷ Chap. 8). Pilkington et al. [64] compared the merits of the integral equation approach and the finite-element approach to the solution of the volume-conductor problem. Many important papers on biophysical basis of electrocardiography were assembled in one volume by Pilkington and Plonsey [65]. Horáček [66, 67] used a numerical model of a three-dimensional, realistically shaped and inhomogeneous human torso to compute image surfaces for various dipole-source locations, and performed as well the analogous computations in a two-dimensional model (❯ Figs. 10.6 and ❯ 10.7).

10.5 Lead Field

The simplicity of Burger's lead-vector concept fades when allowance is made for dipolar sources that are distributed over the entire heart region. Clearly, the size of the heart region relative to its distance from most ECG recording sites on the torso is not negligible, and hence the typical lead vector $\vec{L}$ varies when the dipole-source location shifts; for each given lead, there is a family of lead vectors that takes on a complete set of values $\vec{L}$ for various dipole-source locations. Each such family should be viewed as a vector field $\vec{L}(x, y, z)$, that is, a vector quantity the value of which depends on the coordinates. With this concept in mind, Burger's equation (10.8) can be interpreted more generally; it can be rewritten as

$$V = \vec{L}(x, y, z) \cdot \vec{p} \tag{10.45}$$

allowing a given local current-dipole source to act anywhere in the heart region. According to this interpretation of Burger's equation, the voltage that a local current dipole located at (x_0, y_0, z_0) produces in a lead is the scalar product of the moment of the dipole $\vec{p}$ and the vector field $\vec{L}$ evaluated at (x_0, y_0, z_0). Using the superposition principle, the total contribution of distributed cardiac sources to the lead voltage can be defined as

$$V = \int \vec{L}(x, y, z) \cdot \vec{J}^i(x, y, z)\ dv, \tag{10.46}$$

where $\vec{J}^i(x, y, z)$ is a function defining a distributed impressed current density in the heart region in terms of the current dipole moment per unit volume; the units of $\vec{J}^i$ are Am/m^3, $\vec{L}$ is in $\Omega\, m^{-1}$, and hence, the units of the volume integral are volts. Equation (10.46) is the most general form of Burger's definition of the relationship between cardiac electric sources and the voltage in an electrocardiographic lead.

10.5.1 Lead-Field Derivation

McFee and Johnston provided a physical basis for this operational definition of the lead vector by invoking Helmholtz's reciprocity theorem as follows. Consider a torso-shaped linear volume conductor (❯ Fig. 10.11) with two pairs of electrode sites. The first pair, A and B, which can be located anywhere except in the heart region, can be thought of as the positive terminal (A) and the negative terminal (B) of an electrocardiographic lead. The remaining pair, C and D, separated by a small vector distance $\vec{l}$ directed from D to C, can be arbitrarily located within the heart region; this pair corresponds to the site of the local cardiac electric source.

The reciprocity theorem asserts that the potential difference V_{AB} produced between open-circuited terminals A and B by a current I injected at point C and removed at point D (the condition of normal energization depicted in ❯ Fig. 10.11a) must equal the potential difference V'_{CD} that would be found between points C and D if the same current were injected at point A and removed at point B (the condition of reciprocal energization illustrated in ❯ Fig. 10.11b); this reciprocal current is designated I'. In this case $I' = I$, but in general, it does not have to be so, and the reciprocity theorem is formulated as follows: $V_{AB}/I = V'_{CD}/I'$.

Consider more closely the conditions under reciprocal energization. A source of current I' placed between terminals A and B gives rise to an electric field in the volume conductor that can be characterized at every point by a vector of electric field intensity $\vec{E}'$. By definition, the potential difference between points C and D is given by a line integral along an arbitrary path from D to C (10.5):

$$V'_{CD} = -\int_D^C \vec{E}' \cdot d\vec{l} \tag{10.47}$$

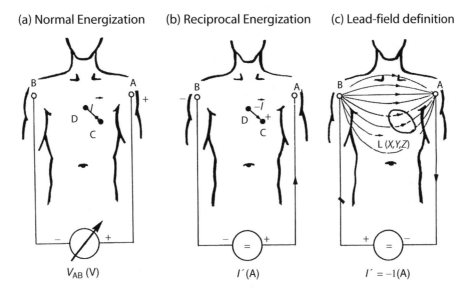

(a) Normal Energization   (b) Reciprocal Energization   (c) Lead-field definition

Fig. 10.11

Lead-field derivation from the reciprocity theorem. The potential difference V_{AB}, produced between open-circuited terminals of an electrocardiographic lead by a current bipole $i\vec{l}$ in the heart region (part (a)), equals the potential difference V'_{CD} produced between the source and sink of the bipole C and D by a reciprocal current $I' = I$ injected into the lead (part (b)). The electric field intensity in the heart region during the lead's reciprocal energization defines the lead field (part (c))

For the small distance between C and D, the field can be considered constant so that the integral becomes simply

$$V'_{CD} = -\vec{E}' \cdot \vec{l}, \tag{10.48}$$

where $\vec{l}$ is the directed distance from D to C.

If the electric field intensity is normalized to a unit reciprocal current the scalar value I' of which is equal to I, and V'_{CD} is replaced with V_{AB} (applying the reciprocity theorem), then

$$V_{AB} = -\left(\frac{\vec{E}'}{I'}\right) \cdot (I\vec{l}) \tag{10.49}$$

This is the desired result; a comparison with the generalized Burger's equation (10.45) clearly shows that the first factor corresponds to the lead vector (measured in $\Omega\,\mathrm{m}^{-1}$) and the second factor is the current dipole moment (units A m). The generalized lead vector can be designated as the lead field

$$\vec{L}(x, y, z) = \frac{\vec{E}'}{-I'} \tag{10.50}$$

Note that the lead field has units $\Omega\,\mathrm{m}^{-1}$; this is a revision of the original definition by McFee and Johnston.

10.5.2 Lead-Field Definition

At any point in the heart region the lead field of a given electrocardiographic lead is defined as a vector field of electric intensity produced by a source of unit current connected to the lead's terminals in the reverse manner (i.e., with current being injected at the negative terminal and removed at the positive terminal as shown in ❯ Fig. 10.11c). Since the electric

◼ Table 10.1

Mean lead field with standard deviations as determined at 1,239 ventricular sites for selected electrocardiographic leads

Lead	$\bar{c}_x$	$\bar{c}_y$	$\bar{c}_z$	$|\bar{c}|$
Homogeneous torso				
I	0.95 ± 0.16	-0.27 ± 0.16	0.07 ± 0.04	**1.00**±0.16
II	0.58 ± 0.10	1.16 ± 0.11	-0.04 ± 0.05	1.31 ± 0.11
III	-0.37 ± 0.16	1.44 ± 0.21	-0.11 ± 0.05	1.50 ± 0.20
aVR	-0.76 ± 0.10	-0.45 ± 0.09	-0.01 ± 0.04	0.89 ± 0.10
aVL	0.66 ± 0.15	-0.85 ± 0.17	0.09 ± 0.04	1.09 ± 0.17
aVF	0.11 ± 0.11	1.30 ± 0.15	-0.08 ± 0.05	1.31 ± 0.14
CT	0.07 ± 0.03	-0.03 ± 0.03	0.21 ± 0.06	0.23 ± 0.05
V_1	-1.07 ± 0.59	-0.22 ± 0.52	-1.21 ± 0.71	1.69 ± 0.95
V_2	-0.13 ± 0.72	-0.55 ± 0.91	-2.26 ± 1.26	2.50 ± 1.44
V_3	0.88 ± 0.88	-0.26 ± 0.79	-2.21 ± 1.15	2.58 ± 1.36
V_4	1.37 ± 0.70	0.07 ± 0.47	-1.44 ± 0.75	2.08 ± 0.95
V_5	1.30 ± 0.50	0.07 ± 0.28	-0.46 ± 0.24	1.41 ± 0.53
V_6	0.85 ± 0.23	0.03 ± 0.16	0.13 ± 0.11	0.88 ± 0.25
V_7	0.56 ± 0.12	0.03 ± 0.12	0.29 ± 0.14	0.64 ± 0.17
V_8	0.33 ± 0.10	0.05 ± 0.11	0.40 ± 0.18	0.54 ± 0.19
V_9	0.08 ± 0.08	0.06 ± 0.11	0.45 ± 0.22	0.48 ± 0.22
V_3 R	-0.98 ± 0.39	0.05 ± 0.20	-0.66 ± 0.26	1.20 ± 0.45
V_4 R	-0.84 ± 0.21	0.09 ± 0.12	-0.36 ± 0.09	0.93 ± 0.22
V_5 R	-0.68 ± 0.10	0.07 ± 0.08	-0.12 ± 0.02	0.70 ± 0.10
X	1.18 ± 0.11	-0.17 ± 0.16	-0.15 ± 0.05	1.21 ± 0.12
Y	0.12 ± 0.04	1.11 ± 0.06	0.07 ± 0.06	1.12 ± 0.05
Z	0.12 ± 0.11	0.17 ± 0.35	1.30 ± 0.34	1.35 ± 0.39
Torso with lungs				
I	0.87 ± 0.10	-0.14 ± 0.11	-0.03 ± 0.04	0.89 ± 0.10
II	0.70 ± 0.08	1.40 ± 0.09	-0.02 ± 0.11	1.57 ± 0.10
III	-0.17 ± 0.10	1.54 ± 0.14	0.01 ± 0.10	1.56 ± 0.14
aVR	-0.79 ± 0.07	-0.63 ± 0.06	0.02 ± 0.07	1.01 ± 0.08
aVL	0.52 ± 0.09	-0.84 ± 0.12	-0.02 ± 0.05	1.00 ± 0.11
aVF	0.26 ± 0.08	1.47 ± 0.11	0.00 ± 0.10	1.50 ± 0.11
WCT	0.07 ± 0.03	-0.01 ± 0.04	0.21 ± 0.07	0.23 ± 0.06
V_1	-1.03 ± 0.64	-0.40 ± 0.52	-1.32 ± 0.81	1.80 ± 1.04
V_2	-0.09 ± 0.73	-0.75 ± 0.97	-2.37 ± 1.31	2.67 ± 1.50
V_3	0.94 ± 0.92	-0.32 ± 0.88	-2.35 ± 1.25	2.75 ± 1.47
V_4	1.45 ± 0.72	0.15 ± 0.54	-1.54 ± 0.79	2.23 ± 1.00
V_5	1.32 ± 0.53	0.21 ± 0.30	-0.56 ± 0.26	1.49 ± 0.56
V_6	0.83 ± 0.24	0.16 ± 0.16	0.05 ± 0.10	0.86 ± 0.24
V_7	0.51 ± 0.12	0.14 ± 0.11	0.23 ± 0.10	0.59 ± 0.14
V_8	0.26 ± 0.05	0.13 ± 0.10	0.36 ± 0.13	0.47 ± 0.13
V_9	-0.01 ± 0.08	0.10 ± 0.09	0.47 ± 0.20	0.49 ± 0.20
V_3R	-0.93 ± 0.44	-0.04 ± 0.21	-0.73 ± 0.34	1.22 ± 0.52
V_4R	-0.79 ± 0.24	0.07 ± 0.13	-0.39 ± 0.14	0.90 ± 0.26
V_5R	-0.64 ± 0.10	0.06 ± 0.08	-0.11 ± 0.04	0.66 ± 0.10

◻ Table 10.1 (Continued)

Lead	$\bar{c}_x$	$\bar{c}_y$	$\bar{c}_z$	$|\bar{c}|$
X	1.12±0.13	−0.07±0.15	−0.26±0.29	1.16±0.15
Y	0.27±0.07	1.34±0.12	0.12±0.09	1.38±0.12
Z	0.03±0.17	0.22±0.38	1.42±0.40	1.48±0.44
Torso with lungs and blood masses				
I	0.80±0.16	−0.12±0.11	0.00±0.12	0.82±0.18
II	0.66±0.15	1.30±0.28	0.04±0.21	1.48±0.28
III	−0.14±0.20	1.42±0.29	0.04±0.21	1.46±0.30
aVR	−0.73±0.12	−0.59±0.15	−0.02±0.13	0.96±0.13
aVL	0.47±0.16	−0.77±0.18	−0.02±0.14	0.92±0.19
aVF	0.26±0.15	1.36±0.28	0.04±0.20	1.41±0.29
WCT	0.07±0.04	0.00±0.05	0.21±0.08	0.23±0.07
V_1	−0.98±0.60	−0.44±0.49	−1.33±0.98	1.80±1.10
V_2	−0.17±0.64	−0.76±0.86	−2.30±1.53	2.61±1.62
V_3	0.77±0.87	−0.35±0.73	−2.22±1.34	2.54±1.50
V_4	1.29±0.81	0.12±0.43	−1.43±0.83	2.02±1.09
V_5	1.21±0.63	0.20±0.25	−0.50±0.29	1.36±0.66
V_6	0.77±0.30	0.16±0.13	0.08±0.13	0.80±0.30
V_7	0.48±0.15	0.14±0.10	0.24±0.13	0.57±0.19
V_8	0.25±0.07	0.13±0.09	0.36±0.15	0.47±0.16
V_9	0.00±0.08	0.10±0.10	0.46±0.22	0.49±0.22
V_3 R	−0.87±0.40	−0.09±0.26	−0.75±0.44	1.21±0.54
V_4 R	−0.73±0.21	0.02±0.18	−0.40±0.21	0.87±0.25
V_5 R	−0.58±0.09	0.03±0.13	−0.13±0.09	0.62±0.10
X	1.02±0.23	−0.05±0.12	−0.21±0.17	1.06±0.25
Y	0.27±0.12	1.23±0.24	0.15±0.20	1.29±0.25
Z	0.06±0.19	0.24±0.34	1.38±0.55	1.45±0.58

Values of the lead-field components $\bar{c}_x$, $\bar{c}_y$, and $\bar{c}_z$ are in relative units, scaled by $|\bar{c}_i|$; absolute units can be restored [68]

intensity vector of the reciprocal field $\vec{E}'$ is by definition the negative of the gradient of the scalar potential, the generalized lead vector can be expressed as

$$\vec{L}(x, y, z) = \frac{\nabla V'}{I'}, \qquad (10.51)$$

and an alternative definition of the lead field can be put forward as follows. At any point in the heart region the lead field of a given electrocardiographic lead is defined as a gradient of the potential distribution V' produced by the source of unit current connected to the terminals of the lead. (Note that the reciprocal current is injected "properly" at the positive terminal and removed at the negative terminal.)

The lead field is an electric field per unit current, or impedance per unit distance ($\Omega\,\mathrm{m}^{-1}$), and hence, Schmitt introduced this concept into electrocardiography as a vectorial transfer impedance $\vec{Z} = \nabla Z$

$$\vec{L}(x, y, z) = \vec{Z}(x, y, z) = \nabla Z \qquad (10.52)$$

Any lead can be described in terms of its lead field or transfer impedance. The lead-field concept can be applied even when the lead terminals are connected to a number of electrodes via a network of resistors. This facilitates synthesis of leads with desired properties; for example, ideal heart-vector leads have uniform lead fields, while lead fields of ideal unipolar leads (with the reference electrode infinitely remote) radiate outwards in straight lines from the exploring electrode with an intensity diminishing inversely with distance squared.

10.5.3 Computed Lead-Field Values

Recently, Horáček et al. [68] used a computer model of a realistic three-dimensional human torso containing lungs and intracavitary blood masses of different conductivities to calculate the lead field for some commonly used electrocardiographic leads. Their torso model is a modification of one described previously [66], with the outer surface modified to simplify the identification of commonly used ECG electrode sites on the model's surface. Three orthogonal components of the lead field were determined at 1,239 ventricular sites for 352 unipolar body-surface leads in the homogeneous torso, in the torso with lungs, and in the torso with lungs and intracavitary blood masses. Mean lead-field values with standard deviations were calculated for commonly used ECG leads from these 1,239 vectors for all three configuration of the torso (❯ Table 10.1). The components of the lead field were calculated in absolute units for unit-dipole sources in the torso of unit conductivity and then normalized by the length of lead vector for lead I and tabulated in relative units. The lead field in absolute units of $\Omega\,m^{-1}$ for unit current dipoles in absolute units of $A \times m$ can be restored by multiplying the values listed in ❯ Table 10.1 by an appropriate factor [68]. The mean lead-field vectors for leads I, II, and III form a characteristic Burger's triangle, with the length of the vectors for leads II and III exceeding that for lead I. The Wilson central terminal has the shortest length of the mean lead-field vector, with only the z-component having a value that is not negligible. The unipolar precordial leads V_2–V_4 have the largest magnitude of the mean lead field. The lead field for Frank's orthogonal leads X, Y, and Z shows excellent orthogonality and reasonably uniform sensitivity for all three leads. These findings are similar in all three configurations of the torso model; however, closer examination reveals that both lungs and intracavitary blood masses exert a noticeable effect on the lead field in specific leads.

10.5.4 Bibliographic Notes

In the early 1950s, several investigators perceived lead properties operationally. Lepeschkin [69] characterized leads in terms of "tubes of influence" and Brody and Romans [54] performed model experiments aimed at finding lead properties through reciprocal energization; a hydrodynamic analogue of reciprocal energization was constructed by McFee et al. [53]. Schmitt [19] introduced the transfer impedance as a vector field characterizing lead properties and McFee and Johnston [16] were the proponents of the lead-field concept based on the reciprocity theorem. Interestingly, the reciprocity theorem, which became a cornerstone of lead-field theory, can be applied to electrocardiography virtually without changing Helmholtz's original wording which was as follows. (The quote is from the article by Helmholtz published in 1853 [32]; translation from German by Frank N. Wilson [16].)

> Every single element of an electromotive surface will produce a flow of the same quantity of electricity through the galvanometer as would flow through that element itself if its electromotive force were impressed on the galvanometer wire. If one adds the effects of all the electromotive surface elements, the effects of each of which are found in the manner described, he will have the value of the total current through the galvanometer.

In present-day electrocardiography, galvanometers have been replaced by amplifiers that measure open-circuit voltage rather than short-circuit current. Further, cardiac electric sources are, to the best of our knowledge, near-ideal current generators. Under such circumstances, the principle of superposition can be applied to sum both input currents and output voltages, and the reciprocity theorem can be restated for double-layer current sources and the lead voltage.

Applications of the lead field to electrocardiography have been discussed in articles by Plonsey [70], Schmitt [71], and others. See also texts by Plonsey [9], Plonsey and Barr [10], and Malmivuo and Plonsey [11].

References

1. Einthoven, W., The different forms of the human electrocardiogram and their signification. *Lancet*, 1912;**1**: 853–861. (Translation: *Am. Heart J.*, 1950;**40**: 195–211).

2. Einthoven, W., G. Fahr, and A. deWaart, Ueber die Richtung und manifeste Groesse der Potentialschwankungen im menschlichen Herzen und ueber den Einfluss der Herzlage auf die Form

des Electrokardiogramms. *Pfluegers Arch. ges. Physiol.*, 1913;**150**: 275–315. (Translation: *Am. Heart J.*, 1950;**40**: 163–211).

3. Wilson, F.N., F.D. Johnston, A.G. Macleod, and P.S. Barker, Electrocardiograms that represent the potential variations of a single electrode. *Am. Heart J.*, 1933;**9**: 447–471.

4. Goldberger E., A simple, indifferent, electrocardiographic electrode of zero potential and a technique of obtaining augmented, unipolar, extremity leads. *Am. Heart J.*, 1942;**23**: 483–492.

5. Wolferth Ch.C. and F.C. Wood, The electrocardiographic diagnosis of coronary occlusion by the use of chest leads. *Am. J. Med. Sci.*, 1932;**183**: 30–35.

6. Wilson F.N., F.D. Johnston, F.F. Rosenbaum, H. Erlanger, Ch.E. Kossmann, H. Hecht, N. Cotrim, R. Menezes de Oliveira, R. Scarsi, and P.S. Barker, The precordial electrocardiogram. *Am. Heart J.*, 1944;**27**: 19–85.

7. Wilson, F.N., F.D. Johnston, F.F. Rosenbaum, and P.S. Barker, On Einthoven's triangle, the theory of unipolar electrocardiographic leads, and the interpretation of the precordial electrocardiogram. *Am. Heart J.*, 1946;**32**: 277–310.

8. Wilson, F.N., A.G. Macleod, and P.S. Barker, *The distribution of the currents of action and of injury displayed by heart muscle and other excitable tissues.* Univ. Mich. Press, Ann Arbor, Mich., 1933.

9. Plonsey R., *Bioelectric Phenomena.* McGraw-Hill, New York, 1969.

10. R. Plonsey and R.C. Barr, *Bioelectricity: A Quantitative Approach.* Plenum Press, New York, 1988.

11. J. Malmivuo and R. Plonsey, *Bioelectromagnetism: Principles and Applications of Bioelectric and Biomagnetic Fields.* Oxford University Press, New York, 1995. see http://butler.cc.tut.fi/malmivuo/bem/bembook/15/15.htm.

12. R.P. Holland and H. Brooks, TQ-ST segment mapping: Critical review and analysis of current concepts. *Am. J. Cardiol.*, 1977;**40**: 110–129.

13. Burger H.C. and J.B. van Milaan, Heart-vector and leads. Part I. *Br. Heart J.*, 1946;**8**: 157–161.

14. Burger H.C. and J.B. van Milaan, Heart-vector and leads. Part II. *Br. Heart J.*, 1947;**9**: 154.

15. Burger H.C. and J.B. van Milaan, Heart-vector and leads: Part III, Geometrical interpretation. *Br. Heart J.*, 1948;**10**: 229.

16. McFee R. and F.D. Johnston, Electrocardiographic leads: I. Introduction. *Circulation*, 1953;**8**: 554–568.

17. McFee R. and F.D. Johnston, Electrocardiographic leads. II. Analysis. *Circulation*, 1954;**9**: 255–266.

18. McFee R. and F.D. Johnston, Electrocardiographic leads. III. Synthesis. *Circulation*, 1954;**9**: 868–880.

19. Schmitt O.H., Lead vectors and transfer impedance. *Ann. N.Y. Acad. Sci.*, 1957;**65**: 1092–1109.

20. Burger H.C., *Heart and Vector: Physical Basis of Electrocardiography.* Philips Technical Library, Eindhoven, The Netherlands, 1968.

21. Frank E., General theory of heart-vector projection. *Circ. Res.*, 1954;**2**: 258–270.

22. Schaefer H. and H.G. Haas, Electrocardiography, in *Handbook of Physiology*, vol. 1. Am. Physiol. Soc., Washington, DC, 1962, pp. 323–415. Vol. 1, Sect. 2 (Circulation).

23. Geselowitz D.B. and O.H. Schmitt, Electrocardiography, in *Biological Engineering*, H.P. Schwan, Editor. McGraw Hill, New York, 1969, pp. 333–390.

24. McFee R. and G.M. Baule, Research in electrocardiography and magnetocardiography. *Proc. IEEE*, 1972;**60**: 290–321.

25. Geselowitz D.B., Electric and magnetic field of the heart. *Annu. Rev. Biophys. Bioeng.*, 1973;**2**: 37–63.

26. Arthur R.M. and D.B. Geselowitz, Effect of inhomogeneities on the apparent location and magnitude of a cardiac current dipole source. *IEEE Trans. Biomed. Eng.*, 1970;**BME-17**: 141–146.

27. Purcell E.M., *Electricity and Magnetism.* McGraw-Hill, New York, 1965. Berkeley physics course – Volume 2.

28. Panofsky W.K.H. and M. Phillips, *Classical Electricity and Magnetism.* Addison-Wesley, Reading, MA, 1962.

29. Courant R. and D. Hilbert, *Methods of Mathematical Physics.* Wiley, New York, 1962. Volume II.

30. Guillemin E.A., *Theory of Linear Physical Systems.* Wiley, New York, 1963.

31. Plonsey R. and Heppner D. Considerations of quasistationarity in electrophysiological systems. *Bull. Math. Biophys.*, 1967;**29**: 657–664.

32. von Helmholtz H.L.F., Ueber einige Gesetze der Verteilung elektrischer Stroeme in korperlischen Leitern mit Anwendung auf die thierisch elektrischen Versuche. *Pogg. Ann. Physiol. Chem.*, 1853;**89**: 222.

33. Oster G.F., A.S. Perelson, and A. Katchalsky, Network thermodynamics: dynamic modelling of biophysical systems. *Quart. Rev. Biophys.*, 1973;**6**: 1–134.

34. Desoer Ch.A. and E.S. Kuh, *Basic Circuit Theory.* McGraw-Hill, New York, 1969.

35. Kaufman W. and F.D. Johnston, The electrical conductivity of the tissues near the heart and its bearing on the distribution of the cardiac action currents. *Am. Heart J.*, 1943;**26**: 42–54.

36. Schwan H.P. and C.F. Kay, Specific resistance of body tissues. *Circ. Res.*, 1956;**4**: 664–670.

37. Burger H.C. and R. van Dongen, Specific electric resistance of body tissues. *Phys. Med. Biol.*, 1961;**5**: 431–437.

38. Rush S., J.A. Abildskov, and R. McFee, Resistivity of body tissues at low frequencies. *Circ. Res.*, 1963;**12**: 40–50.

39. Geddes L.A. and L.E. Baker, The specific resistance of biological material: A compendium of data for the biomedical engineer and physiologist. *Med. Biol. Eng.*, 1967;**5**: 271–293.

40. Rautaharju P.M., The inappropriateness of the commonly used augmentation and lead-recording sequence for ECG analysis. *Pract. Cardiol.*, 1982;**8**: 120–139.

41. Barnard A.C.L., I.M. Duck, M.S. Lynn, and W.P. Timlake, The application of electromagnetic theory to electrocardiology. II. numerical solution of the integral equations. *Biophys. J.*, 1967;**7**: 463–491.

42. Wilson F.N. and R.H. Bayley, The electric field of an eccentric dipole in a homogeneous spherical conducting medium. *Circulation* 1950;**1**: 84–92.

43. Frank E., Electric potential produced by two point current sources in a homogeneous conducting sphere. *J. Appl. Phys.*, 1952;**23**: 1225–1228.

44. Geselowitz D.B. and Ishiwatari H., A theoretical study of the effect of the intracavitary blood mass on the dipolarity of an equivalent heart generator, in *Vectorcardiography, 1965.* North Holland, Amsterdam, 1966, pp. 393–402.

45. Okada R.H., Potentials produced by eccentric current dipole in a finite length circular conducting cylinder. *IRE Trans. Med. Electron.*, PGME, 1956;**7**: 14–19.

46. Okada R.H., The image surface of a circular cylinder. *Am. Heart J.*, 1956;**51**: 489–500.

47. Cornelis J.P.H. and E.H.G. Nyssen, Potentials produced by arbitrary current sources in an infinite- and finite-length circular conducting cylinder. *IEEE Trans. Biomed. Eng.*, 1985;**BME-32**: 993–1000.

48. Plonsey R., Current dipole images and reference potentials. *IEEE Trans. Bio-Med. Electron.*, 1963;**BME-10**: 3–8.

49. Brody D.A., A theoretical analysis of intracavitary blood mass influence on the heart-lead relationship. *Circ. Res.*, 1956;**4**: 731–738.

50. Bayley R.H., J.M. Kalbfleisch, and P.M. Berry, Changes in the body's QRS surface potentials produced by alterations in certain compartments of the nonhomogeneous conducting model. *Am. Heart J.*, 1969;**77**: 517–528.

51. Rudy Y. and R. Plonsey, The eccentric spheres model as the basis for a study of the role of geometry and inhomogeneities in electrocardiography. *IEEE Trans. Biomed. Eng.*, 1979;**BME-26**: 392–399.

52. Wilson F.N., F.D. Johnston, and C.E. Kossmann, The substitution of a tetrahedron for the Einthoven triangle. *Am. Heart J.*, 1947;**33**: 594–603.

53. McFee R., R.M. Stow, and F.D. Johnston, Graphic representation of electrocardiographic leads by means of fluid mappers. *Circulation*, 1952;**4**: 21–29.

54. Brody D.A. and W.E. Romans, A model which demonstrates the quantitative relationship between the electromotive forces of the heart and the extremity leads. *Am. Heart J.*, 1953;**45**: 263–276.

55. Grayzel J. and F. Lizzi, The combined influence of inhomogeneities and dipole location: bipolar ECG leads in the frontal plane. *Am. Heart J.*, 1967;**74**: 503–512.

56. Frank E., Spread of current in volume conductors of finite extent. *Ann. N.Y. Acad. Sci.*, 1957;**65**: 980–1002.

57. Nagata Y., The influence of the inhomogeneities of electrical conductivity within the torso on the electrocardiogram as evaluated from the view point of the transfer impedance vector. *Jap. Heart J.*, 1970;**11**: 489–505.

58. Rush S., An inhomogeneous anisotropic model of the human torso for electrocardiographic study. *Med. Biol. Eng.*, 1971;**9**: 201–211.

59. Frank E., An accurate clinically practical system for spatial vectorcardiography. *Circulation*, 1956;**13**: 737–749.

60. Gelernter H.L. and J.C. Swihart, A mathematical-physical model of the genesis of the electrocardiogram. *Biophys. J.*, 1964;**4**: 285–301.

61. Barr R.C., T.C. Pilkington, J.P. Boineau, and M.S. Spach, Determining surface potentials from current dipoles, with application to electrocardiography. *IEEE Trans. Biomed. Eng.*, 1966;**BME-13**: 88–92.

62. Geselowitz D.B., On bioelectric potentials in an inhomogeneous volume conductor. *Biophys. J.*, 1967;**7**: 1–11.

63. Swihart J.C., Numerical methods for solving the forward problem of electrocardiography, in *The Theoretical Basis of Electrocardiology*, chapter 11, C.V. Nelson and D.B. Geselowitz, Editors. Clarendon Press, Oxford, 1976, pp. 257–293.

64. Pilkington T.C., M.N. Morrow, and P.C. Stanley, A comparison of finite element and integral equation formulations for the calculation of electrocardiographic potentials. *IEEE Trans. Biomed. Eng.*, 1985;**BME-32**: 166–173.

65. Pilkington T.C. and R. Plonsey, *Engineering Contributions to Biophysical Electrocardiography*. Wiley, New York, 1982.

66. Horáček B.M., *The effect on electrocardiographic lead vectors of conductivity inhomogeneities in the human torso*. PhD thesis, Dalhousie University, 1971.

67. Horáček B.M., Numerical model of an inhomogeneous human torso. *Adv. Cardiol.*, 1974;**10**: 51–57.

68. Horáček B.M., J.W. Warren, D.Q. Feild, and C.L. Feldman. Statistical and deterministic approaches to the design of electrocardiographic lead systems. *J Electrocardiol*, 2002; **35**(Suppl): 41–52.

69. Lepeschkin E., *Modern Electrocardiography*, volume 1: The P-Q-R-S-T-U Complex. Williams & Wilkins, Baltimore, 1951.

70. Plonsey R., Reciprocity applied to volume conductors and the ECG. *IEEE Trans. Bio-Med. Electron.*, 1963;**BME-10**: 9–12.

71. Schmitt O.H., The biophysical basis of electrocardiography, in *Proceedings of the 1st National Biophysics Conference*, H. Quastler and H.J. Morowitz, Editors. Yale University Press, New Haven, Connecticut, 1959, p. 510.

72. Horáček B.M. and H.J. Ritsema van Eck, The forward problem of electrocardiography, in *The Electrical Field of the Heart*, P. Rijlant, Editor. Presses Academiques Europeennes, Brussels, 1972, p. 228–238.

11 Lead Systems

Peter W. Macfarlane

P. W. Macfarlane et al. (eds.), *Basic Electrocardiology*, DOI 10.1007/978-0-85729-871-3_11,
© Springer-Verlag London Limited 2012

11.1 Introduction

The extensive theory behind the development of electrocardiographic leads has been dealt with in ❷ Chap. 10. An understanding of some of the concepts embodied in that chapter will be helpful, though not essential, in following the material presented in this chapter. There is no doubt that an experienced cardiologist can make an excellent interpretation of an ECG without a full understanding of the theory of electrocardiographic lead systems, but on the other hand, such an empirical approach to interpretation through pattern recognition could be enhanced with some understanding of lead systems and the relationship between the various leads.

The aim of this chapter is to describe the lead systems commonly used in different areas of electrocardiography and, wherever possible, to indicate comparisons between different types of leads. This can be of important clinical relevance. For example, a bipolar chest lead consisting of one electrode in the V_5 position and the other in the right infraclavicular fossa is often used for exercise testing or ambulatory electrocardiography. However, it is quite wrong to assume that there is a one-to-one correspondence between such a lead and the unipolar lead V_5. In other words, 0.1 mV of ST depression in V5 does not correspond to the same amount of ST depression in the bipolar lead described. This point will be discussed more extensively later in the chapter but has been used here as an illustration of the importance of understanding lead systems and lead theory.

11.2 The 12-Lead ECG

11.2.1 Bipolar Limb Leads

A bipolar lead measures the potential difference between two points-hence the term bipolar. The most commonly used bipolar leads are the bipolar limb leads introduced by Einthoven [1]. ❷ Figure 11.1 shows the circuitry associated with recording these leads. It should be noted that the illustration is didactic and that modern electrocardiographs would incorporate carefully designed electronic circuitry in order to derive these leads (see ❷ Chap. 12), but for the purposes of understanding basic electrocardiography, the illustration is of importance. As explained from a more theoretical standpoint in ❷ Chap. 10, the three bipolar limb leads illustrated which are denoted I, II and III can be represented mathematically as follows:

$$I = E_L - E_R$$
$$II = E_F - E_R$$
$$III = E_F - E_L$$

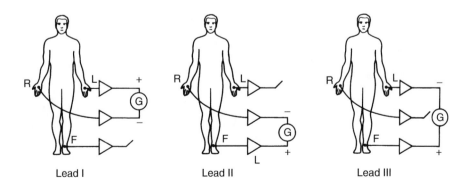

Lead I   Lead II   Lead III

❑ Fig. 11.1
A simplified illustration of the circuitry required to record the three standard limb leads I, II and III. Note the polarity of the connections

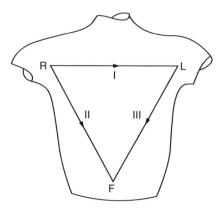

◨ **Fig. 11.2**
The interrelationship of the standard limb leads as depicted by the Einthoven triangle in which the body is assumed to have a triangular configuration from the point of view of its electrical characteristics

where E_L, E_R and E_F denote the potential at the left and right arms and left leg, respectively. In other words, lead I measures the potential difference between the left and right arms, and so on.

Simple combination of the above equations shows that, at any instant in the cardiac cycle, the following relationship holds:

$$I + III = II$$

This is known as Einthoven's law.

It is important to appreciate that with each of these leads is associated a certain direction corresponding to the lead vector (see ❷ Chap. 10). ❷ Figure 11.2 shows the directions associated with leads I, II and III based on the notion of the thorax being a homogeneous conductor, which of course is not the case. The three directions from the Einthoven triangle.

The direction of the lead is of relevance in that, by convention, if the net movement of excitation within the heart is similar to the lead direction, then a positive deflection will be recorded by that lead. Thus, if excitation moves from the right towards the left, lead I would be expected to produce an upward deflection while lead III would produce a negative deflection of lower amplitude based on the concepts illustrated in ❷ Chap. 10 (❷ Fig. 11.3).

It is also of relevance at this juncture to point out that although electrodes may be positioned on the body such that a line joining them is perhaps parallel to lead I, that does not mean to say that they accurately measure the spread of excitation in that direction. This anomaly arises from the inhomogeneities within the thorax. This problem was investigated by Burger and van Milaan [2] who subsequently modified the shape of the Einthoven triangle as shown in ❷ Fig. 10.4. Nevertheless, the idealized shape of the Einthoven triangle as shown in ❷ Fig. 11.2 continues to be used for teaching purposes and for illustrating the approximate relationships between the directions associated with the standard limb leads I, II and III.

11.2.1.1   Limb Electrode Positions

Surprisingly, there is still a debate over the positioning of limb electrodes. For example, in a small study of British hospitals, Turner [3] found that 70% of technicians and nurses used the wrists and ankles for limb electrodes while 16% placed these electrodes on the trunk. The 1975 AHA recommendations [4] stated that the arm electrodes could be on any part of the arm below the shoulders while the left leg electrode should be below the inguinal fold anteriorly and the gluteal fold posteriorly. The "right leg" electrode is required for technical reasons and can in fact be placed anywhere on the body. For convenience, it is usually placed, as the name suggests, on the right leg!!

Later, in 1977, the American College of Cardiology Task Force II which formed part of the 10th Bethesda Conference on Optimal Electrocardiography recommended [5] that the arm electrodes be placed on the wrists and the leg electrodes on the ankles.

The most recent 2007 recommendations for the standardization and interpretation of the ECG [6] drew attention to the 1975 recommendations but also to the paper by Pahlm et al. [7] pointing out that variation in the placement of the arm electrodes can alter ECG morphology and influence computer interpretations of the ECG. Kligfield and Macfarlane showed independently [8] and hence in pooled results that, paradoxically, the potential on the forearm of the left arm was very slightly higher than on the left wrist. Historically, limb potentials were recorded at the wrists and ankles as is evident from ❯ Fig. 1.8 while for many years, plate electrodes were attached to wrists and ankles using straps. This author suggests that many of today's normal limits of ECG measurements were obtained with electrodes limb electrodes on the extremities, i.e., wrists and ankles, and that these positions should continue to be used. Certainly, in the monitoring situation where cardiac rhythm is of concern, electrodes can be shifted to more proximal positions for convenience but it should be appreciated that the ECG morphology will also change. Hence, if ST trending is the reason for monitoring, it should be relative rather than absolute change versus any relevant criterion that is monitored.

11.2.2 Unipolar Limb Leads

A milestone in the development of electrocardiographic leads was the introduction in 1934 of unipolar leads, which are so called because they represent the potential variation at a single point. In order to derive such a lead, Wilson et al. [9] introduced their "central terminal." The circuitry associated with this terminal is shown in ❯ Fig. 11.3 from which it can be seen that potentials at the right and left arms and left leg are summed to form a single potential which, in practice, is relatively constant throughout the cardiac cycle. If E_{wct} denotes the potential at the Wilson central terminal, then $E_{wct} = 1/3 \, (E_R + E_L + E_F)$. The potential E_{wct} is often misnamed the "zero potential" but it should be understood that this is incorrect. ❯ Figure 11.3 shows how the central terminal is used in practice by being connected to one side of a galvanometer with the other side being linked to an exploring electrode P, here shown on the chest. If the potential of the exploring electrode is denoted by E_p, then the potential V_p measured by a unipolar lead is

$$V_p = E_p - E_{wct}$$
$$= E_p - 1/3(E_R + E_L + E_F)$$

It is clear that if E_{wct} provides a relatively constant potential then the unipolar lead basically records the potential variation at the exploring electrode P. The actual level of potential obtained from the central terminal becomes irrelevant since in broad terms it will essentially influence only the baseline level of the unipolar lead. Because the baseline will be adjusted either by the technician during recording or automatically by the currently available electronic techniques, the varying baseline offset potential difference between the central terminal and the exploring electrode in various positions will be unnoticed. The variation of the central terminal potential was investigated by Frank in 1955 [10].

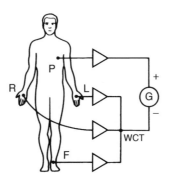

◼ Fig. 11.3

The circuitry used to record a unipolar lead in which it can be seen that the potential difference between a single point on the chest and the Wilson central terminal (WCT) is obtained. Note that the illustration is somewhat didactic in that modern electrocardiographs would employ a different technique to achieve the same end

It should be noted that although a unipolar lead reflects the potential variation at a single point, it is technically a bipolar lead as it measures a potential difference between two terminals, one of which has a relatively constant potential.

If the exploring electrode P is connected to the right arm, then a unipolar limb lead known as VR is obtained. The equation for this lead is as follows:

$$VR = E_R - Ewct$$

Similarly:

$$VL = E_L - Ewct$$
$$VF = E_F - Ewct$$

From the equations presented above, it follows that

$$VR + VL + VF = 0$$

These unipolar limb leads are no longer used but have been replaced by the augmented unipolar limb leads discussed below.

11.2.3   Augmented Unipolar Limb Leads

In 1942, Goldberger [11] modified the Wilson central terminal in order to increase the voltages measured by the unipolar limb leads. The circuitry for one of these leads is shown in ❷ Fig. 11.4. Consider the situation in the case of the unipolar lead VR being modified with the removal of the right arm connection from the Wilson central terminal. In this case, the new central terminal consists of the average of the potentials at the left arm and the left leg. Mathematically, if the potential at the modified terminal is denoted E_{GT}, then it follows that:

$$\begin{aligned}
\text{modified}\quad V_R &= E_R - E_{GT}\\
&= E_R - 1/2\,(E_L + E_F)\\
&= 3/2E_R - 1/2(E_R + E_L + E_F)\\
&= 3/2\,\{E_R - 1/3\,(E_R + E_L + E_F)\}\\
&= 3/2\text{VR}
\end{aligned}$$

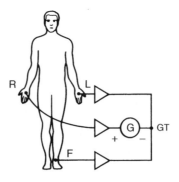

❏ Fig. 11.4
Circuitry used to derive the augmented unipolar limb lead aVR. GT denotes the Goldberger terminal for this particular lead. Note that the right arm electrode, which is effectively the exploring electrode in this particular lead, is connected to the positive terminal of the galvanometer. Again, the illustration is didactic

The modified lead VR became known as an augmented lead because it increased the potential of VR by 50%, and hence the lead was denoted aVR where "a" represented "augmented." Similar considerations apply to the other augmented limb leads denoted aVL and aVF. In summary,

$$aVL = E_L - 1/2(E_F + E_R)$$
$$= 3/2VL$$
$$aVF = E_F - 1/2(E_L + E_R)$$
$$= 3/2VF$$

From this it follows that

$$aVR + aVL + aVF = 0$$

at any instant in the cardiac cycle.

11.2.4 Unipolar Chest Leads

With the use of the Wilson central terminal as shown in ❯ Fig. 11.3, it became possible to measure potentials at varying points on the chest. A committee of the American Heart Association [12] selected six positions on the precordium in order to standardize recordings. The positions of these electrodes, denoted V_1–V_6, are described in ❯ Table 11.1 and are shown in ❯ Fig. 11.5. V_1 and V_2 are at the level of the fourth intercostal space at the sternal borders, V_4 is in the midclavicular line one interspace lower, V_6 is in the left mid-axilla at the same horizontal level as V_4 while V_3 is intermediate to V_2 and V_4, and V_5 is intermediate to V_4 and V_6. These six unipolar chest leads are called V_1–V_6. The AHA recommendations of 1975 stated [4] that V_5 was to be placed at the junction of the left anterior axillary line and the level of V_4. The 1977 ACC 10th Bethesda Report [5] gave a similar position. However, the 2007 recommendations [6] added that if the anterior axillary line is ambiguous, then V_5 should be placed midway between V_4 and V_6.

The directions associated with these leads are shown in ❯ Fig. 11.6. In ❯ Fig. 11.6a the idealized lead directions are shown while in ❯ Fig. 11.6b the theoretically derived directions associated with each lead based on a more realistic model of the torso are indicated [13]. In each case, the vectors can be assumed to lie approximately in the transverse plane.

Some clinicians may wish to record leads an interspace higher or lower than those recommended. There are no specific recommendations in terms of denoting such leads, but occasionally in the literature authors have used 1H to denote a lead

◻ **Table 11.1**
Lead nomenclature (After Sheffield et al. [5])

Electrode	Location of attachment
Right arm (R)	Right wrist
Left arm (L)	Left wrist
Left foot (F)	Left ankle
Right foot (G)	Right ankle
V_1	Right sternal margin, fourth intercostal space
V_2	Left sternal margin, fourth intercostal space
V_3	Midway between V_2 and V_4
V_4	Left midclavicular line, fifth intercostal space
V_5	Left anterior axillary line, V_4 level
V_6	Left midaxillary line, V_4 and V_5 level
V_7 and V_8[a]	Left posterior axillary line and left midscapular line, V_6 level
Leads[a] recorded on right side of thorax, such as V_4R	Right midclavicular line, fifth intercostal space

[a]Optional leads

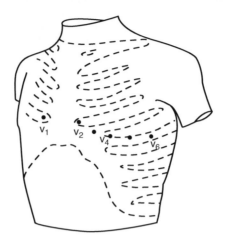

☑ Fig. 11.5

The six positions recommended for the exploring electrode in order to record unipolar chest leads (see ❯ Table 11.1 for further details). By convention, the leads and hence the positions, are denoted V_1–V_6

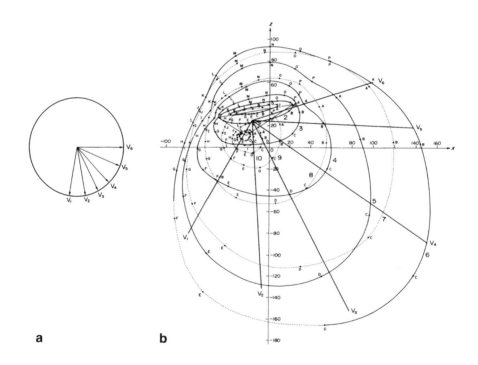

a   b

☑ Fig. 11.6

In (**a**), an idealized description of the directions associated with each of the six precordial leads (that is, the direction in which the component of the resultant cardiac electrical force is measured) is shown. In (**b**), the lead directions of V1 to V6 as derived from Frank's image surface are shown. In this case, the origin of the axes represents the electrical centre of the heart with respect to which the Wilson central terminal is displaced in electrical terms. All lead vectors are drawn from this terminal (at the centroid of the triangle) to the points on the image surface corresponding to the positions of the electrodes on the precordium. The loops 5 and 6 represent different levels of the surface of the thorax separated by two inches approximately at the level of V1 and V4, respectively. Note that leads V1–V6 have different strengths indicated by the length of each lead vector (After Frank [13]. © Mosby, St Louis, Missouri. Reproduced with permission)

recorded one interspace higher, e.g., $V_2 1H$ would denote a lead recorded at the left sternal border in the third intercostal space. Similarly, 1L is sometimes used to denote a lead recorded one interspace lower than that recommended.

11.2.5 Additional Chest Leads

In addition to the internationally accepted six precordial-lead positions, it is not uncommon for additional leads to be recorded on the right side of the chest. For example, routinely in children and in adults with acute inferior myocardial infarction, leads on the right side of the chest which reflect lead positions on the left side of the chest may be recorded. These positions are shown schematically in ❯ Fig. 11.7a. For example, a lead in the midclavicular line at the fifth intercostal space on the right side of the chest (i.e., a reflection of V_4) would be denoted V_4R. The lead intermediate between V_1 and V_4R is denoted V_3R. V_3R and V_4R are perhaps the two most commonly used additional leads. However, on rare occasions V_5R and V_6R may also be recorded.

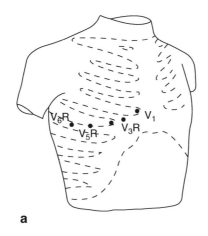

a

■ Fig. 11.7a
Right-sided chest lead positions as used mainly in children and occasionally in the detection of right ventricular involvement in myocardial infarction

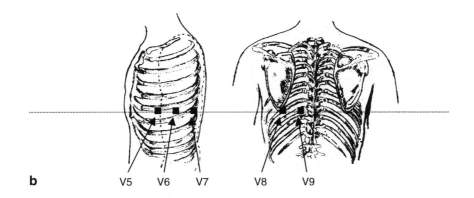

b   V5   V6   V7   V8   V9

■ Fig. 11.7b
Additional left sided chest leads V7–V9. See text for further discussion (Reproduced by kind permission of Ian Bolton, Essex Cardiac Services, England)

To assist in the diagnosis of acute ST elevation myocardial infarction, additional leads are sometimes recorded on the posterior chest. V_7, for example, records the potential at the left posterior axillary line [4, 5], V_8 records the potential in the left midscapular line [4, 5], while V_9 records the potential at the left paravertebral border of the spine [6], with all of these electrode positions being at the level of lead V_6 (❯ Fig. 11.7b).

11.2.6   12-Lead ECG Relationships

The combination of the bipolar limb leads I, II and III, the augmented unipolar limb leads aVR, aVL and aVF, and the six unipolar precordial leads V_1–V_6 is known as the 12-lead ECG. Almost all ECGs recorded worldwide make use of these 12 leads. Additional precordial leads may be recorded as described above, particularly in children, where the six precordial leads are often selected as V_4R, V_1, V_2, V_4, V_5 and V_6.

The limb leads in particular, both bipolar and unipolar, are closely related. In fact, if any two of the six limb leads are recorded simultaneously, the other four can be derived from them. As an example, consider that leads I and II have been recorded. Lead aVF could be calculated from them as follows:

$$\text{aVF} = E_F - 1/2\,(E_L + E_R)$$
$$= 1/2\,(E_F - E_L) + 1/2\,(E_F - E_R)$$
$$= 1/2\text{III} + 1/2\text{II}$$
$$= 1/2\,(\text{II} - \text{I}) + 1/2\text{II}$$
$$= \text{II} - 1/2\text{I}$$

The other limb leads can be expressed in terms of leads I and II as follows:

$$\text{III} = \text{II} - \text{I}$$
$$\text{aVR} = -1/2\,(\text{I} + \text{II})$$
$$\text{aVL} = \text{I} - 1/2\text{II}$$

If an alternative strategy had been adopted whereby leads I and a VF were available, then it can be shown that the following relationships hold:

$$\text{II} = \text{aVF} + 1/2\,\text{I}$$
$$\text{III} = \text{aVF} - 1/2\,\text{I}$$
$$\text{aVR} = -\,(3/4\,\text{I} + 1/2\,\text{aVF})$$
$$\text{aVL} = 3/4\,\text{I} - 1/2\text{aVF}$$

Part of the importance in these relationships is that in computer-based electrocardiography, it is only necessary to record or store two of the limb leads, since the remaining four can be calculated and displayed whenever desired. This has important repercussions in terms of long-term storage on a database where a saving of 33% of data can be achieved by using only the eight independent leads of the 12-lead ECG with the remainder being calculated whenever necessary. In the author's experience, this strategy sometimes creates considerable misunderstanding. The equations described above are totally independent of body habitus. Although the Einthoven triangle is an idealized concept and the Burger triangle represents perhaps a theoretically more exact description of the electrical equivalent of the body, the equations described have been derived from a purely empirical standpoint and are thus independent of body size and internal structure.

The concept of a direction associated with a lead was introduced earlier and the Einthoven triangle (❯ Fig. 11.2) illustrated the directions for the bipolar limb leads. The augmented unipolar limb leads can also be incorporated into the Einthoven triangle as shown in ❯ Fig. 11.8. For example, because the Goldberger terminal for aVF is half of the potential at the right and left arms, it can be regarded as the midpoint on the line joining R and L. The direction associated with aVF is therefore from this midpoint to F, that is, a vertical line in the triangle as shown in ❯ Fig. 11.8.

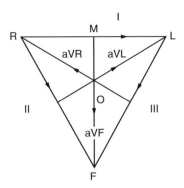

◻ Fig. 11.8
A diagram indicating the approximate directions and strengths associated with the six limb leads. Leads I, II and III have the same strength while leads aVR, aVL and aVF have an equal but different lead strength according to the concept of the equilateral Einthoven triangle; for example, the ratio of the strength of I to aVF is RL/MF. In practice, the six leads have different lead strengths as discussed in the text

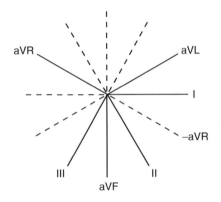

◻ Fig. 11.9
The lead directions of the six limb leads presented in an alternative fashion which incorporates –aVR. This lead is sometimes used in the alternative presentation of leads in the sequence of aVL to III in keeping with the clockwise sequence of the leads shown in the illustration. The *dotted lines* represent the negatively directed axes

Similar considerations apply to the directions associated with aVL and aVR, and these can be combined into a single diagram showing all six lead directions (❷ Fig. 11.9). Note that this diagram shows the approximate direction and strengths associated with each of these leads. The concept of lead strength is discussed in ❷ Chap. 10. It essentially reflects the potential recorded by the lead when a source of unit strength is placed within the thorax and, as such, is used as a relative estimate of the lead capabilities. For example, if there is a potential source within the thorax such that VR measures 1 mV, then aVR would measure 1.5 mV. Theoretically, the relative strengths of aVF and lead I are given by the lengths of the lines MF and RL as shown in ❷ Fig. 11.8. In practice, the actual ratio will be different in view of the shortcomings of the equivalent (equilateral) triangle hypothesis (❷ Fig. 11.2). Langner pointed out some time ago [14] that if a particular source of potential was aligned to produce a maximum potential of one unit in lead III, then the same potential source would produce at most one half of that potential in lead I when similarly reoriented to produce a maximum. In turn, this reflects the ratio of the lengths of the sides RL and FL of the Burger triangle (❷ Fig. 10.3).

❷ Figure 11.9 also shows how the lead directions can be translated to another display known as the hexaxial reference frame. This shows more clearly the relative directions of the different limb leads. It also supports the presentation of the limb leads in a sequence aVL, I, -aVR, II, aVF, III, a practice which is universally adopted in most Scandinavian countries.

This sequence is known as the Cabrera (panoramic) presentation [15, 16]. An illustration can be seen in ❷ Fig. 13.38. While this is a logical sequence for displaying the leads, most cardiologists in other countries have been taught to view the leads in the more conventional sequence I, II, III, aVR, aVL, aVF and an adjustment to the alternative form of display would be likely to prove most difficult. Nevertheless, with the flexibility of microprocessor-based technology incorporated into currently available electrocardiographs, such alternative displays are easily obtainable at the touch of a button.

11.3   Other Bipolar Leads

11.3.1   Bipolar Chest Leads

Another form of lead which is rarely used nowadays is the bipolar chest lead formed by placing one electrode on one of the limbs with the other on any of the precordial positions shown in ❷ Fig. 11.5. If the right arm is used, then a bipolar chest lead derived with the other electrode in the V_1 position would be denoted as CR_1. Similarly, if the limb electrode were on the left leg and the other electrode were applied in the V_6 position, the resulting lead would be denoted CF_6.

Of more interest are bipolar chest leads used for exercise testing or ambulatory monitoring. Most commonly, the positive electrode is placed in the V5 position and the negative electrode is placed at a variety of sites as shown in ❷ Fig. 11.10. Those commonly used include the manubrium (giving lead CM) or the right infraclavicular fossa (giving lead CS5). ❷ Table 11.2 lists the electrode positions, with additional comments on their use in exercise testing.

As mentioned in the introduction, there is, in the author's opinion, considerable misunderstanding over the difference between the unipolar lead V_5 and a bipolar chest lead such as CM_5. The idea of lead strength and direction has now been introduced, and in order to explain the difference between the leads CC_5, CM_5 and V_5, ❷ Fig. 11.11 depicts the lead strength and direction associated with the corresponding lead vectors which have been derived from Frank's image surface [13], a concept described fully in ❷ Chap. 10. It can be seen in the transverse and frontal view that the leads CC_5 and CM_5 both have a longer lead vector than V_5. Thus, the potential measured by CM_5 will be approximately 1.2 times that of V_5 for the same size of electrical force parallel to these axes because the potential measured is directly proportional to lead strength (see ❷ Fig. 10.8). Similarly, CC_5/V_5 is approximately 1.4. The potential measured is also proportional to the component of the electrical force along the direction of the axes (❷ Fig. 10.2) and in this respect ❷ Fig. 11.11 shows that vertically directed electrical forces will have virtually no effect on V_5 and CC_5 while they will influence CM_5. The

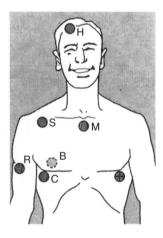

◻ Fig. 11.10

The various electrode positions for recording bipolar chest leads where the positive lead is in the V5 position and the negative lead is in one of a number of other positions shown on the diagram. The code for the electrode positions is explained in ❷ Table 11.2 (After Froelicher et al. [55]. © American College of Chest Physicians, Park Ridge, Illinois. Reproduced with permission)

☐ Table 11.2

Some bipolar leads used in conjunction with stress testing (After Surawicz et al. [50])

Lead	Positive electrode location	Negative electrode location	Comments
CM_5[a]	V_5 position	Manubrium	One of the most sensitive bipolar leads for detecting ST changes
CH_5	V_5 position	Forehead	favored in Sweden, especially bicycle tests
CS_5	V_5 position	right infraclavicular fossa	Detects somewhat more muscle artefact than lead CM_5
CC_5	V_5 position	V_5R position	Bears a closer resemblance to lead V_5 than most bipolar leads
CB_5	V_5 position	low right scapula	Closely resembles lead V_5 but has more muscle artifact than most other bipolar leads
CR_5	V_5 position	right arm	Used in northern Europe and USSR for pre- and postexercise records, usually with 4 to 6 chest lead positions. High muscle artifact level during exercise

[a]The number 5 refers to the position on the chest of a corresponding V lead such as V_5. Thus the positive electrode could be located in any numbered V lead position

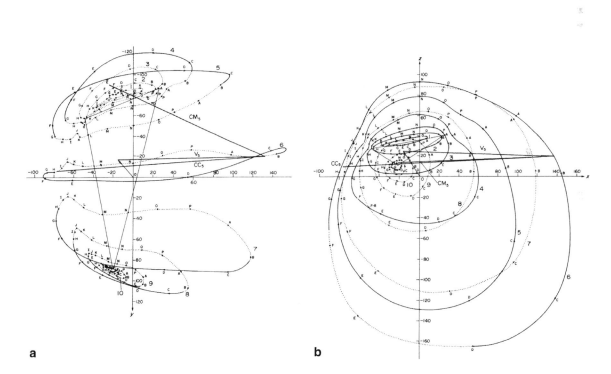

a   b

☐ Fig. 11.11

The projection of the lead vectors for V5, CM5 and CC5 onto (a) the frontal plane; and (b) the transverse plane. The vectors have been derived from Frank's image surface described in ❷ Chap. 10. Note in particular how the frontal view shows quite a divergence in the orientation of the vectors. Since V5 and CC5 are essentially at right angles to the head-to-foot axis, they will not measure any component of an electrical force which is directed along such an axis. The two views summarize a three-dimensional picture from which it can be calculated that the ratio of the lead-vector magnitudes is approximately 1.2: 1 for CM5: V5 and 1.4: 1 for CC5: V5. The tip of the arrow on each view represents the position of the Wilson central terminal in image space (After Frank [13]. © Mosby, St Louis, Missouri. Reproduced with permission) amplitude of CM_5 will be further enhanced by the fact that its lead-vector direction is essentially parallel to the normal mean QRS axis, so that the QRS component will be greater along CM_5 than along the V_5 lead vector. Similarly, lateral ST abnormalities should be larger in CM_5 than V_5.

From the foregoing, it follows that a criterion of, say, 0.1 mV ST depression may lead to a higher percentage of positive findings in CM_5 in any particular comparison with V_5 and the sensitivity and specificity of the test might be completely misinterpreted. Thus, different criteria should be applied to these different leads.

11.3.2 Nehb Leads

In a few countries in Europe (particularly Germany) there are still some cardiologists who make use of the Nehb leads [17]. Essentially, these consist of three bipolar chest leads. The three electrodes are placed on the thorax as shown in ❷ Fig. 11.12. In practice, to record these leads with a single-channel electrocardiograph, the electrode connections used for recording the standard limb leads can be utilized. With this approach, the right arm electrode is placed at the junction of the second rib with the sternum on the right side, the left arm electrode is placed level with the scapular apex on the posterior axillary line, while the left leg electrode is placed on the front of the chest opposite the scapular apex (in proximity to the apex of the heart). The leads recorded are denoted O for dorsal, A for anterior and I for inferior. By using the limb-lead connections, the leads O, A and I would be recorded with the electrocardiograph set up as for leads I, II and III, respectively. Alternatively, the leads are sometimes prefixed with the letter N (after Nehb) giving leads NO, NA and NI. ❷ Figure 11.12 should not be misconstrued as representing three electrodes at the same cross-sectional level of the thorax.

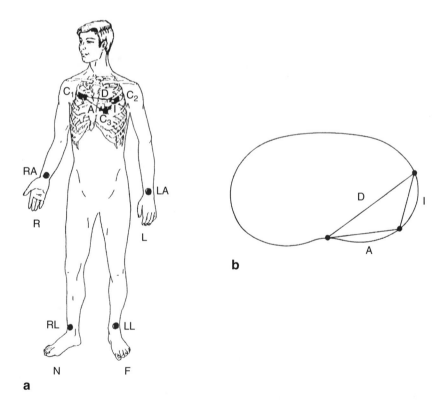

❑ Fig. 11.12

The Nehb-lead system comprising the dorsal lead D, the inferior lead I and the anterior lead A. Note that the three electrodes are not placed at the same level on the thorax as suggested in (**b**) but are at different levels as seen in (**a**) (© Siemens-Elema. Reproduced with permission)

With a multichannel electrocardiograph it is customary to use the $V_1(C_1)$, $V_2(C_2)$ and $V_3(C_3)$ electrode connections to record the Nehb leads. According to the scheme above, V1 replaces the right arm electrode, V2 the left arm electrode and V3 the left leg electrode. For example, lead D records the potential difference between C1 and C2 (see ❷ Fig. 11.12). These leads are also used in experimental work in animals as discussed in the ❷ Chap. 11, ❷ Sect. 11.17.

11.4 Orthogonal-Lead Systems

In earlier chapters, reference has been made to equivalent cardiac generators, and there has been reference to the equivalent cardiac dipole first suggested by Einthoven [1]. As discussed in ❷ Chap. 2, a dipole can be represented mathematically by a vector; that is, an entity having a specific magnitude and direction. In turn, a vector requires three measurements for its definition. In the simplest approach, three such components could be obtained by deriving the projections of the vector onto three mutually perpendicular (orthogonal) axes. ❷ Chap. 2 describes fully how given three components H_x, H_y, H_z in such directions conventionally denoted as X, Y and Z (❷ Fig. 11.13), the resultant vector can be obtained having a magnitude H where

$$H = \left(H_x{}^2 + H_y{}^2 + H_z{}^2\right)^{1/2}$$

and a direction which can be calculated from these three components. By convention, the X component of the vector detects the lateral forces. An electrode array measuring this component is called lead X and by convention produces a positive deflection (similar to lead I) when current flows from right to left within the thorax. Similarly, an electrode array detecting the inferior component is called lead Y and, like aVF, by convention, has a positive deflection when current flows towards the feet. An electrode array detecting current flow in an anteroposterior direction is called lead Z. Most authors

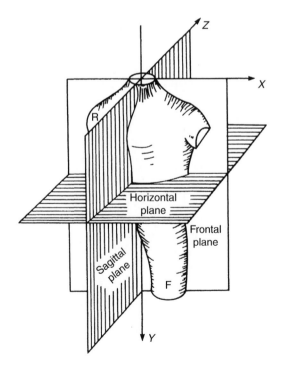

■ Fig. 11.13
The relationship between the various planes and the *X, Y* and *Z* axes (*Circ. Res* 1954; 2: 257. © American Heart Association, Dallas, Texas. Reproduced with permission)

direct lead Z positively to the back, that is, it shows a pattern like an inverted V2. However, this author prefers to direct lead Z positively to the anterior in order to maintain the similarity with V2 and a meaningful discussion in terms of Q waves, and so on.

11.4.1   Uncorrected Orthogonal-Lead Systems

In the 1940s and early 1950s, a number of investigators had the idea of designing lead systems that would measure the three components of the cardiac dipole. These early attempts essentially produced lead systems such that lines joining the electrode positions were mutually perpendicular (see ❷ Fig. 11.14). Examples are the Grishman cube [18], the double cube system of Duchosal [19] and the Wilson tetrahedron system [20]. These systems are essentially no longer in routine use.

The cube system (❷ Fig. 11.14) was a simple arrangement of electrodes such that lines joining the electrode positions lay along the edges of a cube; that is, the three pairs of (bipolar) leads that were formed appeared geometrically orthogonal. The cube system is not used routinely today but still features in research work such as described by Selvester et al. in ❷ Chap. 16, where VCGs derived from the cube system are illustrated.

The tetrahedron system (❷ Fig. 11.14b) is easy to apply with three limb electrodes and one centrally located on the back. The X component was taken as lead I while aVF provided the vertical component Y. The anteroposterior component Z was obtained from the unipolar lead VB. This system is not used nowadays except in animal research. Examples can be found in ❷ Chaps. 9 and ❷ 10 of *Specialized Aspects of ECG*.

Around 1945–55, the theory of electrocardiographic leads was much more intensively investigated as described in ❷ Chap. 10. From such research came an understanding that while electrode systems might appear to be geometrically orthogonal, the equivalent lead-vector orientations were far from orthogonal. Such systems then became known as "uncorrected" orthogonal-lead systems. What was required was a system of electrodes which, in combination, measured as accurately as possible the components of a dipole in three mutually perpendicular directions. In particular, Frank [13] introduced the concept of image space (see ❷ Chap. 10), which allowed assessment of electrocardiographic leads with more precision than had previously been the case.

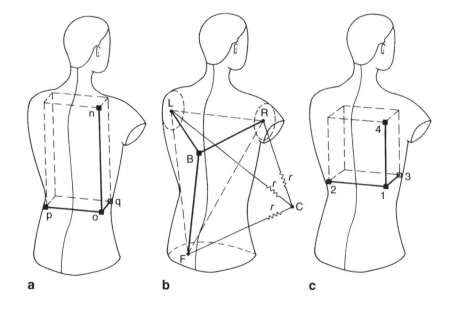

❏ Fig. 11.14

The electrode positions of (a) the Duchosal double cube system; (b) the Wilson tetrahedron; and (c) the Grishman cube (After Frank E, *Circulation* 1954; **10**: 101. © American Heart Association, Dallas, Texas. Reproduced with permission)

11.4.2 Corrected Orthogonal-Lead Systems

The concept behind a corrected lead system was to produce an electrode network that resulted in lead vectors that were of equal magnitude and were mutually perpendicular – at least according to theoretical and modeling studies. It is shown in ❷ Chap. 10 that the potential V measured by a lead is given by the scalar product of two vectors, namely, the cardiac vector H and the lead vector L. Thus,

$$V_{lead} = H\,L_{lead}$$

If L is parallel to the X axis, say, then L has components $(x, 0,0)$ and so

$$Vx = HxLx$$

Thus,

$$Hx = Vx/Lx$$

Similarly,

$$Hy = Vy/Ly$$

and

$$Hz = Vz/Lz$$

The vector magnitude H is calculated from

$$H = \left\{ (Vx/Lx)^2 + (Vy/Ly)^2 + (Vz/Lz)^2 \right\}^{1/2}$$

In order to avoid distortion, it is necessary for $Lx = Ly = Lz = L$. Then,

$$H = \frac{1}{L} \left\{ (V_x)^2 + (V_y)^2 + (V_z)^2 \right\}^{1/2}$$

where L is the common lead strength. A lead system with these characteristics is called a corrected orthogonal-lead system.

11.4.2.1 Frank System

In 1956, Frank [21] published details of what was effectively the first truly corrected orthogonallead system. The term "corrected" implies that the lead vectors associated with the system were indeed orthogonal and, on the basis of tank torso model studies, accurately measured components of "cardiac" electrical activity in mutually perpendicular directions. The electrode positions and the resistor network required to derive the three leads are shown in ❷ Fig. 11.15.

The electrodes A, C, E, I and M should be placed at a level corresponding to the electrical center of the heart. This point is discussed further below. A and I are positioned in the left and right midaxillary lines, respectively. E and M are positioned on the sternum and spine, respectively. C is positioned such that an angle of 45° is produced with respect to the center of the thorax as shown in ❷ Fig. 11.15. This electrode position may need some adjustment in females. Electrode H is usually placed on the back of the neck, although its position is not particularly critical.

It is of passing interest that Frank's electrode position nomenclature was derived very simply from the concept of labeling points around the chest at intervals of 22.5°. Thus, starting from A in the left mid axilla and moving anteriorly, B is 22.5° from A, C is 45° from A. Progressing clockwise in this way, E is 90° from A, I is 180° from A and M is 270° from A.

It can be seen from ❷ Fig. 11.16 that the lead vectors for leads X, Y and Z are essentially mutually perpendicular as required. The length of each lead vector is not the same, with the Y lead vector being the smallest. Frank used shunt resistors of 7.15 R and 13.3 R to reduce the gains of the X and Z leads respectively (see ❷ Fig. 11.15) so that each equaled 136 units. This lead system is therefore "corrected" with respect to both the lead direction and magnitude. The latter is important if the components of the cardiac vector are not to be distorted by an imbalance in the measurement system.

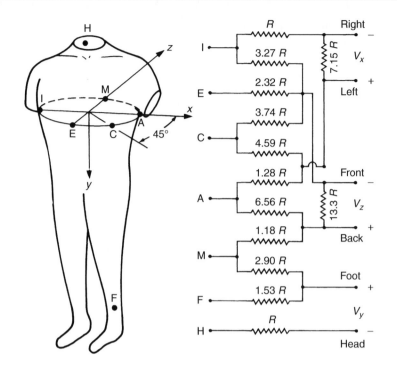

■ Fig. 11.15
Electrodes and circuitry of the Frank-lead system (After Frank [21]. © American Heart Association, Dallas Texas. Reproduced
with permission)

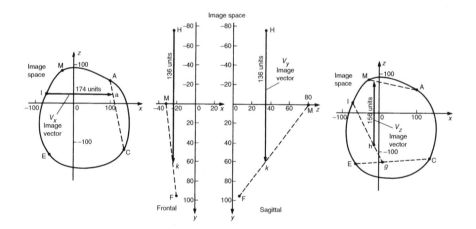

■ Fig. 11.16
The three lead vectors corresponding to leads X, Y and Z of the Frank system as projected onto the transverse, frontal/sagittal
and transverse planes, respectively. It can be seen that the lead vectors are parallel to the desired lead directions although they
do not intersect at a single point (After Frank [21]. © American Heart Association, Dallas, Texas. Reproduced with permission)

An analysis of the resistor network in ❷ Fig. 11.15 leads to the following equations, which show the contribution of each electrode to the potential measured in each lead:

$$Vx = 0.61V_A + 0.171V_C - 0.781V_I$$
$$V_y = 0.655V_F + 0.345V_M - 1.0V_H$$
$$V_z = 0.133V_A + 0.736V_M - 0.264V_I - 0.374V_E - 0.231Vc$$

The Frank system has retained its original popularity wherever vectorcardiography is practised although there are very few medical practitioners nowadays who understand the technique. The only area of controversy in its application has surrounded the use of the fourth or the fifth intercostal space as the reference for siting the precordial electrodes. Frank initially indicated that the electrodes should be placed at a level corresponding to the electrical center of the heart, and described a mechanism for finding such a position [21]. In most early studies the fourth intercostal space was used, and one of the most significant publications on the derivation of normal limits for the Frank XYZ leads [22] arose from the use of the system at the fourth intercostal space. Subsequently the tendency has been for the electrodes to be placed in the fifth intercostal space [23]. Part of this stems from an attempt to combine recording of the 12-lead ECG with the Frank leads. In this case, the C and A electrodes of the Frank system (see ❷ Fig. 11.15) can also be used to record V_4 and V_6, respectively. Thus, compared to recording the 12-lead ECG alone it is necessary to add four electrodes, namely, E, I, M and H if this approach is adopted [24].

11.4.2.2 Axial-Lead System

In 1955, McFee and Parungao [25] introduced what they termed an axial-lead system for orthogonal-lead electrocardiography. This is illustrated in ❷ Fig. 11.17. The $X+$ electrodes in the left anterior axilla are situated approximately 5.5 cm above and below the fifth intercostal space in adults. The $X-$ electrode is situated in the right mid axilla at the level of the fifth intercostal space. The Y lead is a straightforward bipolar lead recorded between the left leg and the neck. The Z lead consists of three electrodes, arranged in the shape of a triangle, with a distance of 6 cm from the centroid, situated approximately at V2, to each of the apices. This measurement is reduced in children. The $Z+$ electrode was positioned behind the triangle on the back at a point corresponding to the centroid as shown in the illustration. In a study of the lead vectors, Brody and Arzbaecher [26] showed that the axial-lead system had the best orthogonality of all corrected orthogonal-lead systems although the strengths of the leads were unequal. Since this is undesirable, Macfarlane introduced a modification [27] in 1969 which equalized the lead strengths. The correction was based on the relative strengths of the X, Y and Z leads as published by Brody and Arzbaecher. As a result, the following equations therefore apply:

$$X \, (\text{modified axial}) = 0.92X \, (\text{axial})$$
$$Y \, (\text{modified axial}) = Y \, (\text{axial})$$
$$Z \, (\text{modified axial}) = 0.66Z \, (\text{axial})$$

The modified axial-lead system was used by Macfarlane in early comparative studies on 12-lead and 3-lead electrocardiography. These showed that there was no significant difference from the diagnostic point of view between 3-lead and 12-lead electrocardiography [28]. For use with children, the system was adapted by reducing the spacing between the triangle of electrodes and the pair of electrodes in the left axilla [29]. A set of templates was constructed for easy application of electrodes.

11.4.2.3 Hybrid-Lead System

Although there were many studies undertaken using orthogonal-lead electrocardiography, it was apparent by the mid-1970s at least that clinicians were reluctant to move towards 3-orthogonal lead systems to the exclusion of the 12-lead ECG.

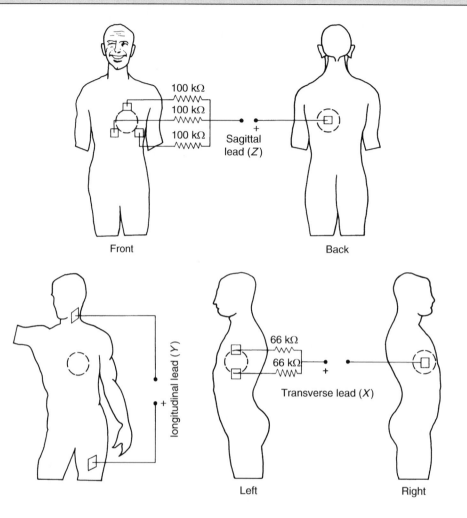

☐ **Fig. 11.17**
The McFee and Parungao axial-lead system. The derivation of the leads is clear from the illustration. Note that each electrode contributes to one lead only (After McFee and Parungao [25]. © Mosby, St Louis, Missouri. Reproduced with permission)

For this reason, Macfarlane designed a new lead system that was aimed at combining the 12-lead and the 3-orthogonal-lead ECG with the minimum number of additional electrodes. The intention was to retain the advantages of the phase relationships of the 3-orthogonal-lead ECG and add them to the information obtained from the 12-lead ECG. The system [30, 31] was also designed by making use of Frank's image space and was intended to produce XYZ leads which had a similar orientation and lead strength to those of the modified axial-lead system previously designed by Macfarlane. The electrode positions of this system are shown in ❯ Fig. 11.18 where it can be seen that there are only two additional electrodes compared to the use of the 12-lead system alone. These electrodes are placed in the V6R position and on the neck:

With the hybrid system, the 12-lead ECG is recorded in the usual fashion. Lead X of the orthogonal-lead ECG is a bipolar lead between V_5 and V_6R. Lead Y is similar to the original axial-lead system and the modified axial-lead system, being a potential difference between the neck and the left leg. Lead Z is obtained by averaging the V_1, V_2 and V_3 potentials and from this subtracting the potential at the neck. The relevant gains are controlled by the use of the resistors as shown in ❯ Fig. 11.18. In this way, the use of a back electrode is obviated while the three potentials $V_1 - V_3$ replace the triangle of electrodes in the axial system. ❯ Figure 11.19 shows how the XYZ lead vectors of the hybrid system relate to those of the original axial system. It can be seen that lead Z is displaced superiorly but still remains parallel to the desired Z direction.

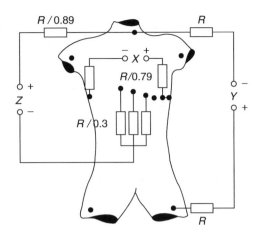

Fig. 11.18
The electrode positions and resistor network of the hybrid-lead system. The 12-lead ECG is derived in the usual way while the corrected orthogonal leads X, Y and Z are derived using the network shown. Note that only two additional electrodes are required compared to the use of the 12-lead ECG alone

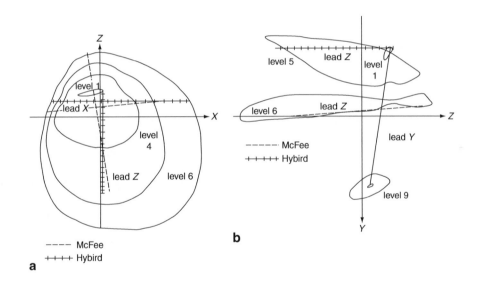

Fig. 11.19
The lead vectors of the hybrid-lead system and the original axial-lead system as seen in (a) the transverse view; and (b) the sagittal view. It can be seen that the hybrid leads are more corrected, i.e. parallel to the X, Y and Z axes, than are the original axial leads. The lead vectors were obtained from analysis of Frank's image surface. The continuous line denotes both the hybrid and axial Y lead vector which is identical in each case

Indeed, it is more corrected than the original axial system at least based on studies using Frank's image space. Likewise, lead X is also parallel to the X axis and is more corrected than the original axial lead. Since lead Y is identical in both cases, only one lead vector can be shown. This is not parallel to the Y axis as would be desired in a perfect orthogonal-lead system.

The hybrid system is no longer used routinely by the author but some normal limits of orthogonal-lead measurements discussed in ❯ Chap. 1 of *Electrocardiology: Comprehensive Clinical ECG* are based on studies with this system.

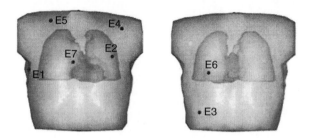

◘ Fig. 11.20

Optimized electrode positioning for the detection of atrial fibrillation using a vectorcardiographic lead system incorporating the electrodes shown (After van Oosterom et al. [32]. © Elsevier. Reproduced with permission)

The lead strengths of the X Y Z leads derived from the hybrid system were equalized via resistors (❯ Fig. 11.18) calculated from modeling studies. The equations for deriving the orthogonal leads are as follows:

$$X = 0.79 \left(V_5 - V_6R \right)$$
$$Y = V_F - V_{neck}$$
$$Z = 0.89 \left\{ \left(V_1 + V_2 + V_3 \right) - V_{neck} \right\}$$

With the use of this system it is necessary to acquire only ten leads I, II, V_1–V_6, V_6R and V_{neck} from which the remaining five can be derived in order to obtain the full 12-lead plus X, Y and Z lead presentation. These ten leads have to be recorded simultaneously for this purpose.

11.4.2.4   Lead Systems for the Characterization of Atrial Fibrillation

van Oosterom and colleagues have recently published details [32] of a vectorcardiographic lead system which they say was dedicated to the analysis of atrial fibrillation. The positions of seven electrodes are shown in ❯ Fig. 11.20. These electrode positions were chosen after extensive mathematical modeling to find leads that best represent atrial activation. The authors were firmly of the opinion that the best lead systems must include at least one electrode on the back. They also presented a series of transformations that allow the standard 12-lead ECG to be derived from the vectorcardiographic leads.

11.5   Derived 12-Lead ECG Systems

11.5.1   The Derived 12 Lead ECG

The reluctance of cardiologists to move from the use of the 12-lead ECG has already been mentioned. In the mid-1970s, the concept of using only three leads for computer analysis of the ECG was attractive in view of the saving in time for measurement and storage requirements. This led Dower and colleagues to introduce the derived 12-lead ECG [33]. By making use of the image space discussed in ❯ Chap. 10, they were able to produce a set of coefficients which allowed the 12-lead ECG to be derived from the XYZ leads.

In mathematical terms, the concept of the derived leads is to express each of the 12 leads as a linear combination of the XYZ orthogonal leads. Mathematically,

$$\text{derived lead} = aX + bY + cZ$$

where X, Y and Z represent the potentials measured by each of these leads respectively, and a, b, c represent coefficients which are fixed from a study of Frank's image space. The values of these coefficients for deriving each of the 12 leads are

⬛ Table 11.3

Transfer coefficients for deriving the 12-lead ECG from the XYZ leads, as obtained by Dower et al. [33]. Note that Z in this case is directed positively towards the back. For convenience, this table is presented in a 3 × 12 format, although it is used as a 12 × 3 matrix in ❯ Sect. 11.6

	I	II	III	aVR	aVL	aVF	V_1	V_2	V_3	V_4	V_5	V_6
X	0.632	0.235	−0.397	−0.434	0.515	−0.081	−0.515	0.044	0.882	1.213	1.125	0.831
Y	−0.235	1.066	1.301	−0.415	−0.768	1.184	0.157	0.164	0.098	0.127	0.127	0.076
Z	0.059	−0.132	−0.191	0.037	0.125	−0.162	−0.917	−1.387	−1.277	−0.601	−0.086	0.230

shown in ❯ Table 11.3. These have been slightly modified compared to an earlier publication [34] and appear in a 3 × 12 format for convenience. As an example, lead I would be derived as follows:

$$\text{lead I} = 0.632\,X - 0.235\,Y + 0.059\,Z$$

Note that this calculation has to be carried out at each sampling instant, that is, the XYZ values represent simultaneous measurements at one particular instant from each of the XYZ leads, and normally, when using computer methods, such measurements are made at least 250 times per second. Thus, the calculation would have to be repeated at this frequency. Note also that if the input from the XYZ leads is in mV, then the resultant calculation also produces mV output values.

An alternative approach is to construct an analog equivalent of the transformation coefficients so that if the XYZ leads are fed as input to electronic circuitry, then there will be a continuous output for each of the leads [35]. Uijen et al. [36], however, suggested that there was an inconsistency between the coefficients of ❯ Table 11.3 and the published hardware implementation [35].

There can be obvious differences between the derived 12-lead ECG and the conventional 12-lead ECG although Dower and colleagues undertook one study [35] which claimed to show that the derived ECG (ECGD) correlated better with the clinical findings than did the actual 12-lead ECG. This is equivalent to saying that in that particular study, the XYZ leads were superior to the conventional 12-lead ECG. An example of the similarity and differences is shown in ❯ Fig. 11.21.

A report by Uijen et al. [36] claimed that the use of a statistically derived transfer matrix gave better agreement between the 12 derived leads and actual data than did either of the Dower transfer matrices. However, the calculation was based on an evaluation of the training set used to develop the transfer matrix and it was noted that there could be wide variations, particularly in V_3 and V_4, between derived and actual leads. The transfer matrix from this group is shown in ❯ Table 11.4.

The value of the derived 12-lead ECG is limited, whatever the method of derivation. No single transfer matrix can be accurate for every patient, and hence the derived 12-lead ECG would require a complete appraisal in terms of normal limits, and so on, before being of more obvious value. Of more interest is the inverse approach described in ❯ Chap. 11, ❯ Sect. 11.6.

11.5.2 The EASI Lead System

Perhaps the most frequently used derived 12 lead system at present is based on the EASI lead system of Dower and colleagues [37]. In this system, only four electrodes are required. These are placed at the Frank positions A, E, and I as well as at the top of the sternum, denoted S. Rearrangement of the electrode nomenclature leads to the descriptor EASI. ❯ Figure 11.22 illustrates this lead system. With the use of these electrodes the three orthogonal leads were derived as follows:

$$X = V_A - V_I$$
$$Y = V_E - V_S$$
$$Z = V_A - V_S$$

The 12 lead ECG was then derived in the usual way described above as a combination of the three "orthogonal" leads. However, Dower did not publish explicit coefficients. Later, Feild et al. published [38] various sets of coefficients derived in

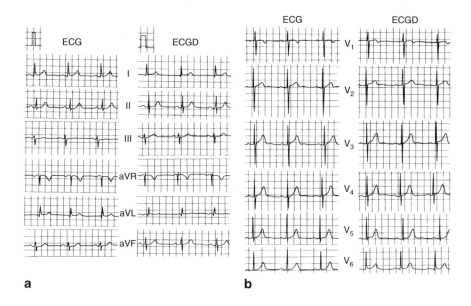

◼ Fig. 11.21
A comparison of the 12-lead ECG recorded in the usual fashion with the derived 12-lead ECG (ECGD). In this example, there is generally good agreement in morphology but differences are apparent on closer inspection; for example, there is more obvious ST elevation in the derived ECG than in the original while there are amplitude differences, e.g. the R wave in aVF in the derived ECG is over 50% larger than in the conventional recording (Reproduced with permission of Dr G Dower)

◼ Table 11.4
Transfer coefficients for deriving the 12-lead ECG from the *XYZ* leads. These values were obtained by Uijen et al. [36]. Note that Z is directed positively to the back

	I	II	III	aVR	aVL	aVF	V₁	V₂	V₃	V₄	V₅	V₆
X	0.79	0.24	−0.56	−0.51	0.67	−0.16	−0.52	−0.15	0.69	1.34	1.09	0.65
Y	−0.24	1.05	1.29	−0.41	−0.77	1.17	−0.06	−0.35	0.38	0.68	0.64	0.52
Z	0.08	−0.01	−0.09	−0.03	0.08	−0.05	−1.04	−1.76	−1.16	−0.49	0.01	0.23

different ways, including a statistical approach based on several thousand actual 12 lead ECGs compared to corresponding 12 lead ECGs derived from the same individuals using the EASI lead system (❯ Table 11.5).

There have been a number of studies that have looked at the accuracy of interpretation of ECGs derived from the EASI lead system and suggested that it is perfectly adequate for several types of applications, e.g. diagnosing acute myocardial infarction [39]. Our own work suggested a propensity for the system to exhibit inferior Q waves when none was present in the true 12 lead ECG [40].

11.5.3   Reduced Lead Sets

An alternative approach to reducing the number of electrodes required particularly for the monitoring situation is to use a reduced number of precordial leads from which the remaining leads can be calculated. Nelwan et al. [41–43] have studied this problem extensively. Essentially there are two approaches to the problem.

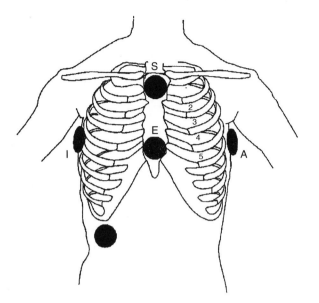

Fig. 11.22

The EASI lead system. The electrodes *A*, *E*, *I* relate to the Frank electrode positions while *S* denotes an electrode at the upper end of the sternum (After Dower [37]. © Elsevier. Reproduced with permission)

Table 11.5

Coefficients for deriving the standard 12 leads from orthogonal leads X, Y, Z obtained using the EASI lead system (Reprinted from [38] with permission)

Lead	AI (X)	ES (Y)	AS (Z)
I	0.701	0.026	−0.174
II	−0.763	−0.002	1.098
III	−1.464	−0.028	1.272
aVR	0.031	−0.012	−0.462
aVL	1.082	0.027	−0.723
aVF	−1.114	−0.015	1.185
V_1	0.080	0.641	−0.391
V_2	1.021	1.229	−1.050
V_3	0.987	0.947	−0.539
V_4	0.841	0.525	0.004
V_5	0.630	0.179	0.278
V_6	0.213	−0.043	0.431

The first is to record a complete 12-lead ECG on an individual. If it is required to monitor the patient using leads V2 and V5 for example (as well as having limb leads available), the missing leads V1, V3, V4 and V6 can each be derived from the remaining leads recorded on that particular patient, namely I, II, V2 and V5. If, for example,

$$V1 = a \, I + b \, II + c \, V2 + d \, V5$$

then a, b, c, d are unique for that individual patient, and the reconstruction is said to be based on a patient specific transformation.

The other approach is to take a group of patients from which a generalized transformation can be developed to enable missing precordial leads to be calculated from a subset such as V2 and V5 plus limb leads as above. The approach to deriving the coefficients a, b, c, d is based on a gathering a training population where all 12 leads are recorded. The optimum values of a, b, c, d are then calculated so that, when applied to all ECGs in the set to produce reconstructed leads, the best correlation is obtained with the original leads. The procedure is repeated for other missing leads. The actual performance accuracy was reported in a separate test set.

Nelwan et al. [42] showed that reconstruction accuracy was high using the generalized approach where the correlation between original and reconstructed leads was approximately 0.93 whereas using a patient specific reconstruction, with up to 4 precordial leads being removed, the correlation increased to 0.97. Thus, as expected, patient specific reconstruction was better than the use of the general transformation.

❯ Figure 11.23 gives an example of general and patient specific reconstruction of leads in an acute situation where recordings have been made at baseline and 24 h later.

It is clear that the patient specific reconstruction is more labor intensive and can only be used effectively in hospital where there is time to make an initial recording, calculate the transformation values and have appropriate equipment that is then able to use the specific transformation for the patient being monitored. In the acute situation, such as recording in an ambulance, the time constraints are such that it would be simpler to use a generalized transformation if a reduced number of leads is to be used, as this is a much faster process. In any event, the full 12-leads must be positioned to derive a patient specific transform so that the main benefit of reduced leads is likely to be in long term monitoring. Nevertheless, the technique does offer an effective approach to reducing the number of leads required to give accurate 12-lead reconstruction and allow ECG interpretation to be made with a high degree of accuracy.

11.6   Derived Orthogonal-Lead ECG

The inverse of the derived 12-lead ECG is the derived orthogonal-lead ECG. Another way of expressing the equation for deriving the ECGD is as follows:

$$D = CL$$

where C is a 12×3 matrix of transformation coefficients (❯ Table 11.3) and L is the 3×1 lead array (the values of XYZ at a particular instant). Multiplication of C and L produces a 12×1 array D containing the derived values of the 12 leads at a particular instant. On the other hand, if it is required to derive the XYZ leads, i.e., L given a knowledge of C and D, then the following equations describe the procedure involved [44].

Let

$$M = C^T C$$

and

$$M^{-1}M = I$$

where I is the identity matrix. Then

$$L = IL = M^{-1}ML$$

$$= M^{-1}C^T CL$$

$$= \left(M^{-1}C^T\right)D$$

The matrix $M^{-1}C^T$ represents an "inverse Dower" transformation and is shown in ❯ Table 11.6. Note that this table shows a 3×8 matrix which was all that was published by Edenbrandt and Pahlm [44]. It indicates that the input D is an 8×1 matrix consisting of the data from the eight independent leads V_1–V_6, I and II. In this implementation, C therefore is an 8×3 matrix where only the 8 independent leads of the 12-lead ECG are used. These authors used V_1–V_6, I and II. Thus, from ❯ Table 11.6,

$$\text{lead } X = -0.172V_1 - 0.074V_2 + 0.122V_3 + 0.231V_4 + 0.239V_5 + 0.194V_6 + 0.156I - 0.010II$$

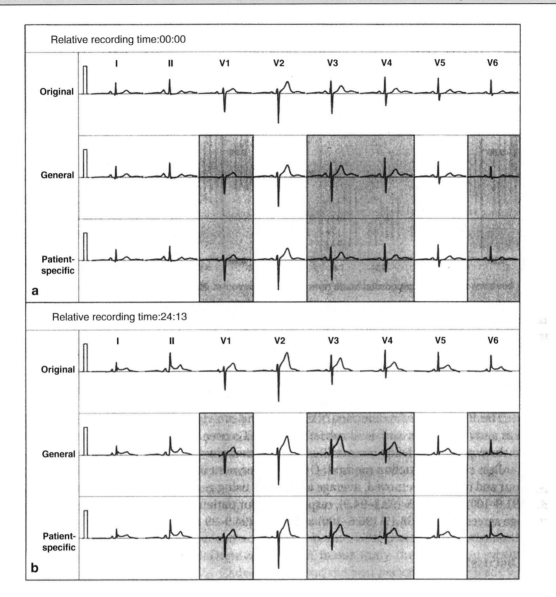

Fig. 11.23
The reconstruction of precordial leads V1, V3, V4 and V6 from 4 other leads, namely I, II, V2 and V5. Two time instants are shown with ❷ 11.23a being a baseline recording while ❷ 11.23b was recorded approximately 24 h later. ST elevation is apparent in **b** (After Nelwan et al. [42]. © Elsevier. Reproduced with permission)

Note in the table that the columns represent the coefficients for V_1–V_6, I and II, respectively.

In an essentially identical manner, Uijen and colleagues [36] derived an inverse matrix, but on this occasion they used their own transfer matrix (❷ Table 11.4) as input to the inverse calculation, with a resulting matrix shown in ❷ Table 11.7. Note in this matrix that leads VR and VL are specified rather than I and II.

A similar approach was adopted by the group of Van Bemmel and the results were published in the 4th progress report of the study sponsored by the European Community on common standards in electrocardiography (CSE) [45]. ❷ Table 11.8 gives the required transfer coefficients. It should be noted that these have been scaled to give the optimum comparison between actual *XYZ* leads and derived *XYZ* leads which were available in the CSE study being directed by Willems [46]. The scaling coefficients are also indicated in the table.

◻ **Table 11.6**

The transfer coefficients for deriving the *XYZ* leads from the 12-lead ECG according to Edenbrandt and Pahlm [44]. The resulting *Z* lead will be directed positively to the back

	V_1	V_2	V_3	V_4	V_5	V_6	I	II
X	−0.172	−0.074	0.122	0.231	0.239	0.194	0.156	−0.010
Y	0.057	−0.019	−0.106	−0.022	0.041	0.048	−0.227	0.887
Z	−0.229	−0.310	−0.246	−0.063	0.055	0.108	0.022	0.102

◻ **Table 11.7**

The transfer coefficients for deriving the *XYZ* leads from the 12-lead ECG according to Uijen et al. [36]. The resulting *Z* lead will be directed positively to the back

	VR	VL	V_1	V_2	V_3	V_4	V_5	V_6
X	−0.52	0.82	−0.01	0.04	0.04	0.05	0.07	0.37
Y	−1.53	−1.09	0.03	−0.02	−0.02	0.03	−0.07	0.08
Z	0.43	−0.01	−0.26	−0.28	−0.14	0.04	−0.15	0.34

◻ **Table 11.8**

The transfer coefficients for deriving the *XYZ* leads from the 12-lead ECG according to the group of Van Bemmel [45][a]

	II	III	V_1	V_2	V_3	V_4	V_5	V_6
X	0.58	−0.82	−1.27	−0.55	0.72	1.86	1.92	1.53
Y	2.58	3.04	−0.71	−0.71	0.10	0.35	0.12	−0.15
Z	−0.80	−1.62	−1.71	−2.26	−2.02	−0.80	0.31	0.97

[a] Scaling: *X* (measured) = 0.134 × *X* (calculated), *Y* (measured) = 0.1565 × *Y* (calculated), and *Z* (measured) = 0.122 × *Z* (calculated)

◻ **Table 11.9**

The transfer coefficients for deriving the *XYZ* leads from the paediatric 12-lead ECG where V4R is used to the exclusion of V3 (from [47])

	I	II	V4R	V1	V2	V4	V5	V6
X	+0.160	−0.013	−0.128	−0.122	+0.009	+0.275	+0.251	+0.185
Y	−0.235	+0.891	+0.073	+0.019	−0.087	−0.065	+0.025	+0.051
Z	−0.023	+0.128	−0.072	−0.278	−0.439	−0.189	−0.016	+0.084

Edenbrandt and Macfarlane published a set of coefficients for deriving the X, Y and Z leads in children [47]. In this age group, V4$_R$ is normally used in preference to V3 as discussed above. Hence the transfer coefficients of ❷ Table 11.3 for example cannot be used. From the image surface data of Frank [13], the coefficients for V4$_R$ were obtained (−0.537, 0.096, −0.272) and these replaced the V3 coefficients in the Dower 12 lead ECG derivation of ❷ Table 11.3. The inverse matrix was then calculated using the method described above. The resulting coefficients are shown in ❷ Table 11.9.

It is unlikely that there will be more intensive investigation of this approach in view of the continued reluctance of cardiologists to study *XYZ* leads or vectorcardiograms. Nonetheless, the approach is inherently attractive in that with the recording of only the eight independent leads of the 12-lead ECG, it then becomes possible to produce all 15 leads of the 12 plus *XYZ* leads. In other words, there is almost a 50% reduction in the storage space required to retain all 15 leads when recorded by standard methods. Although 15 leads can be derived by this approach, there can, of course, be no additional information compared to that contained in the eight independent leads I, II and V_1–V_6.

It should be realized that although from a theoretical standpoint the derived orthogonal leads should resemble the actual *XYZ* leads if they were recorded, they may on occasion be markedly different on account of the use of a single transfer matrix (set of coefficients) being used for subjects of varying build. Proponents of the technique acknowledge this and advocate its use for various reasons. First, no extra electrodes are required to derive the additional X *YZ* leads. Second, the value of such an approach is likely to lie in examining the phase relationships between the different leads as exemplified and studied in vectorcardiography. A simple example is shown later in ❷ Fig. 11.27 where two pairs of leads of similar appearance are shown. However, when these leads are plotted to form a vectorcardiographic loop, two entirely different configurations are seen. This is due to the different timing relationships between the leads, as will be evident from careful study of the data in the illustration.

11.7 The Vectorcardiogram

With the availability of three simultaneously recorded corrected orthogonal leads XYZ, it becomes possible to display the recording in different ways. Clearly, the conventional scalar presentation of the leads is a basic option. On the other hand, the theory of the resultant cardiac vector (dipole) indicates that the magnitude and movement of the vector during the cardiac cycle could be displayed. If it is imagined that the resultant vector increases from zero magnitude and then alters in magnitude and direction throughout the cardiac cycle, the tip of the vector with coordinates (X, Y, Z) (see ❷ Chap. 2) should trace out a loop in space. Conventionally, the projections of this path onto three mutually perpendicular planes have been obtained for study as shown in ❷ Fig. 11.24. The projection on the frontal plane (❷ Fig. 11.13) effectively represents the variation in (X, Y) values throughout the cardiac cycle. Similarly, the sagittal and transverse (horizontal) planes represent changes in the (Z, Y) and (X, Z) coordinates, respectively. Thus, with the use of a graph plotter or equivalent device, for example, it is a simple matter to plot the XY coordinates during the cardiac cycle and obtain the frontal plane loop. Similar procedures can be used to obtain the sagittal and transverse loops as shown in ❷ Fig. 11.25. These loops are known as the vectorcardiogram (VCG). The terminology used to describe vectorcardiographic loops is displayed in ❷ Fig. 11.26. The direction of inscription of the loop can be determined in different ways. For example, if a multicolored plotter is available, the efferent limb can be plotted in a different color compared to the afferent limb. Arrowheads can also be used. Older methods of plotting the loops on an oscilloscope are now largely obsolete, while newer technology, such as the laser printer, will be of increasing value.

The separation of the dots on the plotted loops is arbitrary. Nowadays, however, this may depend on the sampling rate of the computer system used, with dots being typically at 2 or 4 ms intervals. The usefulness lies not only in outlining the direction of inscription but in noting where conduction defects may occur, at which time the separation of the dots becomes reduced. The various aspects of vectorcardiographic interpretation are discussed in the respective clinical chapters.

As an aside, it should be noted that quite independent of any theory of vectorcardiography, it is possible to plot pairs of leads to produce loops. Ideally, however, such leads should have directions which are well separated, otherwise the loop

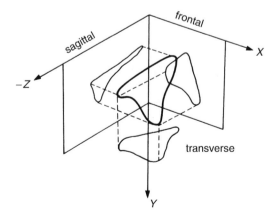

◻ Fig. 11.24
The concept of the projection of a loop in space onto three mutually perpendicular planes. For convenience, the −Z axis is illustrated

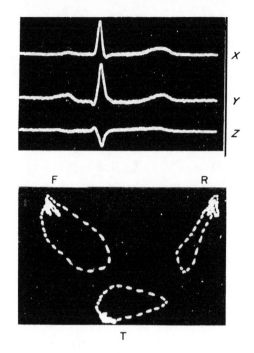

■ Fig. 11.25

An illustration of a VCG obtained in the conventional manner by inputting pairs of leads to opposite points of the oscilloscope. The dashes are separated by 2 ms intervals and inscription is from the thin to the thick end of the dash; for example, there is counterclockwise inscription in the transverse (T) plane (*F* frontal, *R* right sagittal). The corresponding scalar *XYZ* leads are shown with *Z* directed positively to the anterior (= V$_2$)

would tend to a straight line as would be the case with plotting two essentially similar leads. Thereafter, a study of the patterns produced could be undertaken on a purely empirical basis. An understanding of the concept of vectorcardiography and the use of leads with approximately orthogonal directions is still recommended.

To see in a simple way how a vectorcardiographic loop is constructed, the reader should carefully study the example of ❯ Fig. 11.27. The scalar amplitudes of one pair of leads (X, Z) are provided for a small number of instants during the QRS complex for two different cases. For teaching purposes, lead X is identical in the two while appearances in each lead Z are similar but bear a different timing relationship to lead X. The amplitudes of leads X and Z are indicated at corresponding instants in time so that pairs of points (X, Z) can be plotted. In this example, Z is directed positively to the anterior, to resemble V$_1$ or V$_2$. In ❯ Fig. 11.27(a), the direction of inscription of the loop is counterclockwise, which is normal in the transverse plane. In ❯ Fig. 11.27(b), the direction of inscription is clockwise, which is abnormal and would suggest the possibility of right ventricular hypertrophy for various reasons (see ❯ Chap. 3 of *Electrocardiology: Comprehensive Clinical ECG*). Thus, the vectorcardiographic presentation is providing additional information that is not readily seen in the scalar display. The complete VCG would be constructed using the other pairs of leads (X, Y) and (Y, Z) in a similar fashion.

11.8   Derived Vectorcardiogram –12 Lead Vectorcardiography

In ❯ Chap. 11, ❯ Sect. 11.6, the derived orthogonal-lead ECG was introduced. It follows that the derived VCG is simply another form of displaying the derived *XYZ* leads. In ❯ Fig. 11.28, vectorcardiograms are shown which were obtained using the hybrid-lead system and the derived *XYZ* leads based on two forms of inverse Dower transformation [36, 44]. The general similarities can be seen.

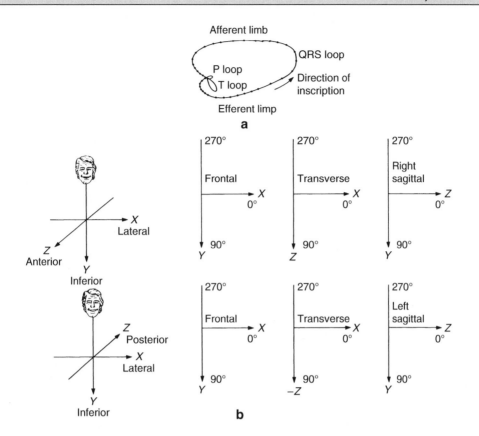

Fig. 11.26

In **(a)**, the terminology used to describe a vectorcardiographic loop is shown. In **(b)**, alternative reference frames for measurement and display of VCGs are displayed. The author prefers lead *Z* directed positively to the anterior so that appearances resemble V1 and V2, as shown at the top of ❷ **Fig. 11.23b**. In addition, by choosing the right sagittal view, all reference frames are similar. An alternative scheme, with *Z* directed positively to the back and with the left sagittal view being used, is shown in the lower part of ❷ **Fig. 11.23b**. In practice, the transverse view is similar to the other scheme, but the VCG as seen in the left sagittal view is a mirror image of that in the right sagittal view

The availability of the derived VCG leads to the possibility of what has been termed "12 lead vectorcardiography" [48]. This topic is discussed more fully in ❷ Chap. 11 of *Specialized Aspects of ECG*. In short, the advantages of vectorcardiography can be utilized by appropriate processing of the 12 lead ECG. While there can be no additional information, the phase relationships between the leads can be utilized to assist with diagnosis as previously illustrated in ❷ Fig. 11.27.

11.9 Interrelationship of the 12-Lead and *XYZ* Lead Electrocardiograms

In schematic form, ❷ Fig. 11.29 shows the relationships between the various leads of the 12 and 3-orthogonal-lead ECGs. As shown above, it is quite possible to derive mathematically one lead set from another. However, on a simpler level it is possible to construct a vector loop manually from a knowledge of the 12-lead ECG and vice versa. The advantage of this lies only in a further understanding of the underlying electrical activity. It goes without saying that estimation of the QRS axis from the 12-lead ECG in the frontal plane is implicitly involved in such a procedure. Indeed, ❷ Fig. 11.27 provides an example of a derivation of a transverse loop given leads *X* and Z, although these equally well could have been called

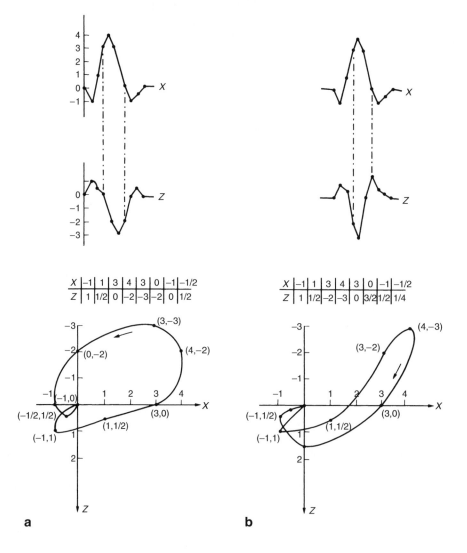

◘ Fig. 11.27
The construction of the transverse plane of the vector loop given simultaneous measurements from leads X and Z. In (**a**), the loop is inscribed counterclockwise; in (**b**), the bulk of the loop is inscribed clockwise. It should be noted that lead X is identical in each example but that the different timing relationships leads X and Z in each case lead to the different loop configurations. Lead Z is directed positively to the anterior in this example so that the rSr′ pattern resembles that often found in V1 or V2. The value of a VCG in such a case should be understood from this example

V_5 and V_1, respectively.

Suppose that leads I and aVF are recorded simultaneously and that a set of amplitudes at corresponding instants in time are obtained as in ❷ Fig. 11.30a. It is then possible to construct a vector loop in the knowledge that this is only an approximation in view of the fact that I and a VF are not electrically orthogonal and have different lead strengths. Nevertheless, using simple graph plotting techniques, a loop can be derived as shown in ❷ Fig. 11.30a. The converse is clearly true in that if the loop represented an actual frontal plane VCG, then the reverse procedure would have produced the scalar leads which in reality would have been X and Y.

The important point to note in this particular illustration is how the crossing of the different axes relates to inscription of the VCG. In general terms, if there is clockwise inscription of the loop as in ❷ Fig. 11.30a, then the lead I axis is crossed

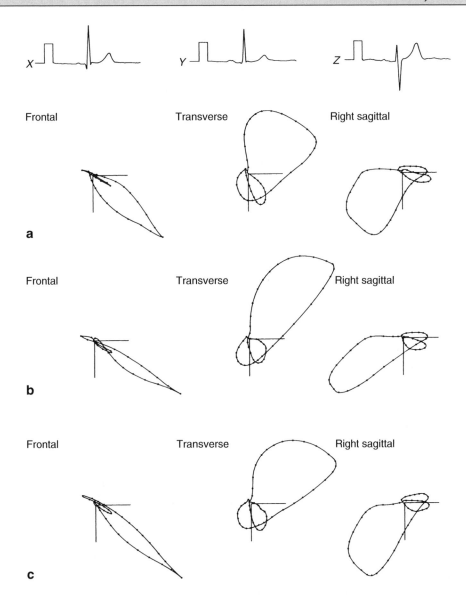

☐ Fig. 11.28
The three vectorcardiographic loops: (**a**), the VCG derived from the hybrid system; (**b**), the VCG on the same patient derived from the inverse Dower technique using the coefficients described in [44] (**c**), the VCG from the same patient using the inverse Dower technique described in [45]. There are some differences in shape but the loops are substantially similar. Lead *Z* is directed positively to the anterior

at a point when the Q wave terminates in aVF and generally prior to the peak value of the R wave in lead I. On the other hand, in a situation where there is counterclockwise inscription (● Fig. 11.30b), the crossing of the aVF axis corresponds to the end of the Q wave in lead I. Warner and colleagues [49] used this type of information, but from leads II and III, in order to improve the diagnosis of inferior myocardial infarction. A point of note here is the value of using multichannel electrocardiographs that permit I and aVF to be displayed simultaneously.

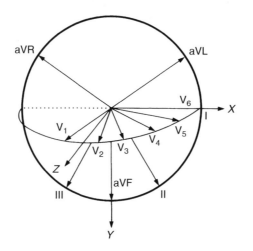

⬛ Fig. 11.29

The interrelationship between the lead vectors of the 12-lead ECG and the orthogonal-lead ECG. These are shown in an idealized form, that is, no allowance is made for torso inhomogeneties, and so on. Lead *Z* is directed positively to the anterior

11.10   Nomenclature

There is considerable variation in the nomenclature of leads, particularly V_1–V_6. The American College of Cardiology in its report [50] on optimal electrocardiography suggested the following guidelines (❱ Fig. 11.31).

I, aVL	lateral leads
II, III, aVF	inferior leads
V_1, V_2	septal leads
V_2–V_4	anteroseptal leads
V_3, V_4	anterior leads
V_5, V_6	anterolateral leads

In ❱ Chap. 4 of *Electrocardiology: Comprehensive Clinical ECG* on myocardial infarction, Selvester et al. argue strongly for terminology based on recommendations of a working group of which he was a member. Their recommendations (corresponding to ❱ Fig. 4 of *Electrocardiology: Comprehensive Clinical ECG* which, for convenience, is shown here as ❱ Fig. 11.32) are based on the anatomical orientation of the heart in the thorax and concern the nomenclature of myocardial regions. However, the electrocardiographer invokes the inverse process by relating changes in various leads to myocardial abnormalities. This being so, the following can be inferred from ❱ Fig. 11.32:

I, aVL, V_5, V_6	posterolateral (apical) leads
II, III, a VF	inferior leads
V_2–V_4	anterior leads

This terminology has evolved from a consideration of coronary arterial distribution and is recommended by Selvester et al. for use in describing myocardial infarction.

Recently, the combination of the ECG and MRI scans has led Bayes de Luna et al. [51] to advocate revised terminology for the location of a myocardial infarction involving the left ventricle. In particular, these authors suggested that the terms "posterior" and "high lateral" should not be used when describing a myocardial infarct and should be replaced by "lateral" and "mid-anterior" respectively (see ❱ Fig. 11.33). It has to be noted that these authors are referring to the position of an infarct and are not necessarily ascribing these names to electrocardiographic leads, but historically, lead descriptors and locations of an infarct are often interchanged.

On the other hand, a writing group of the American Heart Association [52] has recently declined to recommend adoption of the proposed changes until additional data is gathered.

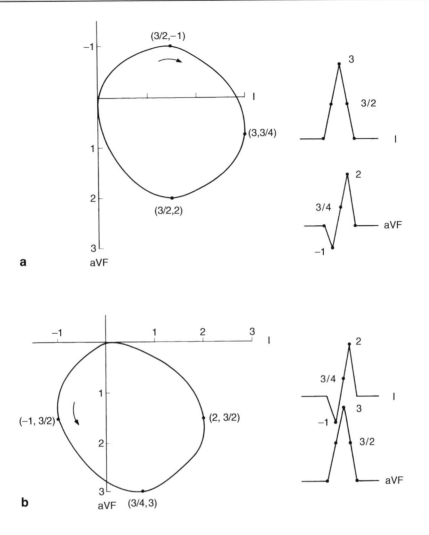

☐ **Fig. 11.30**

Part (a): the construction of a vectorcardiographic loop from leads I and aVF. In this instance, there is clockwise inscription of the vector loop and it can be seen that the termination of the Q wave in aVF is prior to the peak of the R wave in lead I. Part (b): in this example, the relationship of leads I and aVF is such that the derived vectorcardiographic loop has counterclockwise inscription in the frontal plane and, in this case, the end of the Q wave in lead I occurs prior to the peak of the R wave in aVF

The recent series on recommendations for interpretation of the ECG, in paper II [53], lists the following descriptors for the location of a myocardial infarction:

Anterior
Inferior
Posterior
Lateral
Anteroseptal
Extensive anterior
MI in the presence of LBBB
Right ventricular MI

The publication does not define the leads associated with each descriptor.

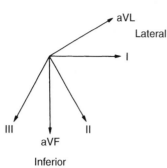
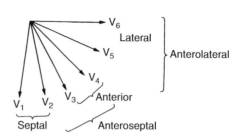

◘ Fig. 11.31
Nomenclature used in the description of various leads

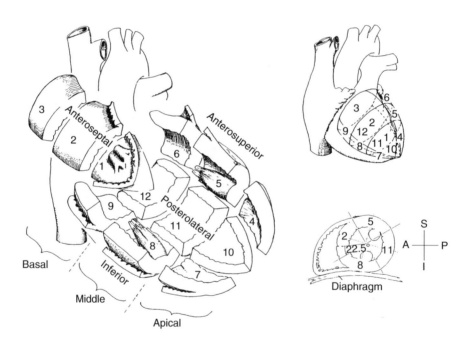

◘ Fig. 11.32
The division of the heart into various regions after Selvester et al. (❷ Chap. 4 of *Electrocardiology: Comprehensive Clinical ECG*) in which their recommendations for terminology can be found

11.11 Exercise ECG Lead Systems

A variety of bipolar chest leads has been used for exercise testing in the past. In the main, these have been a reflection on the use of single-channel equipment and the aim of simplifying the procedure as much as possible. Nowadays, with increased availability of computer-based exercise ECG analysis methods, it is common to utilize the conventional 12-lead ECG for exercise testing.

NAME	ECG PATTERN	INFARCTION AREA (CMR)
SEPTAL	Q in V1-V2	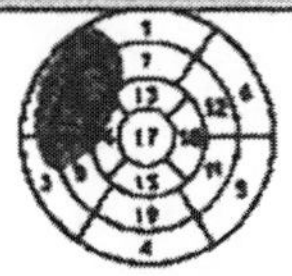
MID ANTERIOR	Q (qs or qr) in aVL and sometimes in I and / or V2-V3	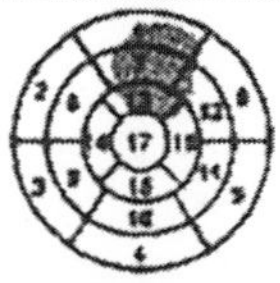
APICAL-ANTERIOR	Q in V1-V2 to V3-V6	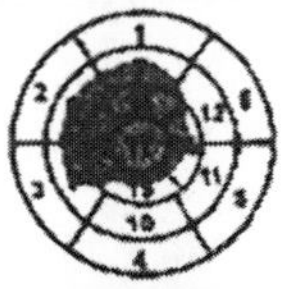
EXTENSIVE ANTERIOR	Q in V1-V2 to V4-V6. aVL and sometimes I	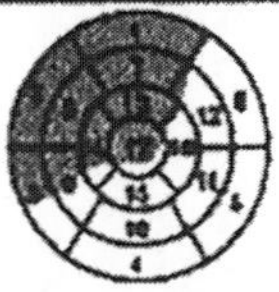
LATERAL	RS in V1-V2 and/or Q wave in leads I. aVL, V6 and/or diminished R wave in V6.	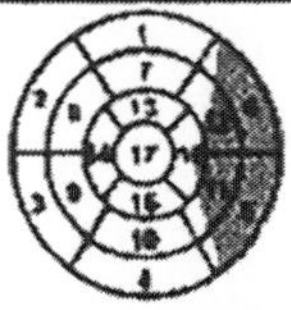
INFERIOR	Q in II, III aVF	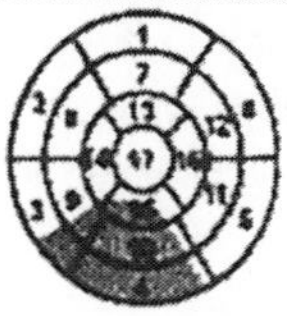

◘ Fig. 11.33
Proposed terminology for describing the location of a myocardial infarction from the 12 lead ECG (After Bayes de Luna et al. [51]. © AHA. Reproduced with permission)

In 1966, Mason and Likar published their recommendations for moving the limb electrodes used to record the 12-lead ECG from the limbs to the thorax [54] for exercise electrocardiography. Their repositioned electrodes are shown in ❷ Fig. 11.34. They compared ECG recordings where the right and left arm electrodes were positioned in the conventional areas of the arm to those obtained from gradually moving the electrodes to progressively proximal positions up the arms and then over the upper anterior chest. Finally, it was recommended that the right arm electrode be moved to a point in the infraclavicular fossa medial to the border of the deltoid muscle and 2 cm below the lower border of the clavicle. The corresponding position was recommended for the left arm electrode as shown in ❷ Fig. 11.34. Further experimentation led to a recommendation that the left leg electrode (denoted LL) be placed in the anterior axillary line halfway between the costal margin and the iliac crest. They suggested that the location of this electrode was not critical; that is, it could be varied by a few centimeters in any direction to avoid skin folds, and so on. Some authors simply regard this reference point as being the left iliac crest [55]. Mason and Likar initially illustrated the right leg electrode as being on the right thigh, but for convenience it is now a matter of routine to place this electrode in the region of the right iliac fossa as recommended by the American College of Cardiology [56].

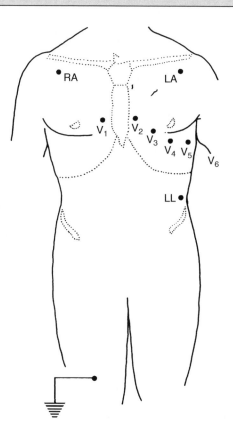

◘ Fig. 11.34
The modified electrode positions for the limbs according to Mason and Likar [54]. See text for further discussion. Note that the right leg (ground) electrode is usually nowadays positioned in the right iliac fossa (After Mason and Likar [54]. © Mosby, St Louis, Missouri. Reproduced with permission)

For a number of years, many investigators used a simple combination of chest electrodes to record a bipolar chest lead during exercise testing. Almost always, the positive electrode was placed in the V_5 position while the negative electrode was placed in a variety of positions that are illustrated in ❷ Fig. 11.10. If the negative electrode were placed on the manubrium, then the lead was denoted CM_5. The full range of positions that have been adopted in the past for the negative electrode is shown in ❷ Fig. 11.10 and listed in ❷ Table 11.2. In ❷ Chap. 4 of *Specialized Aspects of ECG*, there is a discussion of the leads now thought most suited to exercise testing, but for didactic purposes it is instructive to consider further the bipolar leads introduced above.

The configuration of the leads recorded during exercise can vary markedly depending on the position of the negative electrode. This can be seen clearly from scrutiny of ❷ Fig. 11.35. In this illustration, three bipolar leads have been recorded simultaneously and marked differences can be seen in the ST segment. Note here that lead CL is a bipolar lead with the positive electrode on the left leg and the negative electrode on the manubrium. Leads CC_5 and CM_5, which at one stage were commonly used, show entirely different ST changes; in the case of the former, the ST segment is upward sloping whereas in the latter it is flat or slightly downward sloping. Chaitman and colleagues [57], who obtained this illustration, suggested that multiple-lead ECG recording improved the sensitivity and efficiency of maximal treadmill exercise testing. This point is discussed further in ❷ Chap. 4 of *Specialized Aspects of ECG*.

In a separate study, Froelicher et al. [55] assessed CC_5 and CM_5 against the standard lead V_5. They showed that when using visual interpretation, the same criteria could be used for CC_5 and V_5 but different criteria were necessary for interpreting CM_5. ❷ Figure 11.36 shows the different mean slopes before and after exercise in both normal and abnormal responders. Clear differences can be seen between the three leads, with CM_5 showing the most ST deviation.

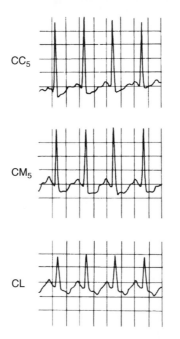

○ Fig. 11.35
An example of three simultaneously recorded leads obtained during exercise. Note the different ST-T configuration in each lead (After Chaitman et al. [57]. © American Heart Association, Dallas, Texas. Reproduced with permission)

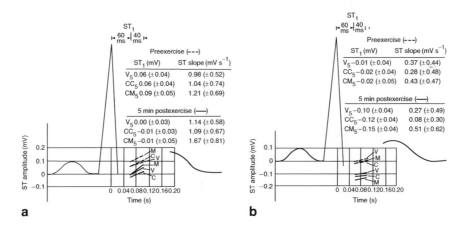

○ Fig. 11.36
The different mean ST amplitudes and slopes before and after exercise for (**a**), a group of 26 normal responders; and (**b**), a separate group of 21 abnormal responders who had three leads simultaneously recorded. M denotes CM5, C denotes CC5 and V denotes V5 (Froelicher et al. [55]. © American College of Chest Physicians, Mark Ridge, Illinois. Reproduced with permission)

On the other hand, CM_5 showed the greatest upward slope of the ST segment. These findings reflect the different strengths and orientations of the lead vectors as discussed in ○ Sect. 11.3 and indicate that different criteria must be used when interpreting different leads. This becomes more feasible in the era of computer averaging of exercise ECG leads where more accurate measurement of ST T changes is now possible.

From ○ Fig. 11.11 it can be seen that the lead strength of CM_5 is greater than V_5 and some additional ST -segment depression would be expected in this lead as confirmed by the data of Froelicher [55]. The lead direction for CM_5, as also would be expected, is quite different to that of CC_5 and V_5, and hence a different ST depression and slope would be expected compared to the other leads which have relatively similar lead-vector directions.

Nowadays, most exercise electrocardiography is 12 lead based with automated analysis of the waveforms. Users should be aware that the averaging techniques used in exercise ECG are of necessity different from those used in a 10 s recording of a resting ECG with some hysteresis involved. Noise can have an effect on the averaging process and scrutiny of the actual recording is recommended in addition to review of the averaged cycles. Furthermore, use of the Mason Likar positions for 12 lead exercise (or resting) electrocardiography results in significant differences in the ECG compared to the standard lead positions and this must always be remembered [7, 58].

11.12   ECG Monitoring in Hospital

It goes without saying that the ECG is used universally for patient monitoring in hospitals. A recent guideline paper set out best practices for hospital monitoring as well as indications for ischemia and QT monitoring among other things [59]. Of relevance to this chapter are the comments on choice of leads for patient monitoring.

The first point to make is that the practice standards acknowledge that for patient monitoring, wrist and ankle electrodes are placed on the torso essentially in the Mason Likar positions [54] described above in 11.11. With 4 electrodes in these positions, a modified version of the six frontal plane leads could be recorded. However, for monitoring purposes, a unipolar chest lead is usually required to assist with rhythm analysis. In this case, conventional circuitry as discussed in 11.2.4 can be used with one to six chest electrodes as desired.

A very simple 3-electrode bipolar system was also included in the hospital monitoring standards [59]. Essentially this used the MCL lead with the third electrode employed as a ground as illustrated in ❷ Fig. 11.37. Many other lead systems that can be used in the monitoring situation such as reduced leads, orthogonal leads and derived 12 leads, have all been discussed at an earlier point in this chapter.

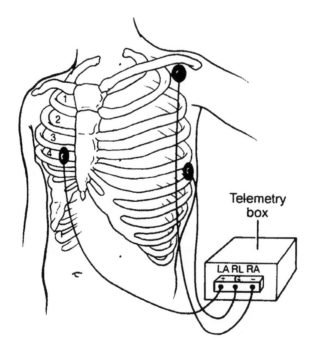

◘ Fig. 11.37
A basic 3 electrode bipolar lead system for recording lead CL_1 i.e. positive electrode placed in V_1 and the negative electrode in the left infraclavicular fossa. The reference electrode, here shown in the V_6 position, could be located anywhere. *LA* left arm, *RA* right arm, *RL* right leg (Reproduced from Circulation 2004; 110: 2721, with permission)

11.13 Body-Surface Mapping Lead Systems

Body-surface mapping was introduced for two reasons. The first reason was to permit a study of the spread of excitation over the thorax. This allowed the normal patterns to be studied and inferences drawn on the time of epicardial "breakthrough" of activation at the right and left ventricles. In addition, empirical study of abnormal patterns together with clinical correlation allowed methods for interpretation of maps to be developed, as discussed in ❷ Chap. 10 of *Cardiac Arrhythmias and Mapping Techniques*. Some investigators use between 16 and 240 electrodes to map the thorax using computer techniques for plotting.

The second reason for mapping is to assess in a mathematical way the total electrical information available, and perhaps relate this via an inverse model to epicardial excitation, etc. (see ❷ Chap. 9). Barr suggested [60] that 24 surface leads would allow the thorax to be mapped so that with the use of a transformation, the ECG data at other points could be estimated. The aim behind this particular study was to derive information on the equivalent cardiac generator and so attack the inverse problem (see ❷ Chap. 9). Kornreich used a 126-lead system to map the body surface and from this concluded that nine independent leads would be adequate to retrieve all of the clinically useful information on the body surface [61, 62]. His array used 18 columns of electrodes with 84 on the anterior chest and 42 electrodes on the back (❷ Fig. 11.38). The group of Taccardi used a 219 irregularly spaced electrode array. Lux et al. [63], as described in ❷ Chap. 9 of *Cardiac Arrhythmias and Mapping Techniques*, also utilized complex mathematical techniques to reduce the number of electrodes required for mapping to a more limited number on which they were able to calculate normal ranges and assess the results of exercise testing.

Mapping systems used for clinical purposes, such as outlining areas of ST elevation following acute myocardial infarction, generally consist of a small array of unipolar chest leads. The differences between the systems essentially relate only to the number of electrodes and hence to their relative spacing on the chest. Maroko et al. in 1972 [64] suggested the use of a 5 × 7 electrode array for ST mapping following myocardial infarction. In 1979, Fox et al. [65] utilized a 4 × 4 array of electrodes for mapping infarcts and also for exercise testing. It was subsequently suggested that this be reduced to a

❏ Fig. 11.38

The 126 electrodes used by Kornreich for mapping. The nine independent leads, which were claimed to contain all of the information for clinical use on the body surface, are also indicated by *circles* **and** *rectangles*

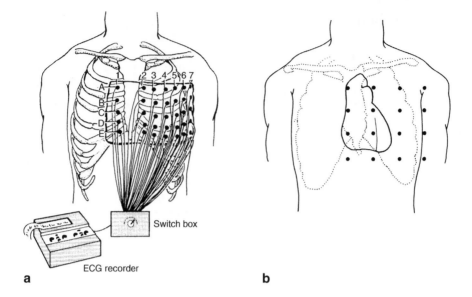

Switch box

ECG recorder

a   **b**

■ Fig. 11.39

In (**a**), the 35 lead mapping system used by Maroko et al. is shown (After Maroko et al. [64]. © American College of Cardiology, New York. Reproduced with permission). In (**b**), the 16-lead array of electrodes used by Fox et al., who subsequently recommended that the rightmost column of electrodes be removed to leave a 12-lead array, is shown (Fox et al., [65]. © British Medical Association, London. Reproduced with permission)

4×3 array [66]. An illustration of these lead systems is shown in ❷ Fig. 11.39. Monro et al. [67] utilized a 24-electrode array that explored both the anterior and posterior chest walls, but in addition, with the use of sophisticated mathematical interpolation techniques, the potentials at any other point on the thorax could be calculated [68, 69]. More recently, the group of Adgey have used 64 anterior (including limb) and 16 posterior electrodes in their work on acute myocardial infarction [70].

The topic of body-surface mapping is under active study in a number of centers. Color displays are now used to present maps (see ❷ Chap. 9 of *Electrocardiology: Comprehensive Clinical ECG*) while commercial mapping systems are becoming increasingly available. Further discussion on mapping can be found in ❷ Chaps. 9 and ❷ 10 of *Cardiac Arrhythmias and Mapping Techniques*, while some early work is summarised in conference proceedings [71, 72].

11.14 Epicardial and Intracardiac Mapping

Cardiac mapping is a term used to describe the recording and display of multiple potentials recorded from the endocardium, the epicardium or transmural sites.

11.14.1 Transmural and Epicardial Mapping

Either for basic research or for clinical purposes, mapping of the spread of cardiac excitation is of value (see ❷ Chaps. 4 and ❷ 10 of *Cardiac Arrhythmias and Mapping Techniques*). Taccardi and colleagues recently described [73] an elegant system for intramural mapping of the dog heart. A form of multi-electrode needle is used with 10 electrodes spaced at 1.6 mm. Up to 56 such needle electrodes together with a sock electrode carrying 242 epicardial electrodes were used. The system allowed recording from up to 1,024 electrodes simultaneously at a sampling rate of 1 KHz. Data were acquired in digital form and processed to produce color coded three dimensional activation maps. An automated system for transmural cardiac mapping has also been described by Witkowski and Corr [74]. For human cardiac mapping, each needle has eight electrodes from which four bipolar signals are recorded. Data are converted into digital form at 2,000 samples s^{-1} and stored on a computer for further processing, e.g., the construction of isochrones of activation or epicardial isopotential maps.

11.14.2 Endocardial Mapping

Another technique for the study of arrhythmias is endocardial mapping. In this case, different intracardiac catheters, e.g., bipolar, quadrupolar or hexapolar, record ventricular electrograms from which relative timings can be obtained. In a ventricular tachycardia (VT), the earliest electrogram is regarded as the site of origin. Bipolar or unipolar electrograms can be recorded in the usual way (see ❷ Chap. 2 of *Cardiac Arrhythmias and Mapping Techniques*). This area has seen an explosion of interest in recent years in relation to the treatment of cardiac arrhythmias. It is discussed fully in ❷ Chap. 3 of *Cardiac Arrhythmias and Mapping Techniques*.

11.14.3 Pace Mapping

Pace mapping has been used to determine the site of origin of a VT [75]. In this case, the tachycardia is maintained by pacing from a particular site. The 12 lead surface ECG recorded during the pacing can be compared with that recorded during spontaneous VT. By changing the site of pacing, the paced ECG which most closely resembles that during spontaneous VT indicates the most likely source of the tachycardia, i.e., the point on the endocardium at which pacing is being undertaken. Epicardial versus endocardial pace mapping has recently been investigated [76] in localizing the site of a VT arising in the right ventricle.

11.14.4 Intracoronary ECG

Although not strictly mapping, a method for recording the intracoronary ECG has recently been described [77, 78]. In practice, the technique can be used to monitor myocardial ischemia during percutaneous transluminal coronary angioplasty. The intracoronary ECG can be obtained by connecting the proximal end of the catheter guidewire as it exits from the balloon catheter to a precordial lead of a surface ECG cable. The Wilson central terminal is used as a reference in the usual way. Friedman et al. [77] filtered the ECG from 0.1 to 100 or 500 Hz, as appropriate. They obtained best results when a short segment of the guidewire protruded beyond the distal lumen of the balloon catheter. DeMarchi et al. [78] recently used the technique in a study which showed that, in patients with chronic stable angina pectoris, after all known determinants of infarct size were taken into account, susceptibility to ischemia is greater in the left than in the right coronary artery region.

11.15 Ambulatory Monitoring Leads

Ambulatory monitoring may be carried out for different purposes, and to a certain extent, the leads selected may reflect the purpose of the test. Perhaps the most common requirement for undertaking ambulatory recording is to investigate cardiac rhythm. For many years, single channel recordings were made on account of cost and availability of equipment. In such cases, a bipolar lead such as CS_5 was, and still is, often employed. More recently, multichannel recording equipment has now become readily available, as have replay facilities that display the recorded leads simultaneously. The use of this approach assists in discriminating artifact from genuine ectopic beats and pauses. The recording of multiple leads also provides an additional safety factor in the event of malfunction of one channel or perhaps detachment of one electrode, which is a common occurrence.

The American Heart Association (AHA) established a task force of the Committee on Electrocardiography to report on the practice of ambulatory electrocardiography. The recommendations [79] included suggestions for electrode placement for two-channel recording. It is clear that the subcommittee did not wish to be dogmatic about recommended positions since they acknowledged that different positions would be required based on the varying need for undertaking a 24-h recording. The recommendation for two-channel recording was based on a five-electrode system, one of which is a ground electrode with the other two pairs each forming a bipolar lead. The recommended electrode positions are as follows.

(a) V_1 *type lead.* The positive electrode should be in the fourth right intercostal space, 25 mm from the sternal margin while the negative electrode should be in the lateral third of the left infraclavicular fossa.

(b) V_5 *type lead.* The positive electrode should be in the fifth left intercostal space at the anterior axillary line and the negative electrode should be 25 mm below the inferior angle of the right scapula on the posterior torso. The fifth electrode, the ground. electrode, should be placed in the lateral third of the right infraclavicular fossa.

The subcommittee pointed out that the use of individual negative or reference electrodes contributes to the redundancy of the two-lead recording system in that if a common reference electrode were to fail, both channels would be of no use. The electrode positions are illustrated in ❷ Fig. 11.40. With the appropriate circuitry, unipolar precordial leads and limb leads could be recorded using the Mason-Likar electrode positions (❷ Fig. 11.34). Indeed, there are now commercially available ambulatory monitors that record a full 12 lead ECG in digital form for 24 h.

A second reason for undertaking ambulatory electrocardiography may be to evaluate symptoms that are possibly related to myocardial ischemia. In this case, assuming that equipment with the appropriate characteristics is available (see ❷ Chaps. 12 and ❷ 1 of *Specialized Aspects of ECG*) the recording is aimed at assessing ST-segment changes. The AHA committee noted previous suggestions that a pair of leads approximating V_3 and aVF may detect more ST-segment shifts in patients with unstable angina [80]. In another study [81], Quyyumi et al. utilized two bipolar leads to assess ST changes in patients with varying severity of coronary artery disease. In this case a CM_5 lead and an inferior lead said to resemble aVF were used. The latter was obtained with one electrode positioned at the xiphisternum and the other at the

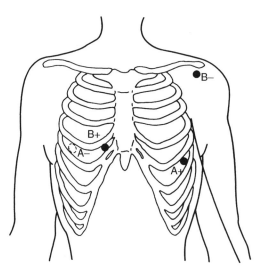

❏ **Fig. 11.40**

The recommended electrode positions for two-channel ambulatory ECG recording according to the subcommittee of the American Heart Association [79], A+ and A− are the positive and negative electrodes for the V5 type lead (not the same as V5) and B+ and B− are the electrodes for the V1 type lead)not the same as V1). The *open circle* denotes an electrode on the back. See text for a full description of electrode positions

left sternoclavicular joint. Further discussion on ambulatory monitoring can be found in ❯ Chap. 1 of *Specialized Aspects of ECG*.

A more recent set of ACC/AHA guidelines [82] on ambulatory electrocardiography concentrated more on the indications for ambulatory ECG than the technique itself.

11.16   Esophageal Leads

The use of an esophageal lead, for detection of atrial electrical activity in particular, is well established, having been introduced in the 1930s [83]. A more recent development in this area has been the availability of a pill electrode designed by Arzbaecher [84]. This device resembles an ordinary pharmaceutical capsule and is connected to a thin wire claimed to be "threadlike." The pill is swallowed by the patient with water and is allowed to descend into the esophagus. If sufficient length of the wire is used by the technician undertaking the procedure, the electrode will be positioned below the level of the atrium. The other end of the electrode is connected to a small amplifier unit which in turn is linked to lead I cables of an ordinary electrocardiograph.

The technician can then monitor the signal recorded by the pill electrode and withdraw the electrode gradually, i.e., raise the level of the electrode until it is behind the atria. This is recognized by the high-amplitude atrial signal which can be seen in the lead I position of the electrocardiograph. With the use of a multichannel machine, it is possible to record another lead simultaneously for timing purposes even though this additional lead may not be a perfect derivation in view of the fact that the left and right arm connections are linked to the pill electrode. It should be noted that the capsule containing the electrode actually dissolves so that the electrode is then exposed for the ECG recording. ❯ Figure 11.41 shows an esophageal ECG recording together with one other lead (lead II).

One report [83] suggested that the esophageal ECG may be diagnostic in 86% of cases where the surface ECG is inconclusive for rhythm determination. Furthermore, the esophageal ECG was used during 24-h ambulatory monitoring and proved valuable in 41% of patients.

Although the esophageal ECG is normally used for clarification of arrhythmias, it has been used for ischemia detection. Machler et al. [85] in their study concluded that the clinical relevance of the esophageal ECG is that it provides a convenient technique with high sensitivity, for monitoring intraoperative myocardial ischemia and detecting atrial activity during cardioplegia. The technique is not commonly used nowadays though research reports occasionally appear, e.g., for diagnosing paroxysmal supraventricular tachycardia [86].

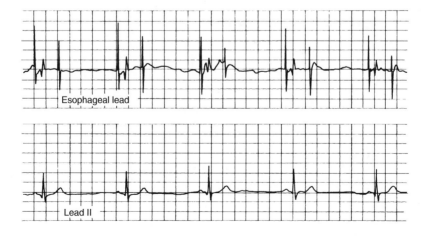

◼ Fig. 11.41

A two-channel recording showing an esophageal lead and lead II. In these simultaneously recorded leads, the atrial activation can be seen clearly (the large deflection) in the esophageal lead, where atrial bigeminy can be detected. In lead II, i.e., the surface ECG, the second P wave is essentially hidden in the T wave (Reproduced with permission of Dr. Arzbaecher)

11.17   Fetal ECG Lead Systems

Fetal ECG recording has been practised for many years to assess the status of the unborn child, principally by heart-rate analysis during labor. In earlier times, it was also used to assess whether the fetus was still alive and occasionally to confirm the presence of twins. The advent of noninvasive ultrasound Doppler telemetry has perhaps diminished the usefulness of the fetal ECG (FECG), but on account of reservations over the safety of ultrasound in fetal monitoring, and in view of the possibility of analyzing the morphology of the FECG, there has been continued interest in fetal electrocardiography.

There are two approaches to recording the fetal ECG. The first is to utilize surface electrodes placed on the abdomen of the mother. Most commonly, a bipolar lead in a vertical direction is used, with the electrodes being placed near the umbilicus and above the mons pubis. Electrodes can be connected to lead I of an ordinary electrocardiograph with the other limb electrodes also being connected to the mother. With a high gain setting, it is normally possible to record the fetal ECG together with the maternal ECG signal. However, the amplitude of the FECG is relatively small compared to the maternal ECG and may on occasion be difficult to separate from background noise. Signal-processing techniques are required, as discussed in ❷ Chap. 8 of *Electrocardiology: Comprehensive Clinical ECG*.

The second approach to FECG recording during labor is to attach an electrode directly to the fetal scalp. Another electrode, forming the second part of the bipolar lead, can be clipped to the perineum or placed in cervical/vaginal secretions. An indifferent electrode can be attached to a maternal limb. A higher quality FECG signal is obtained with this technique, but computer-based signal processing techniques are still required to facilitate analysis [87].

A different type of abdominal-lead system has also been described by Oostendorp et al. [88]. The 32 electrodes are arranged on the maternal abdomen and back in order to display, after appropriate signal processing, the potential distribution generated by the fetal heart; that is, a "fetal body-surface map" can be produced.

The European Community supported research into this topic, some aspects of which were presented in a series of articles [89]. A much more recent Cochrane review [90] noted that hypoxaemia during labor can alter the morphology of the fetal ECG, notably the relation of the PR to RR intervals, and elevation or depression of the ST segment. Techniques have therefore been developed to monitor the fetal ECG during labor as an adjunct to continuous electronic fetal heart rate monitoring with the aim of improving fetal outcome and minimizing unnecessary obstetric interference. The review concluded that there was some justification for the use of fetal ST analysis when a decision has been made to undertake continuous electronic fetal heart rate monitoring during labor. However, the advantages need to be considered along with the disadvantages of needing to use an internal scalp electrode, after membrane rupture, for ECG waveform recordings.

11.18   Comparative Electrocardiography

Because the ECG is of interest in many investigations assessing the efficacy of new therapeutic agents, the use of lead systems in various animals is introduced. First of all, the reader is referred to ❷ Chap. 9 of *Specialized Aspects of ECG* where the dog ECG is discussed extensively. For this reason, no further reference to ECG lead systems in dogs is given here. ❷ Chap. 10 of *Specialized Aspects of ECG* also discusses the ECG lead systems in mammals, but it is worth considering the ECG in rats in this chapter in view of the use of the rat as an experimental model. The Nehb leads have been introduced above in ❷ Sect. 11.3 and for rats and guinea pigs a modification introduced by Sporri [91] is commonly used. In this case the electrode placements are as follows:

(a) on the right scapula,
(b) over the apex of the heart, and
(c) over the lumbar vertebra

Using a conventional electrocardiograph, these leads would be connected, respectively, to the right arm, left leg and the left arm electrodes. This would allow leads D, A and I (alternatively called J) to be recorded. This modification of the Nehb leads is now referred to as the Nehb-Sporri lead system.

It is also possible to record a form of VCG in the rat using an uncorrected lead system. In this case, the X component would be measured by lead I with the positive electrode being on the left foreleg and the negative electrode on the right foreleg, the Y component would be recorded using aVF, i.e., the left and right leg electrodes would be used as with the

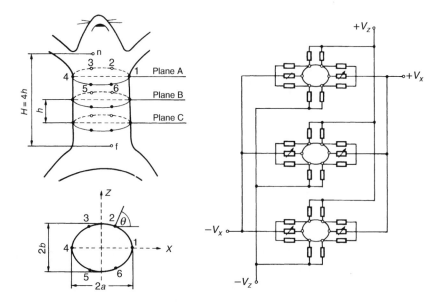

⬛ **Fig. 11.42**
The modified form of the Nelson-lead system used by Schwartze and Thoss [93] for recording the VCG in rats. A total of 20 electrodes is used, from which the three vector components can be derived

12-lead ECG, while the Z component would be obtained using a bipolar lead with electrodes placed on the sternum and the thoracic vertebrae. This system is uncorrected in that the lead strengths would be unequal and therefore considerable distortion of the VCG would ensue.

Yamori et al. [92] have utilized the Takayasu-lead system in order to record the ECG from rats. The X lead is a straightforward bipolar lead with large electrodes on each side of the thorax, the Y lead is a bipolar lead between the base of the tail and the bridge of the nose, and the Z lead is also a bipolar lead with a large electrode on the sternum and another over the thoracic vertebrae.

The Frank system [21] has been used in rats by Schwartze and Thoss [93]. These authors also make use of a modified form of the Nelson-lead system [94]. This is illustrated in ❯ Fig. 11.42. The theory is based on earlier work of Gabor and Nelson [95], which theorized that the components of the resultant cardiac dipole M could be determined as follows:

$$M_x = \sigma \iint V \, dy \, dz$$

$$M_y = \sigma \iint V \, dx \, dz$$

$$M_z = \sigma \iint V \, dx \, dy$$

where σ is the electrical conductivity of the body and the integrations are over the body surface. Since surface integration is not feasible, discrete approximations are required. Eifrig et al. [96] used three planes with six surface electrodes on each (❯ Fig. 11.42) together with a foot and neck electrode. Then,

$$M_x = \frac{\sigma HP}{24} \sum_{\alpha=A,B,C} \left(V_1^\alpha - V_4^\alpha + (V_2^\alpha + V_6^\alpha - V_3^\alpha - V_5^\alpha) \cos \theta \right)$$

$$M_y = \sigma D(V_f - V_n)$$

$$M_z = \frac{\sigma HP}{24} \sum_{\alpha=A,B,C} (V_2^\alpha + V_3^\alpha - V_5^\alpha - V_6^\alpha) \sin \theta$$

where V_i^α is the potential at point i on plane α, V_f and V_n are the foot and neck potentials and H, P and D are the body length, circumference and cross-sectional area, respectively; θ is the angle between the X axis and the normal to the boundary (❷ Fig. 11.42). Angle θ depends on b/a, the semimajor and minor axes of the thorax cross section, assumed to be elliptical. In practice, the summations are achieved by the resistor network shown in ❷ Fig. 11.42, where adjustable potentiometers allow the index b/a to be incorporated. The net effect is that V_x, Y_y and V_z are recorded via the resistor network to give

$$M_x = \sigma K_x V_x, \quad K_x = \frac{3HP}{24}(1 + 2\cos\theta)$$

$$M_y = \sigma K_y V_y, \quad K_y = D(V_y = V_f - V_n)$$

$$M_z = \sigma K_z V_z, \quad K_z = \frac{3HP}{24}\sin\theta$$

The use of such a technique allowed Eifrig et al. [96] to study the relationship between the development of body weight and the dipole moment.

Driscoll [97] reviewed the normal rat ECG and pointed out that the appearances of the rat ECG among other things depended on the form of restraint being used to position the rat during recording. Some authors record the ECG with the rat lying on its back normally under anesthesia; alternatively, others restrain the rat perhaps in a cylindrical device. The important point to realize is the difference in ECG appearances depending on the approach adopted.

Electrocardiograms can be recorded from baboons using the conventional 12-lead or 3-orthogonal-lead ECG. Hermann and Herrmann [98] utilized the 12-lead ECG in their studies. Ruttkay-Nedecky and Cherkovich [99] used the axial-lead system described in ❷ Sect. 11.4.2.2 in their studies of baboons.

References

1. Einthoven, W., G.E. Fahr, and A. De Waart, Uber die Richtung und die manifeste Grosse der Potentialschwankungen im menschlichen Herzen und iiber den Einfluss der Herzlage auf die Form des Elektrokardiogramms. *Pflug. Arch.*, 1913;**150**: 275–315. (Translation: Hoff H E. Sekelj P. On the direction and manifest size of the heart on the form of the electrocardiogram. *Am. Heart J.* 1950;**40**: 163–211.)

2. Burger, H.C and J.B. van Milaan, Heart vector and leads. I, II and III. *Br. Heart J.* 1946;**8**: 157–161, 1947;**9**: 154–160, 1948;**10**: 229–233.

3. Turner AM, 12 Lead recordings: Implications of an inconsistent approach. *Cardiology News* 2006;**9**: 10–12.

4. Pipberger, H V., R.C. Arzbaecher, A. Berson et al., Recommendations for standardization of leads and of specifications of instruments in electrocardiography and vectorcardiography. A report of the committee on electrocardiography of the AHA. *Circulation*, 1975;**52**(August Suppl): 11–31.

5. Sheffield, L.T., R. Prineas, H.C. Cohen, A. Schoenberg, and V. Froelicher, Optimal electrocardiography-1977. Task force II: Quality of electrocardiographic records. *Am J. Cardiol.*, 1978;**41**: 146–157.

6. Kligfield, P., L.Gettes, J.J. Bailey et al., Guidelines for the standardization and interpretation of the electrocardiogram, Part 1. The electrocardiogram and its technology. *Circulation*, 2007;**115**: 1306–1324.

7. Pahlm, O., W.K. Haisty, L. Edenbrandt et al., Evaluation of changes in standard electrocardiographic QRS waveforms recorded from activity compatible proximal lead positions. *Am. J. Cardiol.*, 1992;**69**: 253–257.

8. Kligfield, P. and P. Macfarlane, Non equivalence of proximal and distal arm electrode placement in routine electrocardiography. *J. Electrocardiol.*, 2005;**38**(Suppl): 36 (Abs).

9. Wilson, F.N., F.D. Johnston, A.G. MacLeod, and P.S. Barker, Electrocardiograms that represent the potential variations of a single electrode. *Am. Heart J.*, 1934;**9**: 447–458.

10. Frank, E., Determination of the electrical center of ventricular depolarization in the human heart. *Am. Heart J.*, 1955;**9**: 670–692.

11. Goldberger, E., A simple, indifferent, electrocardiographic electrode of zero potential and a technique of obtaining augmented, unipolar, extremity leads. *Am. Heart J.*, 1942;**23**: 483–492.

12. Committee of the American Heart Association for the Standardization of Precordial Leads. Standardization of precordial leads. (a) Supplementary report. *Am. Heart J.*, 1938;**15**: 235–239. (b) Second supplementary report. *J. Am. Med. Assoc.*, 1943;**121**: 1349–1351.

13. Frank, E., The image surface of a homogeneous torso. *Am. Heart J.*, 1954;**47**: 757–768.

14. Langner, P.H., Jr., An octaxial reference system derived from a nonequilateral triangle for frontal plane vectorcardiography. *Am. Heart J.*, 1955;**49**: 696–704.

15. Anderson, S, O. Pahlm, R. Selvester et al., Panoramic display of the orderly sequenced 12-lead ECG. *J. Electrocardiol.*, 1994;**7**: 47–352.

16. Cabrera, E., *Electrocardiographie clinique. Theorie et pratique.* Paris: Masson, 1959.

17. Nehb, W., Zur Standardisierung der Brustwandableitungen des Elektrokardiogramms. Mit Bemerkungen zum Friihbild des Hinterwandinfarkts und des Infarktnachschubs in der Vorderwand. *Klin. Wochenschr.*, 1938;**17**: 1807–1811.

18. Grishman, A. and L. Scherlis, *Spatial Vectorcardiography.* Philadelphia, Pennsylvania: Saunders, 1952.

19. Duchosal, P.W. and R. Sulzer, *La vectocardiographie.* Basel: Karger, 1949.

20. Wilson, F.N., F.D. Johnston, and C.E. Kossmann, The substitution of a tetrahedron for the Einthoven triangle. *Am. Heart J.*, 1947;**33**: 594–603.

21. Frank, E., An accurate, clinically practical system for spatial vectorcardiography. *Circulation.* 1956;**13**: 737–749.

22. Draper, H.W., C.J. Peffer, F.W. Stallmann, D. Littmann, and H.V. Pipberger, The corrected orthogonal electrocardiogram and vectorcardiogram in 510 normal men (Frank lead system). *Circulation.* 1964;**30**: 853–864.

23. Nemati, M., J.T. Doyle, D. McCaughan, R.A. Dunn, and H.V. Pipberger, The orthogonal electrocardiogram in normal women. Implications of sex differences in diagnostic electrocardiography. *Am. Heart J.*, 1978;**95**: 12–21.

24. Teppner, U., S. Lobodzinski, D. Neubert, and M.M. Laks, A technique to evaluate the performance of computerized ECG analysis systems. *J. Electrocardiol.*, 1987;**20** (Suppl.): 68–72.

25. McFee, R. and A. Parungao. An orthogonal lead system for clinical electrocardiography. *Am. Heart J.*, 1961;**62**: 93–100.

26. Brody, D.A. and R.C. Arzbaecher. A comparative analysis of several corrected vectorcardiographic leads. *Circulation.* 1964;**29**: 533–545.

27. Macfarlane, P.W., A modified axial lead system for orthogonal lead electrocardiography. *Cardiovasc. Res.*, 1969;**3**: 510–515.

28. Macfarlane, P.W., A.R. Lorimer, and T.D.V. Lawrie, 3 and 12 lead electrocardiogram interpretation by computer. A comparison of 1093 patients. *Br. Heart J.*, 1971;**33**: 266–274.

29. Macfarlane, P.W., E.N. Coleman, and A. Simpson, Modified axial lead system in children. *Br. Heart J.*, 1977;**39**: 1102–1108.

30. Macfarlane, P.W., A hybrid lead system for routine electrocardiography, in *Progress in Electrocardiology*, P.W. Macfarlane, Editor. Tunbridge Wells, Pitman Medical, 1979, pp. 1–5.

31. Macfarlane, P.W., M.P. Watts, and T.D.V. Lawrie, Hybrid electrocardiography, in *Optimization of Computer ECG Processing*, H.K. Wolf, and P.W. Macfarlane, Editors. Amsterdam, North-Holland, 1980, pp. 57–61.

32. van Oosterom, A., Z. Ihara, V. Jacquemet, and R. Heokema, Vectorcardiographic lead systems for the characterization of atrial fibrillation. *J. Electrocardiol.*, 2007;**40**: 343.e1–343.e11.

33. Dower, G.E., H. Bastos Machado, and J.A. Osborne, On deriving the electrocardiogram from vectorcardiographic leads. *Clin. Cardiol.*, 1980;**3**: 87–95.

34. Dower, G.E., A lead synthesizer for the Frank system to simulate the standard 12-lead electrocardiogram. *J. Electrocardiol.*, 1968;**I**: 101–16,252.

35. Dower, G.E. and H. Bastos Machado, Progress report on the ECGD, in *Progress in Electrocardiology*, P.W. Macfarlane, Editor. Tunbridge Wells, Pitman Medical, 1979, pp. 264–271.

36. Uijen, G.J.H., A. van Oosterom, and R.T.H van Dam, The relationship between the 12-lead standard ECG and the *XYZ* vector leads, in *Proc. 14th Int. Congr. Electrocardiology*, E. Schubert, Editor. Berlin, Academy of Sciences of the DDR, 1988, pp. 301–307.

37. Dower, G.E., A. Yakush, S.B. Nazzal, R.V. Jutzy, and C.E. Ruiz, Deriving the 12-lead electrocardiogram from four (EASI) electrodes. *J. Electrocardiol.*, 1998;**21**(Suppl): 182–187.

38. Field, D.Q., C.L. Feldman, and B.M. Horacek, Improved EASI coefficients: Their values, derivation and performance. *J. Electrocardiol.*, 2002;**35**(Suppl): 23–33.

39. Sejersten, M., G.S. Wagner, O. Pahlm, J.W. Warren, C.L. Feldman, and B.M. Horacek, Detection of acute ischemia from the EASI-derived 12 lead electrocardiogram and from the 12-lead electrocardiogram acquired in clinical practice. *J. Electrocardiol.*, 2007;**40**: 120–126.

40. Suraweera, J., E. Clark, and P.W. Macfarlane, EASI derived 12 Lead ECG v. Conventional 12 Lead ECG, in Computer Applications in Electrical Engineering, Recent Advances, India, IITR, Roorkee, 2005, pp. 1–4.

41. Nelwan, S.P., J.A. Kors, and S.H. Meij, Minimal lead sets for reconstruction of 12-lead electrocardiograms. *J. Electrocardiol.*, 2000;**33**: 163–166.

42. Nelwan, S.P., J.A. Kors, S.H. Meij, J.H. van Bemmel, and M.L. Simoons, Reconstruction of the 12-lead electrocardiogram from reduced lead sets. *J. Electrocardiol.*, 2004;**37**: 11–18

43. Nelwan, S.P., S.W. Crater, and S.H. Meij et al., Assessment of derived 12-lead ECGs using general and patient-specific reconstruction strategies at rest and during transient myocardial ischemia. *Am. J. Cardiol.*, 2004;**94**: 1529–1533.

44. Edenbrandt, L. and O. Pahlm, Vectorcardiogram synthesized from a 12 lead ECG: Superiority of the Inverse Dower Matrix. *J. Electrocardiol.*, 1988;**21**: 361–367.

45. Willems, J.L., *Common Standards for Quantitative Electrocardiography. 4th Progress Report.* Leuven: Aceo, 1984, 199–200.

46. Willems, J.L., P. Arnaud, J.H. Van Bemmel et al., Assessment of the performance of electrocardiographic computer programs with the use of a reference data base. *Circulation.* 1985;**71**: 523–534.

47. Edenbrandt, L., A. Houston, and P.W. Macfarlane, Vectorcardiograms synthesized from 12 lead ECGs: a new method applied in 1792 healthy children. *Pediatr. Cardiol.*, 1994;**15**: 21–26.

48. Macfarlane, P.W., L. Edenbrandt, and O. Pahlm, *12 Lead Vectorcardiography.* Oxford: Butterworth-Heinemann, 1995.

49. Warner, R., N.E. Hill, P.R. Sheehe, S. Mookherjee, C.T. Fruehan, and H. Smulyan, Improved electrocardiographic criteria for the diagnosis of inferior myocardial infarction. *Circulation.* 1982;**66**: 422–428.

50. Surawicz, B., H. Uhley, R. Borun et al., Task force I: Standardization of terminology and interpretation. *Am. J. Cardiol.*, 1978;**41**: 130–145.

51. Bayes de Luna, A., G. Wagner, Y. Birnbaum et al., A new terminology for left ventricular walls and location of myocardial infarcts that present Q waves based on the standard of cardiac magnetic resonance imaging. *Circulation.* 2006;**114**: 1755–1760.

52. Wagner, G., P.W. Macfarlane, H. Wellens et al., Recommendations for the standardization and interpretation of the electrocardiogram. Part VI. Acute ischemia/infarction. *J. Am. Cell. Cardiol.*, 2009;**53**: 1003–1011.

53. Mason, J.W., E.W. Hancock, and L.S. Gettes, Recommendations for the standardization and interpretation of the electrocardiogram: II: Electrocardiography diagnostic statement list. *Circulation.* 2007;**115**: 1325–1332.

54. Mason, R.E. and I. Likar. A new system of multiple-lead exercise electrocardiography. *Am. Heart J.*, 1966;**71**: 196–205.

55. Froelicher, V.F., Jr., R. Wolthius, N. Keiser et al., A comparison of two bipolar exercise electrocardiographic leads to lead V_5. *Chest.* 1976;**70**: 611–616.

56. Sheffield, L.T., R. Prineas, H.C. Cohen, A. Schoenberg, and V. Froelicher, Task force II: Quality of electrocardiographic records. *Am. J. Cardiol.*, 1978;**41**: 146–157.

57. Chaitman, B.R., M.G. Bourassa, P. Wagniart, F. Corbara, and R.J. Ferguson, Improved efficiency of treadmill exercise testing using a multiple lead ECG system and basic hemodynamic exercise response. *Circulation.* 1978;**57**: 71–79.

58. Papouchado, M., P.R. Walker, M.A. James, and L.M. Clarke, Fundamental differences between the standard 12-lead electrocardiograph and the modified (Mason-Likar) exercise system. *Eur. Heart J.*, 1987;**8**: 725–733.

59. Drew, B.J., R.M. Califf, M. Funk et al., Practice Standards for electrocardiographic monitoring in hospital settings. *Circulation.* 2004;**110**: 2721–2746.

60. Barr, R.C., M.S. Spach, and G.S. Herman-Giddens, Selection of the number and positions of measuring locations for electrocardiography. *IEEE Trans. Biomed. Eng.*, 1971;**18**: 125–138.

61. Kornreich, F, The missing waveform information in the orthogonal electrocardiogram (Frank leads). I. Where and how can this missing waveform information be retrieved? *Circulation.* 1973;**48**: 984–995.

62. Kornreich, F. and D. Brismee, The missing waveform information in the orthogonal electrocardiogram (Frank leads). II. Diagnosis of left ventricular hypertrophy and myocardial infarction from "total" surface waveform information. *Circulation.* 1973;**48**: 996–1004.

63. Lux, R.L., C.R. Smith, R.F. Wyatt, and J.A. Abildskov, Limited lead selection for estimation of body surface potential maps in electrocardiography. *IEEE Trans. Biomed. Eng.*, 1978;**25**: 270–276.

64. Maroko, P.R., P. Libby, J.W. Covell, B.E. Sobel, J. Ross, Jr., and E. Braunwald, Precordial S T segment elevation mapping: An atraumatic method for assessing alterations in the extent of myocardial ischemic injury. *Am. J. Cardiol.*, 1972;**29**: 223–230.

65. Fox, K.M., A.P. Selwyn, and J.P. Shillingford, Projection of electrocardiographic signs in praecordial maps after exercise in patients with ischaemic heart disease. *Br. Heart J.*, 1979;**42**: 416–421.

66. Fox, K.M., J. Deanfield, P. Ribero, D. England, and C. Wright, Projection of ST segment changes on to the front of the chest. Practical implications for exercise testing and ambulatory monitoring. *Br. Heart J.*, 1982;**48**: 555–559.

67. Monro, D.M., R.A.L. Guardo, P.J. Bourdillon, and J. Tinker, A Fourier technique for simultaneous electrocardiographic surface mapping. *Cardiovasc. Res.*, 1974;**8**: 688–700.

68. Monro, D.M., Interpolation by fast Fourier and Chebyshev transforms. *Int. J. Numer. Meth. Eng.*, 1979;**14**: 1679–1692.

69. Monro, D.M., Interpolation methods for surface mapping. *Comput. Programs Biomed.*, 1980;**2**: 145–157.

70. Menown, I.B.A., J. Allen, J.M. Anderson, and A.A.J. Adgey, Early diagnosis of right ventricular or posterior infarction associated with inferior wall left ventricular acute myocardial infarction. *Am. J. Cardiol.*, 2000;**85**: 934–938.

71. Yamada, K., K. Harumi, and T. Musha, Editors. Advances in Body Surface Potential Mapping, *Proc. Int. Symp. Body Surface Mapping.* Nagoya: University of Nagoya Press, 1983.

72. van Dam, R.T.H. and A. van Oosterom, Editors. *Electrocardiographic Body Surface Mapping.* Dordrecht: Nijhoff, 1986.

73. Taccardi, B., B.P. Punske, F. Sachse, F. Tricoche, P. Colli-Franzone, L.F. Pavarino, and C. Zabawa, Intramural activation and repolarization sequences in canine ventricles. Experimental and simulation studies. *J. Electrocardiol.*, 2005;**38**(Suppl): 131–137.

74. Witkowski, F.X. and P.B. Corr, An automated simultaneous transmural cardiac mapping system. *Am. J. Physiol.*, 1984;**247**: H661–668.

75. Holt, P., P.V.L. Curry, P.B. Deverall, C. Smallpiece, and A.K. Yates, Ventricular arrhythmias-An accurate guide to their localisation. *Br. Heart J.*, 1981;**45**: 615–616.

76. Bazan, V., R. Bala, F.C. Garcia, et al., 12 lead ECG features to identify ventricular tachycardia arising from the epicardial right ventricle. *Heart Rhythm.*, 2006;**10**: 1132–1139.

77. Friedman, P.L., T.L. Shook, J.M. Kirshenbaum, A.P. Selwyn, and P. Ganz, Value of the intracoronary electrocardiogram to monitor myocardial ischemia during percutaneous trans luminal coronary angioplasty. *Circulation*, 1986;**74**: 330–339.

78. DeMarchi, S.F., P. Meier, P. Oswald, and C. Seiler, Variable signs of ischemia during controlled occlusion of the left and right coronary artery in humans. *Am. J. Physiol.*, 2006;**291**: H351–H356.

79. Sheffield, L.T., A. Berson, Bragg-Remschel, et al., Recommendations for standards of instrumentation and practice in the use of ambulatory electrocardiography. *Circulation*, 1985;**71**: 626A–636A.

80. MacAlpin, R.N., Correlation of the location of coronary arterial spasm with the lead distribution of ST segment elevation during variant angina. *Am. Heart J.*, 1980;**99**: 555–564.

81. Quyyumi, A.A., L. Mockus, C. Wright, and K.M. Fox, Morphology of ambulatory ST segment changes in patients with varying severity of coronary artery disease. Investigation of the frequency of nocturnal ischaemia and coronary spasm. *Br. Heart J.*, 1985;**53**: 186–193.

82. Crawford, M.H., S.J. Bernstein, P.C. Deedwania, J.P. DiMarco, K.J. Ferrick, A. Garson Jr., L.A. Green, H.L. Greene, M.J. Silka, P.H. Stone, and C.M. Tracy, ACC/AHA guidelines for ambulatory electrocardiography: executive summary and recommendations: A report of the American College of Cardiology/American Heart Association Task Force on Practice Guidelines (Committee to Revise the Guidelines for Ambulatory Electrocardiography). *Circulation*, 1999;100:886–893.

83. Schnittger, I., I.M. Rodriguez, and R.A. Winkle, Esophageal electrocardiography: A new technology revives an old technique. *Am. J. Cardiol.*, 1986;**57**: 604–607.

84. Arzbaecher, R., A pill electrode for the study of cardiac arrhythmia. *Med. Instrum.*, 1973;**12**: 277–281.

85. Mächler, H., A. Lueger, S. Huber, P. Bergmann, P. Rehak, and G. Stark, The Esophageal-ECG: New applications with a new technique. *Internet J. Thoracic Cardiovasc. Surgery*, 1997;**2**(2).

86. Li, Y., L. Rao, S.G. Baidya, Y. Feng, J. Zhang, and J. Yang, The combined use of esophageal electrocardiogram and multiple right parasternal chest leads in the diagnosis of PSVT and determination of accessory pathways involved: A new simple noninvasive approach. *Int. J. Cardiol.*, 2006;**113**: 311–319.

87. Jenkins, H.M.L., Technical progress in fetal electrocardiography-A review. *J. Perinat. Med.*, 1986;**14**: 365–370.

88. Oostendorp, T.F., A. van Oosterom, H.W. Jongsma, and P.W.J. van Dongen, The potential distribution generated by the fetal heart at the maternal abdomen. *J. Perinat. Med.*, 1986;**14**: 435–444.

89. Advances in fetal electrocardiography (Symposium). *J. Perinat. Med.*, 1986;**14**: 345–452.

90. Neilson, J.P., Fetal electrocardiogram (ECG) for fetal monitoring during labor, Cochrane Database of Systematic Reviews 2006, Issue 3. Art. No.: CD000116. DOI: 10.1002/14651858.CD000116.pub2

91. Sporri, H., Der Einfluss der Tuberkulose auf das Elektrokardiogramm. (Untersuchungen an Meerschweinchen und Rindern.) *Arch. Wiss. Prakt. Tierheilkd.*, 1944;**79**: 1–57.

92. Yamori, Y., M. Ohtaka, and Y. Nara, Vectorcardiographic study on left ventricular hypertrophy in spontaneously hypertensive rats. *Jpn. Circ. J.*, 1976;**40**: 1315–1329.

93. Schwartze, H. and F. Thoss, Applicability of two different lead systems in studies of the electrical activity of the hearts in newborn guinea pigs. *J. Electrocardiol.*, 1981;**14**: 9–12.

94. Nelson, C.V., P.R. Gastonguay, A.F. Wilkinson, and P.C. Voukydis, A lead system for direction and magnitude of the heart vector, in *Vectorcardiography* 2, I. Hoffman, R.I. Hamby, E. Glassman, Editors. Amsterdam, North-Holland, 1971, pp. 85–97.

95. Gabor, D. and C.V. Nelson, Determination of the resultant dipolt of the heart from measurements on the body surface. *J. Appl. Phys.*, 1954;**25**: 413–416.

96. Eifrig, T., H. Schwartze, and A. Joel. Experiences with the Nelson lead system in physiological animal experiments, in *Electrocardiology '81*, Z. Antaloczy, I. Preda, Editors. Amsterdam, Excerpta Medica, 1982, pp. 461–464.

97. Driscoll, P., The normal rat electrocardiogram (ECG), in *The Rat Electrocardiogram in Pharmacology and Toxicology*, R. Budden, D.K. Detweiler, G. Zbinden, Editors. Oxford, Pergamon, 1981, pp. 1–14.

98. Hermann, G.R. and A.H.W. Herrmann. The electrocardiographic patterns in 170 baboons in the domestic and African colonies at the primate center of the Southwest Foundation for Research and Education, in *The Baboon in Medical Research* H. Vagtborg, Editor. Austin, Texas, University of Texas Press, 1965, pp. 251–264.

99. Ruttkay-Nedecky, I. and G.M. Cherkovich, *The Orthogonal Electrocardiogram and Vectorcardiogram of Baboons and Macaques.* Bratislava: VEDA, 1977.

12 ECG Instrumentation: Application and Design

S.M. Lobodzinski

P. W. Macfarlane et al. (eds.), *Basic Electrocardiology*, DOI 10.1007/978-0-85729-871-3_12,
© Springer-Verlag London Limited 2012

12.1   Introduction

This chapter addresses the theory and practice of ECG recording and processing. The current state of the art and latest technical developments in the field of electrocardiography are discussed with respect to:

1. Formation and characterization of ECG signals
2. Biopotential ECG sensors
3. ECG signal recording
4. ECG recording standards
5. Patient safety standards
6. ECG signal processing

The emphasis lies on the treatment of biopotential sensors (electrodes) and in particular on recent developments in this domain. Other topics like instrumentation and signal processing are treated at an introductory level, mainly defining concepts and terminology, with numerous references to the available high quality textbooks and publications in the literature. The brief section on the formation and characterization of basic ECG features includes ample references to the other chapters in this Volume, which describe this topic in greater detail (❷ Chaps. 5–8). In Appendix Section entitled "Basic Digital ECG Signal Processing" some signal processing methods are described by A. van Oosterom, restricted to topics that are highly specific to the ECG.

For additional reading on the material discussed, the reader is referred to the related chapter by the late Christoph Zywietz in the first edition of this book [1], as well as to an overview by E. McAdams in the Encyclopedia of Medical Devices and Instrumentation [2].

12.2   Formation and Characterization of the ECG Signal

The electrical activity of the heart generates an electrical potential field on the body surface. Given the anatomy of the heart and the chest, the potentials at locations on the body surface represent composite electrical activity from the entire heart. A body surface electrocardiogram (ECG) is the manifestation of this electrical activity. It provides a measure of the potential difference between two points on the body surface as a continuous function of time, or between the two terminal points of a network sensing the potential field (❷ Chaps. 10 and ❷ 11). The ECG is routinely measured using standard ECG electrodes. Commonly, ten such electrodes are used, four of which are placed on or near the limbs and six of which span the chest, primarily on the left side. As discussed in ❷ Chaps. 10 and ❷ 11, only nine of these electrodes are involved in documenting the potential field generated by the heart, the tenth electrode (usually attached to the right leg) serving as a means for reducing the interference from external electric fields. From the nine electrodes, at most eight independent signals can be extracted. Hence, those forming the standard set of 12 ECG leads contain some redundancy.

12.2.1   Formation of the ECG

A brief summary of the sequence of events involved in electrical activation of the atria and the ventricles that give rise to the ECG is presented below. A more complete handling of this topic, with increased detail, is given in ❷ Chaps. 4–7.

As the heart undergoes depolarization and repolarization, electrical currents spread throughout the body that acts as an electric volume conductor (❷ Chap. 2). If a piece of living myocardium is placed in a bath containing a saline solution, which conducts electric currents, and if the terminals of a voltmeter are placed in the bath on either side of the muscle segment, no potential difference is observed between the sensors when the muscle is in its polarized, resting state (❷ Fig. 12.1a). The reason for this is discussed in ❷ Sect. 6.2.1. If the left side of the muscle is stimulated electrically a self-propagating transmembrane potential gradient is produced. A wave of depolarization will sweep through the tissue from left to right (❷ Fig. 12.1b). Midway through this depolarization process, cells on the left part of the tissue (depolarized cells) are negative *on the outside* relative to their inside, whereas the cells ahead of the front, the right, are still polarized (positive on the outside), thus creating a potential difference between the two terminals of the voltmeter. Through the labeling of these two terminals by the signs as shown, the recorded voltage is, by convention, assigned a positive value (upward

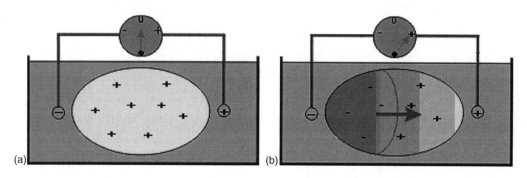

◻ Fig. 12.1

Schematic diagram of an *elliptically shaped* section of myocardial tissue placed inside a saline-filled container. The *signs drawn* inside the ellipses indicate the potential difference on the outside of the surface bounding the tissue with reference to the intracellular potential. (a) Equilibrium of the potential; all myocytes in their fully polarized state: potential difference observed in the external medium is zero. (b) Situation during a propagated activation. The potential in the external medium is positive ahead of the wave front with respect to that behind it. The *small circles* denote the two electrodes mentioned in the text. The one carrying the "+" label may be interpreted as the sensing electrode, the other one as the reference electrode (see ❷ Chap. 10). Voltage differences between these electrodes result in an upward deflection if the polarity of the difference is concomitant with the signs labeling the electrodes

deflection in the recording). After the wave of depolarization has swept across the entire muscle mass, the outsides of all cells are negative with respect to their interior, and once again, no potential difference exists between the two sensors. This formulation ignores the field produced by currents originating from the repolarization processes that have already started in the part of the tissue that depolarized first.

12.2.2 Formation of ECG Wave Forms

The entire process of depolarization and repolarization of the myocardium is illustrated in the ❷ Fig. 12.2, which is a crude representation of the electrical events that occur in the atria. A more comprehensive treatment of the subject is given in ❷ Chap. 5.

During the resting, polarized state, no potential difference is measured between the sensing electrode (labeled as positive) and the reference electrode (labeled as negative). When the sino-atrial node fires, a wave of depolarization spreads out over the atria. During this period, some of the muscle mass overlaying the polarized myocytes temporarily remain positive on the outside, while the part overlaying the depolarized myocytes is negative. This potential gradient in the external medium is sensed as a potential difference between the two electrodes. Once the entire myocardium is depolarized completely, there is once again no potential difference, and the voltage difference sensed by the electrodes is zero just as it was in the polarized state. During repolarization, again starting in the SA-nodal region and then moving across the atria, there will be a potential gradient, but this time the polarity is reversed, causing a downward deflection. Finally, when all of the cells are repolarized, the measured voltage difference will once again be zero until a subsequent activation is initiated.

The cardiac activation creates an electric potential field throughout the body as well as on its surface (❷ Fig. 12.3). The human body may be considered as a resistive, piecewise homogeneous and linear volume conductor (❷ Chap. 2). The electric potential differences measured between specific points on the outer surface of the volume conductor, i.e., on the body surface, are referred to as electrocardiograms, or "the" ECG.

The entire electric activity of the heart may be represented by equivalent electric current generators. Several models of such generators have been formulated, each differing in their complexity and their direct link with the underlying electrophysiology.

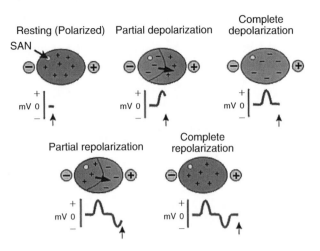

Fig. 12.2

The entire process of depolarization and repolarization that is representative of the electrical events that occur in the atria. The ± signs drawn inside the ellipses denote the polarity of the voltage just outside the myocardium with respect to the intra-cellular potential of the myocytes

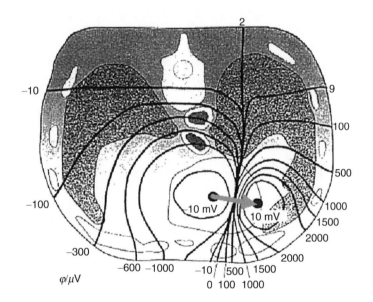

Fig. 12.3

Transverse cross section of the thorax showing regions having different electric conductivity (bone, lung, muscle) (From R. Hinz [3]). *Isopotential lines* illustrate the type of potential field generated by a single dipole

A classic example of this is the single current dipole, generally placed at the center of gravity of ventricular mass (❯ Fig. 12.3). Other major source descriptions are discussed in ❯ Chaps. 2 and ❯ 5–8.

Several basic rules emerge from the modeling of potential fields for interpreting observed potential differences in terms of the sources of cardiac electric activity:

1. A wave of depolarization traveling toward the sensing electrode results in a positive deflection in the ECG trace.
2. A wave of repolarization traveling away from the sensing electrode results in a positive deflection.

■ Table 12.1

Sources of electric signals observable on the body surface [6]

Source	Signal amplitude range	Signal frequency range (Hz)
Heart, electrocardiogram, ECG	0.5–4 mV	0.01–250
Brain, electroencephalogram, EEG	10–5,000 μV	0–150
Gastrointestinal tract, Electrogastrogram, EGG	10–1,000 μV	0–1
Nerve potentials, electroneurogram, ENG	0.01–3 mV	0–10,000
Skeletal muscles, electromyogram, EMG	0.1–5 mV	0–10,000

3. A wave of depolarization or repolarization traveling perpendicular to the axis of an electrode pair results in a biphasic deflection of equal positive or negative voltages at each electrode, and, hence, no deflection.
4. The instantaneous amplitude of the measured potentials depends upon the orientation of the lead relative to the mean electric vector.
5. The voltage amplitude is directly related to the mass of tissue undergoing depolarization or repolarization.

Rules 1–3 are derived from the volume conductor model described above. Rule 4 takes into consideration that, at any given point in time during depolarization in the atria or ventricles, there can be many separate waves of depolarization traveling in different directions relative to the electrode locations. The ECG reflects the time course of the average, instantaneous direction and magnitude (i.e., a mean electrical vector) of all depolarization waves present. Rule 5 simply states that the amplitude of the wave recorded by the ECG is directly related to the mass of the muscle undergoing depolarization or repolarization. For example, when the mass of the left ventricle is increased by hypertrophy, the amplitude of the QRS complex is increased in certain leads, provided that the local source strength (impressed current per unit volume of tissue) remains the same (❷ Chap. 2). Note however, that such simple rules apply strictly only if the observation point is located close to the source of the electric activity.

12.2.3 Other Sources of Electric Signals Inside the Body

In addition to the heart, there are other sources of electric activity present inside the body. The major ones are included in ❷ Table 12.1. These generators produce electric signals at various locations within the volume conductor that add to the electrocardiogram. It is important to note that the EEG, EGG and EMG signal amplitudes and the range of their frequency spectra overlap with that of the ECG signal [6].

12.2.4 Characteristics of Composite ECG Signals

The amplitudes of the ECG signal components as measured on the body surface vary with time and range from 0.1 to 5 mV. Significant components in their frequency spectra lie in the range between 0.05 and 250 Hz. The ECG waveforms generally exhibit small but distinct beat to beat variations. In patients with implanted pacemakers, narrow voltage pulses appear superimposed on the ECG signal. These must be identified to differentiate them from the ECG signals in order to prevent an incorrect heart rate evaluation.

The bandwidth of the ECG is defined as the frequency range between low and high frequency cutoffs (−3 dB) of the magnitudes of their Fourier amplitude spectrum [6]. For accurate recording of ECGs, the dynamic input range and the bandwidth of the recording system are of major importance and should at least extend to the highest peak-to-peak amplitude and the highest frequency component in the ECG signal, respectively.

12.3 Biopotential Sensors

A biopotential sensor is a device that responds to the presence of electric charges in living tissues by producing an analog electrical input signal to the instrumentation amplifier. Biopotential sensors carry out a complex transducer function, in which the charge of the ions carrying the current inside the body is transferred to that of the electrons constituting the sensor output current. A common, time-sanctioned practice is to refer to all biopotential sensors as "electrodes."

The word "electrode" was coined by Michael Faraday in 1834 from a combination of the Greek words *elektron* (meaning amber, and from which the word electricity is similarly derived) and *hodos*, a way [4]. It signifies a conductor used to make contact with a non-metallic part of a circuit such as an electrolyte. As an example, we consider a "wet" biopotential sensor, commonly referred to as a "disposable ECG electrode," shown in ❷ Fig. 12.4. It comprises an electrochemically active gel in contact with the skin, an electrode connecting clip that is coated with a layer of Ag/AgCl on the inside, mounting flexible foam pad with adhesive and many other electro-mechanical parts not directly involved in conversion of a flux of ions into an electric current carried by electrons. Together, the layer of the gel and the metal electrode perform the transducer function. Since electrochemical sensors also utilize metallic electrodes, we shall use the terms biopotential sensors and electrodes interchangeably where appropriate.

Modern biopotential sensors include electrochemical, capacitive, optical and impedance transducers capable of sensing changes in the immediate electric field caused by the electrical activity of the heart.

There are many types of biopotential sensors in use today that are used for recording electrocardiograms. Those discussed in this chapter are used in clinical and research based electrocardiology. Special devices, such as needle electrodes and microelectrodes used for measurement of intracellular and extracellular electrical activity, are not treated here.

Electrochemical biopotential sensors share two major components:

1. an electrochemical electrode, which may be metallic, carbon, composite electro-conductive film, etc.
2. the electrolyte, which may be an electrolytic medium or gel such as is used with surface electrodes, or it may be the body fluids that come into contact with an electrode such as the perspiration that accumulates under a dry electrode applied to skin containing sweat glands.

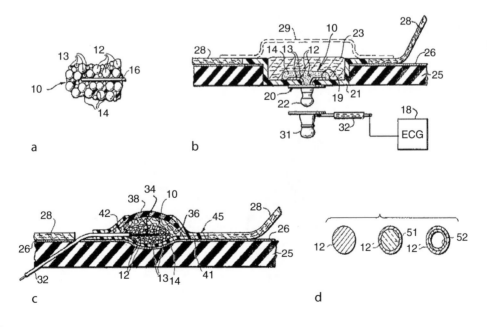

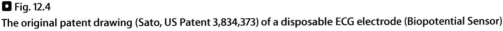

❏ Fig. 12.4
The original patent drawing (Sato, US Patent 3,834,373) of a disposable ECG electrode (Biopotential Sensor)

The biopotential sensors that require a direct contact with the skin are referred to as Galvanic Sensors, i.e., they are involved in an electrochemical reaction with electrolytes inside the body. In order to achieve a better understanding of the working principles of galvanic biopotential sensors, some details about the electrode–electrolyte interface are discussed first. This is followed by a discussion of the sensor–skin interface.

12.3.1 The Sensor–Electrolyte Interface

12.3.1.1 Electrochemical Reactions

The electrodes used in biopotential sensors comprise metallic atoms M. They are in contact with an electrolyte, a solution comprising cations of the electrode metal M^+ and anions A^-. When an electrode comes into contact with an electrolyte, an electrochemical reaction is initiated; it can be described as:

$$M \leftrightarrow M^{n+1} + n^{e-} \tag{12.1}$$

$$A^{m-} \leftrightarrow A + m^{e-} \tag{12.2}$$

where n is the valence of M and m is the valence of A. Equation (12.1) tells us that the metal in the electrode at the interface oxidizes to form a cation and one or more free electrons. The cation is then discharged into the electrolyte and the electron remains as a charge carrier in the electrode. Equation (12.2) describes the anion reaction. The anion in contact with the electrode–electrolyte interface can be oxidized to a neutral atom, giving off one or more free electrons to the electrode. The reactions described by (12.1) and (12.2) are reversible. Since the electrolyte contains cations discharged from the electrode, the charge distribution is not neutral. The potential set up by the electrolyte in a direct contact with the electrode is known as the half-cell potential (❷ Fig. 12.5).

When two aqueous ionic solutions of a different concentration are separated by an ion-selective semi-permeable membrane, an electric potential exists across the membrane. Its value follows from the Nernst equation as

$$E_{cell} = E_{cell}^0 - \frac{RT}{nF} \ln Q$$

R – gas constant
T – temperature in Kelvin
Q – thermodynamic reaction quotient
F – Faraday's constant
n – number of electrons transferred

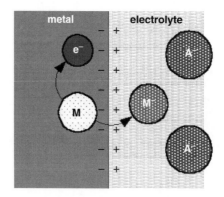

❏ Fig. 12.5
Charges at a metal–electrolyte interface

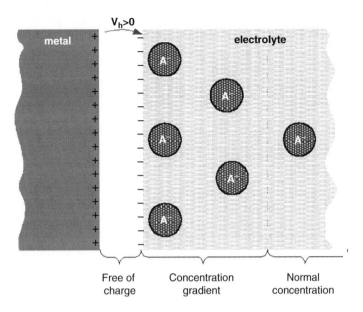

V_h>0

metal

electrolyte

Free of charge | Concentration gradient | Normal concentration

🔲 **Fig. 12.6**

A double layer potential at the electrode surface for a metal with a positive half-cell potential (Courtesy of Prof. R. Hinz [3])

The quantity Q, the thermodynamic reaction constant, is like a dynamic version of the equilibrium constant in which the concentrations and gas pressures are the instantaneous values in the reaction mixture [5].

For the general oxidation–reduction reaction we have

$$\alpha A + \beta B \leftrightarrow \gamma D + ne^{-1} \tag{12.3}$$

Each ion has an equilibrium potential associated with it whereby the diffusive forces and the electrical forces balance. The Nernst equation for the so-called half-cell potential set up at the interface is

$$E = E^0 + \frac{RT}{nF} \ln \left[\frac{a_C^\gamma a_D^\delta}{a_A^\alpha a_B^\beta} \right] \tag{12.4}$$

E^0 – Standard half-cell potential
E – Half-cell potential
a – Ionic activity (generally same as concentration)
n – Number of valence electrons involved

When a pair of the biopotential sensors is connected to the instrumentation amplifier, a small current may flow through the sensor–electrolyte interface. Any such net transient current crossing the interface interferes with the static equilibrium of the half-cell potential. If the current flow is from electrode to electrolyte, the oxidation reactions dominate, whereas if it is in the opposite direction, the reduction reactions dominate (❷ Fig. 12.6).

Different metals exhibit different half-cell potentials when in contact with an electrolyte, as illustrated in ❷ Fig. 12.7.

12.3.1.2 Impedance of the Interface

The electrode–electrolyte interface is highly complex and non-linear in nature and strongly depends on the electrode metal, its contact area, the makeup of an electrolyte, surrounding temperature, and the density and the frequency of the current passing through the interface.

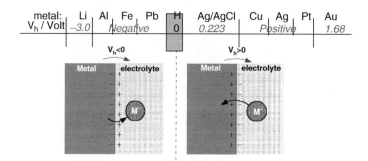

⬤ Fig. 12.7

Half-cell potentials of various metals in contact with the electrolyte

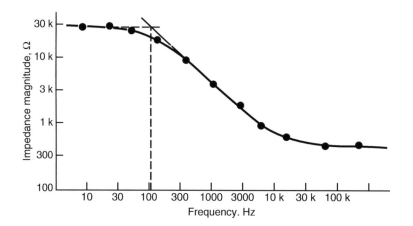

⬤ Fig. 12.8

Experimentally determined magnitude of the electrode–electrolyte interface impedance as a function of frequency (From [6])

Electrode impedances can be difficult to measure with high accuracy on living subjects. The term electrode impedance really refers to the impedance at each electrode interface and does not include the impedance of the biological material between the electrodes. Frequently, however, the term is used to describe the total impedance of the circuit between the electrode terminals. An example of the frequency dependency of an experimentally observed electrode impedance is shown in ❷ Fig. 12.8.

A simple, linearized equivalent circuit of the interface, including a voltage source in series with an impedance of the interface, is depicted in ❷ Fig. 12.9.

Capacitance

The presence of a charge distribution at an electrode–electrolyte interface produces not only an electrode potential but also a capacitance. Conceptually, two layers of charge of opposite sign as shown in ❷ Fig. 12.5, separated by a distance, form a capacitance. The distance between the layers of charge is molecular in dimension; therefore the capacitance per unit area is quite large [6]. In combination with R_d the capacitance C_d shown in ❷ Fig. 12.9 is usually taken to approximate the experimentally observed frequency dependency of the interface. In fact this dependency is slightly more complex [7]. The resistance R_d in the series-equivalent circuit models the ability of an electrode–electrolyte interface to conduct direct current (DC).

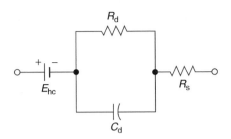

□ Fig. 12.9

A linearized equivalent circuit of the electrode–electrolyte interface. E_{hc} is the half-cell potential, R_d and C_d make up the impedance associated with the electrode–electrolyte interface, and R_s is the series resistance associated with the resistivity of the electrolyte (From [6])

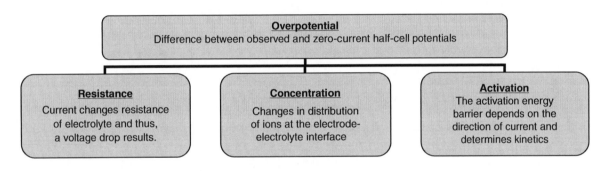

□ Fig. 12.10

Sources of the overpotential in electrochemical electrodes

Series Resistance

The series resistance R_s shown in ❷ Fig. 12.9 is associated with the resistivity of the electrolyte. Its magnitude is (approximately) inversely proportional to the square root of the surface area of the electrode, and also inversely proportional to the conductivity of the electrolyte (or body tissues in the application to the ECG).

12.3.1.3 Electrode Polarization

As discussed above, when two biopotential sensors placed in direct contact with the tissue are connected to the instrumentation amplifier, a very small current will flow through both electrodes and the input impedance of the amplifier. Any current flowing between a pair of biopotential sensors will alter the half-cell potential, effecting the polarization of the electrodes. The difference between the half-cell potential in the presence of current passing the interface and the equilibrium zero-current potential is known as the overpotential [8]. The contributing terms, as identified in ❷ Fig. 12.10, are

$$V_P = V_R + V_C + V_A \tag{12.5}$$

12.3.2 Polarizable and Non-polarizable Biopotential Sensors

We distinguish between two types of electrochemical sensors: polarizable and non-polarizable. This classification is based on what happens to a sensor electrode when a current passes it into the electrolyte. The theoretical polarizable electrodes are those in which no actual charge crosses the electrode–electrolyte interface when a current is applied. In reality, due to the capacitance present at the interface, the displacement current will be present at the interface. The theoretical non-polarizable electrodes are those in which current passes freely across the interface, requiring no energy to make the transition. The overpotentials are not present on non-polarizable electrodes. In practice neither truly non-polarizable nor polarizable sensors can be produced, and hence most practical biopotential sensors may only approximate either of the two types.

12.3.2.1 Polarizable Electrodes

Electrodes made of inert metals such as platinum or stainless steel have difficulty in oxidizing and dissolving. Their characteristics therefore closely approximate those of theoretically polarizable electrodes but only within an electrode potential range called the "double-layer range." In these electrodes, the current passing between the electrode and the electrolyte primarily changes the concentration of ions at the interface, so the major part of the overpotential observed in this type of electrode is the result of the concentration type of overpotential (❷ Fig. 12.10). ❷ Figure 12.11 shows a stainless steel electrode (Fe) in contact with an electrolyte. The electrochemical reaction at the electrode–electrolyte interface is described as:

$$Fe \leftrightarrow Fe^+ + e^-$$ (12.6)

We note that there is no charge crossing the stainless steel–electrode interface. Stainless steel is subject only to the displacement current, and therefore the electrode behaves like a capacitor. The behavior of polarized electrodes can be modeled by an RC network, also shown in ❷ Fig. 12.11.

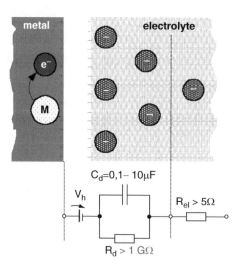

❏ Fig. 12.11

A polarizable, metal electrode such as made of stainless steel or iridium in contact with electrolyte. A metal electrode is subject to the displacement current only and therefore the electrode behaves like a capacitor (the very high resistance of R_d effectively blocks ion exchange between the electrode and the electrolyte). V_h is the half-cell potential, C_d is the make up the impedance associated with the electrode–electrolyte interface, and R_{el} is the resistance associated with the resistivity of the electrolyte

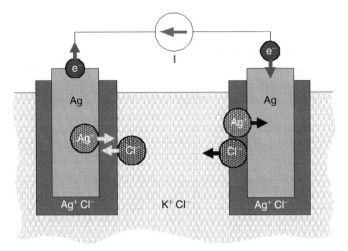

◘ Fig. 12.12

Ag/AgCl electrodes submerged in an electrolyte. A current *I* flows through the electrolyte containing ions of Cl⁻ and K⁺. The electrons from electrode (a) flow to the electrode (b), the electrode (a) discharges a silver cation into the electrolyte (oxidation reaction) and the electrode (b) absorbs the silver cation from the electrolyte (reduction reaction)

12.3.2.2   Non-Polarizable Electrodes

Perfectly non-polarizable electrodes allow a free passage of current across the electrode–electrolyte interface, and hence exhibit no accumulation of overpotential. The examples of electrodes closely approximating the characteristics of a theoretically non-polarizable electrode include Ag/AgCl and mercury/mercurous chloride (Hg/Hg_2Cl_2). These electrodes comprise the metal surface coated by a slightly soluble metal chloride layer. The behavior of Ag/AgCl is governed by two chemical reactions, described by (12.7) and (12.8) and illustrated in ❷ Fig. 12.12. The first involves the oxidation of silver atoms on the electrode surface to silver ions in the electrolyte solution at the interface. The second reaction occurs immediately after the formation of silver ions. These ions combine with chloride cations already in the solution and form the ionic compound – silver chloride [6]. Since silver chloride is only slightly soluble in water, most of it precipitates from the solution on to the silver electrode, where it forms a silver chloride deposit [9].

$$Ag \leftrightarrow Ag^+ + e^- \, (\text{oxidation}) \tag{12.7}$$

$$Ag^+ + Cl^- \leftrightarrow AgCl \, (\text{reduction}) \tag{12.8}$$

In summary, both the polarizable and non-polarizable electrodes are non-linear, exhibit a reactive behavior, alter the half-cell potential, cause resistive loss and are frequency dependent. A single sensor electrode–electrolyte interface can be modeled by a half-cell potential in series with a resistor–capacitor network; the magnitudes of both depend on the type of metal, its surface area, surface condition, any electric current density passing through the electrode and the type of electrolyte involved as well as its concentration.

12.3.3   The Sensor–Skin Interface

The ECG can be regarded as the potential difference between a pair of biopotential sensors placed on the surface of the body. Therefore the current flowing between two biopotential sensors applied to the skin must also pass the layers of the skin and the underlying tissues. The sensor–skin interface is critical for the sensing of biopotentials, since the electrically charged ions from the body volume conductor must pass through the skin to the body surface to engage in oxidation and reduction reactions at the electrode interface. In this section we shall discuss skin anatomy and its electrical properties [10].

12.3.3.1   Anatomical Details of the Skin

❯ Figure 12.13 shows the main features of the skin. The most superficial layer is called the epidermis and consists of the stratum corneum (SC), the stratum lucidum (seen only on "frictional surfaces"), the granular layer, the prickle cell layer, and the basal or germinating layer. The surface of the corneum (i.e., surface of the skin) is composed of dead cells, while at its base, healthy living cells are to be found. Between these two sites there are transitional cells. This layer is also called the horny layer. Blood vessels are present in the dermis whereas eccrine sweat gland secretory cells are located at the boundary between the dermis and the panniculus adiposus, also referred to as the hypodermis and the superficial fascia. The excretory duct of the eccrine sweat glands consists of a simple tube made up of a single or double layer of epithelial cells; this ascends to and opens out on to the surface of the skin. It is undulating in the dermis but then follows a spiral and inverted conical path through the epidermis to terminate in a pore on the skin's surface. Cholinergic stimulation via fibers from the sympathetic nervous system constitutes the major influence on the production of sweat by these eccrine glands.

From an examination of ❯ Fig. 12.14, it can be appreciated that the epidermis ordinarily has a high electrical resistance due to the thick layer of dead cells with thickened keratin membranes. This aspect is not surprising, since the function of the skin is to provide a barrier and protection against abrasion, mechanical assaults, and so on. The entire epidermis (with the exception of the desquamating cells) constitutes the barrier layer, a permeability barrier to flow. Experiments show its behavior to be that of a passive membrane.

The corneum is penetrated by the aforementioned sweat ducts from underlying cells. As these ducts fill, a relatively good conductor (sweat can be considered the equivalent of a 0.3% NaCl salt solution and, hence, a weak electrolyte) emerges, and many low-resistance parallel pathways result. A further increase in conductance results from the hydration of the corneum due to the flow of sweat across the duct walls, a process that is facilitated by the corkscrew duct pathway

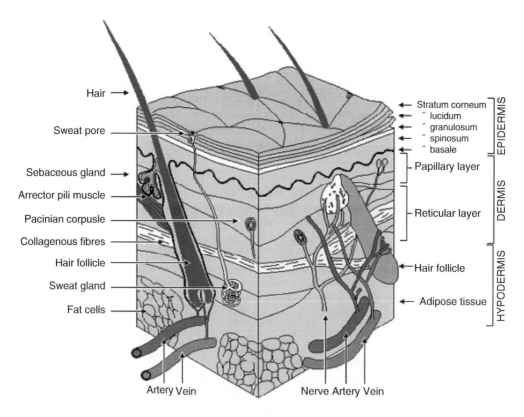

◼ Fig. 12.13

Main features of the skin. Section of smooth skin taken from the sole of the foot. Blood vessels have been injected (Redrawn from [11])

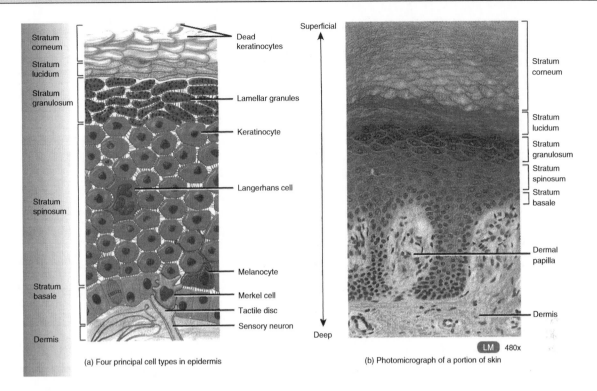

Stratum corneum — Dead keratinocytes

Superficial

Stratum lucidum

Stratum granulosum — Lamellar granules

Keratinocyte

Langerhans cell

Stratum spinosum

Stratum basale — Melanocyte

— Merkel cell

— Tactile disc

Dermis — Sensory neuron

Deep

Stratum corneum

Stratum lucidum

Stratum granulosum

Stratum spinosum

Stratum basale

Dermal papilla

Dermis

LM 480x

(a) Four principal cell types in epidermis

(b) Photomicrograph of a portion of skin

☐ Fig. 12.14
Skin layers involved in the passage of the ions

and the extremely hydrophilic nature of the corneum. As a consequence the effective skin conductance can vary greatly, depending on present and past eccrine activity. It should be noted that the loading of ducts with sweat can already be taking place before any (observable) release of sweat from the skin's surface and/or noticeable diffusion into the corneum. The exertion of sweat modifies the electric properties of the skin. These changes produce transient and non-linear changes in the skin impedance.

Just like the electrode interface, the electric properties of the skin can be modeled by equivalent capacitor and resistor networks. Their properties are based on measurements of the electric current flowing across the skin resulting from a rectangular voltage pulse applied between two electrodes on either side of the skin. It is believed that there are two parallel current pathways, one crossing the lipid-corneocyte matrix (m) of the SC, and the other going through the appendages (a). An equivalent electrical model of this system is shown in ❷ Fig. 12.15. The elements in the model are as follows.

Lipid-Corneocyte Matrix Pathway
From an electrostatic point of view, the m-subsystem of the SC can be considered as a dielectric with a resistance (R_m) of 105 Ωcm^2 and a capacitance (C_m) of 0.03 $\mu F/cm^2$ [12, 13].

The Corneocytes
The corneocytes (❷ Fig. 12.14) contain water and small ions resulting in an equipotential domain within these compartments. Thus, the potential drop across the SC occurs predominantly across the lipid domains between the corneocytes [13]. Such lipid domains can be described by parallel resistors and capacitors placed in a series, passing through the SC. There are on average 15–20 corneocyte layers in the SC, each separated by lipid domains of 0.05 mm thickness [14, 15].

The effective thickness of this non-conducting layer is 1 mm, yielding an effective dielectric constant of 15–20. This value is intermediate between that for lipids (2–3) and water (80) and is reasonable for hydrated lipid bilayers. This estimate suggests that the voltage drop is concentrated across lipid bilayers that are oriented "normal" to the electric field.

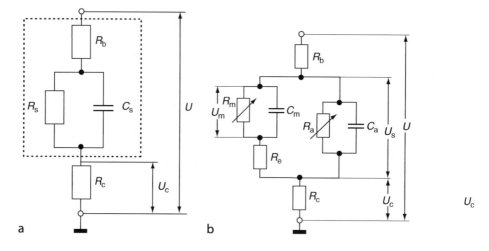

Fig. 12.15

The equivalent electrical circuit of an outermost layer of skin. (a) An integral model where R_b, R_s, and R_c are the resistances of bulk solution, skin, and measuring resistor, correspondingly; C_s is skin capacitance. (b) A more detailed version, including two parallel pathways. R_m and C_m refer to the lipid-corneocyte matrix, and R_a and C_a refer to the appendages

The SC matrix resistance (R_m) and capacitance (C_m) introduced in this way are frequency independent. If the time constant $(\tau_m = R_m C_m)$ of the network is small compared with that of the fluctuations of the processes involved, the equivalent scheme of the SC can be reduced to a simple voltage divider that includes four resistors in sequence, the bulk (R_b), epidermal (R_e), measuring (R_c), and matrix (R_m) resistances (❷ Fig. 12.15b).

12.3.3.2   Equivalent Circuits for the Interface

It is possible to create dedicated versions for polarizing and non-polarizing sensor–skin interfaces, similar to the simplified equivalent circuits for an electrode–electrolyte interface shown in ❷ Fig. 12.15. The version shown in ❷ Fig. 12.16 represents an example of the polarizing interface (steel-skin), and ❷ Fig. 12.17 that of a non-polarizing interface (Ag/AgCl). An inspection of ❷ Figs. 12.16 and ❷ 12.17 reveals that in addition to the resistive and capacitive components, and previously discussed half-cell potential E_{hc}, there are two other sources of potentials present in the model: one at the electrolyte gel/electrolyte–skin interface E_{se} and the other at the gel/electrolyte–sweat duct/follicle channels' interface E_p.

12.3.3.3   Practical Considerations

The physical size of the components and the properties of the electrolyte will govern their impedances; for this reason it is difficult to specify the magnitudes of the electromotive forces, reactances, and resistances. Nonetheless, a few general statements can be made regarding the characteristics of impedance–frequency measured between the electrode terminals. In the previous discussion, it was shown that the impedance of an electrode–electrolyte interface decreases with increasing frequency (❷ Figs. 12.8 and ❷ 12.9). Similarly, the capacitive nature of the electrical model for living tissue also indicates that its impedance decreases with increasing frequency. Therefore the impedance measured between the terminals of a pair of sensors applied to living tissue is high in the lower frequency region, decreases with increasing frequency, and approaches a relatively constant value when the reactances in the circuit become small with respect to their associated resistances. In general, with electrodes having a small surface area, the zero-frequency (i.e., direct current: DC) impedance is largely dependent on the electrode area.

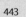

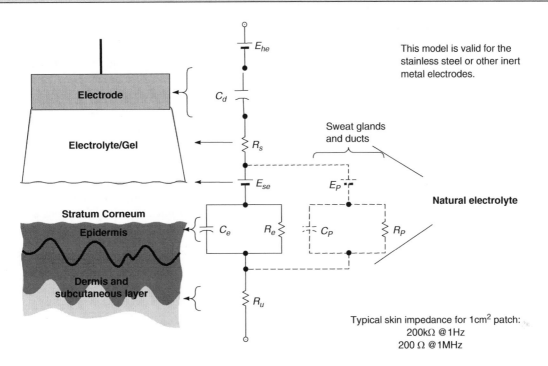

Fig. 12.16
The electrical model of a polarizing sensor in contact with the surface of the skin

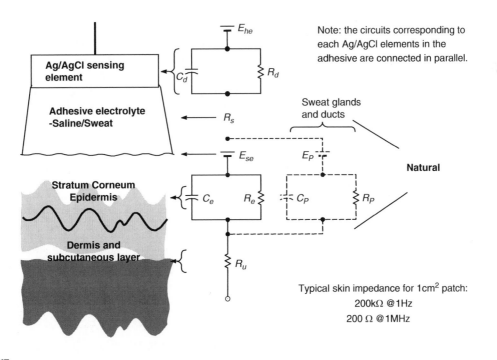

Fig. 12.17
The electrical model of a non-polarizing sensor in contact with the surface of the skin

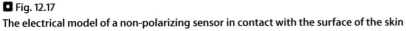

As mentioned previously, there may be a DC potential appearing across the electrode terminals in the absence of a bioelectric event. For example, if the two half-cell potentials of the electrodes are unequal, a constant potential will be present whose magnitude and polarity depend on the relative magnitudes of the two half-cell potentials. This offset potential is of considerable importance when direct-coupled recording techniques are employed.

12.3.3.4   Measurement Artifacts at the Galvanic Sensor–Skin Interface

As discussed in ❷ Sect. 12.3.1, when a polarizing electrode is in contact with an electrolyte, a double layer of charge forms at the interface [6, 16]. If the electrode is moved with respect to the electrolyte, this mechanically disturbs the distribution of the charge at the interface and results in a momentary change of the half-cell potentials until equilibrium can be re-established. If a pair of electrodes is placed in an electrolyte and one of these is shifted while the other remains stationary, a potential difference appears between the terminals of the two electrode cables. This potential is known as a motion artifact and can be a serious cause of interference in the measurement of biopotentials. The major components of this noise lie in the lower frequency range.

The electrode–electrolyte interface is not the only source of motion artifacts. The equivalent electric models in ❷ Figs. 12.16 and ❷ 12.17 show that E_{hc}, E_{se} and E_p can also cause motion artifacts due to movement of the sensor electrode.

The sensor itself is also a source of measurement noise, which depends on the electrode material (thermal noise), electrode impedance, electrode area, electrolytic gel, the patient, and the placement site. In the frequency band from 0.5 to 500 Hz, root-mean-square electrode noise is usually less than 1 μV for sensors placed face-to-face and ranges from 1 to 15 μV for sensors on the body surface. The spectral density of the noise is highest at low frequencies and it is always higher than the thermal noise from the real part of the electrode impedance. There is a high correlation between electrode offset voltage and electrode noise [17].

12.3.4   Survey of Biopotential ECG Sensors

The need for handy, easy-to-apply sensors with low offset voltage and low impedance, low artifact pickup, high stability of electrical properties and minimal skin irritation has resulted in the design of a number of different electrode types with varying modes of operation. Some typical examples and their advantages and disadvantages are as follows. A more comprehensive description of the theory and design of biopotential sensors can be found in [18, 19].

Most widely used present day ECG sensors utilize the electrolytic gel as a layer between the metallic electrode and the skin. These are commonly referred to as "wet-gel electrodes." Some variations of these sensors for applications in CCU monitoring are made of carbon, to render them X-ray transparent.

Due to the low cost of disposable wet-gel ECG sensors, reusable metal electrodes are less frequently used.

In specific applications dry ECG sensors with built-in amplifiers have been integrated into the sensor housings. Such sensors are referred to as "active electrodes."

Of late, major progress has been made in the development of new materials such as hydrogels, conductive polymers, spike electrodes, capacitive electric field pickups, impedance and optical probes for use in biopotential sensor design.

Offset voltage, low noise, low impedance, short-term stability (during the measurement) and sensor longevity on the body surface remain the design goals. Other important design parameters include considerations of possible biotoxicity of the sensor materials in direct contact with the body, skin irritation and shelf life.

12.3.4.1   Metal Electrodes

Metal electrodes are traditionally made of German silver (a nickel-silver alloy) or stainless steel [6]. Before being attached to the body, their surface is covered with an electrolytic paste or gel. These electrodes are of the "wet" type. They involve the use of an electrolytic paste or gel forming a conductive medium between the skin and the electrode.

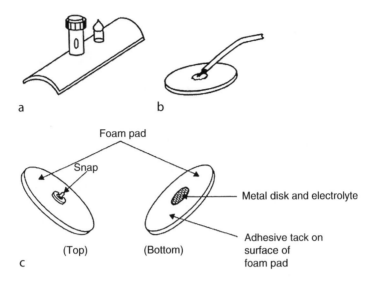

◘ Fig. 12.18

(a) Metal-plate electrode used for application to limbs. (b) Metal-disk electrode applied with surgical tape. (c) Disposable foam-pad electrodes, often used with electrocardiograph monitoring apparatus (From [6])

A typical stainless steel ECG electrode is made of stainless steel grade 304 or 316. Low half-cell potentials can be achieved in stainless steel electrodes if potassium citrate EDTA or sodium sulfate is used in the liquid gel. The electrochemical reactions that govern the operation of a stainless steel electrode include O_2 reduction and H_2 production at the cathode, coupled with O_2 production and formation of metal oxides at the anode, which cause much larger polarization effects than in the Ag/AgCl electrodes. Typical parameters: offset (mV) = 1–50, impedance 800–2,200 Ω and polarization 400–1,200 mV [20].

The large plate electrodes (3–5 cm), which were introduced in 1917 [21], are made of stainless steel, German silver (an alloy of nickel, copper and zinc), nickel or nickel-plated steel. To obtain a stable offset voltage and allow electrode-skin impedance, the metal electrode should be separated from the skin by a film of electrolyte paste.

Metal electrodes of the type shown in ❷ Fig. 12.18(a) are usually fixed by rubber straps. These electrodes are well suited for the limb leads, but not for the pre-cordial leads. For the latter, the accuracy of localization is poor and the unstable skin–electrode interface produces motion artifacts in the ECG signal.

The smaller metal disk electrodes of the type shown in ❷ Fig. 12.18(b) are made of nickel, a silver alloy sometimes coated with silver chloride or sintered material containing Ag/AgCl. In ECG recording these electrodes have diameters of 1–2 cm. A self-adhesive variation of the metal electrode for monitoring applications is shown in ❷ Fig. 12.18(c).

Metal electrodes are rarely used in clinical applications today due to their poor noise immunity and high cost, and due to concerns of cross-infection. The use of electrode paste or gel in routine clinical electrocardiography is a cumbersome procedure. Skin preparation of, and gel application to, each patient for each electrode is time consuming, and the multiple-use electrodes need to be cleaned regularly to maintain low noise and low electrode skin impedance. In long-term applications, gel or paste tends to dry out or may irritate the skin (❷ Table 12.2).

12.3.4.2   Pre-Gelled Galvanic Electrochemical ECG Sensors

A serious source of motion artifacts in solid metal reusable electrodes is caused by variations in a double layer of charge at the electrode–electrolyte interface. To minimize the measurement artifacts common in metallic electrodes, Ag/AgCl electrodes have been developed. Furthermore, in an effort to stabilize the skin–electrode interface, floating ECG sensors

◼ Table 12.2

Summary of the metal electrodes properties

Advantages	Disadvantages
Reusable	Poor noise immunity
Infinite shelf life	Not suitable for long-term applications
	Require liquid gel
	Possibility of cross infection
	Require sterilization
	Require cleaning
	Variable electrode–skin contact area
	Leaking gel causing excessive baseline drift
	High cost

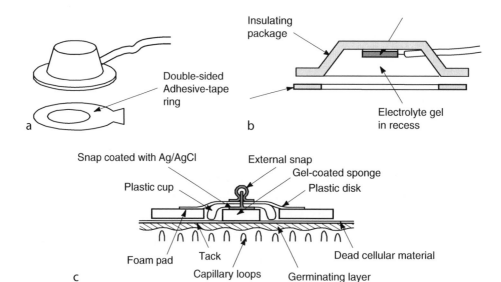

◼ Fig. 12.19

Pre-gelled ECG sensor assembly. The sensor comprises a metal snap coated with Ag/AgCl, which is embedded in an electrolytic gel filled cavity (From [6])

have been devised. Their advantage is high artifact immunity, due to the absence of a direct contact of the sensor metallic electrode with the skin. The single use foam-pad floating sensors are routinely used in rest, stress and monitoring ECG applications. There are many designs of floating sensors, which include metal electrodes and carbon electrodes with Ag/AgCl coated surfaces.

Another type of a pre-gelled ECG sensor comprises of a mesh woven from fine silver-coated wire, with a flexible lead wire attached (❷ Fig. 12.19) [22]. Adhesive electrolytic gel is applied to the mesh. Other models employ a carbon-filled silicone-rubber compound in the form of a thin film strip or disk, which is used as the contact element of the sensor. The lead wire is attached to the surface of the film strip. Such sensors are particularly suitable for the monitoring of newly born infants since the flexible sensors adapt very well to the curvature of a small chest. The thin silver film is X-ray translucent, so that these electrodes do not need to be removed for radiography.

A number of ultra flexible electrodes that use silver-coated nylon gauze and elastomeric materials, such as carbon-filled rubber and vinyls, silver-filled silicone rubber and silver-plated particle-filled elastomers have also been described in [23].

◘ **Table 12.3**

Summary of the pre-gelled ECG sensor properties

Advantages	Disadvantages
Reasonable noise immunity	Limited shelf life
Single use application	Poor longevity on the body surface
Commonly available from multiple sources	Require skin preparation
Low cost	Not suitable for long-term applications
	Prone to motion artifacts
	Skin irritation
	Poor skin adhesion, especially in hair and sweat

A flexible electrode system where conductive elastomers were used as the electrode element was described in [24]. The electrodes were developed for arrhythmia monitoring of high-risk patients in a field study involving telephone transmission of the ECG [25].

Patten [26] and Roman [27] described "spray-on" electrodes, which were applied directly to the skin. First, the electrode gel was rubbed into the skin with a toothbrush and the skin was then wiped dry with gauze. Subsequently, a film of conductive adhesive was painted or sprayed on the skin, forming a conducting spot of about 20 mm in diameter. A silver-plated copper wire was attached to the skin by conductive adhesive glue. After drying, a coat of insulating cement was applied, to cover the electrode. ECGs from spray-on sensors have been recorded successfully during 100 h in flight and on the ground for air force personnel, indicating that a sufficiently long-term stability of the skin–electrode contact can be obtained (❯ Table 12.3) [18].

12.3.4.3   ECG Sensors for Long-Term Monitoring and Stress Testing

Hospital applications require around the clock ECG monitoring patients during a typical 5-day hospital stay in post acute myocardial infarction (AMI) and coronary artery bypass grafting (CABG). A complete set of 12-lead ECG signals is required for an accurate assessment of acute and old coronary events. An onset of an acute myocardial ischemia usually manifests itself by the development of ST-segment and T-wave changes. ST-segment depression measured by an electrode overlying the injured area is believed to indicate subendocardial involvement, with less extensive myocardial injury. ST-segment elevation reflects transmural involvement, with greater extent of myocardial injury. Clinical decisions concerning treatment are based on ST-segment shifts in the body surface electrocardiogram. It is therefore very important to provide high fidelity ECG signals, since the detection of ST elevation myocardial infarction (STEMI) affects the choice of drug therapy and any accompanying procedures such as percutaneous coronary intervention [28].

Ambulatory applications are predominantly 24 h ECG Holter recordings, interpreted by computer-aided interpretation systems and read over by physicians. There is a growing need for longer term monitoring. Recently, Hindricks et al. [29] have demonstrated that 7 day Holter monitoring of patients after ablation for AF showed intermittent recurrence of AF not detectable by a 24-h procedure. In all ECG applications, signal morphology and rhythm analysis reveal the presence of acute and chronic heart disease.

12.3.4.4   Challenges Encountered in the Current Practice of ECG Monitoring

The traditional electrochemical ECG sensors described above suffer from the potential disadvantages inherent in wet systems, such as skin irritation, loss of electrical contact due to the drying of the paste or lead wires falling off, poor shelf life, etc. Success and failure of these gel- or paste-based electrodes is largely dependent on the hydration level of the skin. Long-term monitoring requires that the sensors and patient cables stay on the body surface for prolonged periods of time. The electrode-wire management imposes a significant burden on patients and caregivers.

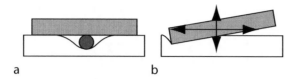

a   b

⬛ Fig. 12.20

(a) Loss of contact area and increase of contact impedance due to hair. (b) Loss of contact and increase of artifacts due to charging effects caused by motion of electrode relative to skin (Adopted from Anna Karilainen, Stefan Hansen, and Jörg Müller, Dry and capacitive electrodes for long-term ECG-monitoring. *8th Annual Workshop on Semiconductor Advances for Future Electronics and Sensors*, 1995)

Such wires need to be temporarily detached and then reattached each time a patient is bathed, leaves the bed, or is transported to another department, because current wired ECG monitoring requires a patient to be attached to a monitor by wires. Electrodes are frequently disposed of with each detachment, and new electrodes are applied with the reattachment. In addition to the demand on staff time and materials costs associated with these attachments and detachments, the current wired ECG systems also frequently generate false alarms due to movement of the lead wires and to artifacts due to inconsistent placement of the electrodes. These false alarms require a nurse to attend to the patient, and frequently involve detachment and reattachment of wires. Owing to significant difficulties in obtaining clean signals from wired ECGs in ICE/CCU and ambulatory (Holter) settings, at the present time 12-lead ECG monitoring is rarely used [30].

There is an increasing need for more reliable ECG monitoring technology and new methodology for long-term ECG monitoring.

In ambulatory monitoring, the shaving of a patient before application of the electrodes is often necessary. In long-term monitoring applications, even shaving does not produce stable results because of hair re-growth within a few days. A slightly invasive mechanical abrasion of the skin routinely performed in ambulatory care does not solve the problem because skin regenerates within about 24 h. A shift of the rigid electrodes relative to the skin caused by unavoidable movement of the patient (❯ Fig. 12.20) during long-term monitoring results in random variations of electrode contact area, which may cause severe motion artifacts.

A recent study suggests that reusable ECG electrodes may provide a reservoir for multidrug-resistant bacteria [31]. The author studied 100 selected ECG electrodes that had been reprocessed and were ready for use in new patients. He found one or more antibiotic-resistant pathogens on 77% of the electrodes. In a different study, in the burns ICU at a university medical center, contaminated ECG electrodes were found to have renewed vancomycin-resistant enterococcal (VRE) infections. It was found that in 18% of the cases studied, the ECG electrode cultures tested positive for VRE. In one case, rekindled VRE infection due to electrodes contaminated by a former burns patient were tracked. The present day standards of the Joint Commission on Accreditation of Healthcare Organizations (JCAHO) call for at least one activity in the infection control process to be aimed at preventing the transmission of infections.

12.3.5 Biopotential Fiber Sensors

A newly-developed biopotential fiber sensor (BFS) technology [32] aims at significantly reducing the size of the ECG sensors, eliminates the pastes and gels by the introduction of new sensor materials and does away with patient cables. A typical BFS sensor assembly combines the functions of the sensor itself, a lead wire and a patient cable.

12.3.5.1 Principle of Operation

An equivalent circuit of a galvanic biosensor, shown in ❯ Fig. 12.16, suggests that in order to minimize the impedance of the skin–sensor interface, the resistive contributions from electrolyte/gel and the skin itself must be minimized. A key issue in sensor design is the identification of transport pathways that allow body electrolyte molecules to pass through the

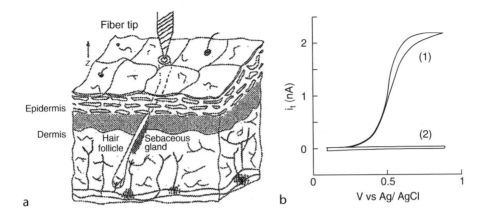

⬛ Fig. 12.21

(a) Schematic drawing illustrating the fiber tip positioned directly above the opening of a hair follicle. (b) Voltammetric response of a 20 μm-radius fiber tip positioned directly above a hair follicle opening in hairless mouse skin (curve 1) and 150 μm away from the opening (curve 2) (From [34])

skin. This can be accomplished by increasing the permeability of the skin and reduction of the gel/electrolyte resistance. Recent studies of the dependence of skin permeability on the contact area show that an array of smaller reservoirs is more effective in increasing transdermal electrolyte transport than a large single reservoir of the same total area. Karande [33] showed that Mannitol transport per unit area into and across the skin increased with a decrease in the area in contact with the skin. Mannitol permeability increased approximately sixfold with a decrease in the reservoir size from 16 to 3 mm in the presence of 0.5% SLS in PBS (phosphate buffered saline) as a permeability enhancer. Similar results were obtained when oleic acid was used as an enhancer. The molecular transport across the skin is also affected by hair follicles, which offer low resistance pathways for transport across the stratum corneum.

White [34] reported on studies of molecular transport in skin using scanning electrochemical microscopy (SECM) to investigate and quantify transport in artificial and biological skin and other membranes. ❷ Figure 12.21 shows the steady-state voltammetric response of the fiber tip when it is positioned directly above a hair follicle opening (curve 1) and at a lateral distance of ~ 150 μm from the opening (curve 2). In this experiment, the redox-active molecule is transported across skin by diffusion alone and is detected by oxidation at the fiber tip. The sigmoidal-shaped voltammetric curve recorded above the hair follicle (curve 1) corresponds to the oxidation of molecules that have diffused across the skin sample through the hair follicle. The magnitude of the tip voltammetric current is proportional to the local rate at which the molecule permeates the skin. The fiber tip current decreases to background levels (curve 2) when the tip is moved away from the pore opening, demonstrating that the diffusive flux of the molecules is localized to the hair follicle. The sites of highly diffusive flux are independently identified as hair follicles using a dye staining technique in which colloidal Prussian blue is precipitated at the opening of the follicle. Similar experiments using small organic and inorganic redox species, with different charges ($z = +1, 0$, and -1) indicate that hair follicles in skin act as the primary route for transdermal transport. The BFS takes advantage of both the follicular transdermal transport mechanism and enhancing arrays, which lower the skin permeability without the need for mechanical skin preparation.

12.3.5.2 Technology

The sensing fibers were developed by chemically impregnating the surface of synthetic acrylic fibers by metal molecules. The outer conductive layer of the fiber completely surrounded the inner part of the host fibers.

The fiber characteristics are: diameter: 20 μm; thickness of the electrically conductive layer: 30–100 nm; electrical resistance: 10^{-2} Ω cm.

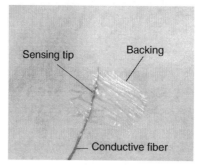

◾ Fig. 12.22
BFS applied to the body surface

The biopotential fiber sensors were made up of the conductive bundle comprising about 100 individual fiber strands coated with an Ag/AgCl ink. The Ag was deposited electrochemically on the exposed sections of the fibers. The Ag surface was chlorinated to AgCl. The chlorination process was performed in a solution of $KCl/AgNO_3$ (1 M, pH 1) at a constant current of 0.2 mA. For the realization of the thin-film sensor a rapid dipping technique was used. As a result, the Ag/AgCl ink was deposited on the outer layer of the fibers. The resulting sensors were treated for 2 h at 120°C. The Ag/AgCl layer of the sensor tip was further coated with a 5 μm layer of the conductive adhesive mixed with skin permeability enhancers (Parker Laboratories, Fairfield, NJ). The non-sensing surface areas of the fibers were coated with a 2.5 μm thick Parylene C layer. The uncoated ends of the conductive fibers were bonded by conductive epoxy (Creative Materials) to gold-plated contact pins of a standard DB-15 connector. The sensing areas of the fibers were applied directly to the unprepared skin and covered by thin transparent dressing (3 M, Tegaderm) as shown in ❷ Fig. 12.22.

12.3.5.3   Electric Performance

The following tests on the electric performance of BFSs were carried out; the results were compared with the ANSI/AAMI EC 12:2,000 standard for disposable ECG electrodes.

Environment: All tests were performed at 23 ± 5°C, relative humidity less than 10%.

- Average value of AC Impedance (kΩ) at 10 Hz. Test Conditions: The impedance of a pair of sensors connected surface-to-surface was determined by applying 20 μA p-p sinusoidal current and observing the amplitude of the resulting voltage across the sensors.
- DC offset voltage [mV]. Test Conditions: BFS's sensor pair connected surface-to-surface, continuous 200 nA DC current applied.
- Offset Voltage [mV]. Test Conditions: BFS sensor pair connected surface-to-surface, after 1-min stabilization.
- Combined offset instability and internal noise [μV]. Test Conditions: Sensor pair connected surface-to-surface, after 1-min stabilization, in the band of 0.15–100 Hz, for 5 min.

The results of the test are shown in ❷ Table 12.4. All measured parameters were comparable to wet-gel electrodes and well below the limits specified by the AAMI EC:12 standard [37] (❷ Table 12.5).

12.3.5.4   Clinical Testing

Due to their very small mass and excellent flexibility, biopotential fiber sensors can be attached directly to the skin, as shown in ❷ Fig. 12.23. An example of an exercise ECG recorded from BFS in a subject running up the stairs is shown in ❷ Fig. 12.24.

Table 12.4

Electric characteristics of BFS as compared to wet-gel electrodes and ANSI/AAMI EC12:2,000 limits

	Lead-lok wet-gel	BFS typical	ANSI/AAMI EC 12 Limits
DC offset voltage (mV)	0.15	0.11	Not more than 100
AC impedance @ 10 Hz (Ω)	51	22	Not more than 2,000
DC offset @ 5 s cap dis (mV)	0.7	0.4	Not more than 100
Recovery slope @ 30 s interval (mV/s)	0.0	0.0	Not more than 1.0
AC impedance after defibrillation (Ω)	49	18	Not more than 3,000

Table 12.5

Summary of the BFS sensor properties

Advantages	Disadvantages
Excellent noise immunity	May require more time to apply
Single use application	
Suitable for long-term applications	
No skin preparation required	
Excellent adhesion to the skin, especially in hairy chests	
Suitable for pediatric applications	
Long shelf life	
Low cost	

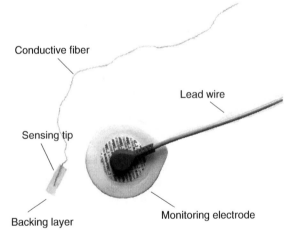

Fig. 12.23

BFS compared to a standard wet-gel monitoring electrode with an attached lead wire

12.3.6 Active ECG Sensors

A considerable research effort went into the development of "active sensors" that incorporate a high impedance amplifier into the sensor itself and required no wet gel or paste as a medium between the sensor electrode and the skin [35]. The placement of an electronic amplifier on the sensor itself is based on the idea that a high impedance amplifier is able to detect a signal from a high impedance source with a minimum of signal distortion, and then drive the signal through a long cable with a minimum of interference by virtue of the low output impedance of the amplifier [36].

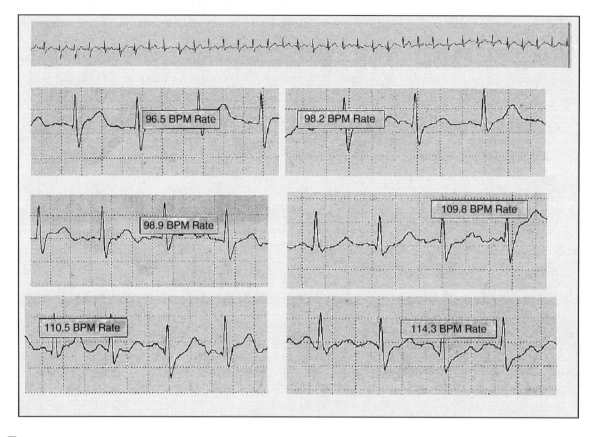

Fig. 12.24
Upper trace: A full disclosure strip of a subject walking vigorously. *Below*: Exercise ECGs recorded at 40 s intervals from a subject running up the stairs. King of Hearts ECG Monitor (Instromedix). Speed: 25 mm/s, Gain: 10 mm/mV, Highpass Filter: OFF, Lowpass Filter: 100 Hz

The idea of having the first amplifier stage integrated with the electrode probably goes back as far in time as the introduction of the transistor. Over the past years, researchers have described the realization of several prototypes, and in most cases these indeed offered the advantages in signal quality that were promised originally by the interference theory [37].

Advances in solid-state electronic technology have made it possible to record surface biopotentials utilizing electrodes that can be applied directly to the skin without abrading the skin or requiring the use of an electrolytic gel. These electrodes are not based on an electrochemical electrode–electrolyte interface. Rather, these electrodes are active and contain a very high impedance-converting amplifier [38]. In this way, biopotentials can be detected with minimal or no distortion. Burke [39] described an active biopotential sensor that utilizes a very low-power preamplifier, intended for use in the pasteless-electrode recording of the ECG. The input signal range of the amplifier was reported to be 100 μV to 10 mV. The amplifier provides a gain of 43 dB in a 3-dB bandwidth of 0.05 Hz to 2 kHz with a defined high input impedance of 75 MΩ. It uses a driven common electrode to enhance the rejection of common-mode interfering signals, including low-frequency motion artifacts, achieving a common-mode rejection ratio (CMRR) of greater than 80 dB over its entire bandwidth (❯ Sect. 12.4.1.2). The amplifier has a power consumption of 30 μW operating from a 3.3 V battery.

Valchinov [40] described an active sensor assembly developed for the measurement of small biopotentials on the body surface (❯ Fig. 12.25). This active sensor features an adjustable anchoring system designed to reduce the electrode-skin contact impedance, its variation and motion artifacts. This is achieved by increasing the electrode-skin tension and

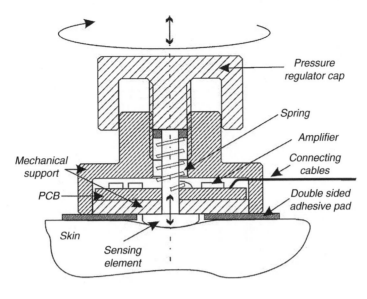

■ **Fig. 12.25**
An active sensor assembly with an anchoring system

decreasing its relative movement. Additionally the sensing element provides local constant skin stretching thus eliminating the contribution of the skin potential artifact. The electrode is attached to the skin by a double-sided adhesive pad, where the sensor is a stainless steel element, 4 mm in diameter. The front-end operational amplifiers (op-amps, ❷ Sect. 12.4.1.1) of the biopotential amplifier is incorporated in the sensors, thus avoiding the use of extra buffers. The biopotential amplifier features two selectable modes of operation: semi-AC mode with a −3 dB bandwidth of 0.32–1,000 Hz and AC-mode with a bandwidth of 0.16–1,000 Hz. The average measured DC electrode-skin contact impedance of the proposed electrode was 450 kΩ, with electrode tension of 0.3 kg/cm^2 on an unprepared skin of the inner forearm. The peak-to-peak noise voltage, with the input terminals connected to a common mode, was 2 μVp-p referred to the input.

The common-mode rejection ratio of the amplifier was 96 dB at 50 Hz, measured with imbalanced electrode impedances.

Although active electrodes offer the advantage of not requiring some of the preparation needed with conventional electrodes, they have certain inherent disadvantages. One problem is that many previously described designs, including DC biased transistor amplifiers, differential amplifiers, and amplifiers with gains above unity are not compatible with commonly-used ECG equipment unless some adjustment or modifications are made to the front-end of the electrocardiograph. Even with unity-gain, DC-biased transistor amplifiers that are capacitively coupled at the output cannot be conveniently used with different types of electrocardiographs without the risk of linear distortion caused by an impedance mismatch with the different electrocardiograph inputs, and without large transient DC offsets arising when switching leads (❷ Table 12.6).

Defibrillation voltages, static charge accumulation on the skin and clothes, and other medical equipment may cause potentials up to 25,000 V in contact with the input of the electrode amplifier, resulting in permanent failure of the device if not protected. Some designs made use of input resistors or unspecified current limiters for device and patient protection, but failed to show a means for compensating for the degradation of input impedance to the device as a result of parasitic capacitance coupling to ground through the resistor or current limiter. However, a means for adequately protecting the electronic circuitry from repeated exposure to high voltages, without compromising the essential electrical characteristics of the amplifier input, has not yet been devised.

Most active sensors are bulky in size due to the additional electronics and power sources required and they are typically more expensive to produce owing to the electronic assembly required. As of today, there has not yet been a breakthrough in the application of an active sensor to commercially available ECG recorders.

◻ Table 12.6

Summary of the active ECG sensor properties

Advantages	Disadvantages
Reasonable noise immunity	Limited shelf life
Single use application	Poor longevity on the body surface
Commonly available from multiple sources	Require skin preparation
Low cost	Not suitable for long-term applications
	Prone to motion artifacts
	Skin irritation
	Poor skin adhesion, especially in hair and sweat

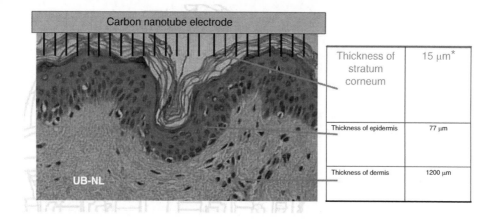

◻ Fig. 12.26

The principle of operation of the CNT biopotential sensor

12.3.6.1 Carbon Nanotube Active Biopotential Sensor

The experimental carbon nanotube (CNT) biopotential sensors [41] utilize a penetrating brush-like structure to provide an electrical contact with the skin (❷ Fig. 12.26). The nanostructure is designed to limit penetration of the stratum corneum of the skin in order to avoid direct contact with the dermis and prevent the risk of infection.

The principle of operation of the CNT biosensor named ENOBIO is similar to the spike electrodes described before. The sensor is shown in ❷ Fig. 12.27. The carbon nanotubes, which form a brush-like structure, are coated with silver and then treated with chloride to form an Ag/AgCl type of electrode interface. ENOBIO also features a high impedance amplifier built into the sensor assembly. The amplitude spectral density of the noise signal from the sensor was found to be 1.4 μV RMS in the range of 0.1–100 Hz (❷ Table 12.7).

12.3.7 Paste-Less Electrodes

The other "dry electrodes" reported in the literature comprise either metallic, ceramic or carbon-filled rubber assemblies, which are firmly attached to the body surface [42–44].

Direct skin contact dry ECG sensors for long-term monitoring have been devised. The sensors were embedded in a chest belt. The sensors, which are made of carbon-loaded rubber, are placed into a garment using a thermal molding process [24]. The ECG signal is passed from the body surface to the module PCB by means of a very thin and flexible shielded cable, anchored in the rubber of each sensor (❷ Table 12.8).

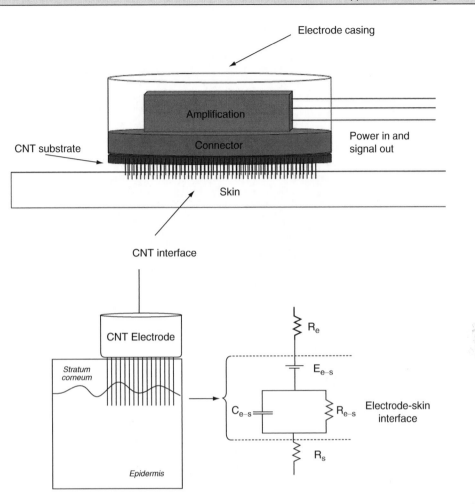

■ Fig. 12.27
CNT ENOBIO active biopotential sensor

■ Table 12.7
Summary of the ENOBIO sensor properties

Advantages	Disadvantages
Potentially better noise immunity	Experimental device
	May mechanically abrade the skin
	Nanotubes are potentially toxic
	Not compatible with existing ECG instruments
	Very costly
	Skin irritation
	Poor skin adhesion, especially in hair and sweat

Table 12.8

Summary of the properties of the "dry" sensors

Advantages	Disadvantages
Reasonable noise immunity	Higher noise levels than wet sensors
Longer shelf life	Relatively high cost
Suitable for long-term applications	Not widely avilable
No skin irritation	

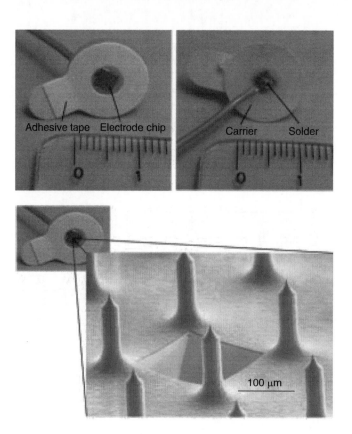

Fig. 12.28

Micromachined spiked electrode for measurement of biopotentials. The spikes are placed in the center of the adhesive foam collar, which affixes the assembly to the surface of the skin

12.3.7.1   Biopotential Sensors with Spiked Electrodes

In 2001, the Microsystem Technology Group of the Royal Institute of Technology (Stockholm,Sweden), in collaboration with the Datex-Ohmeda Division of Instrumentarium Corporation (Helsinki, Finland), presented the concept and fabrication of a micro-machined biopotential electrode, which requires neither electrolytic gel, nor skin preparation, nor an on-chip pre-amplification [45]. The principle of this electrode is based on the penetration of the living epidermis (LE) by micro-scaled spikes (i.e., micro needles). The skin penetrating system reduces the isolating influence of the stratum corneum (SC) on the electrode–skin impedance and brings the electrode into direct contact with the electrically conductive LE (❷ Fig. 12.28). The thickness of the SC, e.g., on the forehead or the forearm, is 10–20 μm. The thickness of the LE varies greatly locally but is approximately 150 μm.

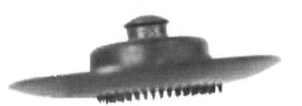

◘ Fig. 12.29
Commercial Spiked Electrode Biosensor [46]

The biopotential sensors with spiked electrodes were evaluated for their potential in long-term monitoring applications [45]. The authors of the paper observed a significant dependency of the electrode–skin–electrode impedance (ESEI) on the electrode size (i.e., the number of spikes) and the coating material of the spikes.

Electrodes larger than $3 \times 3\,mm^2$ coated with Ag/AgCl have sufficiently low ESEI to be well suited for recording of the biopotentials. The maximum measured ESEI was $4.24\,k\Omega$ and $87\,k\Omega$, at 1 kHz and 0.6 Hz, respectively. The minimum ESEI was $0.65\,k\Omega$ and $16\,k\Omega$ at the same frequencies. The ESEI of spiked electrodes was stable over an extended period of time.

The arithmetic mean of the generated offset voltage was 11.8 mV immediately after application of the ESEI to the skin and 9.8 mV after 20–30 min. A spectral study of the generated potential difference revealed that the AC part was unstable at frequencies below approximately 0.8 Hz, thus making them unsuitable for some diagnostic ECG applications. The spiked electrodes have found applications in EEG monitoring, where a low frequency response is not required.

A commercial version of the spike electrode for ECG monitoring applications as shown in ❷ Fig. 12.29 has been marketed by the Orbital Research Corporation.

12.3.8 Electrical Performance Testing for Disposable Electrochemical Biopotential Sensors

Regulatory agencies such as FDA in the US, EMEA in Europe and PMDA in Japan have adopted performance standards for disposable ECG electrodes exemplified by ANSI/AAMI EC12:2,000. They focus specifically on test methods and establish the minimum performance standards (ST) as discussed below.

12.3.8.1 AC Impedance

Human skin impedance varies from a few hundred to hundreds of thousands of ohms. Electrode impedance is important, because the higher the impedance, the more impedance imbalance is likely to occur between electrodes, thereby lowering the common-mode-rejection ratio (CMRR; ❷ Sect. 12.4.1.2) of the ECG amplifier and leading to increased AC interference. The 2 kΩ level specified in the standard represents a compromise, assuring the user of a low probability of interference problems caused by the electrode, while at the same time providing a generous flexibility in electrode design. In the monitoring applications, skin impedances are reduced to 1 kΩ or less by vigorous skin preparation (for example, ambulatory monitoring and stress testing).

Although ECG monitors incorporate protective devices to absorb overloads caused by defibrillation or electrosurgery currents, if the electrode's impedance is high, a substantial amount of heat may be generated at the skin–electrode interface, raising the probability of electrode failure as well as patient injury. The AC impedance requirement for purposes of quality assurance is specified by both a mean value and a permissible upper limit.

The measurement of impedance at 10 Hz, as currently specified in ST, has become an industry standard. The fact that currently marketed electrodes provide adequate performance, supports the adequacy of the 10-Hz measurement as a bench-mark for electrode performance. However, the AC impedance may not be a direct indicator of the sensor performance, since tests carried out by the Utah Biomedical Testing Laboratory (UBTL) indicated that the effective impedance of an electrode type, when tested on unprepared human skin, did not correlate well with the bench-test measurements of impedances for electrodes joined gel-to-gel. However, a 99% correlation was established between the results of tests on prepared (abraded) skin and those obtained using the bench test.

12.3.8.2   DC Offset Voltage

Because the input buffer amplifiers of cardiac monitors saturate under conditions of excessive DC offset voltage, a reasonable limit must be established regarding the offset voltage contributed by the electrodes.

The maximum allowable DC offset voltage was originally specified at 300 mV, based on the data gathered during the UBTL study [47]. The American National Standard on Cardiac monitors, heart rate meters, and alarms requires that cardiac monitors be capable of tolerating up to 300 mV offsets (AAMI, 1992). A 100 mV offset voltage limit for disposable ECG electrodes would provide reasonable assurance that electrodes conforming to this limit would be acceptable for use with most cardiac monitors. The 100 mV limit for ECG electrodes provides a sufficient operating margin to accommodate increases in electrode offset voltages caused by unequal potentials at the skin–electrode interface, defibrillation overloads, pacemaker currents, and/or ECG amplifier bias current.

The 100 mV offset voltage limit is adequate for accommodating the offset tolerance capabilities of currently available cardiac monitors, most of which can tolerate offsets of at least 200 mV. A DC offset voltage well below 100 mV would be beneficial, since emerging evidence links high offset voltages with motion artifact and other types of interference [48].

12.3.8.3   Combined Offset Instability and Internal Noise

At a 1977 conference on "Optimal Electrocardiography" convened in Bethesda, Md., by the American College of Cardiology, the Task Force on Quality of Electrocardiographic Records reserved its highest rating for baseline drift to those records exhibiting drifts of less than 0.1 mV/s [49]. Recordings exhibiting baseline drifts of 0.1–0.4 mV/s, while judged to be less desirable by the task force, were not considered unacceptable. Although electrocardiographic recording devices generally filter the signals to reduce or eliminate baseline drift, a contribution to the drift rate from the electrode–electrolyte interface of less than 150 V/s is desirable to ensure a minimal contribution by the electrode to the baseline wander.

12.3.8.4   Defibrillation Overload Recovery

After a defibrillation attempt, the ECG is important to the clinician in determining whether the heart has been returned to normal sinus rhythm. For this reason, the ECG trace must return within 5–10 s to an input offset voltage within the range that can be tolerated by cardiac monitors so that the condition of the patient can be assessed as rapidly as possible. During the next 30 s, the offset drift with time should not vary by more than 1 mV/s in order to display a clinically useful ECG. The prolongation of recovery time may also occur, due to the very high input impedance of the monitoring devices.

As many as 20–25 defibrillation attempts for an individual patient have been reported, suggesting the maximum number of consecutive defibrillation overloads that the electrode must absorb. However, this high number of attempts is unusual. An overload of 2 millicoulomb represents a worst-case condition that would be encountered only if the defibrillator paddles are placed in immediate contact with the ECG electrodes. Even if the electrodes are 10 cm (4 inches) away from the paddles, the overloads are likely to be reduced by only 50%. In most clinical situations, where skin preparation is sub-optimal, the circuit impedance will probably be much higher than the average of 1.5 kΩ encountered in UBTL animal testing [47]. On this basis, four consecutive discharges, delivered at 15–30 s intervals, should provide an adequate criterion for judging the performance of the electrode.

12.3.8.5   Bias Current Tolerance

When subjected to DC bias currents, the reactants involved in the chemical reactions occurring at the electrode–electrolyte interface can become depleted, which causes significant variations in the electrode half-cell potential. The ST demands that the compatibility of electrodes with the 200 nA bias current allowed for cardiac monitors must be demonstrated. Older monitors can have higher bias currents, so that a higher bias current tolerance for electrodes might be desirable.

12.3.9   Safety Requirements for Electrodes

12.3.9.1   Biological Response

Certain materials, if used in the fabrication of ECG electrodes, could cause skin sensitivity or skin irritation problems, especially if skin abrasion prior to electrode application is used to enhance the transfer of the ECG signal. The biocompatibility is defined in industry-wide standards such as ANSI/AAMI/ISO 10993:1997. Presently, no universal system exists to grade biocompatibility. Current practice relies on the expert who evaluates the test results and determines whether or not the material is biocompatible in the intended application. The determination of biocompatibility does not necessarily require testing in each new design. The expert, using his/her professional judgment, may decide that, based on the availability of biocompatibility data for the components, in conjunction with an evaluation of the intended application of the new design, additional testing is not required [50].

12.3.9.2   Preattached Lead Wire Safety

Historically, many electrodes with preattached lead wires were connected to the patient cable by means of male pins. There have been incidents where these pins were inserted into detachable power cords, thus applying full-line voltage to the patient. To ensure patient safety, the leadwire/patient-cable connector must not be permitted to make contact with a possibly hazardous potential, or a conductive surface that may be at ground potential, thereby compromising patient isolation.

12.3.9.3   Electrode Adhesiveness

The ability of an electrode to adhere satisfactorily to the skin over the expected period of use is an important feature of its performance. During the development of the initial 1984 standard, a study of the adhesiveness characteristics of disposable ECG electrodes, by the UBTL, did not yield a suitable bench test for evaluating adhesion performance; that is, a bench test that would correlate well with adhesiveness as observed clinically [47].

Over the last 10 years, progress has been made in identifying adhesive tests that can indicate how well certain adhesive systems will perform in ECG electrode applications [50].

12.3.9.4   ECG Cables and Lead Wire Standards

In 1995, the AAMI standard (ANSI/AAMI EC53:1995) on ECG cables and lead wires was published, addressing specific design requirements. It covers cables and patient lead wires used for surface electrocardiographic (ECG) monitoring in cardiac monitors as defined in the ANSI/AAMI EC13-1992 standard: Cardiac monitors, heart rate meters, and alarms. It covers both disposable and reusable lead wires, with certain sections applicable to both types, and certain sections applicable to one only.

This standard defines a safe common interface at the cable yoke and lead wire connector (no exposed metal pins). Specified are standards for: cable labeling, manufacturing, cleaning, disinfection, chemical resistance and sterilization exposure. Performance requirements (trunk cable and patient lead wires) include the following: dielectric voltage withstand, sink current, defibrillation withstand, cable and lead wire noise, flex life of instrument connector, cable yoke, patient lead wire connector, patient end termination flex relief, tensile strength of cable connections, number of connector mate/unmate cycles, contact resistance, connector retention force and patient lead wire resistance.

This standard also incorporates by reference the DIN 42–802 standard (Connector, touch proof, for electromedical application, 1990). Devices that comply with this standard also meet the FDA mandatory standard 21 CFR Part 898, "Medical Devices; Establishment of a Performance Standard for Electrode Lead Wires and Patient Cables."

The scope of EC53 excludes ECG cables and lead wires that are used in applications that may require special characteristics, such as ambulatory ECG devices, telemetry units, the operating room and the cardiac catheterization lab. The cables and patient lead wires included in the scope of EC53 also relate to other applications than ECG monitoring, such as respiration monitoring by impedance pneumography. The cable and patient lead wires should meet all of the requirements of this standard, unless a requirement is specifically excluded for that device by the standard.

12.3.10   Non-Contact Biopotential Sensors

A desire to replace wet ECG sensors prompted the research toward the development of the non-contact sensors that work on the principle of the displacement current in the body. These are referred to in the literature as insulated, capacitive or impedance probes. Richardson [51] and Lopez used an anodized aluminum disk as the electrode, though in a patent application they claim the use of any conductive material such as "copper, aluminum, or stainless steel having an insulation on its outer or skin contacting surface." In this particular case, the insulating coating was produced using an anodizing process. They maintained that the aluminum oxide can be used so that the film will be "free from pores or grain structure." To produce the film, they immersed the electrode in a standard sulfuric acid anodizing bath for 1.1 h. The process was finalized by dying the oxide, and immersing the electrode in hot water for oxide sealing.

To obtain the dimensions of the insulating layer, they measured the capacitance on the basis of which they calculated the thickness. For the said electrode, the resistance was greater than 4 GΩ and the capacitance was 5,000 pF.

Richardson et al. [51] concluded that "the production of motion artifacts caused by change in coupling capacity limits the use of this type of electrode." This is a major problem with a capacitive electrode-skin junction. With any kind of movement, the capacitance will change because the contact area will change. Despite many years of research, the capacitive insulated sensors have not yet exhibited the same consistency and signal to noise ratio (SNR) as the pre-gelled wet biopotential sensors.

The efforts to realize active insulated electrodes have been prompted by significant research and development in the area of sensor dielectrics. A number of materials have been investigated regarding thin-film capacitor fabrication in sensors of active hybrid electrodes. Some of the materials typically considered for use include silicon monoxide (SiO), silicon dioxide (SiO_2), silicon nitride (Si_3N_4), diamond-like carbon (DLC), and tantalum pentoxide (Ta_2O_5). In practice, deposited dielectric films thinner than 500–700 angstrom (Å) have a fairly high pinhole density and the yields are poor. Pinholes lead to resistive shorts between the electrodes placed in the vicinity of each other and increase the leakage current. Thick dielectric films, or films with a thickness greater than 20,000 Å, also may exhibit problems because of the high internal stress levels found in these films. High compressive forces cause the films to peel off; however, large tensile forces can be relieved by crazing, i.e., the production of fine cracks in the film. These factors thus have limited the thickness of the dielectric material to between 800 and 10,000 Å.

The progress in development of low noise Giga Ohm impedance probes [52] has further enabled research activities in the field of non-contact biopotential sensors.

12.3.10.1   Low Invasive Measurement of Electrocardiogram for Newborns and Infants

In 2003, a group of Japanese researchers reported on the development of a non-contact biopotential sensor for ECG applications in neonatal monitoring [53]. Here, thin silk fabric is used as an insulator between the skin and the sensor. The authors demonstrated that it is feasible to measure the ECG signal through silk with a capacitive sensor if the impedance of the capacitive probe is of the order of 10^{12} Ω at 10 Hz. Consequently, the input impedance of the measurement system

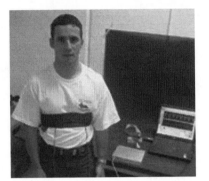

■ Fig. 12.30
This photo shows through-clothing biosignal recording

has to be higher or at least equal to 10^{12} Ω to detect stable ECG signal. Although the capacitive sensors produced stable ECG signals, they were attenuated at the high frequency range and could not be used for diagnostic purposes.

12.3.11 Recent Developments and Trends

Recent breakthroughs have been made in the form of miniature insulated biopotential sensors [53]. They can measure the electric potential on the skin without resistive electrical contact and with very low capacitive coupling. This has been made possible by a combination of circuit design and the use of a new, low-dielectric material. These sensors enable through-clothing measurements, and results from 40 subjects have shown them to be capable of a higher than 99% correlation with gold standard conventional electrodes. The capacitively coupled non-contact sensor (CCNS) utilizes high impedance, low noise probe technology that measures low frequency electric potentials in free space, i.e., without physical contact to any object. The process of biopotential recording through the clothing is shown in ❯ Fig. 12.30.

The CCNS produced signals that are morphologically very similar to the electrocardiogram recorded from the standard Ag/AgCl electrodes as shown in ❯ Fig. 12.31.

The first version of the CCNS biopotential sensor, including all amplification electronics, resulted in an approximately 1 inch square and 0.35 inch thick module (❯ Fig. 12.32).

12.3.11.1 A Prototype Biopotential Sensor Shirt

A non-invasive, zero prep time biopotential shirt system utilizing CCNS was developed for use with firemen. The shirt offers the first non-contact system of its kind, allowing an instantaneous biosignal collection (❯ Fig. 12.33).

In another development, common cotton was used as an insulator in between a capacitive sensor and the body. A sheet of conductive fabric was substituted for the conventional metal plate to realize a deformable coupling surface corresponding to the contour of the body [53] as shown in ❯ Fig. 12.34.

The measurement system involved is as shown in ❯ Fig. 12.35 (see also ❯ Sect. 12.4). It comprised of two buffer circuits, a differential highpass filter, an instrumentation amplifier, a lowpass filter, a highpass filter, a band elimination filter, an inverting amplifier, an A/D converter, and a personal computer. Two buffer circuits with high input impedance of 1000GΩ were employed for matching of the high impedance at the coupling involving cloth and the low impedance required by the subsequent circuitry. The differential highpass filter circuit (cutoff frequency: 0.05 Hz) was inserted in front of an instrumentation amplifier to reduce the low frequency component in the detected signal effectively prior to amplification. The cutoff frequency of the lowpass filter was set to 100 Hz. The notch filter was used in order to reduce 50 Hz interference. The total gain of the device was 60 dB.

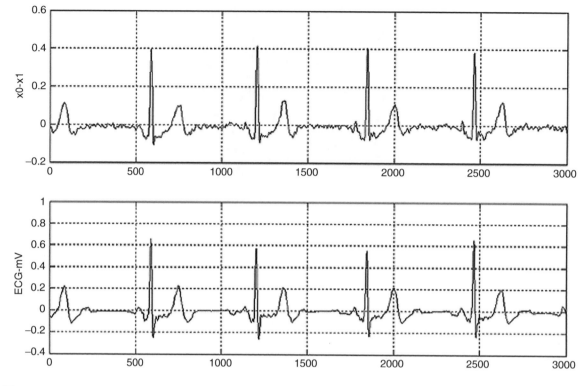

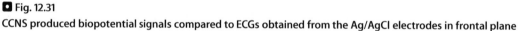

☐ Fig. 12.31

CCNS produced biopotential signals compared to ECGs obtained from the Ag/AgCl electrodes in frontal plane

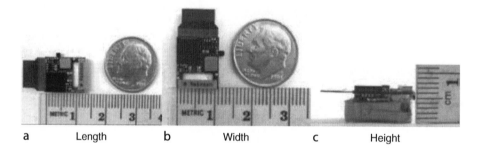

a   Length   b   Width   c   Height

☐ Fig. 12.32

The CCNS sensor assembly ($13\,mm \times 11\,mm \times 7\,mm$)

12.3.11.2   High Impedance Biopotential Optical Sensor

In 2003, Kingsley [54] reported on the development of a new non-contact ultra high input impedance biopotential sensor, which he named Photrode (❷ Fig. 12.36). The resistive part of its impedance can be as high as 10^{14} Ω, while the capacitive component is commonly a few picofarads. This allows the system to make non-contact capacitively-coupled measurements of ECG signals through clothing. The sensor requires no surface preparation or conductive gel. The Photrode is an optical modulator that employs an electro-optic material, in this case lithium niobate, to modulate the intensity of the light transmitted by the device. Unmodulated light from a laser or super-luminescent light emitting diode (SLD) enters the sensor and intensity-modulated light exits the device. The Photrode is a "Plug-N-GO" component that uses commercial fiber optic connectors at its pigtailed interfaces. A special type of single-mode fiber called a polarization-maintaining fiber

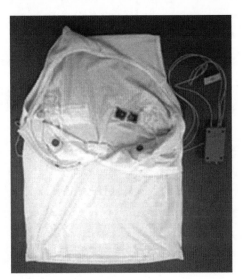

■ Fig. 12.33
A prototype biopotential sensor shirt for real time measurement of the electrocardiogram

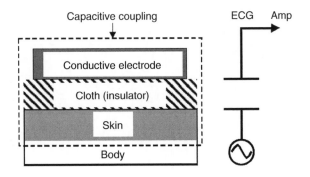

■ Fig. 12.34
A model of a capacitive biopotential sensor coupled to the body surface through cloth

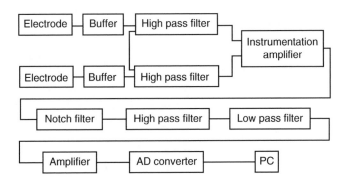

■ Fig. 12.35
Block diagram of the ECG measurement system for capacitive biopotential sensors

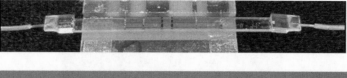

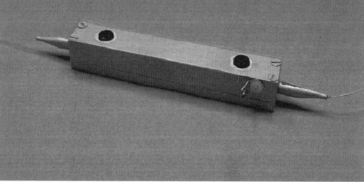

◘ Fig. 12.36

Photograph showing a prototype packaged PhotrodeTM designed for ECG and EEG signal monitoring. The *upper picture* **shows the bare optical chip, about 5 cm in length**

◘ Table 12.9

Summary of the non-contact displacement current biopotential sensors

Advantages	Disadvantages
Reasonable noise immunity	Non-standard ECG signal
Multiple use application	Not compatible with standard ECG instrumentation
Excellent longevity on the body surface	High cost
Requires no skin preparation	
Suitable for long-term applications	

connects the device to the light source. A second, single mode fiber conveys the modulated light to an optical receiver, where the signal is converted back to the electronic circuitry, where the ECG signal is processed in a similar fashion to the small voltages that would normally be obtained from a conventional electrode (◗ Table 12.9).

12.3.11.3 Electroactive Fabrics and Wearable ECG Devices

Promising recent developments in material processing, device design and system configuration have enabled the scientific and industrial community to focus their efforts on the realization of smart textiles. All components of a wearable ECG system (sensors, electronics and power sources) can be made from polymeric materials, to be woven directly into textile structures (sensing micro-fibers) or printed or applied onto fabrics (flexible electronics). In particular, intrinsic sensing, dielectric or conductive properties, lightness, flexibility and the relative low cost of many electroactive polymers makes them potentially suitable materials for the realization of such systems.

The use of "intelligent materials" enables the design and production of a new generation of garments incorporating distributed sensors and electrodes [55, 56]. Wearable non- obtrusive systems will permit the user to perform everyday activities with minimal training and discomfort.

A shirt was functionalized with CLR piezo-resistive fabric sensors used to monitor respire trace (RT), and conductive fabrics used as electrodes to detect the ECG [57].

To record the ECG signals, two different square-shaped fabrics (1×1 cm) were used: the first was made with steel threads wound round acrylic yarns, the second with a layer of acrylic/cotton fabric coupled with a layer containing stainless steel threads. In order to assess their performances, the signal originating from an Ag/AgCl electrode (Red Dot by 3 M) was recorded simultaneously with the signal detected by the fabric electrode.

12.3.11.4 Trends

The recent advances in miniaturization of ECG devices, as well as mobile computing, have fostered a dramatic growth of interest in wearable sensor technology.

The interest in wearable ECG systems stems from the need to monitor patients over extensive periods of time and reinforces the "doctor is always with you" paradigm since the usual clinical or hospital monitoring of the electrocardiogram provides only a brief window on the status of the patient. Practical wearable ECG systems require to be quite non-obtrusive devices that allow physicians to overcome the limitations of ambulatory technology and provide a response to the need for monitoring individuals over weeks or even months. They will rely on wireless, miniature sensors enclosed in patches or bandages, or in items that can be worn, such as personal jewellery or underwear.

Wearable ECG sensors and systems have evolved to the point that they can be considered ready for clinical application. This is due not only to the tremendous increase in research efforts devoted to this area in the past few years but also to the large number of companies that have recently started investing in the development of wearable products for clinical applications. The current upward trend in the use of this technology suggests that soon wearable ECG systems will be part of routine clinical evaluations. Wearable devices that can intermittently or continuously monitor and record good quality ECG signals will offer an important solution to the limits imposed by traditional monitoring schemes [58, 59].

12.4 ECG Signal Recording and Basic Processing

As discussed in ❯ Chap. 10, ECG leads are the signals that represent the time course of the electric potential differences that are observed between any two terminals of a configuration of electrodes attached to the body surface. In its most simple form, a lead represents the potential difference between the ends of the two electric wires connected to the two sensors attached to the body surface (❯ Fig. 12.37).

For most lead configurations the potential difference generated by the heart is typically of the order of 1 mV and, for subsequent display and interpretation of the signal, amplification is needed. Connecting the two wires to a modern electronic amplifier will generally not affect the voltage difference present.

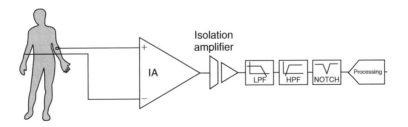

❑ **Fig. 12.37**
ECG Signal processing chain. The biopotentals measured by the sensors are applied to the front-end of an instrumentation amplifier (*IA*). For safety reasons the front-end is often isolated from other processing circuits by an isolation amplifier that limits current flow from the recording equipment to the patient. The ECG signal is band limited by a combination of a low-pass filter (LP) and a highpass (HP) filter that minimize signal aliasing (Appendix Section "Sampling Theorem and Analog Filters") and cut off the DC voltage, respectively. A notch filter of 50–60 Hz is frequently used to minimize the power line interference

Next to amplification, ECG measurement and recording systems perform some basic signal pre-processing steps. These may be carried out in analog and/or digital signal processing modules. The need for such signal processing steps and the way in which these are implemented are discussed in the next sub-sections as well as in Appendix Section entitled "Basic Digital Signal Processing." This section treats the most basic notions and principles only. For a more comprehensive treatment of signal analytical methods the reader is referred to the textbooks dedicated to this topic, in particular to ❯ Chap. 7 of: Bioelectrical Signal Processing in Cardiac and Neurological Applications by L. Sörnmo and P. Laguna [60].

12.4.1 Amplification and Analog Signal Processing

The potential difference between the two input terminals of the amplifier shown in ❯ Fig. 12.37 does not signal just the potential field generated by the heart's electric activity. It also includes contributions of several other sources, the most important ones being: the sum of the two half-cell DC voltages (hundreds of mV) at the sensors (❯ Sect. 12.3.3), the contributions of other bioelectric sources within the patient (muscular activation) and the interference from electromagnetic fields surrounding the patient, e.g., generated by the power line, RF or radio frequencies, electro-surgery devices etc.

The electric part of the electromagnetic field is passed to the body by currents flowing through the (small) capacitance between the power lines and body surface, returning to the "earth" or "ground" of the power line via similar such capacitances. This sets up a potential difference with respect to earth that is common to both electrodes.

12.4.1.1 Front-End of the Amplifier

The first stage of the instrumentation amplifier (IA in ❯ Fig. 12.37), its front-end, serves to raise the signal amplitudes to some desired level and also to reduce the representation of any potential that both sensors may have in common relative to the ground of the power supply of the recording equipment. Its basic design is shown in ❯ Fig. 12.38.

The triangles shown represent standard operational amplifiers. These have a very high amplification factor; the resistors shown set the actual, overall amplification of the configuration. Ideally, the potential at the output of the second stage shown should be proportional to $V_{ab} = V_a - V_b$ and be completely independent of the mean value of V_a and V_b, the

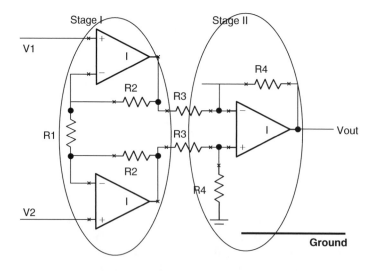

□ Fig. 12.38
First two stages of an ECG instrumentation amplifier

value the sensing electrodes a and b have in common. By using highly accurate, identical values for the resistors having a common label, a high rejection of the common, mean potential can be achieved.

12.4.1.2   Common Mode Rejection

An outline of the complexity of power line (50/60 Hz) interference, as well as of methods for minimizing its contribution to the ECG signal, is shown in ❷ Fig. 12.39.

The capacitances C_{pw}, C_{ca}, C_{ab} couple the body, lead wires and the power supply to other sources of the electromagnetic interference such as 50/60 Hz power lines.

The potential differences at the ECG sensors with reference to "ground" that arise from the capacitive coupling to the mains are almost identical. This creates a common component that, ideally, would not be present between the two terminals of the ECG lead. However, the recording equipment is generally also coupled to the ground of the power line, be it capacitively or galvanically. The provision shown in ❷ Fig. 12.38, referred to as the right leg drive, aims at minimizing any incomplete rejection of the common mode interference achieved by the front-end discussed in ❷ Sect. 12.4.1.1.

The right leg drive demands the incorporation of an additional electrode (sensor). Its position may influence the quality of the common mode rejection. However it does not, or at least should not, affect the observed wave forms related to the electric activity of the heart. Ten electrodes (wires) are attached to the patient when recording the standard 12-lead system. Besides the right leg electrode, three of the remaining nine electrodes, viz. the three electrodes placed on the other extremities are involved in the definition of Wilson's Central Terminal serving as the reference for the cardiac potential fields. As discussed elsewhere, e.g., ❷ Chap. 11, the maximum number of independent signals contained in the standard 12-leads is eight.

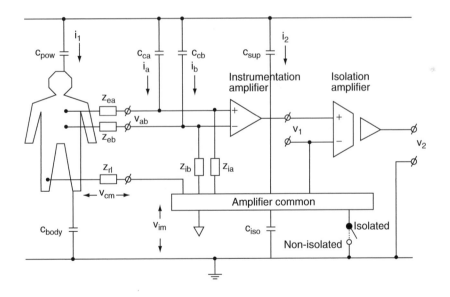

◘ Fig. 12.39

A simplified diagram illustrates the environmental sources of interference in ECG measurement. C_{pw}, C_{ca}, C_{ab}, and C_{sup} capacitances couple the sources of electromagnetic energy to the body, lead wires, and power supply respectively. C_{body} and C_{iso} capacitors provide a path to ground for AC leakage currents. V_{im} is the potential between the ECG amplifier common and ground, V_{cm} is a common mode potential on the body surface. I_1, i_a, i_b and i_2 are the AC interference currents. Z_{ea} and Z_{eb} are the equivalent skin–sensor impedances, Z_{rl} is the impedance of the ECG common, the right leg. The Z_{ib} and Z_{ia} are the input impedances of the instrumentation amplifier. V_1 and V_2 denote the non-isolated and the isolated ECG signals respectively (From [61])

12.4.1.3 The Isolation Amplifier

The isolation amplifier indicated in ❯ Fig. 12.37 is included for safety reasons. It isolates the patient from other processing circuits by limiting current flow from the recording equipment to the patient. It demands a galvanically isolated, battery powered front-end. The coupling to the main recording equipment may be achieved by using fiber glass transmission or, RF transmission.

12.4.1.4 The Highpass Filter

The most common disturbance encountered in the ECG signal is the one caused by changes in the half-cell potentials at the sensor–skin interface, which also affect the electrode impedance (❯ Fig. 12.40). This may be due to motion artifacts, temperature changes, changes in skin moisture (perspiration) and leaking gel or paste [55, 56]. This is particularly important in stress testing, respiration and monitoring applications, since the sensors tend to peel off and the skin contact under the sensors change when patients move. The resting ECG signals often show the artifacts caused by respiration or by muscle tremor at low temperatures. Additionally, poor skin preparation on subjects with hairy chests may create noise due to poor sensor adhesion and high skin–sensor impedance interface.

Even during the resting state, the changes at the sensors may give rise to potential fluctuations in the ECG that are larger than the ECG itself. Fortunately, under these conditions the changes have a low frequency spectrum, with frequencies lower than those present in the ECG. The observed effect on the ECG is that of a slowly wandering baseline. This permits the reduction of the so-called baseline wander by means of highpass filtering in the frequency domain of the signal (Appendix Section "Sampling Rate"), a procedure generally carried out in the front-end of the amplifier. Its most simple form of implementation is that of including capacitors in the wires connecting the sensors to the amplifier. The cutoff frequency used depends on the particular application involved.

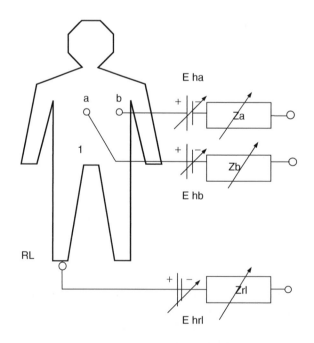

☐ Fig. 12.40

Sources of measurement artifacts in ECG signal acquisition. Eha, Ehb and Ehrl denote the variable sensor half-cell potentials, Za, Zb and Zrl the skin–sensor impedances

Even during the resting state, the changes at the sensors may give rise to potential fluctuations in the ECG that are larger than the ECG itself. Fortunately, under these conditions the changes have a low frequency spectrum, with frequencies lower than those present in the ECG. The observed effect on the ECG is that of a slowly wandering baseline. This permits the reduction of the so-called baseline wander by means of highpass filtering in the frequency domain of the signal (Appendix Section "Sampling Rate"), a procedure generally carried out in the front-end of the amplifier. Its most simple form of implementation is that of including capacitors in the wires connecting the sensors to the amplifier. The cutoff frequency used depends on the particular application involved.

12.4.1.5 The Lowpass Filter

An additional undesirable component in the ECG is the one generated by the electric activity of skeletal muscles. This interference hinders in particular the interpretation of the ECG during exercise-stress testing, or long-term (holter) monitoring. Here, major parts of the frequency spectrum lie above those of the ECG signals, and a lowpass filter can be used to reduce their effect (❯ Fig. 12.37).

Another application of this lowpass filter is that of reducing the influence of the aliasing effect (Appendix Section "Sampling Filters and Analog Filters) that crops up when digitally processing the signals originating from the analog amplifier.

12.4.1.6 Strategies for Ensuring a High Signal Quality ECG Acquisition

Great care must be exercised in the selection of the instrumentation amplifier and in particular of the components at its front-end. Here, very high input impedance, low noise instrumentation amplifiers, involving precision laser trimmed resistors are used for obtaining a high common-mode rejection ratio (CMRR). In addition, most modern front-end designs utilize active elimination of the common mode interference [56, 61, 62] by applying common mode noise signals in the opposite phase to the right leg drive (ECG common), as shown in ❯ Fig. 12.39 and, a more basic variant, in ❯ Fig. 12.41 [63].

Interfering electric signals from muscles and the internal organs form a composite signal with the ECG and cannot be easily filtered out without affecting the bandwidth of the ECG. Good skin preparation and the relaxation of subjects usually results in lower muscle tremor and baseline shifts.

The power line frequency 50/60 Hz and its harmonics, RF and radio frequency interference are usually eliminated by careful shielding of the lead wires, patient cables and signal filtering [64].

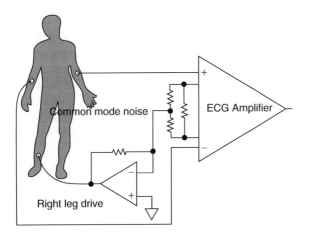

◨ **Fig. 12.41**
Right-leg drive circuit used in ECG front-end designs that minimize common mode "noise"

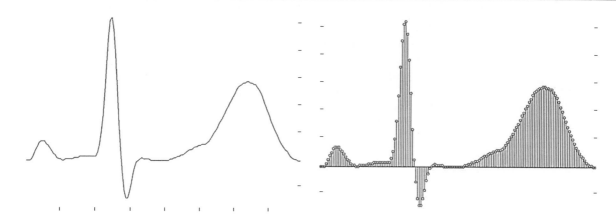

◼ Fig. 12.42

Left: original analog ECG; *right*: a digitized variant. Time interval shown: 640 ms

APPENDIX: Basic Digital ECG Signal Processing

A. van Oosterom

Department of Cardiomet, University of Lausanne, Lausanne, Switzerland

Conversion to Digital Data

Modern ECG systems utilize microcomputers or dedicated digital signal processors (DSP) for ECG signal display, storage, analysis and transmission. This requires that all analog lead voltages must be converted to numbers, i.e., their digital equivalents.

Analog to Digital ECG Signal Conversion

The values of continuous time-domain ECG signals at discrete time intervals can be extracted by means of an electronic device: the analog-to-digital converter (ADC). An example of the result of this procedure is shown in **❷** Fig. 12.42. The ECG signal on the left depicts the continuous, analog signal, the one on the right its digitized variant.

The individual, documented numbers representing the instantaneous signal values are referred to as the samples of the signal, the intervals between the subsequent samples being at the sampling interval T_s, which is 4 ms for the example shown in **❷** Fig. 12.42 (right panel). An alternative, equivalent specification is the sampling rate $f_s = 1/T_s$, the number of samples taken per second. Its unit is sps, s^{-1}, or less accurately, Hz.

The display of the result of the AD conversion used in **❷** Fig. 12.42 has been chosen to emphasize the fact that the result of the digital signal conversion does not specify signal values in between the subsequent samples. The display used in practice usually does not show the vertical lines that mark the individual samples. Instead, the subsequent values of the samples are connected by continuous line segments found by means of an interpolation procedure based on neighboring sample values. Note, however, that the actual information stored is that specified by the sample values only.

Sampling Rate

The amount of detail present in the analog signal that is retained in the digitized signal depends critically on the length of the sampling interval or, equivalently, on the sampling rate. The sampling interval dominates the accuracy with which derived signal features like peak amplitudes and their timing in the analog version of the signal can be recovered from the digital data.

For any duration P of a signal segment to be stored, the number of samples N_s is

$$N_s = P/T_s = D \times f_s \qquad (12.9)$$

The use of higher sampling rates imposes not only a greater demand on the quality of the AD converter but also on the storage capacity of the digital device. This number is multiplied by the number of signals that one may wish to record simultaneously. This poses the question of which sampling rate should be used.

The required sampling rate is linked to the amount of detail that might be contained *within* a sampling interval: the higher this information is expected to be, the higher the sampling rate should be. The "amount of information" is a notion that requires to be specified before the required sampling rate can be selected. The commonly-used specification makes use of the representation of the signal in the so-called frequency domain, a domain based on the theory of the Fourier series. A brief description of this theory is as follows.

Any biological signal recorded over a restricted period of time P can be represented by a constant A_0 to which is added a weighed sum of sinusoidal wave forms having frequencies that are integer multiples of the basic frequency $f_b = 1/P$. The sinusoids having frequencies $f_k = k \times f_b$ ($k = 1, 2, 3, \ldots$) are called the harmonics of the basic frequency. For $k = 1$, this identifies the sinusoid at the basic frequency as the first harmonic of the signal.

The constant A_0 is the mean value of the signal over the period P. This constant component can be interpreted as having zero frequency, and is referred to as the DC component of the signal. The mean value of the sum of the sinusoids is zero, since, for each harmonic, integer numbers of complete sinusoids are contained within the segment P, and the mean value over time of a complete sinusoid is zero.

By specifying A_0 and the amplitudes A_k for each of the harmonics, as well as a set of individual phase shifts φ_k the entire wave form can be represented at any desired precision, provided that the number of harmonics included is sufficiently large. This shifts the question of specifying the amount of information to: what is the number of harmonics needed? The answer to this question evolves from performing a Fourier analysis of the signal. Applied to sampled signals, this analysis can be carried out by means of the discrete Fourier transform (DFT), from which the amplitudes A_k are computed. The plot of the amplitudes A_k as a function of the frequency $f_k = k \times f_b$ results in the so-called amplitude spectrum. The squared amplitudes form the basis of the so-called power spectrum.

For biological signals, invariably the spectra tend to zero for high values of f_k. Performing a reconstruction of the signal (Fourier synthesis) on the basis of the first K harmonics results in a signal that is almost a replica of the original signal, provided that a sufficiently high value of K is used. If this is possible for a finite number of K, the signal is said to be band limited to frequency f_K.

For progressively lower values of K, the reconstruction results in increasingly larger deviations between the original and the resynthesized signal. Based on this type of analysis the maximum frequency content of the signal is defined as f_K. The final step in the procedure follows from a result stemming from communication theory. It states that for a signal that is band limited at frequency f_K, the number of samples needed for a perfect, i.e., error free, resynthesis should be at least $2 \times K + 1$. This result relates to the fact that the synthesis of the signal requires the specification of the values of K amplitudes, K phases and the DC component. This puts the minimal required sampling rate at

$$f_s \geq \frac{2K+1}{P}; \ 2K\frac{1}{P} = 2K f_b = 2f_K, \qquad (12.10)$$

expressed in words, the minimal required sampling rate f_s of a signal having harmonics up to the frequency f_K should be at least twice f_K. The variable f_s is known as the Nyquist rate [65]. Correspondingly, the highest frequency possible in a DFT spectrum is $f_K = f_s/2$.

Sampling Theorem and Analog Filters

No ECG signal is truly and perfectly band limited. Signal component at frequencies above f_K may be judged to be unrelated to the heart's electric activity, but rather to the activity of, for example, skeletal muscles. This would allow the suppression of such signal components by means of analog lowpass filters (➋ Fig. 12.37) prior to the AD conversion step, with their cutoff frequency set at f_K. It prevents the influence of such high frequency components on the sampled signal. Without the inclusion of the filter, the Fourier spectrum, of the signal sampled at the then too low sampling rate, will include contributions of the signal components above f_K. This effect is known as aliasing; it is reduced by the inclusion of the analog lowpass filter.

In practice the signals are often sampled at frequencies that are much higher (up to 5 times) than the minimum value required by the sampling theorem (12.2). This facilitates the subsequent display of the data as well as their analysis.

Basic Digital Signal Processing

After AD conversion, the analog signal $x(t)$ is replaced by a series of numbers

$$x(t) \Rightarrow [x_1, x_2 \ldots x_i \ldots x_N] \tag{12.11}$$

with x_i the value of the sample of the analog signal taken at time $t = t_i$ and N the total number of samples taken. Subsequent digital signal processing procedures are applied to this series. These include:

1. filtering, now by digital filters,
2. identification of timing of onsets and endpoints of signal wavelets,
3. timing of extreme values (peak amplitudes of the signal, like R wave, etc.,
4. extraction of extreme values and slopes,
5. suppression of any power line interference that may remain after the analog filtering,
6. the specification and/or correction of the baseline of the signal.

Some of these procedures affect the wave form of the signal. When inspecting any ECG signal presented on a monitoring device one should be aware of the fact that what is seen may not be the same as what is sensed by the electrodes. Below, a few examples of this are demonstrated. The wave forms shown relate to the signal of lead V3 from a healthy subject, sampled at 1 ms intervals. In their display the subsequent samples are connected by straight line segments. The input signal is shown in ➋ Fig. 12.43. It depicts the output of the AD converter. The setting of the analog filters (➋ Fig. 12.37) were lowpass at 500 Hz, and highpass at 0.2 Hz. With the healthy subject at rest in the supine position, the baseline wander, although clearly present, was small.

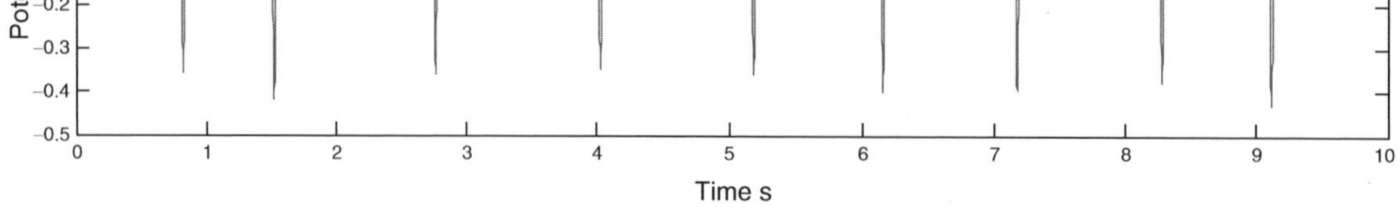

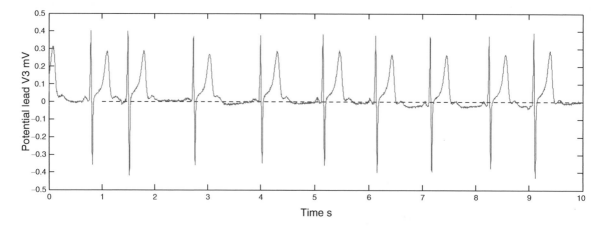

Fig. 12.43
Output of an AD converter; 10 s episode from a recording of lead V3

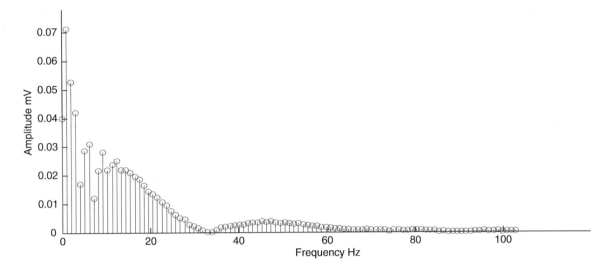

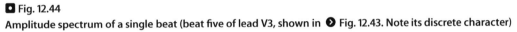

□ Fig. 12.44
Amplitude spectrum of a single beat (beat five of lead V3, shown in ❷ Fig. 12.43. Note its discrete character)

Amplitude Spectrum

The amplitude spectrum of the signal during the full duration of a single beat (beat five in ❷ Fig. 12.43), determined by means of the discrete Fourier transform (DFT), is shown in ❷ Fig. 12.44.

Although the output of the DFT computed over the P = 972 ms duration of the beat, taken from samples at 1 ms intervals, contains frequencies up to $f_K = f_s/2 = 0.5^*1{,}000 = 500$ Hz, only the lower-frequency part of the spectrum is shown here, the amplitudes of the higher frequencies are much smaller than those below 100 Hz. This indicates that the sampling rate used for this signal is more than adequate. As discussed in the previous subsection, the frequency resolution is $f_b = 1/P = 1.029$ Hz.

For intra-cardiac signals, the fast down-stroke of the observed electrograms may demand higher sampling rates. A correct representation in the frequency domain of fast signal segments demands the inclusion of spectral components of high frequencies.

The display method chosen for ❷ Fig. 12.44 emphasizes the nature of spectra obtained by using the DFT. In that method, the implied signal representation beyond the period analyzed is that of an infinite periodic repetition of the segment analyzed, thus typifying the method as computing a Fourier series representation rather than a Fourier transform. In most ECG spectra figuring in the literature, this aspect is hidden as a result of the method employed of connecting the individual spectral values by means of continuous line segments.

As discussed in ❷ Sect. 12.4.1, the output of the analog amplifier usually includes a highpass filter, which blocks any DC component present in the sensor output. When computed over an infinitely long period, the mean value of the output of the amplifier will therefore be zero. However, this does not apply to a much smaller signal period, even if this period contains a full beat. In ❷ Fig. 12.44 this can be seen in the non-zero component of the spectrum at zero frequency.

Additional Filtering

In their digital form, AD-converted analog signals may be processed by numerical methods that resemble those of analog filters. Such filtering may be required for completing an incomplete job performed in the analog amplifier, or to extract, or emphasize some signal features. Since digital signals may be stored easily in digital memory, the filtering procedure for a digital signal value x_i may incorporate preceding signal values $x_{i-1}, x_{i-2}, \ldots$ as well as later ones $x_{i+1}, x_{i+2}, \ldots$.

In online applications, the length of the sample string x_{i+1}, x_{i+2}, ... depends on the delay between the occurrence of the event and the time of observation on a monitor. The sharpness of the cutoff of the various filters needs to be tuned to the particular type of application. For a full discussion of the design of such filters the reader is referred to the general literature on this topic [60].

Here, some simple filters are discussed and their effect is illustrated when they are applied to the signal shown in ❷ Fig. 12.43. In the notation used, x_i refers to the data used as input of the filter, y_i to its output. The filter parameters used may not correspond to desirable practical settings, but are chosen to clearly illustrate the nature of the effect of the filter. The values shown relate to a sampling rate of 1,000 sps.

Recursive LP Filter

The most simple form of a digital lowpass (LP) filter is defined by the recipe: take $y_0 = 0$, followed by computing for $i = 1, ..., N$,

$$y_i = \alpha x_i + (1 - \alpha) y_{i-1} \tag{12.12}$$

As can be seen, the output of the filter depends on the instantaneous input value (x_i) as well as on the value of the preceding output value (y_{i-1}). The latter property classes the recipe as an example of a recursive filter. On-line implementation demands just the storing of this preceding output value. The value of α sets the cutoff frequency, the frequency where the amplitude of a sinusoidal signal applied to the filter is reduced by a factor of $1/\sqrt{2}$ (the -3dB point).

The application of this filter to beat 5 of the reference signal (❷ Fig. 12.43) is shown in ❷ Fig. 12.45. The output signal is drawn by a solid line, the dashed line represents the input signal. The value of α was set at 0.2073, resulting in -3B point at 33 Hz, the frequency corresponding to the local minimum in the amplitude spectrum around 33 Hz (❷ Fig. 12.44).

The typical effect of the application of a LP filter can be seen to be:

1. reduction of noise,
2. reduction of the amplitude at sharply peaked signal segments,

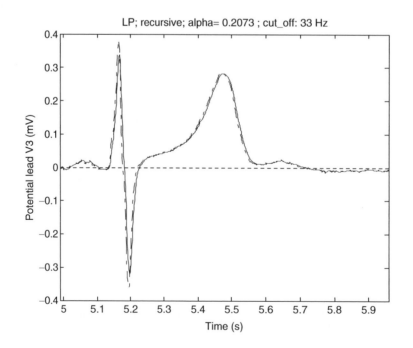

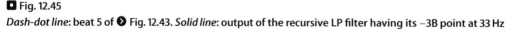

❑ **Fig. 12.45**

Dash-dot line: beat 5 of ❷ Fig. 12.43. *Solid line*: output of the recursive LP filter having its -3B point at 33 Hz

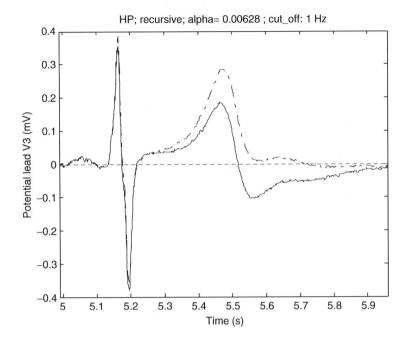

Fig. 12.46
Dash-dot line: beat 5 of ❷ Fig. 12.43. *Solid line*: output of the HP filter

3. a reduction of the slope of the fast deflection (R-S segment)
4. a delay in the timing of the signal, as is always the case for recursive filters.

All these effects are more pronounced if the cutoff frequency is set at a lower value.

Recursive HP Filter

The output of a simple form of a digital highpass (HP) filter is found by, after initializing: $v_0 = 0$, $y_0 = 0$, followed by iterating for $i = 1, \ldots, N$,

$$y_i = x_i + v_{i-1}$$
$$v_i = \alpha x_i + (1 - \alpha)v_{i-1} \tag{12.13}$$

This may be viewed as the subtraction of a lowpass-filtered version of the input signal (12.4) from the input itself.

The LP filter can be seen to leave the fast signal segments (QRS) relatively unaffected, but the pronounced effect on the slower parts (the STT segment) should be well noted. The filter forces the mean value of the output to be zero.

The application of this filter to beat 5 of the reference signal (❷ Fig. 12.43) is shown in ❷ Fig. 12.46. As in ❷ Fig. 12.45, the output signal is drawn by a solid line, the dash-dot line represents the input signal. The value of α was set at 0.00628 (sampling interval 1 ms), resulting in −3B point at 1 Hz. This value is close to the basic frequency of the signal segment (1.029 Hz).

Lowpass Moving Average Filter

The final example of simple digital filters is the lowpass moving average filter. Its recipe is

$$y_i = \frac{1}{W} \sum_{k=-W/2}^{W/2} x_{i+k} \tag{12.14}$$

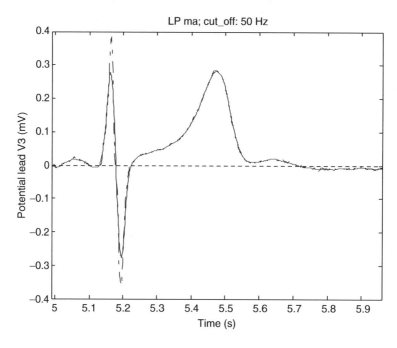

■ Fig. 12.47

Dash-dot line: beat 5 of ❯ Fig. 12.43. *Solid line*: output of the LP moving average filter; *W* = 20

It represents the moving average (sliding average) of *W* input values (an integer number). Since this does not involve previous output values (like y_{i-1}), it is a called a non-recursive filter. In contrast to the previous examples, this filter demands not just a single stored value, but rather: *W* values within the sliding window. The value of *W* determines the filter properties, in particular its cutoff frequency.

In the formulation given here the input includes samples related to later sampling moments and so it cannot be implemented in real time. A major, more general and highly valuable feature of the filter is that it does not produce phase-shift distortion. When using a sampling rate of 1,000 sps, and *W* = 20 the filter has a complete suppression of signal components at frequencies that are integer multiples of 50 Hz. This implies that, in addition to its lowpass character, the filter also suppresses completely any 50 Hz power line interference. The performance of this filter to beat 5 of the signals shown in ❯ Fig. 12.43 is presented in ❯ Fig. 12.47. The value of 50 Hz lowpass may high enough for some applications (compare ❯ Fig. 12.45). Note that, like the recursive filter, it produces some attenuation at the sharp peaks of the signal, but no delay, clearly: the off-line application.

Baseline Correction/Definition

As discussed in ❯ Sect. 12.4.1.5, bioelectric potentials observed by means of electrodes are contaminated by the half-cell potentials. The magnitudes of these potentials are much larger than those of the ECG, are unknown, and may change slowly in time: the so-called baseline "wander" or "drift." The common way of treating this problem is by including a highpass filter in the first stage of the amplifier (❯ Fig. 12.37). The resulting signal is referred to as an AC-recording (AC = alternating current). This produces an output signal that, when computed over a very long time, has zero mean value, i.e., the DC component of the signal is zero. If more rapid perturbations of the contact potential occur, the baseline of the signal, i.e., the values in the observed signal that should be assigned a zero value, must be specified on a beat-to-beat basis. Even if the dynamic range of the input stage would be wide enough to encompass the full range of sensor potentials (allowing a DC recording in spite of the presence of the half-cell potentials) the subseqent shift to a zero level remains to be defined.

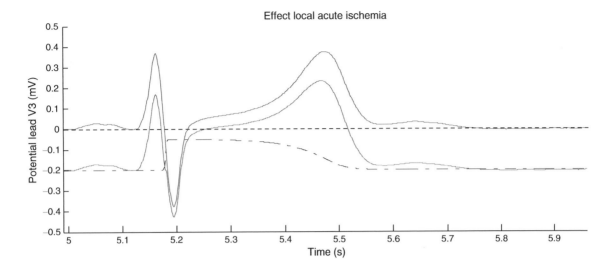

Fig. 12.48

Upper trace: lead V3, beat 5 of ❯ Fig. 12.43. *Dash-dot trace*: expression of the contribution to lead V3 due resulting from acute ischemia in the myocardium close to electrode V3. *Lower*, continuous trace: sum of the previous two traces: the DC representation of lead V3 during the ischemic period

The treatment of the problem is generally referred to as baseline correction. However, this is a somewhat misleading term since it assumes that the signal level that should be specified as zero is self evident, which is, in fact, not the case. The problem involved is illustrated by the following examples.

The ECG records differences in the potential field generated at different locations on the thorax. This potential field is uniform over the thorax (thus resulting in zero ECG potential differences) if all myocytes have the same transmembrane potential (❯ Sect. 12.2.1). In healthy myocardial tissue, the time instant at which this situation is most closely approximated is just before the beginning of atrial depolarization: the onset of the P wave. The signal of lead V3 shown in ❯ Fig. 12.43 is the (unprocessed) output of an AC-coupled amplifier. Beat 5 of this signal is shown as the upper trace of ❯ Fig. 12.48. For this healthy subject and this particular beat, the onsets of the P waves were close to zero, and so only a minor shift would be required to refer this signal to zero baseline.

For the entire segment shown in ❯ Fig. 12.43 an optimal baseline definition can be carried out by fitting a continuous function (e.g., a cubic spline) to the signal values at the onsets of the P waves of all beats. Subtraction of this function from the trace of ❯ Fig. 12.43 then produces the optimal baseline, provided that baseline wander or other recording artifacts are not too extreme.

The problem of baseline definition is more pressing for recordings taken during periods of acute ischemia. During ischemia, the transmembrane potential (TMP) of the myocytes within the region change: the resting potential decreases (tends to zero), the upstroke of the TMP is reduced. The size of these changes varies during the various stages of ischemia [66]. The coupling of the intra-cellular domains of neighbouring myocytes I in the ischemic region and myocytes H in the healthy region and differences in the TMPs of these myocytes result in a current flow. For the ventricular myocardium, there is a intracellular current flow from cells I to H during the time interval between the end of the T wave and the onset QRS interval. In the extracellular domain there is a return flow of current, flowing in the opposite direction, since charge is conserved. Hence, in the extracellular domain, this can be expressed by an equivalent current sink at the borders of the ischemic zone, which lowers the value of the nearby extracellular potential field [66].

In ❯ Fig. 12.48 the effect of this current sink on the potential of lead V3 is simulated by a downward DCshift of 0.2 mV. During the activation of the tissue surrounding the ischemic zone the potential difference between the regions is smaller and as a consequence the loading effect is smaller. In this simulation, ❯ Fig. 12.48, the contribution to the potential of lead V3 was set to −0.05 mV. During repolarization the contribution of the sink slowly returns to −0.2 mV. The time course of the contribution of the current sink is shown by the dash-dot line shown in ❯ Fig. 12.48. The addition this contribution to the signal of the non-ischemic situation (the upper trace) results in the type of wave form for the V3

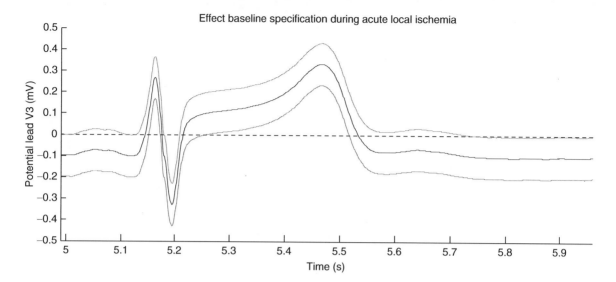

Fig. 12.49

Lower trace: DC variant of lead V3, beat 5 of ❯ Fig. 12.43 during ischemia (*lower* continuous trace of ❯ Fig. 12.48). *Middle trace*: zero mean variant of the *lower trace*, as would result from AC coupling. *Upper trace*: a variant of the *lower* trace in which zero baseline is defined at the beginning and the end of the entire beat

signal that can be expected during the ischemic period (the lower solid trace in ❯ Fig. 12.48). Note that between the end of the T wave and the moment of depolarization around the ischemic-zone (R-S segment) the signal is lowered by 0.2 mV and the remaining part by 0.05 mV, followed by a slow return to the (depression) of −0.2 mV at the perceivable end of the repolarizing phase.

Standard ECG recordings do not reveal the baseline depression shown in the lower solid trace in ❯ Fig. 12.48. The presence of the highpass filter results in a signal that has a zero mean value over the interval indicated (middle trace in ❯ Fig. 12.49). A (subsequent) baseline "correction" to the onset of the P wave then results in the upper trace of the same figure. Note that as a result of the current sink formed by the ischemic source, the actual baseline depression is seen to be expressed as an elavation of the ST-segment, merely as a result of the definition of the baseline. This phenomenon cleary hinders a direct intrepetation of the ECG features in terms of the underlying source-sink configurations associated with electrophysiology.

References

1. Zywietz, C., Technical Aspects of Electrogram Recording, in *Comprehensive Electrocardiology; Theory and Practice in Health and Disease*, P.W. Macfarlane and T.D. Veitch-Lawrie, Editors. New York, Pergamon Press, 1989, pp. 353–404.
2. McAdams, E., Bioelectrodes, in *Encyclopedia of Medical Devices and Instrumentation*, J.G. Webster, Editor. New York, Wiley, 2006, pp. 120–166.
3. Hinz, R., *Private Communication*. 2007.
4. Faraday, M., *On Electrical Decomposition*. Philosophical Transactions of the Royal Society, London, 1834.
5. Hill, J.W. and D.K. Kolb, *Chemistry for Changing Times*, 9th ed. New Jersey: Prentice-Hall, 2001.
6. Webster, J., ed. *Medical Instrumentation, Application and Design*, 3rd ed. New York: John Wiley and Son, 1998.
7. de Boer, R.W. and A. van Oosterom, Electrical properties of platinum electrodes: impedance measurements and time-domain analysis. *Med. Biol. Eng. Comput.*, 1978;**16**: 1–10.
8. Fisher, C., Electrode Dynamics, *Oxford Chemistry Primers*, Vol. 34. Oxford: Oxford University Press, 1998.
9. Liebman, J.F., *Structural Chemistry*. New York: Springer, 2004.
10. Scott, E.R., et al., Transport of ionic species in skin: contribution of pores to the overall skin conductance. *Pharm. Res.*, 1993;**10**(12): 1699–1709.
11. Ebling, F., R. Eady, and I.M. Leigh, Anatomy and organization of human skin, in *Textbook of Dermatology*, R.H. Champion and J.L. Burton, Editors. Oxford, Blackwell, 1992.
12. Grimnes, S., Psychogalvanic reflex and changes in electrical parameters of dry skin. *Med. Biol. Eng. Comput.*, 1982;**20**(6): 734–740.

13. Edelberg, R., Electrical properties of skin, in *Biophysical Properties of the Skin*, H.R. Elden, Editor. New York, Wiley, 1992.

14. Holbrook, K.A. and G.F. Odland, Regional differences in the thickness (cell layers) of the human stratum corneum: an ultrastructural analysis. *J. Invest. Dermatol.*, 1974;**62**: 415–422.

15. Swartzendruber, D.C., et al., Organization of the intercellular spaces of porcine epidermal and palatal stratum corneum: a quantitative study employing ruthenium tetroxide. *J Cell Tissue Res.*, 1995;**279**(2): 271–276.

16. Harrison, S.A.B. and D.F. Lovely, Identification of noise sources in surface recording of spinal somatosensory evoked potentials. *Med. Biol. Eng. Comput.*, 1995;**33**(3): 299–305.

17. Fernandez, M. and R. Pallas-Areny, Ag–AgCl electrode noise in high-resolution ECG measurements. *Biomed. Instrum. Technol.*, 2000;**34**(2): 125–130.

18. Geddes, L.A., *Electrodes and the Measurement of Bioelectric Events*. New York: Wiley-Interscience, 1972.

19. Swanson, D.K., et al., *Biomedical Electrode Technology*. New York: Academic Press, 1974.

20. Godin, D.T., P.A. Parker, and R.N. Scott, Noise characteristics of stainless-steel surface electrodes. *Med. Biol. Eng. Comput.*, 1991;**29**: 585–590.

21. Pardee, H.E.B., Concerning the electrodes used in electrocardiography. *Am. J. Physiol.*, 1917;**44**: 80–83.

22. Way, T.J., *Non-invasive, Radiolucent Electrode*. US Patent 5356428, 1994.

23. Rositano, X., Ultra-soft dry electrodes for electrocardiography. *Med. Instrum.*, 1973;**7**(1): 76.

24. Ryu, C.Y., S.H. Nam, and S. Kim, Conductive rubber electrode for wearable health monitoring, in *IEEE Annual International Conference*. Engineering in Medicine and Biology 27th Annual Conference, Shanghai, China, 2005.

25. Trank, J., R. Fetter, and R.M. Lauer, A spray-on electrode for recording the electrocardiogram during exercise. *J. Appl. Physiol.*, 1968;**24**(2): 267–268.

26. Patten, C.W., F.B. Ramme, and J. Roman, *Dry Electrodes for Physiological Monitoring*. Washington, DC: National Aeronautics and Space Administration, 1966.

27. Roman, J., *Flight Research Program III – High-Impedance Electrode Techniques, Nasa Technical Note D-3414 Supplement*. Washington, DC: National Aeronautics and Space Administration, 1966.

28. Wehr, G., et al., A vector-based, 5-electrode, 12-lead monitoring ECG (EASI) is equivalent to conventional 12-lead ECG for diagnosis of acute coronary syndromes? *J. Electrocardiol.*, 2006;**39**(1): 22–28.

29. Hindricks, G., et al., Perception of atrial fibrillation before and after radiofrequency catheter ablation. Relevance of asymptomatic arrhythmia recurrence. *Circulation*, 2005;**112**: II63–II68.

30. Jernberg, T., B. Lindahl, and L. Wallentin, ST-segment monitoring with continuous 12-lead ECG improves early risk stratification in patients with chest pain and ECG nondiagnostic of acute myocardial infarction. *J. Am. Coll. Cardiol.*, 1999;**34**: 1413–1419.

31. Jancin, B., Cell Phones ECG Leads Are Nosocomial Pathways. *Obst. Gyn. News.*, 2003.

32. Lobodzinski, S.M. and M.M. Laks, Biopotential fiber sensor. *J. Electrocardiol.*, 2006;**39**(4 suppl): S41–S46.

33. Karande, P., A. Jain, and S. Mitragotri, Relationships between skin's electrical impedance and permeability in the presence of chemical enhancers. *J. Control. Release.*, 2006;**110**(2): 307–313.

34. White, H., Electrochemical imaging of molecular transport in skin. *The Electrochemical Society Interface*, 2003;**12**: 29–33.

35. MettingVanRijn, A.C., et al., Low cost active electrode improves the resolution in biopotential recordings, in Proceedings of 18th *Annual International Conference of IEEE Engineering in Medicine Biology*. Amsterdam, IEEE Engineering and Medicine Biology, 1996.

36. Hagemann, B., G. Luhede, and H. Luczak, Improved active electrode for recording bioelectric signals in work physiology. *Eur. J. Appl. Physiol. Occup. Physiol.*, 1985;**54**: 95–98.

37. Padmadinata, F.Z., et al., Microelectronic skin electrode. Sens. actuators, 1990;**B1**: 491–494.

38. MettingVanRijn, A.C., A. Peper, and A.C. Grimbergen, Amplifiers for bioelectric events: a design with a minimal number of parts. *Med. Biol. Eng. Comput.*, 1994;**32**: 305–310.

39. Burke, M.J. and V.D.T. Gleeson, Biomedical Engineering, Issue Page(s): A micropower dry-electrode ECG preamplifier. *IEEE Trans. Biomed. Eng.*, 2000;**47**(2): 155–162.

40. Valchinov, E.S. and N.E. Pallikarakis, An active electrode for biopotential recording from small localized bio-sources. *BioMed. Eng. Online*, 2004;**3**(25): 1.

41. Ruffini, G., et al., *ENOBIO – First tests of a dry electrophysiology electrode using carbon nanotubes*, in *IEEE EMBS Annual International Conference*. New York City, USA, 2006.

42. Bergey, G.E., R.D. Squires, and W.C. Sipple, Electrocardiogram recording with pasteless electrodes. *IEEE Trans. Biomed. Eng.*, 1971;**18**: 206–211.

43. Gondron, C., et al., Nonpolarisable dry electrode based on NASICON ceramic. *Med. Biol. Eng. Comput.*, 1995;**33**: 452–457.

44. Ko, W.H. and J. Hynecek, Dry electrodes and electrode amplifiers, in *Biomed Electrode Technol*, A.C. Miller and D.C. Harrison, Editors. London, U.K, Academic Press, 1974, pp. 169–181.

45. Griss, P., et al., Characterization of micrimachined spiked biopotential electrodes. *IEEE. Trans. Biomed. Eng.*, 2002;**49**(6): 597–604.

46. www.orbitalresearch.com/PDFs/dry-electrode-technology_v. DF.pdf.

47. Schoenberg A.G., Klingler D.R., Baker C.D., Worth N.P., Booth H.E., Lyon P.C. Final report: *Development of test methods for disposable ECG Electrodes*. UBTL Technical Report No. 1605—005, Salt Lake City, UT, 1979.

48. Huigen, E., A. Peper, and C.A. Grimbergen, Investigation into the origin of the noise of surface electrodes. *Med. Biol. Eng. Comput.*, 2002;**40**: 332–338.

49. Sheffield, L.T., et al., Optimal electrocardiographic: task force II – quality of electrocardiographic records. *Am. J. Cardiol.*, 1978;**4**(1): 146–157.

50. *Pressure Sensitive Tape Councel.* 1979, UBTL: Salt Lake City (Utah).

51. Richardson P.C., The insulated electrode: A pasteless electrocardiographic technique, 20th *Proc. Annu. Conf. Eng. Med. Biol.*, Boston, Mass., 1968.

52. Prance, R.J., An ultra-low-noise electrical-potential probe for human-body scanning. *Meas. Sci. Technol.*, 2000;**11**: 1–7.

53. Lee, J.M., et al., Evaluating a capacitively coupled, noncontact electrode for ECG monitoring, in *NATO Research and Technology Organisation (Human Factors and Medicine Panel) meeting*

in cooperation with the Advanced Technology Applications for Combat Casualty Care conference. St. Petersburg, FL, 2004.

54. Kingsley, S.A., et al., Photrode optical sensor for electrophysiological monitoring. *Aviat. Space. Environ. Med.*, 2003;**74**(11): 1215–1216.

55. Pallás-Areny, R., Interference-rejection characteristics of biopotential amplifiers: A comparative analysis. *IEEE Trans. Biomed. Eng.*, 1988;**35**: 953–959.

56. Winter, B.B. and J.G. Webster, Reduction of interference due to common mode voltage in biopotential amplifiers. *IEEE Trans. Biomed. Eng.*, 1983;**30**: 58–62.

57. McAdams, E.T., J. McLaughlin, and J.M. Anderson, Wearable and implantable monitoring systems: 10 years experience at University of Ulster. *Stud. Health. Technol. Inform.*, 2004;**108**: 203–208.

58. Led, S., J. Fernandez, and L. Serrano, Design of a wearable device for ECG continuous monitoring using wireless technology, in *26th Annual international Conference of IEEE Engineering in Medicine and Biological Society*, San Francisco, 2004.

59. Chun, H., et al., IT-based diagnostic instrumentation systems for personalized healthcare services. *Stud. Health. Technol. Inform.*, 2005;**117**: 180–190.

60. Sörnmo, L. and P. Laguna, *Bioelectrical Signal Processing in Cardiac and Neurological Applications.* Amsterdam: Elsevier Academic Press, 2005.

61. MettingVanRijn, A.C., A. Peper, and C.A. Grimbergen, High quality recording of bioelectric events. Part 1: Interference reduction, theory and practice. *Med. Biol. Eng. Comput.*, 1990;**28**: 389–397.

62. Thakor, N.V. and J.G. Webster, Ground-free ECG recording with two electrodes. *IEEE Trans. Biomed. Eng.*, 1980;**BME-27**: 699–704.

63. Winter, X., et al., Driven-right-leg circuit design. *IEEE Trans. Biomedical. Eng.*, 1983;**30**(1): 62–66.

64. Huhta, J.C. and J.G. Webster, 60-Hz Interference in electrocardiography. *IEEE Trans. Biomed. Eng.*, 1973;**20**: 91–101.

65. Nyquist, H., Certain topics in telegraph transmission theory. *Trans. AIEE*, 1928;**47**: 617–644.

66. Janse, M.J., et al., Flow of injury current and patterns of excitation during early ventricular arrhythmias in acute regional myocardial ischemia in isolated porcine and canine hearts; evidence for two different arrhythmogenic mechanisms. *Circ. Res.*, 1980;**47**: 151–165.

Index

Note: The page numbers that appear in bold type indicates a substantive discussion of the topic.